D1034113

Butterworths Guides to Information Sources

Information Sources in the
Medical Sciences

Third Edition

Butterworths Guides to Information Sources

A series under the General Editorship of
D. J. Foskett, MA, FLA
and
M. W. Hill, MA, BSc, MRIC

This series was known previously as 'Information Sources for Research and Development'. Other titles available are:

Information Sources in Agriculture
edited by G. P. Lilley

Information Sources in the History of Science and Medicine
edited by P. Corsi and P. Weindling

Information Sources in Education and Work
edited by E. H. K. Dibden and J. C. Tomlinson

Use of Chemical Literature (Third edition)
edition by R. T. Bottle

Use of Engineering Literature
edited by K. W. Mildren

Use of Mathematical Literature
edited by A. R. Dorling

Use of Physics Literature
edited by H. Coblans

Use of Reports Literature
edited by C. P. Auger

Use of Social Sciences Literature
edited by N. Roberts

Butterworths Guides to Information Sources

Information Sources in the
Medical Sciences

Third Edition

Editors
L. T. Morton, FLA
Consultant Librarian, British Postgraduate Medical Federation
(formerly Librarian, National Institute for Medical Research,
London)

S. Godbolt, BA, FLA
Librarian, Charing Cross Hospital Medical School, London

Butterworths
London Boston Durban Singapore Sydney Toronto Wellingon

First published as *Uses of Medical Literature* 1974
Second edition 1977
Third edition as *Information Sources in the Medical Sciences* 1984

© **Butterworth & Co (Publishers) Ltd 1984**

British Library Cataloguing in Publication Data
Information sources in the medical sciences.—3rd ed.
 —(Butterworths guide to information sources)
 1. Medicine—Bibliography
 I. Morton, Leslie T.   II. Godbolt, S.
 016.61   Z6658

 ISBN 0–408–11473–8

Library of Congress Cataloging in Publication Data
Main entry under title:
Information sources in the medical sciences

 (Butterworths guides to information sources)
 Rev. ed. of: Use of medical literature. 1977.
 Includes index.
 1. Medical literature—Addresses, essays, lectures.
 2. Medical—Bibliography—Addresses, essays, lectures.
 I. Morton, Leslie Thomas.   II. Godbolt, S.   III. Series.
 [DNLM: 1. Bibliography of medicine. ZWB 100 U84]
 R118.6.154 1983   610′.7   83–7781
 ISBN 0–408–11473–8

Typeset by Phoenix Photosetting, Chatham
Printed in Great Britain at the University Press, Cambridge

Series Editors' Foreword

Daniel Bell has made it clear in his book *The Post-Industrial Society* that we now live in an age in which information has succeeded raw materials and energy as the primary commodity. We have also seen in recent years the growth of a new discipline, information science. This is in spite of the fact that skill in acquiring and using information has always been one of the distinguishing features of the educated person. As Dr Johnson observed, 'Knowledge is of two kinds. We know a subject ourselves, or we know where we can find information upon it.'

But a new problem faces the modern educated person. We now have an excess of information, and even an excess of sources of information. This is often called the 'information explosion', though it might be more accurately called the 'publication explosion'. Yet it is of a deeper nature than either. The totality of knowledge itself, let alone of theories and opinions about knowledge, seems to have increased to an unbelievable extent, so that the pieces one seeks in order to solve any problem appear to be but a relatively few small straws in a very large haystack. That analogy, however, implies that we are indeed seeking but a few straws. In fact, when information arrives on our desks, we often find those few straws are actually far too big and far too numerous for one person to grasp and use easily. In the jargon used in the information world, efficient retrieval of relevant information often results in information overkill.

Ever since writing was invented, it has been a common practice for men to record and store information; not only facts and figures, but also theories and opinions. The rate of recording accelerated after the invention of printing and moveable type, not because that in itself could increase the amount of recording but because, by making it easy to publish multiple copies of a document and sell them at a profit, recording and distributing information became very lucrative and hence attractive to more people. On the other hand, men and women in whose lives the discovery of the handling of information plays a large part usually devise ways of getting what they want from other people rather than from books in their efforts to avoid information overkill. Conferences, briefings, committee meetings are one means of this; personal contacts through the 'invisible college' and members of one's club are another. While such people do read, some of them voraciously, the reading of published literature, including in this category newspapers as well as books and journals and even watching television, may provide little more than 10% of the total information that they use.

Computers have increased the opportunities, not merely by acting as more efficient stores and providers of certain kinds of information than libraries, but also by manipulating the data they contain in order to synthesize new information. To give a simple illustration, a computer which holds data on commodity prices in the various trading capitals of the world, and also data on currency exchange rates, can be programmed to indicate comparative costs in different places in one single currency. Computerized data bases, i.e. stores of bibliographic information, are now well established and quite widely available for anyone to use. Also increasing are the number of data banks, i.e. stores of factual information, which are now generally accessible. Anyone who buys a suitable terminal may be able to arrange to draw information directly from these computer systems for their own purposes; the systems are normally linked to the subscriber by means of the telephone network. Equally, an alternative is now being provided by information supply services such as libraries, more and more of which are introducing terminals as part of their regular services.

The number of sources of information on any topic can therefore be very extensive indeed; publications (in the widest sense), people (experts), specialist organizations from research associations to chambers of commerce, and computer stores. The number of channels by which one can have access to these vast collections of information are also very numerous, ranging from professional literature searchers, via computer intermediaries, to Citizens' Advice Bureaux, information marketing services and information brokers.

The aim of the Butterworths Guides to Information Sources is to bring all these sources and channels together in a single convenient form and to present a picture of the international scene as it exists in each of the disciplines we plan to cover. Consideration is also being given to volumes that will cover major interdisciplinary areas of what are now sometimes called 'mission-oriented' fields of knowledge. The first stage of the whole project will give greater emphasis to publications and their exploitation, partly because they are so numerous, and partly because more detail is needed to guide them adequately. But it may be that in due course the balance will change, and certainly the balance in each volume will be that which is appropriate to its subject at the time.

The editor of each volume is a person of high standing, with substantial experience of the discipline and of the sources of information in it. With a team of authors of whom each one is a specialist in one aspect of the field, the total volume provides an integrated and highly expert account of the current sources, of all types, in its subject.

D. J. Foskett
Michael Hill

Preface to the third edition

Previous editions of this book were published under the title *Use of Medical Literature*. For this third edition the title has been changed to reflect the broader scope of the work. Each chapter has been revised to take account of important new publications and information services. Three additional chapters have been added, dealing with audio-visual materials, with the literature of general practice, and with information for patients and public. As the chapter on historical and biographical sources deals with medicine in general, chapters devoted to medical and surgical specialties include information on historical works.

We are indebted to the contributors whose excellent work ensured the success of the previous editions and who have so enthusiastically collaborated in the production of the present volume. We are most grateful to Miss Christine Gammon for expert clerical assistance. We would also like to thank the series editors (Mr Douglas Foskett and Mr Michael Hill), the editorial staff of Butterworths, and many of our library colleagues for their help and advice during the preparation of this edition.

L.T.M.
S.G.

Preface to the first edition

This book attempts to provide a comprehensive guide to the general and specialist literature covering the medical sciences. It is intended for clinicians, medical scientists, librarians and information scientists; it should prove particularly useful to workers moving into a new and unfamiliar field of research. Besides describing published work within the subject field, it includes a chapter on mechanized information services and another on the organization of personal index files.

Limitations of space have not permitted a separate chapter for every branch of medicine but readers will find that several of the contributors have covered their subject very broadly. For example, Miss Read's chapter on Clinical Medicine deals with most of the clinical specialties and Dr Postlethwaite's contribution on Medical Microbiology includes such subjects as epidemiology, infectious disease, and some aspects of public health. Occasional overlapping is to be expected in a book for which most of the contributors have designed their chapters to be self-contained guides to their respective subjects.

It will be noticed that works quoted are predominantly in the English language, a reflection of the increasing international use of English in the medical and scientific literature.

I am grateful to the contributors who have collaborated as a team to produce this book. It is hoped that the results of their labours will prove a worthy addition to the series on Information Sources for Research and Development. Thanks are due also to the editors of the series, Dr Bottle and Mr Foskett, and to the publishers, Butterworths, for help and advice during the planning stages.

L.T.M.

Contributors

E. S. Brooke, ALA
Librarian, Institute of Child Health, University of London

D. H. Calam, MA, D Phil, C Chem, FRSC
Head, Chemistry Section, National Institute for Biological Standards and Control, London

M. A. Clennett, BA, ALA
Librarian, British Dental Association, London

R. J. Dannatt, BA, ALA
Librarian, Welsh National School of Medicine, Cardiff

E. J. Freeman, BA, ALA
Librarian and Deputy Director, Wellcome Institute for the History of Medicine, London

R. E. Gann, BA, Dip Lib, ALA
Assistant Regional Librarian (Patient Care), Wessex Regional Library Information Service

V. J. Glanville, ALA
Formerly Librarian, London School of Hygiene and Tropical Medicine

S. Godbolt, BA, FLA
Librarian, Charing Cross Hospital Medical School, London

S. Gove, BSc, Dip Lib, ALA, FZS
Assistant Librarian in Charge, Thane Library of Medical Sciences, University College, London

H. R. Hague, BA, MA (Librarianship), ALA
Assistant Librarian, Charing Cross Hospital Medical School, London

D. N. H. Hamilton, MB, PhD, FRCS Glasgow
Department of Surgery, Western Infirmary, Glasgow

M. Hammond, Dip Soc
Librarian, Royal College of General Practitioners, London

M. C. Jones, BA, AKC, ALA
Information Officer/Librarian, British Life Assurance Trust for Health and Medical Education, London

L. T. Morton, FLA
Consultant Librarian, British Postgraduate Medical Federation (formerly Librarian, National Institute for Medical Research, London)

C. Norris, MA (Cantab)
MEDLARS Section, British Library Lending Division, Boston Spa, Wetherby, W. Yorkshire

D. C. Roberts, FRC Path, MRCS, MI Biol, MI Inf Sci, LRCP
Head, Research Data Unit and Registry and Information Service for Experimental Tumours, Imperial Cancer Research Fund, London

A. M. Rodger, BA, ALA
Librarian, Royal College of Physicians and Surgeons of Glasgow, Glasgow

J. F. B. Rowland, MA, MI Inf Sci
Assistant to the Director of Information Services, Royal Society of Chemistry, Nottingham

D. W. C. Stewart, BA, ALA,
Librarian, Royal Society of Medicine, London

F. M. Sutherland, MA, FLA
Formerly Librarian, British Medical Association, London

R. B. Tabor, L Th (Hons), ALA
Regional Librarian, Wessex Regional Health Authority, Southampton

H. E. Taylor, BA, Dip Lib Stud, ALA
Assistant Regional Librarian (Psychiatry), S. W. Thames
Regional Health Authority

P. C. Want, ALA
Librarian, Royal College of Obstetricians and Gynaecologists,
London

B. H. Whyte, MA, ALA
Formerly Librarian, Public Health Laboratory Service, London

Contents

1

Libraries and their use

L. T. Morton and S. Godbolt

Today's doctor or medical scientist requires more information than ever before. Medical education and training have increased in complexity and are followed by specialization and possibly also research. The need for both the researcher and the practitioner to keep abreast of current developments necessitates using libraries and being conversant with the literature.

Despite upheavals and financial stringency the modern medical library, large or small, provides the key to a network of sophisticated and comprehensive services. The user may expect to find information in a variety of non-print formats, such as tape-slide and video. In larger libraries a terminal, through which many databases may be interrogated, is now essential equipment, and smaller libraries can provide advice on access and availability of computerized information retrieval services.

Microfiche library catalogues and the transformation of familiar reference tools such as *British Books in Print* (UK) or *Books in Print* (US) into microfiche as well as hard copy format necessitate machines for their use. This equipment is well designed and easy to use. Reader printers are likely to be available in these libraries, which may have journal runs as well as catalogues in microfiche form. Even the smallest library is likely to possess a photocopier and larger libraries may have two or more.

Use of the library is free to its membership but certain services, such as inter-library loans, online searching and photocopying may be charged for. However, hours of work in manual searching can be saved for a relatively small cost. Photocopying, too, is cheap and offers the convenience of copies for personal files or perusal when the library is closed. Users should bear in mind their responsibilities under copyright law to make no more than one copy of one article from any single issue of a periodical. Most libraries ask for a declaration to be signed stating that the copy is only for use for the purposes of private study or research. Self-service copying is common and for their own convenience users should always check that the article reference on the copy is complete.

Great emphasis has been placed in recent years, formally and informally, on the importance of reader services and user education. The staff are the most valuable resource in any library and getting to know staff members with special responsibilities for reference and advisory functions so that they are aware of particular interests and needs is an important aspect of good library use.

Library publications designed to assist users to exploit available services are numerous and range from lists of the library's periodicals to newsletters and/or accessions lists, bulletins and other information leaflets.

A very thorough and lucid review of the biomedical literature and its use is provided by *Coping with the Biomedical Literature. A Primer for the Scientist and the Clinician* edited by K. S. Warren (Praeger, 1981). It contains contributions from twelve distinguished American biomedical scientists and librarians. It is divided into four sections which deal, respectively, with the structure, production, utilization and sources of biomedical information.

Medical libraries in Great Britain and Ireland

Britain is well equipped with medical libraries. The Royal Colleges, the medical societies, and the teaching and research institutes have, between them, accumulated a rich storehouse of literature probably unsurpassed elsewhere. In recent years this has been considerably augmented by the British Library. A key to this storehouse is provided by the *Directory of Medical and Health Care Libraries in the United Kingdom and Republic of Ireland* (1982), which gives information on about 500 libraries.

London

The greatest concentration of libraries is in London and includes the libraries of the Royal Society of Medicine, the British Medical

Association, the Wellcome Institute for the History of Medicine, and the Royal Colleges.

The Royal Society of Medicine was founded as the (Royal) Medical and Chirurgical Society in 1805. In 1907 it was combined with other medical societies (and their libraries) and assumed its present name. Its library is one of the largest postgraduate medical collections in Europe, with about 450 000 volumes and taking 2100 current journals. The library is available to members of the Society; others may have reference facilities on written introduction by a member. There is also a Library (Scientific Research) Section intended to accommodate employees of private and public companies, and of certain other groups, who wish to use the library to assist their employers in the furtherance of medical research. The library provides full reference and postal services.

The British Medical Association is the representative body of the medical profession in Britain. Its library, founded in 1887, now has over 100 000 volumes and takes some 1100 current periodicals. Reference and postal services are available to its members; others may use it at the discretion of the Librarian. It also offers institutional membership, with restricted service facilities, to libraries within the National Health Service.

One of the finest collections of medico-historical material in the world is that in the Wellcome Institute for the History of Medicine. The Institute was founded by the generosity of the late Henry S. Wellcome. It has some 300 000 volumes besides manuscripts, *incunabula,* prints, autograph letters, etc. It frequently arranges exhibitions on medico-historical topics. It is available for reference purposes to all interested in the history of medicine and science. Readers' tickets are available on application to the Librarian.

The formation of the British Postgraduate Medical Federation (University of London) in 1945 led to the establishment of a number of specialist postgraduate institutes. The Federation also incorporated two existing institutes – the Institute of Cancer Research and the (Royal) Postgraduate Medical School at Hammersmith Hospital (30 000 vols, 770 current periodicals). The latter has since become an independent school of London University. Both these establishments already had good libraries and the majority of the new institutes have since assembled sound, specialized collections in the care of experienced librarians. They include the Cardiothoracic Institute (at the National Heart Hospital and Brompton Hospital), and the institutes of Child Health, Dental Surgery, Dermatology, Laryngology and Otology, Neurology, Obstetrics and Gynaecology, Ophthalmology, Orthopaedics, Psychiatry and Urology. Another postgraduate school of the University of

London is the London School of Hygiene and Tropical medicine, which has 83 000 volumes and takes 1300 current journals.

All these libraries are intended primarily for the use of the institutes or associated hospital staff, although others are usually allowed reference facilities.

Undergraduate medical schools in London have good libraries, most of which cater both for the hospital medical staff and for the postgraduate research staff. Several of the librarians, like their provincial colleagues, give instruction in the use of medical libraries and the full exploitation of the literature, and by doing so make an important contribution to the early training of research workers.

The combined library resources of the University of London Library at Senate House and those of its constituent Schools and Colleges are vast. The work of co-ordinating these is carried on by the Library Resources Co-ordinating Committee (LRCC), whose staff is based at the University Library. Formally constituted in 1973 following the Humphreys Report of 1971, initiatives of major importance have been undertaken by LRCC working in co-operation with the librarians throughout the University. The creation of the London University Union List of Serials (ULISES), for example, has ensured more effective utilization of academic library resources for the user. The twelfth edition of the list was issued in December 1982 on microfiche and included 128 000 holdings of 72 000 titles contributed by 48 libraries. The work is ongoing. The University Library has itself built up a good collection of medical journals. In the nearby Thane Library of Medical Sciences at University College there is an important collection covering the basic medical sciences, with 70 000 volumes and 600 periodicals on anatomy, physiology, biochemistry, biophysics and pharmacology. It is designed for the use of its academic and research staff and its students.

The Royal Colleges maintain valuable libraries. The Royal College of Physicians of London was founded in 1518, but most of its original library was lost in the Great Fire of 1666. Its present collection of about 48 000 volumes is rich in historical material. It also has a working collection of modern books and periodicals. Fellows and Members of the College and all *bona fide* research workers may use it.

The Royal College of Surgeons of England (1800) has a fine specialist collection including 590 current journals and 160 000 books. It is a reference library; it does not lend to individuals although books and journals less than 50 years old may be lent to other libraries. The Royal College of Obstetricians and Gynaecologists, founded in 1929, has developed a library of both historical and contemporary publications in its subject field. It is available to Fellows and Members of the College and to suitably introduced and qualified persons for reference only. The Royal College of General Practitioners inaugurated a medical recordings service (now the Graves Medical Audiovisual Library, an independent charity) and maintains a bibliographical service on general practice publications. The Royal College of Pathologists is building up a historical library covering pathology, microbiology and related subjects.

The principal medical research institute in Britain is the Medical Research Council's National Institute for Medical Research (1913) at Mill Hill, London. Its library of 71 000 volumes and 700 current journals serves the scientific staff of the MRC at the Institute and elsewhere. Others wishing to use it may apply to the Director. The MRC also has small libraries in a number of its research units in various parts of the country. It has more recently established its Clinical Research Centre at Northwick Park Hospital, Harrow, which is equipped with a rapidly expanding library of clinical material, now containing 36 000 volumes and receiving 750 current journals.

Other research establishments, such as the Imperial Cancer Research Fund and the National Institute for Biological Standards and Control, have good libraries, and several of the pharmaceutical houses maintain libraries of good standing.

The Library of the Department of Health and Social Security was founded in 1834. It now takes 1600 journals and contains a total of 200 000 volumes. It is concerned with all aspects of public health and social welfare and is available to staff, postgraduate students or accredited research workers for reference only.

Under a scheme of specialization operated by the public libraries of London, the Marylebone Road branch of Westminster City Libraries maintains a medical collection including a good selection of periodicals. This library is, appropriately, near Harley Street. It is open to the public and lends (books only). London is also fortunate in having a subscription medical library, maintained by H. K. Lewis and Co. Ltd., the medical publishers and booksellers. This has about 30 000 titles and well in excess of 100 000 volumes, including multiple copies of most books. Printed catalogues of the library are available.

Besides the postgraduate institute libraries already mentioned, some other London libraries dealing with particular subjects are worth noting. The British Dental Association has the principal library covering this subject in the country. It lends books and journals to members and journals only to other libraries. A smaller library is at the Royal Dental Hospital. The most important pharmaceutical library is that of the Pharmaceutical Society of Great Britain. Fellows, members, and other *bona fide* qualified persons may use it; books may be borrowed only by fellows and members. The School of Pharmacy (University of London) has a good library in its field.

Provinces

Some excellent medical libraries are maintained in the provincial medical schools. The need for continuing medical education has led, in recent years, to the establishment of a number of postgraduate medical centres. These are sited mainly in non-teaching hospitals in the provinces. Their aim is to provide a suitable, adequately equipped location for the postgraduate teaching of hospital staff and general medical and dental practitioners, and at the same time to cater for consultants, junior hospital staff and general practitioners who wish to meet to discuss problems of common interest. The first purpose-built postgraduate medical centre was opened in 1963; since then these centres have rapidly proliferated and the *Directory of Postgraduate Medical Centres 1982* records 382, including some in psychiatric and teaching hospitals. All but a handful of these centres have only small libraries. Standards of library provision vary considerably; in some cases a regional organization has been or is being developed, covering all libraries within the area administered by the Regional Health Authority and backed up by the university medical library.

Medical societies, too, have been active in the provinces, but most of their libraries have now been incorporated in local hospital or university libraries. An important exception is the library of the Liverpool Medical Institution, founded about 1773, which now contains more than 30 000 volumes and subscribes to 200 current journals.

Scotland

Edinburgh University has a modern medical library of about 63 000 volumes and 820 current sets of journals. Notable medical collections are available in the other universities – Aberdeen, Dundee, Glasgow and St. Andrews. Strathclyde is building up a library covering the biological sciences.

The Royal College of Physicians of Edinburgh has a fine library of both historical and modern material amounting to about 270 current periodicals and 200 000 volumes. The smaller, more specialized library at the Royal College of Surgeons of Edinburgh contains about 32 000 volumes. In Glasgow, the Royal College of Physicians and Surgeons has a good modern library supported by a rich historical collection, together totalling 200 000 volumes. These college libraries are usually available to fellows and members, with restricted use by others.

A subscription library similar to Lewis's Library, but on a smaller scale, is maintained by Donald Ferrier Ltd of Edinburgh. This includes medicine, dentistry, veterinary medicine and science in its subject coverage, and contains about 30 000 volumes.

For further information on medical libraries in Scotland, *see* Bunch (1975).

Ireland

In Belfast the Queen's University Medical Library is housed in the Institute of Clinical Science. The Northern Ireland Health and Social Services Library was recently incorporated with it, and the medical library now provides a province-wide service for the social services' teaching units, nursing schools, district hospital medical collections and postgraduate medical schools, besides catering for the needs of the medical staff and students of the University and members of the medical profession in Northern Ireland.

In Eire the Royal College of Surgeons in Ireland, University College Dublin (National University of Ireland) and the Irish Dental Library, all in Dublin, have notable collections.

National Libraries

The British Library was formed in 1973 by the amalgamation of several existing libraries, including the British Museum Library. Two sections are of particular usefulness in medicine and science – the British Library Lending Division and the Science Reference Library.

The British Library Lending Division, at Boston Spa, Yorkshire, is one of the best sources for modern medical and scientific literature in Britain. Its stock includes all significant serials in all subjects and languages (56 000 are currently received), all important English language and foreign monographs, report literature and conference proceedings. It makes use of a number of 'back-up' libraries, including the Royal Society of Medicine, to obtain material not on its own shelves, as a result of which some major libraries not previously able to take much part in interlibrary lending can now make a useful contribution. It incorporates the National Central Library, which was the recognized national centre for the loan of books between libraries covering all subject fields, and which, besides its own large collection, could call on many general and special libraries both in Britain and abroad. It was, in fact, a clearing house through which it was possible to borrow almost any book or journal. It built up union catalogues of the holdings of many of the outlying libraries it used.

The British Library Science Reference Library was formed by expanding the former Patent Office Library with scientific literature from the British Museum and with newly acquired material. Life science subjects, including a medical collection, are housed at the Aldwych Branch, 9 Kean St, Drury Lane, London WC2.

The professional organization for medical librarians in Britain is the Medical, Health and Welfare Libraries Group of the Library Association. Its meetings include an annual week-end conference, usually in one of the large cities with well-established medical libraries. It is responsible for several publications and in other ways does its best to promote the interests of medical libraries and their users.

For language and other reasons British medical libraries have a close affinity with their American counterparts. Some of the areas of difference between American and British experience are skilfully defined by Gaskell (1970).

North American libraries

The United States has a wealth of medical libraries. The *Directory of Health Sciences Libraries in the United States* (1979) lists 2775 and gives details of stock, strength of personnel, etc.

The most important medical library in the world is the National Library of Medicine, in Bethesda, Maryland. Founded in 1836 as the Library of the Surgeon General's Office, US Army, it now possesses well over a million volumes and takes more than 10 000 current periodicals. It is rich in historical material; its catalogues of *incunabula* and early printed books and its other publications are described elsewhere in this volume. It is responsible for the compilation of the *Index Medicus,* and for MEDLARS, perhaps the two most valuable contributions to medical information services in the world today. It has generously arranged the decentralization of MEDLARS, which is now available in suitably equipped centres in and outside the US. One of these centres is the British Library Lending Division. The National Library of Medicine also offers the usual reference and interlibrary loan facilities. Its functions and responsibilities are outlined by Cummings (1981) and its long and fascinating history has been fully documented by Miles (1982).

The second largest American medical library is the Francis A. Countway Library at Harvard Medical School. This was formed by the amalgamation in 1965 of Harvard Medical School Library (1783) with the Boston Medical Library (1807). This amalgamation resulted in a library of more than 600 000 volumes and 5000 current periodicals.

The library of the New York Academy of Medicine has an exhaustive collection of contemporary medical literature and is also richly endowed with historical material in all branches of medicine, together with collections of portraits, manuscripts, letters, medals, stamps, etc. It contains more than half a million volumes.

Other important American collections that may be mentioned here are those of the College of Physicians of Philadelphia; Yale Medical Library; the Mayo Clinic; Johns Hopkins School of Medicine; the State University of New York, Downstate Medical Center; the Biomedical Library at the Center for the Health Sciences, University of California at Los Angeles; the National Institutes of Health at Bethesda, Maryland; the Cleveland Health Sciences Library; and the Medical section of the John Crerar Library, Chicago. Some recent developments in health science libraries in North America are described by Campbell (1981).

The professional organization for medical librarians in the US is the Medical Library Association (MLA), founded in 1898. Its objectives are to foster medical libraries, to encourage the training and continuing education of medical librarians, and to operate an exchange of duplicate material. It is responsible for a number of important publications, including the quarterly *Bulletin of the Medical Library Association*, the most important serial publication in the field; *Medical Reference Works 1679–1966: a Selected Bibliography* by Blake and Roos (1967) with several supplements; and the *Handbook of Medical Library Practice* (4th edn, 3 vols, Medical Library Association, 1982–4). MLA holds an annual meeting for the presentation of papers and the discussion of its organizational affairs.

Canada's principal medical libraries are at the Academy of Medicine, Toronto; McGill Medical Library, Montreal; the Department of National Health and Welfare, Ottawa; the W. K. Kellogg Health Sciences Library at Dalhousie University, Halifax; the Health Sciences Centre Library at London, Ontario; and the McMaster University Health Sciences Library at Hamilton, Ontario.

Other libraries

In France the Institut National de la Santé et de la Recherche Médicale (INSERM) plays an important part in the provision of biomedical documentation. It is responsible for operating the MEDLARS service in France. Mention should be made of the collections of the Bibliothéque de la Faculté de Médecine de Paris and the Académie de Médecine, Paris. Although German libraries suffered considerably during the war, large medical libraries are established at Heidelberg, Göttingen, Munich and Cologne. The Deutsches Institut für Medizinische Dokumentation (DIMDI) operates a MEDLARS service at Cologne.

Switzerland is fortunate in being the home of the World Health Organization, in which the need for an adequate library and reference service to support the technical work of WHO has been recognized since its foundation. The first books and periodicals were acquired by 1946, since when the collection has grown steadily. The WHO library in Geneva now contains over 100 000 volumes, having inherited at an early stage the library of the Office International de l'Hygiène Publique. It currently receives about 3000 periodicals on an exchange, gift or subscription basis. Its special collections include one on the history of international health and an extensive collection of WHO unpublished documents and reports.

A distinguishing feature of the WHO library has been its use as a training centre for future medical and scientific librarians. In 1974 it initiated a global health literature programme for the improvement of medical library services and, particularly, the development of regional medical libraries. A provisional service was started to respond especially to the needs of developing countries. A MEDLARS service is operated by the WHO library.

There is a modern library for the Faculty of Medicine of the University of Geneva. The universities of Basle and Zürich have extensive medical collections.

In the Scandinavian countries the Karolinska Institutet in Stockholm has the largest collection of current medical literature. Its Biomedical Documentation Centre operates a MEDLARS service for Scandinavia and the Biomedical Department of Göteborg University is also well provided. An outstanding medical library in Norway is that in the Biomedical Department of the University Library, Oslo. The State Hospital and Ullevål Hospital in Oslo and Haukeland Hospital in Bergen are also well equipped. The largest collection of medical literature in Denmark is in the Second Department of the University Library at Copenhagen, and in Finland the Central Medical Library at Helsinki is the most important. There is excellent collaboration between the medical libraries in Scandinavia.

Fine collections exist in Russia, Italy and elsewhere, and Thornton (1966) should be consulted for information on these and other foreign libraries. The development of medical libraries in the Third World has been documented by McCarthy (1981).

Arrangement

A large part of the stock of a modern medical library consists of periodicals. These are usually kept together, arranged in subject or alphabetical order. Current issues are usually segregated for the benefit of readers who regularly monitor the incoming literature. Besides the usual catalogue, most libraries provide a handlist of their current periodicals.

Catalogues

A library catalogue is most commonly found on cards or microfiche, but may also be available in book, loose-leaf (sheaf catalogue), computer print-out or microform. The catalogue may be in the form of:

(1) An author catalogue, with some entries arranged under the names of authors, institutions, and sometimes series titles.
(2) A subject catalogue, with its entries grouped together under subject headings, arranged alphabetically or in a classified order. Most libraries have both author and subject catalogues of their books.
(3) These may be brought together in one sequence and amplified with certain other entries to form a dictionary catalogue.

Main entries in catalogues usually include a classification symbol or shelf mark to indicate the location of the item concerned. The periodicals catalogue is often separate.

Classification

The National Library of Medicine has introduced a classification scheme developed from that of the Library of Congress, Washington (*National Library of Medicine Classification*, 1978). This classification permits specific entry, bringing together in one place material on all aspects of a particular topic. A combination of letters and figures is employed in the notation. Material concerning the preclinical sciences is arranged under the letters QS–QZ and material on medicine and related subjects under the letter W. The synopsis of classes is as follows:

Preclinical Sciences

QS	Human anatomy	QW	Bacteriology and immunology
QT	Physiology	QX	Parasitology
QU	Biochemistry	QY	Clinical pathology
QV	Pharmacology	QZ	Pathology

Medicine and Related Subjects

W	Medical profession	WJ	Urogenital system
WA	Public health	WK	Endocrine system
WB	Practice of medicine	WL	Nervous system
WC	Infectious diseases	WM	Psychiatry
WD 100	Deficiency diseases	WN	Radiology
WD 200	Metabolic diseases	WO	Surgery
WD 300	Diseases of allergy	WP	Gynaecology
WD 400	Animal poisoning	WQ	Obstetrics
WD 500	Plant poisoning	WR	Dermatology
WD 600	Diseases caused by physical agents	WT	Geriatrics. Chronic diseases
WD 700	Aviation and space medicine	WU	Dentistry. Oral surgery
WE	Musculoskeletal system	WV	Otorhinolaryngology
WF	Respiratory system	WW	Ophthalmology
WG	Cardiovascular system	WX	Hospitals
WH	Haemic and lymphatic systems	WY	Nursing
WI	Gastrointestinal system	WZ	History of medicine

An example of subdivision (WG Cardiovascular system) is:

WG	Cardiovascular system
WG 200	Heart, general works
WG 201	Anatomy. Histology. Embryology
WG 202	Physiology. Mechanism of the heart beat
WG 205	Cardiac emergencies
WG 220	Congenital heart disease

One advantage of this scheme is its simplicity. Another is that the National Library of Medicine publishes *NLM Current Catalog* quarterly, with annual cumulations (*see* page 56) in which entries are given NLM classification numbers and subject headings. New medical books published in the US sometimes contain the NLM classification number.

Another scheme designed for medical libraries is the Barnard classification, devised by a former librarian of the London School of Hygiene and Tropical Medicine for his own library in 1936. He subsequently revised it to make it suitable for all types of medical libraries (Barnard, 1955). Like the NLM scheme, it provides for specific entry – one place for each topic, under which all its aspects are brought together. The scheme has 26 main classes, symbolized by the letters of the alphabet:

Main Classes (alternative notation, 1955)

A	Generalia
B	Natural sciences, including anatomy and physiology
C	General medicine
D	History of medicine
E	Epidemiology, medical statistics and medical geography
F	Specific diseases and their causative agents, including immunology, bacteriology, parasitology and medical entomology
G	Pathology and haematology
H	Diagnosis and clinical medicine
I	Materia medica, pharmacy and therapeutics
J	Hygiene, public health, social medicine, and medical jurisprudence
K	Aviation medicine
L	Tropical, military and naval medicine
M	Industrial medicine
N	Locomotor system
O	Cardiology and angiology
P	Neurology and psychiatry
Q	Ophthalmology
R	Otorhinolaryngology and respiratory system
S	Gastro-enterology and endocrinology
T	Dermatology, urology, and sexology
U	Gynaecology, obstetrics, paediatrics, and geriatrics
V	Surgery
W	Dentistry (odontology and stomatology)
X	Veterinary science
Y	Agriculture (plant and animal industry)
Z	Geography, anthropology, and sociology

An example of subdivision (O Cardiology and angiology) is:

O	Cardiology and angiology
OA	Blood pressure
OB	Hypertension
OBJ	Heart failure

Some important medical libraries in Britain use the Dewey decimal system or its modification, the Universal Decimal Classification (UDC). In the schemes the whole field of human knowledge is divided into ten main classes:

000	Generalities	600	Technology (applied sciences)
100	Philosophy	700	The arts. Fine and decorative arts
200	Religion	800	Literature
300	Social sciences	900	General geography and history and their
400	Languages		auxiliaries
500	Pure sciences		

These are further subdivided by adding figures to the right of the main number, giving decimal subdivision. A decimal point is added after the third figure. An advantage of these two decimal systems is that they permit infinite expansion within each subject field to accommodate new subjects or to expand existing ones. A disadvantage is that they separate material dealing with different aspects (anatomy, physiology, disease, etc.) of an organ, system or region. In the UDC the classification numbers can be very long and unwieldy.

In the Dewey system the class 600 is devoted to Technology (applied sciences) and its first subdivision, 610, is allocated to Medicine. An example of subdivision is:

600	Technology (applied sciences)
610	Medical sciences. Medicine
611	Human anatomy, cytology, tissue biology
611.1	Cardiovascular organs
611.11	Pericardium
611.12	Heart
612	Human physiology
612.1	Blood and circulation
616	Diseases
616.1	Diseases of cardiovascular system
616.11	of cardiac membranes
616.12	of heart

The subdivisions .1 to .8 are the same in anatomy (611), physiology (612) and diseases (616). The UDC has the same framework.

A few other classification schemes may be met in medical libraries – for example, the Library of Congress and the Bliss schemes, designed to cover all fields of knowledge, and the Cunningham and Boston schemes, intended for use in medical libraries. Some libraries have invented their own schemes to meet their particular needs.

Co-operation

The continuous growth of scientific literature, the proliferation of periodicals and the interconnection of one discipline with another make it impossible for any one library to be completely independent. Other sources must be tapped.

The most recent trend in Britain and in the US has been similar – the development of library networks; approaches are varied but the objectives are common. On both sides of the Atlantic attempts are being made through co-ordination and co-operation to improve standards of service to the user by making more effective use of existing local and regional resources. Wessex Regional Library and Information Service provides a good example of a well-developed service which includes back-up from a major resource collection, that of the Wessex Medical Library, which is a part of the Southampton University Library. There are four Thames Regional Health Authority Librarians and regional schemes at different stages of development now cover a significant part of the UK.

Apart from the facilities offered at a national level by the British Library, a good deal of co-operation is practised informally between individual libraries. Rapid loans of books and journals, and the supply of photocopies are possible in Britain, where the telephone and Telex may produce the required item within a matter of hours. Many libraries compile and regularly revise handlists of their periodicals, and circulate them to other libraries to encourage inter-library lending. Although the efficient and expanding services offered by the British Library and the National Library of Medicine in recent years have, to some extent, superseded this friendly co-operation, a considerable amount of help is still given to readers through this source.

References

Barnard, C. C. (1955), *A Classification for Medical and Veterinary Libraries,* 2nd edn, London, H. K. Lewis

Bunch, A. J. (1975), *Hospital and Medical Libraries in Scotland,* Glasgow, Scottish Library Association

Campbell, J. M. (1981), Some recent developments in health science libraries in North America. In: *Medical Librarianship,* p. 284, edited by M. Carmel, London, Library Association

Cummings, M. M. (1981), The National Library of Medicine. In: *Coping with the Biomedical Literature* edited by K. S. Warren, New York, Praeger

Directory of Health Sciences Libraries in the United States (1979), Chicago, American Medical Association

Directory of Medical and Health Care Libraries in the United Kingdom and Republic of Ireland (1982), 5th edn, London, Library Association

Directory of Postgraduate Medical Centres 1982, London, Council for Postgraduate Medical Education

Gaskell, E. (1970), British Medical Libraries. In: *Handbook of Medical Library Practice,* 3rd edn, p. 381, edited by G. L. Annan and J. W. Felter, Chicago, Medical Library Association

McCarthy, C. (1981), Third World medical libraries. In: *Medical Librarianship,* p. 297, edited by M. Carmel, London, Library Association

Miles, W. D. (1982) *A History of the National Library of Medicine,* Washington DC, US Govt. Printing Office

National Library of Medicine Classification (1978), 4th edn, Washington, US Dept. of Health, Education and Welfare

Thornton, J. L. (1966), *Medical Books, Libraries and Collectors,* 2nd edn, p. 318, London, A. Deutsch

Warren, K. S. (ed) (1981), *Coping with the Biomedical Literature. A Primer for the Scientist and Clinician,* New York, Praeger

2

Primary sources of information

R. J. Dannatt

One of the earliest large-scale surveys of a representative group of scientists (Halbert and Ackoff, 1959) showed that on average more time was spent in scientific communication than in any other activity. The mean 33 per cent of total time identified in the survey included time spent in both oral and print communication. As a prelude to this chapter on primary sources of information, it seems worthwhile to consider first the importance of oral communication, so far as it is known, and how it relates to communication mechanisms which operate through the published literature. The work done in this field has usually considered communication in science and technology, but much of it carries significance for medicine as well.

Personal contacts

De Solla Price (1963) has postulated the existence of 'invisible colleges': informal groupings of 100–200 scientists, active in research, who communicate verbally with each other at conferences, colloquia, summer schools and by long-distance telephone while adding to the cumulating structure of the scientific literature only belatedly and more from convention than need. The colleges clearly have much in common with the Information Exchange Groups (IEG) sponsored by the National Institutes of Health in the early sixties, whose aim was the free circulation of unrefereed memoranda among members and the encouragement of informal comment, without prejudice to later publication of the same material in the literature. The subject scope of the seven experimental IEGs was quite limited, as for instance Haemostasis and Immunopathology, but even so memberships were generally between 500 and 1000. More recent examples of invisible colleges are the Connective Tissue groups and the European Iron Club. The latter is an informal grouping of research workers and clinicians with an interest in iron metabolism, about 100 in number, who meet once every year.

A recurrent theme in studies of communication has been that it is a complex and often idiosyncratic process in which the individuals are concerned to safeguard their sense of autonomy and creativity against the pressure of both other people's words and other people's writings. Information discovered by chance, whether during casual conversation with colleagues or while browsing in the literature, may be valued more highly than information sought specifically or deliberately because it seems to have been elicited spontaneously. It is possible that communication studies carried out by means of interviews emphasize the importance of personal contacts and chance because this is a natural response in the interview situation, whereas studies carried out by questionnaire, often associated with libraries, emphasize rather the systematic scanning and searching of the literature.

More recent studies of the invisible college concept (Meadows, 1974) have shown that it, too, is a complex process which varies according to the subject field in which communication is taking place. These studies emphasize the importance of local research groups, often based on one scientific centre, whose 'internal' communication system provides a necessary backing to the longer range contacts between individuals. While the existence of certain individuals, often prominent members of research teams, is fundamental to the invisible college, the same individuals also have a range of contacts outside the college and in addition communicate extensively by means of the literature.

These findings seem to confirm work that has been done on the diffusion of information in industrial R and D laboratories (Allen, 1969) and on the communication of drug information to physicians (Herman and Rodowskas, 1976). Allen showed that certain individuals in each organization functioned as 'gatekeepers' – intermediaries through whom other members of the staff contacted individuals outside the organization and kept in touch with the published literature. The implication here is that though much of the flow of information in industrial laboratories is through personal contacts, the literature is being monitored nonetheless by means of the gatekeepers. In an analogous way, surveys of the process by which drug information is disseminated in communities of physicians have tended to show that in respect of new drugs, at least, the process is dependent on a few individuals who advise their colleagues while at the same time keeping in touch with both professional (including published) sources of information and commercial ones.

In biomedical fields such as cancer research, where the pace of investigation and achievement is at its most rapid, communication by means of personal contacts has been described as both 'instantaneous' and accurate (Thomas, 1978). This is due to the greater openness of present day research, which is itself due to a heightened awareness on the part of researchers that so much still awaits discovery. Communication in technology is of interest because it is possible that medicine has more affinities with technology than with science. De Solla Price (1965, 1970) has distinguished between science and technology on the basis of the pattern of citation in scientific and technological papers. Bibliographies in science are longer and exhibit a higher proportion of references to the recent literature than those in technology – a measure of this being the percentage of references to papers less than five years old in the total number of references included in a bibliography. This value may range from 70 to 90 per cent for a science with a rapidly cumulating literature such as biochemistry (where the number of references per paper is normally about 30) to figures of less than 40 per cent in engineering. In an analysis of papers published in *The Lancet* and *British Medical Journal* between 1900 and 1970, Liepa (1971) showed that the increase in the proportion of scientifically oriented papers during the period was matched by an increase in the proportion of papers carrying bibliographies. It would be interesting to see a further analysis to show whether there was a parallel increase in the 'immediacy' of the references listed in the bibliographies published during this period.

In a large-scale survey of British publications in all fields, Earle and Vickery (1969) showed that bibliographies in medical books and periodicals are, on average, five times longer than those in engineering, and some two and a half times longer than those in other technologies, such as agriculture. It can therefore be argued that by De Solla Price's test much of present-day laboratory and clinical medicine, as well as anaesthetics, pathology, obstetrics, epidemiology and pharmacology, is akin to science. In surgery, and especially its various branches such as orthopaedic or plastic surgery, bibliographies are both shorter and conform more to the technological pattern. One senses, too, that in these fields the paper being written is less important than the particular prosthesis or technique of skin grafting under discussion. Another of the distinctions between science and technology made by De Solla Price is that in the former it is the literature that develops and cumulates while in the latter the literature is subservient and it is a 'state of the art' that cumulates. There may be some significance in the fact that the *Journal of Bone and Joint Surgery* is published in two sections, an American and a British, with the implication that the journals contribute towards a national art rather than international knowledge.

Making use of Wood and Hamilton's survey of mechanical engineers working in the UK (1967), it seems likely that surgeons rate personal contacts higher as an information source than documentary sources, such as original papers or reviews, while workers in other branches of medicine rate personal contacts relatively lower. The success of the various 'Clinical Librarian' experiments during the seventies seems to indicate the readiness of doctors in the typical clinical setting to accept verbal information, either from a clinical librarian or from a colleague, and also their ultimate reliance on the published literature. Greenberg (1978) reports that no significant differences were found in the experiment at Yale–New Haven Hospital between the use made of clinical librarian services across a range of medical fields, which included surgery, paediatrics and psychiatry. The results of a clinical librarian experimental project in Britain are reported by Childs (1982), Moore (1982) and Wilkin (1982).

The periodical literature

One of the most valuable and largely unforeseen consequences of our increased awareness of oral communication in science and technology has been increased understanding of the way the literature operates and the ends it serves. The view that the function of the periodical literature is the communication of information was put by Bernal (1939) in his now classic *Social Function of Science*. He voiced quite clearly the indifference of science to linguistic or national barriers and the need of practitioners, at all levels, for the data, information on techniques, conceptual frameworks and new ideas that the literature conveys (Bernal, 1959).

Characteristically, he saw the literature as part of a system having properties such as 'sluggishness' and 'waste' and was one of the first to propose ways by which the system could be improved. This is in contrast to the view (Ziman, 1968) that the fact of publication is less important than the processes of comment, modification and evaluation that each account of new work passes through during publication (the refereeing process) and thereafter, and that ends with assimilation into the corpus of scientific knowledge. While allowing that the literature embodies great quantities of data and information, this view allows also for the fact that much of it may be unimportant or unoriginal; value resides not in the literature but in the consensus of ideas that experienced scientists create out of it. De Solla Price (1965, 1967) has described the periodical litera-ture as having today a merely archival function in contrast to the function of primary communication performed verbally and through agencies such as the invisible colleges. Hence his view that scientists are motivated to add to the published literature but not any longer to read it. The literature, while accounting only for about 20 per cent of overall scientific communication, is neverthe-less useful partly for the purpose of reviewing the relationships and significance of new advances, partly as a means whereby the inex-perienced can obtain access to problems of current research and partly as a record of achievement which interacts with technology and the general culture of the time. This view of the periodical literature as archive emphasizes the permanent need of all scien-tists for access to it.

Publication in the periodical literature has been the prime way scientists claim priority for their work; the public availability of this literature is the chief guarantee that the recognition awarded them, however much or little it may amount to, emanates from their peers and is real (Hagstrom, 1965). The growth of team research, often giving rise to multiple authorship, and the custom of publishing a description of a research project for accounting purposes has undoubtedly eroded this particular aspect of the liter-ature, but it still exists. It was assumed at their inception that memoranda distributed within Information Exchange Groups (IEGs) would eventually be published in the normal way, thus safeguarding the right of authors to recognition. Whether the cir-culation of a memorandum gave priority or not was an early cause of embarrassment, but what ended the IEG experiment, apart from its cost, was the refusal of a number of important biochemical journals to accept any paper for publication that had previously existed as an IEG memorandum (Thorpe, 1967). In the same way, the indifference which most scientists feel for the research report literature is due not so much to a low opinion of reports as to a respect for the traditional primacy of the 'open' literature. One may note in passing that in medicine and in engineering there are ways of establishing priority, and of thereby obtaining recognition, that are additional to the way established within science of first publishing in the literature. These are, in medicine, the first accurate and complete description of a disease or physical condition and, in engineering, the successful patenting of a new mechanism or process.

It has been left to the journal editors such as Fox (1965), Maddox (1967) and Ingelfinger (1974) to emphasize that periodicals, in addition to their other functions, must stimulate their readers and provide an outlet for argument, criticism, speculation and comment. In medicine, especially, they must also meet the needs of the developing specialty and of education in general, which means the publication of papers with a factual rather than an experimental content addressed by the expert to the less well qualified. *The Lancet, Nature* and *New England Journal of Medicine (NEJM)* have deliberately set out to combine the function of 'recorders' of advances in knowledge with the function of medical or scientific 'newspapers'. Review periodicals are covered in Chapter 3, but the point is perhaps worth making here that they can be grouped with the 'newspapers' rather than the 'recorders'.

The Council of Biology Editors has accepted (Zwemer, 1970) a formal definition of the scientific periodical which stresses, among others, the following characteristics:

(1) It should contain first disclosures, i.e. first accounts of new work.
(2) Papers should provide sufficient detail for observations to be assessed, experiments repeated and ideas evaluated.
(3) It should be permanent.

Developments in biomedical communication

In biomedicine, as in other fields, it seems clear that the historical development of periodicals has been in the direction of perfecting them as a means by which knowledge can be enlarged and consolidated while at the same time providing a mechanism for the reward, through peer recognition, of individual contributing authors. The outcome of this historical process is the primary journal as we now know it – a package made up of a varying number of the basic and now perfected units of information, or scientific papers. It seems equally clear that the orientation of periodicals towards what Ziman aptly called public knowledge, with the attendant concern to prefer the publication of first disclosures and to aim at archival permanence, has meant that the other important function of the literature – communication – has become neglected. What seems to have happened is that the immense strength of the scientific tradition, as demonstrated in the cumulating structure of the scientific archive, has resulted in a widespread feeling that papers with a different aim – that of education, or speculation, or case report – must still be as self-contained and formal as the archival literature proper. We may smile at the drug advertisements, each with its carefully composed list of references, but were it not for the strength of the archive tradition they could dispense with them and get on with the business of telling doctors how good the drugs are!

Wyatt (1972) has taken this line of argument a stage further and, in a detailed analysis of the events, discussions and publications leading up to the discovery of the helix structure of DNA in 1953, suggests that the progress of discovery itself was slower and more erratic than it need have been had an earlier paper on DNA in 1948 been less reticent, or the reviews of it less cautious. He has also analysed the network of citations linking the various papers published between 1948 and 1953 and shows that there are several serious discontinuities; he concludes, pessimistically, that new information is unrecognized until it is transformed into knowledge. Perhaps the often documented part played by chance in the process of discovery is so large simply because the literature as a source of information is so unresponsive. An account of the events, some accidental, leading up to the discovery of the mechanism of poliomyelitis infection (Bodian, 1976) gives some support to this. Shephard (1973) has documented the history of a paper reporting some unusual cases of poisoning in the US which was refused publication by four major national journals (some refereed) before being accepted, unchanged, by a local medical journal. It appears that the paper was not well written in the first place, but it seems likely that a further reason for the rejections was the paper's limited scope. Nevertheless it was, as Shephard points out, the first original case report in America of this particular type of poisoning. The continuing importance of case reports in clinical medicine is shown by the fact that research into a new method of publishing and storing them forms one of the recommendations of the recent Medical Information Review Panel (Cockerill, 1981)

The Information Exchange Groups were a significant experiment in communication because they were devised by scientists rather than by documentalists or scientific management. The proposal that unrefereed and unedited communications should be circulated to loosely defined groups of co-workers was both made and received with enthusiasm (Green, 1964). Membership of the groups rose rapidly, as did the number of memoranda in circulation. There is an interesting parallel here with the informal distribution of preprints, reprints and reports of research, in addition to discussions of work in progress at meetings and seminars, which exists on an extensive scale in psychology (Garvey and Griffith, 1965). Posen and Posen (1969) have shown that the demand for reprints of some quite representative papers published in the earliest years of *Current Contents, Life Sciences* and long before the appearance of *Current Contents, Clinical Practice* can run well into three figures, while requests for a reprint of a particular review article on alkaline phosphatase were as high as 1246. A reprint, once received, can be thought of as a personal communication and it may be that the demand for reprints is higher than the demand, within an equivalent time, for the same papers as part of the normal periodical literature. If so, this and the popularity of reprint and memorandum circulation systems, such as the IEG, may be due to the individual scientist's wish to participate, both as giver and receiver, in an informal – even personal – information system within which a degree of inefficiency and waste is taken for granted.

Significantly, perhaps, one of the more effective recent developments in communication is also in the biomedical field: the International Research Communications System (IRCS). In this the basic unit of information is a short paper of 1000 words (more if no tables are included) with a bibliography of not more than ten references. The papers, which may report research or patient care – but in either case factually – are submitted with a small fee and if acceptable to a board of editors and referees are published within about a month as separates. They also form contributions to one or more of a series of 32 IRCS Medical Science journals, published monthly or bimonthly, and may also contribute to a further IRCS Medical Science *Key Reports* series. It is evident that IRCS papers lend themselves to packaging in a range of formats and very recently a new one has been added, an online format. Papers will now be available, except for their illustrations, in advance of publication in any other format as part of a computer database held in the USA by Bibliographic Retrieval Services. The database exists currently from 1982 and papers can be obtained either directly in the form of printout or alternatively by requesting, via the terminal, a copy of the printed separate. There are obvious parallels between this mode of communication and the synopsis journal mode, which, however, has not been experimented with in medicine. In synopsis journals each paper exists in two versions: a short one of 800 to 1000 words which is published in the normal way and a full length version made permanently available in some more easily stored but less convenient format, such as microfiche, mini-print or even on disc – in which case it is only accessible online.

The traditional communication system in science is held together by two groups of people: the authors, who generate new information but who as readers equally consume it, and the referees. The traditional rewards of recognition and status can only be given by the consumers of new information and, therefore, the referee's function is really to distance and screen new information during its transmission from author to consumer. This preliminary validation is nevertheless essential for the health of the system, but there is also a basic rule underpinning the whole – that of the 'first disclosure'. It follows, therefore, that any weakening of the reporting tradition shows itself either in a weakening of the basic rule or in a weakening of the author–consumer and referee relationship. In biomedicine especially there are now indications that the rule is not being observed, or rather that its importance to the system is no longer understood. Relman (1977) describes two occasions in which a paper submitted to *New England Journal of Medicine* was already being considered, with substantially the same content and the same authors, by two other journals. The two papers were both in effect published three times over a short period without any of the editors, or referees, having been apprised of the situation.

One aspect of these two instances of triplicate publication that Relman does not discuss is the part that may have been played by the co-authors, since both papers had several authors. It seems likely that co-authorship, now so common, dilutes 'authorship' to the point at which the first disclosure rule loses significance. Any recent issue of *New England Journal of Medicine* or *The Lancet* shows a list of original articles with an average of six or more authors for each. Durack (1978) showed that the number of papers with a single author published in *NEJM* had declined to four per cent by 1977 and that the average authorship in *NEJM* for that year was between four and five per paper. The question that needs to be asked, one feels, is whether the multiple publication of new work is a help or a hindrance to its dissemination. This question is not answered definitively by referring to the danger of choking the communication system; it is well known, for instance, that the same information is multiplied many times in the pre-publication mode of communication in science.

It may also be significant that the role of referees in biomedicine is being questioned and especially their traditional anonymity (Ingelfinger, 1974). Furthermore, certain journals of high standing such as *The Lancet* make little use of referees. A recent innovation in *Nature* is the publication of Matters Arising. These are short commentaries on papers already published in the journal which are submitted jointly by the original paper's author and the author of the commentary. The significance of this development is that it seems to show a weakening of the referee role, since the first author is effectively functioning as referee for the second. The editor of *British Medical Journal* criticizes refereeing from the point of view of its unreliability in selecting for originality and merit (Lock, 1982).

In contrast to what appears to be a trend in medicine towards publishing for dissemination, the trend in science seems strongly towards preserving the traditional system of publishing for knowledge through the quality control mechanisms of first disclosure, refereeing and peer review. A recent study of the scientific information system in the UK conducted by the Royal Society (Rowland, 1982) showed that nearly all British scientists were in favour of refereeing and that most thought the important characteristic of a journal chosen for publication purposes was its scientific standard and reputation. There was little enthusiasm for developments which, potentially at least, dilute the first disclosure principle by two-part publication, i.e. synopsis journals or 'letters' journals – and still less for the publication of all new papers as separates. This study of the scientific information system was conducted by means of a questionnaire. In a recent article Ziman (1982) reiterates his belief in the communication system as the 'core institution' of science and in its absolute dependence on the 'public social apparatus' of authoritative refereeing, open publication and collective review.

Medical journals

Journals comprising the primary literature of medicine are basically of three types: journals devoted to news, opinion and comment; journals devoted to original contributions; and review journals. Original contributions in medicine are normally reported once only and at full length, but journals publishing preliminary communications (normally about 2500 words), such as *Biochemical and Biophysical Research Communications,* are beginning to make their appearance. The three basic types of journal are not mutually exclusive; the *New England Journal of Medicine* contains, for example, original contributions as well as case reports and editorial comment, while about 60 per cent of the review articles listed in *Bibliography of Medical Reviews* do not appear in specific review periodicals. Certain journals with, primarily, a review function, such as *Obstetrical and Gynecological Survey* and the *Year Book* series, also publish extended abstracts of original papers appearing elsewhere. English language review journals in medicine are comparatively recent in origin, the earliest *Year Books* appearing in the mid-thirties and the first formal review journals, *Progress in Allergy* and *Advances in Internal Medicine,* several years later. German journals in the *Ergebnisse* series were first published between 1892 and 1902.

The Lancet, one of the oldest medical journals, first appeared in 1823. Liepa (1971) sampled issues of this and the *British Medical Journal* decennially from 1900 to 1970 and has shown that the decline of 16 per cent in the number of clinical studies being published by the end of this period was matched by an increase of 22 per cent in the number of experimental studies. More specifically, she found that surgical and pathological papers diminished by 19 per cent and 15 per cent, respectively, while papers in biochemistry and drug therapy increased by 12 per cent and 18.5 per cent. Articles in the field of social medicine increased during the period by seven per cent. In addition to the apparent change in orientation, there has been a great increase in the volume of periodical publishing in medicine, particularly in the sixties and seventies. Webb (1970) analysed papers in 19 primary journals in biochemistry between 1958 and 1967 and found that the doubling time for the total number of papers in this field was 6.9 years. The doubling time for pages or words was 5.2 years – a more realistic figure from the point of view of the reader wishing to keep up to date and one which shows, incidentally, that in spite of editorial policies papers are tending to become longer rather than shorter. A recent year (1977) of the Source Data listing in *Journal Citation Reports* shows that nearly half of the world's journals that publish more than 1000 articles a year, general journals such as *Nature* excluded, were biomedical ones.

The volume of publishing in medicine is giving rise, inevitably, to change in the proportion of the primary literature devoted to original contributions, to commentary and to review. The review journals have grown relative to the recorders because, especially in the more clinical fields, they play such an active and essential part in promulgating therapy and in advancing the 'state of the art'. If scientific knowledge cumulates, only occasionally to be reformed, it is probably truer of knowledge in medicine to say that it constantly updates. De Solla Price (1981) makes the point that the clinical literature, unlike the scientific, is not self-validating (since revising a 'state of the art' is an end in itself) and that the functions of evaluation and validation must therefore be performed separately. It is noticeable that in medicine there are a number of newer journals, for instance *Cancer Surveys* or *Life Chemistry Reports*, whose aim is to review a section of the overall field in depth and thereby to arrive at a definitive update. These publications represent a development of the traditional review journal, a further development being the creation of knowledge bases. The *Hepatitis Knowledge Base*, for instance (Bernstein, 1980), is more authoritative than any single review since it is based on a large number of them (40), with additional input from other experts; yet it still maintains links with the contributing papers by quoting data from them and citing them in full. Developing the medical journal in this direction necessitates computer storage of the material and interrogation of it online.

Guides to journals

General guides are often presented from the viewpoint of the availability of periodicals on subscription while other guides cover particular applications, such as inter-library borrowing. Perhaps the most useful general guide to medical periodicals is *Ulrich's International Periodicals Directory*. This is published every year and there is also *Irregular Serials and Annuals*, a separate biennial publication listing less frequent periodicals and annuals. A supplement to both these publications is entitled *Ulrich's Quarterly*. The *Directory* is confined to periodicals currently in print and now incorporates an International Standard Serial Number (ISSN) for each title. Periodicals in *Ulrich* are listed under general headings such as Medical Sciences and Biology, divided to cover special areas such as Dentistry or Genetics. *World Medical Periodicals* is a listing of all medical, dental and veterinary journals in print at the time of the latest edition (1961, plus *Supplement*, 1968) with the addition of a number of journals which ceased publication between 1900 and 1950. Unlike *Ulrich* it is an alphabetical listing, but there is an Index to the entries by subject. *World Medical Periodicals* and its *Supplement* indicate that about 6000 periodicals were being published during the sixties in medicine generally. A more selective list of journals but one still representative of all specialties is the *List of Journals Indexed in Index Medicus*. This is published each year with the January issue of *Index Medicus* (also separately) and comprises currently about 2700 titles. In addition to subject representation, other criteria used in drawing up the *List* are: sponsorship of a journal by a recognized professional organization or national academy, existence of an active and high-level editorial board and freedom from sectional or promotional bias. *BIOSIS* (BIOSciences Information Service) and *Excerpta Medica* also publish lists of the journals from which papers are chosen and abstracted. The BIOSIS list, published annually, includes an American Standard abbreviation for each title plus a coden (further abbreviation to 6 upper case letters), if available. A listing of some 300 of the more important medical journals from the point of view of authors seeking publication has been published with the title *Writer's Guide to Medical Periodicals*, compiled by Lane and Kammerer (1975). This includes information, not previously available, on the average rejection rates of most of the periodicals listed.

Both *Ulrich* and the separately published version of the *Index Medicus* list include listings of journals according to subject. The latter is more detailed and is carried out at the level of specialties such as orthopaedics or nephrology. Subject guidance to medical periodicals may also be obtained from the list of journals held by a library specializing in the field, for instance the *Periodical Holdings* of the Institute of Psychiatry, or by consulting the subject index in *World Medical Periodicals* or a national listing such as *British Medical Periodicals*. The latter covers current British journals of repute and includes notes on subject scope, with additional information on subscription costs, date of first publication, frequency, and publishers and their addresses. The last edition appeared in 1980.

Guides to abstract journals and indexes in medicine are dealt with in Chapter 3. Review articles, as noted earlier, tend to be dispersed throughout the medical literature, but a list of review journals proper can be found in *List of Annual Reviews of Progress in Science and Technology*, published by Unesco. Fifty-three review journals are identified in medicine and a further 45 in special fields such as surgery and paediatrics. Apart from obscure journals, the one category less easily covered by lists is new journals. *Ulrich* gives coverage in the *Directory* and the information is updated in the *Quarterly*. The National Library of Medicine *Current Catalog* lists new journals quarterly and British titles are recorded in *British Medicine*. The first issue of all new British periodicals is listed in the weekly *British National Bibliography*, where details of publisher, subscription and frequency are given. *Serials in the British Library*, No 1 – (June 1981 –; quarterly) lists new periodicals, British and foreign, with details which include publisher, price, frequency, abbreviated key title, location and holdings. It has wider coverage than indicated by its title as it includes new periodicals held in a number of British libraries.

Usage

Because periodicals are not themselves units of information, but merely packages, comparative studies of the use of periodicals are of little interest to first-hand readers. Few doctors or biomedical scientists work in isolation and the 'pecking order' of the current journals in a research field is one of the least disputed of its characteristics (Royal Society, 1981). Use studies are, however, of great interest to librarians since their work is, to a considerable extent, the management and handling of information packages, not that of the units of information – or papers – themselves.

Records of the consultation of periodicals either in or between libraries form the usual material for studies of use, though the scale of consultation must obviously be large enough to sustain any subsequent comparisons between titles or ranking. The alternative material for studying use is a very different record of the consultation of a periodical: the citation. In the search for quantifiable acts of use from which generalizations can be made, it is extremely easy to lose sight of the basic fact that a citation is a rather specific linking of one unit of information with another. The consultation of periodicals in or between libraries on the other hand includes other linkings of equal importance from the usage point of view. It covers the use of the package directly, for instance to look up a particular periodical's instructions to authors. It also covers a wider spectrum of the readers of periodicals since use studies based on citation are necessarily limited to readers who are also authors; often, indeed, authors writing from some interdisciplinary viewpoint. From the librarian's point of view it is not unfair to say that the overall rankings of periodicals based on frequency of citation in the *Science Citation Index* source journals and reported in *Journal Citation Reports* and elsewhere (Garfield, 1972, 1976a) are of limited use precisely because the database is so general. The more specific studies that have been published from time to time such as the analysis of citations in a number of pathology journals (Garfield, 1976b) are of more practical interest. It may well be, of course, that an overall ranking based on interdisciplinary citation turns out *not* to be so different from one based on citation in one particular field of one particular discipline!

The phenomena of 'self-citation' and 'self-derivation' play a part in all use studies based on citation since they vary considerably from one discipline to another. Earle and Vickery (1969) showed that self-citation in medicine, the extent to which medical publications (books included) cite publications in medicine, is quite high (61 per cent), but less high than self-citation in science generally (70 per cent) and much less so than in technology (81 per cent). Self-derivation in medicine, the extent to which medical references derive from medical sources, was 70 per cent, again lower than in science (78 per cent), but higher than in technology (62 per cent). The implication is that medicine is not less but more interdisciplinary than science and therefore that a ranking of periodicals by interdisciplinary citation in science favours general periodicals slightly less than should be the case for medicine.

The closest equivalent to a usage study based on borrowing from a British medical library is a survey carried out at the National Lending Library for Science and Technology (NLLST) in 1967 (Wood and Bower, 1969). The assumption is made in this survey, as in other NLLST and British Library Lending Division (BLLD) surveys, that borrowing within a certain field from a national library can be equated with borrowing within the same field from a local library. In the context of medicine this assumption seems questionable, one reason being an apparent disparity between the population of borrowers from the national library and the population of borrowers in a normal medical library. Less than a quarter of the libraries requesting items from the NLLST at the time of this survey were medical ones, the majority being industrial, research establishment and general university libraries. It is well known that in medicine the availability of libraries (and hence the availability to practitioners of the national library) is generally poor; in this field, more perhaps than in any other today, an older tradition of buying the literature either oneself or through one's employer still persists.

Scales (1976) has compared rankings of most frequently cited periodicals obtained from the *Science Citation Index* database with rankings of periodicals carrying similar dates of publication as most frequently borrowed from NLLST. She found many differences between the two rank lists so produced. Titles common to both the 50 most borrowed and the 50 most cited lists totalled 16 only. The conclusion is drawn that since inter-library borrowing is a measure of 'actual' use, citation frequency must therefore be unreliable as such a measure. Some consideration is, however, given in this paper to the question of whether the pattern of borrowing from a national library through inter-library loan is a true reflection of literature needs generally. This question has been taken up in a later survey of the usage of periodicals at the BLLD in 1980 (Clarke, 1981) in which a rank list of titles most frequently borrowed was found to be substantially different from one produced five years earlier. The point is conceded that 'core lists' of periodicals do not seem to have any lasting validity and that this may be due to the effect of changing local circumstances on the demand relationship between client libraries and a central interlending one. The Clarke survey reported in passing that medical libraries accounted in 1980 for 14 per cent of overall requests for periodicals at BLLD. Since this figure excluded some university medical libraries it may well be that the total demand on BLLD from medical libraries exceeds 20 per cent. One wonders what proportion of the total usage at BLLD is represented by medicine as a subject. It is probably safe to assume that this usage is greater than that represented by the social sciences (13 per cent), but there is no breakdown in this paper (nor in the British Library *Annual Reports*) of the overall science and technology figure of 80 per cent approximately.

A refinement of the citation method of estimating usage was employed by Raisig (1966) to produce a rank list of all biomedical periodicals being published between 1951 and 1960. In this the final ranking was derived not from numbers of citations as such, but from the number of citations per article published in the given period, essentially the same method as the one used in *Journal Citation Reports* under the heading 'Impact Factor'. The advantage of ranking periodicals by impact factor is that it eliminates the bias introduced by periodicals which publish a large tally of papers every year (since more papers means potentially more citations) and at the same time the bias introduced by the existence in some years of a few papers in a few journals carrying very high citation counts. These papers may well be the first ones to describe a promising technique, for instance in pathology, or a new statistical method as in epidemiology. The disadvantage of ranking by impact factor is that it unduly favours review periodicals, since these inevitably contain a number of very frequently cited articles. A further point is that ranking by impact factor lends itself to viewing the usefulness of periodicals in terms of cost effectiveness, but this in turn raises the question of 'cost effectiveness to whom?'

In addition to the assessment of usage by means of library borrowing statistics or citation counts, usage may of course be predicted intuitively on a basis of the 'best' periodicals in a given field or with a given group of users in mind. An example of this is the 99 periodicals chosen for inclusion in *Abridged Index Medicus* in 1970. Appendix 2 at the end of this chapter comprises this listing together with, for comparison, a list based on British inter-library borrowing (Wood and Bower, 1969) and one based on frequency of citation in a group of pathology journals (Garfield, 1976b). The 'overlap' between the last two lists is about 50 per cent if allowance is made for some self-citation in pathology. The inclusion of *Science* in the *Abridged Index Medicus* list and its ranking in the other two lists illustrates the importance of wide-ranging periodicals in both medicine generally and in a specific medical field.

Research reports

As a form of primary communication, reports are of much less significance in medicine than in other areas of science, or in technology. Not only is there a long-standing tradition of publication in the conventional literature, but the somewhat less Government-controlled institutional research in medicine than, for instance, in atomic energy or space research has meant less demand for the 'instant publication' that reports provide. The Medical Research Council's research reports and the American Public Health Service's equivalents are published not as communications directly from a research establishment, with merely an identifying code and serial number, but as normal publications of the respective state publishing systems. As such they are better organized bibliographically and much more easy to acquire. The beginnings of a research report literature can, however, be seen in the field of aerospace medicine, particularly in the US. Documents in this field carry prefixes such as ARU (US Army Aeromedical Research Unit) and SAM-TR (USAF School of Aerospace Medicine, Technical Report) and are often available only on microfiche.

Theses

Theses, like conference papers, must be considered primary sources of information since the research projects written up in them may not receive publication in any other form. Part or parts of a thesis are sometimes rewritten and published as a periodical article, but the thesis remains a first and often fuller statement of results. As such it may be of great importance to a research worker commencing study in a new field and to others as a source of ideas. It is said that both Germany and Japan have a blanket order for copies of all the theses handled by University Microfilms, amounting to about 90 per cent of all American doctoral dissertations. A copy of all theses submitted and accepted for higher degrees is deposited in the University, Faculty of Medicine or Medical School Library, as appropriate, where it is normally available on inter-library loan. Some universities also deposit a copy of each of their doctoral theses with the British Library Lending Division. In the UK about 8000 theses a year are accepted for the award of higher degrees and a guide to these is Aslib's *Index to Theses accepted for Higher Degrees by the Universities of Great Britain and Ireland and the Council for National Academic Awards.* Theses are listed by subject with an index by author. An indirect guide to theses in progress is *Research in British Universities, Polytechnics and Colleges,* since this lists research projects under the names of academic staff immediately responsible. This publication appears annually in three volumes of which the second, *Biological Sciences*, includes medicine. Arrangement is by broad subject areas and each volume has name and subject indexes.

Dissertation Abstracts International is basically a guide to American and Canadian doctoral theses, though recently theses from a small number of European universities have been included and policy is to widen the European coverage as much as possible. It is published in two parts, the second being science and engineering, including biology and health science. The details of theses entered include a summary of 400–600 words and the names of both the author and supervisor of the thesis. *Dissertation Abstracts International* is now searchable online as one of the DIALOG databases under the name *Comprehensive Dissertation Index.* Both University Microfilms and Aslib are making attempts to improve bibliographical access to British theses, chiefly by proposing ways in which the abstracts submitted with theses can be collected and published separately. Abstracts of British theses are now usually available from the Aslib Library.

Translation facilities

The significance of foreign-language publications in academic work generally has been examined by Hutchins, Pargeter and Saunders (1971) and some interesting conclusions were arrived at regarding this significance in medicine as distinct from science and other non-humanities subjects. Surveys of borrowing, both local and non-local, photocopying, library consultation and citation were carried out at Sheffield University and these were backed by a number of interviews. It was found that the use made of foreign language materials was lower in the faculty of medicine than, on average, in other non-humanities faculties – in particular the use made of Russian-language publications, either in the original or in cover-to-cover translation, was very much lower. It was also found that the tendency for French-language publications to be most frequently used after those in English was not confirmed in medicine. German-language publications proved slightly more important here than French.

The Sheffield study of the 'language barrier' recommended that universities should provide facilities for 'outline translations' and that a translation centre for the UK should be set up to provide full translations of foreign-language publications where necessary. Both Aslib and the International Translations Centre at Delft maintain indexes of translations complete and in progress from most languages into the chief European ones, and can put individuals interested in a translation of a particular item in touch with the library or other organization which has undertaken it. The International Translations Centre publishes a monthly *World Transindex* and the American equivalent of this, published by the US National Translations Centre, is *Translations Register-Index*. The Aslib index of translations into English covers both British and American work and is at present growing by about 10 000 items a year.

Both Aslib and the Institute of Linguists maintain lists of qualified and experienced translators in all fields including medicine. The Institute's list is published as *Index of Members of the Translators' Guild* and is arranged primarily by subject, but has also a list of translators by geographical location.

Current awareness

The prime importance of current awareness for doctors and other hospital medical staff, for dentists and for general practitioners was established in a recent survey conducted in the UK (Ford, 1980). Not only was 'keeping up to date' mentioned most often by respondents to the survey questionnaire as a reason for seeking information, but, more significantly, it was ranked as most important among a range of information needs by all groups except the hospital dentists. Second place in terms of the importance of information needs was occupied for most respondents by 'clinical problems'. The Ford report included an account of a separate survey of the information needs of some paramedical hospital staff (physiotherapists) in which the paramount importance of keeping up to date was again emphasized, clinical problems coming second in the ranking.

Medical libraries often issue bulletins listing references of current interest which makes it easier for their readers to keep up to date. Inevitably, the coverage of the primary literature in these is dependent on the range of journals received in the library, while compilation is dependent on the prompt arrival of current issues. The advantage of locally produced current-awareness bulletins is that they may select from the medical literature papers of special interest, as for instance in dentistry, or carry out some editing of the titles which are not self-explanatory. Current awareness is a small and fairly self- contained segment of the total documentation field and in it the publications and methods recommended by librarians, more perhaps than in other segments such as retrieval, seem out of step with the methods favoured and used by biomedical scientists, if not also by doctors. We recommend using the secondary literature (*see* Chapter 3) – a surrogate literature designed to facilitate handling and scanning, yet reasonably complete; our scientific clients resolutely prefer the primary (Royal Society, 1981). The reason for this can only be a difference in what is held to be the most important characteristic of 'current' information. As librarians, we believe this to be scope, since all libraries aim at completeness in some sense or other, but our users are more concerned that current information should provide stimulus.

References

Allen, T. J. (1969) *Admin. Sci. Quart*, **14**, 12
Bernal, J. D. (1939), *The Social Function of Science*, Routledge
Bernal, J. D. (1959), In *Proceedings of the International Conference on Scientific Information*, vol 1, National Academy of Sciences
Bernstein, L. M. (1980), *Ann. Intern. Med*, **93**, 169
Bodian, D. (1976), *Johns Hopkins Med. J.*, **138**, 130
Childs, S. (1982), *The Experiences of a Clinical Librarian in Medicine*, British Library
Clarke, A. (1981), *Interlending Review*, **9**, 111
Cockerill, P. E. (1981) *Information and the Practice of Medicine: Report of the Medical Information Review Panel*, British Library
De Solla Price, D. J. (1963), *Little Science, Big Science*, Colombia University Press
De Solla Price, D. J. (1965), *Technology Cult.*, **6**, 553
De Solla Price, D. J. (1967), In *Communication in Science*, Little, Brown
De Solla Price, D. J. (1970), In *Communication among Scientists and Engineers*, D. C. Heath & Co.
De Solla Price, D. J. (1981), In *Coping with the Biomedical Literature* edited by K. S. Warren, Praeger
Durack, D. T. (1978), *N. England J. Med.*, **298**, 773
Earle, P. and Vickery, B. (1969), *Aslib Proc.*, **21**, 237

Ford, G. (1980), *The Use of Medical Literature,* British Library
Fox, T. (1965), *Crisis in Communication,* Athlone Press
Garfield, E. (1972), *Science,* **178,** 471
Garfield, E. (1976a), *Nature,* **264,** 609
Garfield, E. (1976b), *Pathol. Annu,* **11,** 335
Garvey, W. D. and Griffith, B. C. (1965), *Am. Psychol.,* **20,** 157
Green, D. E. (1964), *Science,* **148,** 1543
Greenberg, B. (1978), *Bull. Med. Libr. Assoc.,* **66,** 319
Hagstrom, W. O. (1965), *The Scientific Community,* Basic Books
Halbert, M. H. and Ackoff, R. L. (1959), In *Proceedings of the International Conference on Scientific Information,* vol 1, National Academy of Sciences
Herman, C. M. and Rodowskas, C. A. (1976), *J. Med. Educ.,* **51,** 189
Hutchins, W. J., Pargeter, L. J. and Saunders, W. L. (1971), *The Language Barrier: A Study in Depth of the Place of Foreign Language Materials in the Research Activity of an Academic Community,* Sheffield University
Ingelfinger, F. J. (1974), *Amer. J. Med.,* **56,** 686
Liepa, D. (1971), *MSc Thesis,* Postgraduate School of Librarianship and Information Science, Sheffield University
Lock, S. (1982), *Brit. Med. J.,* **285,** 1224
Maddox, J. (1967), *Nature,* **214,** 1077
Meadows, A. J. (1974), *Communication in Science,* Butterworths
Moore, A. (1982), *The Clinical Librarian in the Department of Surgery,* British Library
Posen, S. and Posen, J. S. (1969), *J. Med. Educ.* **44,** 648
Raisig, L. M. (1966), *Bull. Med. Libr. Ass.,* **54,** 108
Relman, A. S. (1977), *N. England J. Med.,* **297,** 724
Rowland, J. F. B. (1982), *J. Doc.,***38,** 94
Royal Society. (1981), *A Study of the Scientific Information System in the United Kingdom,* The Society
Scales, P. A. (1976), *J. Doc.,* **32,** 17
Shephard, D. A. E. (1973), *IEEE Trans. Prof. Comm.,* **PC 16,** 143
Thomas, L. (1978), *Science,* **200,** 1459
Thorpe, W. V. (1967), *Nature,* **213,** 547
Webb, E. C. (1970), *Nature,* **225,** 132
Wilkin, A. (1982), *The Evaluation of a Clinical Library Experiment,* British Library
Wood, D. N. and Bower, C. A. (1969), *Bull. Med. Libr. Assoc.,* **57,** 47
Wood D. N. and Hamilton, D. R. L. (1967), *The Information Requirements of Mechanical Engineers,* Library Association
Wyatt. H. V. (1972), *Nature* **235,** 86
Ziman, J. M. (1968), *Public Knowledge,* Cambridge University Press
Ziman, J. M. (1982), *Times Higher Ed. Suppl.,* No 518
Zwemer, R. L. (1970), *Fed. Proc.,* **29,** 1595

Appendix 1

Guides to periodicals and other publications

BioSciences Information Service: Serial sources for the BIOSIS database. Annual. BioSciences Information Service, Philadelphia

British Medical Periodicals: Supplement to *British Medicine 1980, No 9.* British Council, London

British Medicine. Monthly. Pergamon, Oxford

Dissertation Abstracts International. Monthly. University Microfilms, Ann Arbor

Index to Theses accepted for Higher Degrees by the Universities of Great Britain and Northern Ireland and the Council for National Academic Awards. Twice yearly. Aslib, London

Institute of Linguists: Index of members of the Translators' Guild. 1980. The Institute, London

Institute of Psychiatry: Periodicals Holdings. Regularly updated. The Institute, London

Irregular Serials and Annuals. 7th edn., 1982. Bowker, New York

Journal Citation Reports. Published with *Science Citation Index.* q.v.

Lane, N. D. and Kammerer, K. L. (1975), *Writer's Guide to Medical Periodicals,* Ballinger, Mass.

List of Annual Reviews of Progress in Science and Technology, 2nd edn., 1969. UNESCO, Paris

List of Journals Abstracted by Excerpta Medica. Annual. Excerpta Medica, Amsterdam

List of Journals Indexed in Index Medicus. Annual. National Library of Medicine, Bethesda

Research in British Universities, Polytechnics and Colleges. Annual. British Library, Boston Spa

Science Citation Index. Every 2 months. Institute for Scientific Information, Philadelphia

Serials in the British Library. Quarterly, British Library

Translations Register-Index. Monthly. National Translations Centre, Chicago

Ulrich's International Periodicals Directory. Annual. Bowker, New York

Ulrich's Quarterly. Quarterly. Bowker, New York

World Transindex. Monthly. International Translations Centre, Delft

World Medical Periodicals. 3rd edn., 1961, World Medical Association, New York

World Medical Periodicals. Supplement to 3rd edn., 1968. World Medical Association, New York

Appendix 2

Biomedical periodicals selected (a) as representing in 1970 all fields of clinical medicine, (b) as most frequently borrowed by other libraries from the British Library Lending Division in 1967, (c) as most promptly and frequently cited in 1972 by a group of 21 pathology journals selected from the *Science Citation Index* database.

Title of Journal	*(a) Selected for* Abridged *Index Medicus*	*(b) Ranking as most frequently borrowed from BLLD*	*(c) Ranking in* SCI *pathology study*
Acta Medica Scandinavica	Yes		72
Acta Neuropathologica			63
Acta Pathologica et Microbiologica			
Scandinavica			6
Acta Physiologica Scandinavica		29	
American Heart Journal	Yes	60	65
American Journal of Anatomy			59
American Journal of Cardiology	Yes		
American Journal of Clinical Nutrition	Yes		
American Journal of Clinical Pathology	Yes	11	13
American Journal of Digestive Diseases	Yes	48	
American Journal of Diseases of			
Children	Yes		69
American Journal of Human Genetics	Yes		
American Journal of Medical Sciences	Yes	29	19
American Journal of Medicine	Yes	48	
American Journal of Obstetrics and			
Gynecology	Yes	1	47
American Journal of Ophthalmology	Yes		
American Journal of Pathology	Yes	34	1
American Journal of Physical Medicine	Yes		
American Journal of Physiology	Yes	8	35
American Journal of Psychology	Yes		
American Journal of Public Health and			
the Nation's Health	Yes		
American Journal of Roentgenology	Yes		
American Journal of Surgery	Yes	60	
American Journal of Tropical Medicine			
and Hygiene	Yes		
American Review of Respiratory			
Diseases	Yes	60	
Anatomical Record		29	43
Anaesthesia	Yes		
Anesthesiology	Yes		
Annals of Internal Medicine	Yes	34	38
Annals of the New York Academy of			
Sciences		2	24

Title of Journal	(a) Selected for Abridged Index Medicus	(b) Ranking as most frequently borrowed from BLLD	(c) Ranking in SCI pathology study
Annals of Otology, Rhinology and Laryngology	Yes		
Annals of Physical Medicine	Yes		
Annals of Rheumatic Diseases		22	
Annals of Surgery	Yes		
Annals of Thoracic Surgery	Yes		
Applied Microbiology			66
Archives of Dermatology	Yes		
Archives of Environmental Health	Yes	27	
Archives of of General Psychiatry	Yes		
Archives of Internal Medicine	Yes		48
Archives Internationales de Pharmacodynamie et de Thérapie		19	
Archives of Neurology	Yes		73
Archives of Ophthalmology	Yes	48	
Archives of Otolaryngology	Yes		
Archives of Pathology	Yes		9
Archives of Physical Medicine and Rehabilitation	Yes		
Archives of Surgery	Yes		
Arthritis and Rheumatism	Yes	48	
Atherosclerosis			53
Australian Journal of Experimental Biology and Medical Science		60	
Beiträge zur Pathologie			40
Biochemical Journal			29
Biochemical Pharmacology		41	
Biochemica et Biophysica Acta			33
Blood	Yes	60	26
Brain	Yes		
British Heart Journal	Yes		
British Journal of Experimental Pathology		34	22
British Journal of Haematology			49
British Journal of Radiology	Yes		
British Journal of Surgery	Yes		
British Medical Journal	Yes	19	21
Bulletin of the World Health Organization		60	
Canadian Medical Association Journal	Yes	48	75
Cancer	Yes		14
Cancer Research		22	28
Chemical and Pharmaceutical Bulletin		41	
Circulation	Yes		54
Circulation Research		9	45
Clinica Chimica Acta		34	55

Title of Journal	(a) Selected for Abridged Index Medicus	(b) Ranking as most frequently borrowed from BLLD	(c) Ranking in SCI pathology study
Clinical Chemistry		34	
Clinical Pharmacology and Therapeutics	Yes	60	
DM: Disease a Month	Yes		
Diabetes	Yes		
Diseases of the Chest	Yes	60	
Endocrinology	Yes		64
Experimental Cell Research			30
Experimental Molecular Pathology			41
Federation Proceedings			36
GP	Yes		
Gastroenterology	Yes	22	51
Gut	Yes		
Histochemie			67
Immunology			50
Journal of Allergy	Yes		
Journal of the American Dietetic Association	Yes		
Journal of the American Geriatric Association	Yes		
Journal of the American Medical Association	Yes	6	25
Journal of Applied Physiology	Yes	48	
Journal of Bacteriology			39
Journal of Biological Chemistry		12	17
Journal of Bone and Joint Surgery	Yes		
Journal of Cell Biology			2
Journal of Clinical Endocrinology and Metabolism	Yes	41	
Journal of Clinical Investigation	Yes	16	18
Journal of Clinical Pathology	Yes	19	20
Journal of Comparative Pathology			70
Journal of Dental Research		41	
Journal of Endocrinology		60	
Journal of Experimental Medicine	Yes	27	5
Journal of General Microbiology			61
Journal of Gerontology	Yes		
Journal of Histochemistry and Cytochemistry			23
Journal of Hygiene		16	
Journal of Immunology	Yes	29	16

Title of Journal	(a) Selected for Abridged Index Medicus	(b) Ranking as most frequently borrowed from BLLD	(c) Ranking in SCI pathology study
Journal of Infectious Diseases	Yes		62
Journal of Investigative Dermatology	Yes	16	
Journal of Laboratory and Clinical Medicine	Yes	6	27
Journal of Laryngology and Otology	Yes		
Journal of Medical Education	Yes		
Journal of Medicinal Chemistry		48	
Journal of the National Cancer Institute		41	32
Journal of Nervous and Mental Diseases	Yes		
Journal of Neuropathology and Experimental Neurology			31
Journal of Neurosurgery	Yes	48	
Journal of Nutrition		41	
Journal of Obstetrics and Gynaecology of the British Commonwealth	Yes		
Journal of Oral Surgery	Yes		
Journal of Pathology			8
Journal of Pediatrics	Yes	34	56
Journal of Pharmaceutical Sciences		14	
Journal of Pharmacy and Pharmacology		12	
Journal of Pharmacology and Experimental Therapeutics		10	
Journal of Physiology		22	71
Journal of Surgical Research		60	
Journal of Thoracic and Cardiovascular Surgery	Yes		
Journal of Trauma	Yes		
Journal of Ultrastructural Research			34
Journal of Urology	Yes		74
Klinische Wochenschrift			68
Laboratory Investigation		14	7
Lancet	Yes	5	4
Medical Clinics of North America	Yes		
Medical Journal of Australia		41	
Medical Letter on Drugs and Therapeutics	Yes		
Medicine (Baltimore)	Yes		
Nature			3
Neurology			58
New England Journal of Medicine	Yes	4	12
New York State Journal of Medicine		48	

Title of Journal	(a) Selected for Abridged Index Medicus	(b) Ranking as most frequently borrowed from BLLD	(c) Ranking in SCI pathology study
Obstetrics and Gynecology	Yes	22	
Pediatrics	Yes		60
Pharmacological Reviews		48	
Pharmazie		48	
Physical Therapy	Yes		
Physiological Reviews	Yes		
Plastic and Reconstructive Surgery	Yes		
Postgraduate Medicine	Yes		
Postgraduate Medical Journal		60	
Presse Médicale		60	
Proceedings of the National Academy of Sciences USA			37
Proceedings of the Royal Society of Medicine		29	
Proceedings of the Society for Experimental Biology and Medicine		3	10
Progress in Cardiovascular Diseases	Yes		
Public Health Reports	Yes		
Radiology	Yes		
Scandinavian Journal of Clinical and Laboratory Investigation		60	
Science	Yes	34	11
Southern Medical Journal		48	
Surgery	Yes		
Surgery, Gynecology and Obstetrics	Yes	60	
Surgical Clinics of North America	Yes		
Thrombosis et Diathesis Haemorrhagica			44
Transplantation			57
Verhandlungen der Deutschen Gesellschaft für Pathologie			52
Virchows Archiv			15
Virology			46
Zeitschrift für Zellforschung und Mikroskopische Anatomie			42
TOTALS	99	73	75

3

Indexes, abstracts, bibliographies and reviews

F. M. Sutherland

Since the fifteenth century, the printed book, and subsequently the periodical, have been the principal means for communicating scientific knowlege over the barriers of space and of time. Until the mid-nineteenth century, the number of publications in the field of medicine was comparatively small, and individual doctors were able, by personal contact with their fellows, and by their own reading, to keep abreast of current developments. Bibliographies and guides to the literature had been compiled since the sixteenth century, but they were private efforts by enthusiasts and would not have been regarded by the ordinary medical practitioners as publications essential to their needs.

In the early years of the nineteenth century, the changes wrought on the political and economic scenes by the French and Industrial Revolutions were matched by equally fundamental changes in the sphere of science. In medicine, the pace and scope of research quickened, and the communication of the results of that research led, inevitably, to an increase in the volume of publications. The growth of specialization in medicine produced a like effect, with the proliferation of books and journals devoted to particular subjects. By the 1860s, it was no longer possible for the individual worker to read all the literature which might be of interest. By the same token, it was no longer possible for the individual bibliographer, working alone, to compile and publish guides to that literature. The production of such guides required, to an ever-increasing degree, resources in finance, manpower, and, ultimately, in machines, which could only be deployed by organizations and governments. The indexing of medical publications not only became essential for medical progress, but also developed into the institutional and commercial affair which it is today.

The guides to medical literature which have evolved during the past hundred years fall into two distinct categories.

The first, in the form of indexes, catalogues and book lists, draw attention to the existence of publications without elaborating on their contents. The primary test of their efficiency is the comprehensiveness of their coverage of the literature and the speed with which they announce its publication; a secondary test is the ease with which the information contained in them can be made available by retrospective searching. In their earliest form they sought to cover both books and periodicals, but the differing techniques involved in indexing the two types of literature meant that the marriage was never an entirely happy one, and this led ultimately to the physical separation of periodical indexes and book lists, which, at the present time, is more or less complete.

The second category of guide to the literature goes beyond the mere listing of titles, and, in the form of abstracts or reviews, provides a summary of content to a varying degree of detail. The summary may be quite brief, and be meant purely as an indication to the reader of the importance of the publication and whether the original should be consulted; alternatively, it may seek to be a substitute for that original by outlining all its salient features. Review articles, which collect together and summarize recent information on specific subjects, are a collective form of abstract; if they are based on adequate coverage of the literature and are the product of expert and critical authorship, they can perform an extremely useful function. As with indexes and book lists, the effectiveness of abstracts and reviews is dependent on their comprehensiveness, the rapidity of their production and their adaptability for retrospective searching.

Indexes

The detailed story of the modern indexing of medical literature begins in 1865, when John Shaw Billings, an American army doctor, was given responsibility for the library of the Surgeon General's Office in Washington. It is, perhaps, a strange fact that modern medical bibliography owes much of its origin to the US where, in the nineteenth century, resources in medical literature were meagre as compared with those in the countries of Western Europe. It was, however, this very lack of resources, which

Billings himself experienced when writing his graduation thesis, that convinced him of the necessity not only for adequate libraries, but also for adequate bibliographical procedures to exploit the contents of those libraries (Marson, 1969). With the same energy that was being used to develop all other aspects of American life at the time, Billings proceeded to create, out of the comparatively small library at the Surgeon General's Office, one of the greatest collections in the world, and his first step to exploit the contents of that collection, for the benefit of the medical profession at large, was the *Index-Catalogue*.

Index-catalogue of the Library of the Surgeon General's Office

A detailed history of the *Index-Catalogue* can be found in Rogers and Adams (1950). To obviate possible confusion later in this chapter, it must be emphasized that the Library of the Surgeon General's Office has undergone several changes of title, being called, at a later date, the Army Medical Library and the Armed Forces Medical Library, and it is known today as the National Library of Medicine.

In 1876 Billings had outlined his intentions by issuing an author and subject catalogue of his library in dictionary form under the title of *Specimen Fasciculus of a Catalogue of the National Medical Library*, but the first volume of the *Index-Catalogue* proper did not appear until 1880, when Congress appropriated the necessary funds.

As the name *Index-Catalogue* implies, both book and periodical literature were covered. Books were listed under authors' names and under subject headings; journal articles were listed under subject headings only. Under subject headings useful cross-references were made to kindred topics and sub-headings were provided where the amount of material justified it.

The main author and subject entries were arranged alphabetically in dictionary form, the first volume of 1880 covering the letters A to BERLINSKI. Volumes appeared annually until 1895, when the alphabet was completed in 16 volumes. Some 679 669 subject references had been published, and the Surgeon General's Library itself had grown to 308 000 volumes. It is important to note, however, that much of the older literature had still to be acquired by the Library, and references to these older books must be sought in later series of the *Index-Catalogue*.

Billings himself retired from the Library in 1895, but the work was carried on by his successors in the form of further series, the details of which are as follows:

1st Series: vols 1–16 (1880–1895)
2nd Series: vols 1–21 (1896–1916)
3rd Series: vols 1–10 (1918–1932)
4th Series: vols 1–11 (A-Mn) (1936–1955)
5th Series (Selected Monographs): vols 1–3 (1959–1961)

Nearly 540 000 books and pamphlets and 2 556 000 journal articles are recorded in these different series.

As to the extent to which the *Index-Catalogue* covered the whole field of medical literature, Billings was careful to emphasize, in his preface to the first volume of the 1st Series, that it was not a complete medical bibliography but rather a catalogue of a single collection, and indeed as an index to that one collection it had certain limitations. All books, pamphlets and theses received entries, but the indexing of periodicals were selective, aiming to include 'the principal original papers in medical journals and transactions'. Secondary material, which was regarded as worthless, was omitted. It must not be forgotten, however, that the Surgeon General's Library had already become one of the world's greatest medical libraries, and that, even with the selective indexing of periodicals, the *Index-Catalogue* forms a published guide to the medical literature of its day that was as comprehensive as could reasonably be expected.

It suffered, however, from the two fundamental defects of being arranged alphabetically and of covering both book and periodical literature. The alphabetical arrangement meant that insertions or supplements were not possible, and that publication in series was inevitable. Even in the 1st Series, authors and subjects, whose entries began with the letter A and which just missed inclusion in the first volume, had to wait some 15 years before they appeared in the 2nd Series. The inexorable increase in the volume of publication, particularly in periodical form after 1900, made such delay ever worse and, ultimately, unacceptable.

By the 1920s, the number of entries awaiting publication had become so large that, in 1926, the decision was taken, beginning with volume 6 of the 3rd Series, to omit subject entries for material published after 1925. In 1932 the decision was reversed, and some of the missing material from the period 1926–1932, under the letters Ge–Z, is to be found in the volumes of the 4th Series. For complete coverage of those years, however, use of the *Index-Catalogue* must be supplemented with *Index Medicus* and *Quarterly Cumulative Index Medicus* (*see* pages 49 and 52).

The final crises for the *Index-Catalogue* came immediately after World War II. The effects of the increase in publication of scientific literature were exacerbated by the inflow of a backlog of

A chronology of the Index-Catalogue

1880 — 1961

Index-Catalogue of the Library of the Surgeon General's Office: a dictionary catalogue of serials and monographs in 5 series

1st series: 16 vols, 1880–1895
2nd series: 21 vols, 1896–1916
3rd series: 10 vols, 1918–1932
4th series: 11 vols, 1936–1955, A–Mn only
5th series: 3 vols, 1959–1961, selected monographs published up to 1950 only

1950   1954   1955   1959   1960   1965   1966

Armed Forces Medical Library Catalog: 6 vols, 1955

National Library of Medicine Catalog: 6 vols, 1960

National Library of Medicine Catalog: 6 vols, 1966

National Library of Medicine Current Catalog

Computer generated CATLINE. Appears quarterly and cumulates annually and quinquennially. Lists monographs and serials under name, title and subject.

overseas publications, from the war years. By 1950 there were 1 750 000 subject entries from the period 1920–1950 still awaiting publication, and it was estimated that by 1958 the *Index-Catalogue* would be withholding from publication more references than it had published over the whole period since 1880. The prudent decision was made to cease publication with volume 11 (Mh–Mn) of the 4th Series. Entries for monographs published up to 1950 were subsequently published, under both authors and subjects, in a 5th Series of three volumes.

Although, by its design, the *Index-Catalogue* proved inadequate to meet the needs of the medical community for up-to-date indexing, it is now an invaluable mine of historical information, recording, as it does, a total of about 3 000 000 journal articles, books and pamphlets from the earliest times up to 1950. It forms a bibliographical tool without equal in any other subject field. But above all it established in the US a pioneering tradition for the comprehensive indexing of medical literature, which has been carried forward to the present day.

Index Medicus

Before describing the successors to the *Index-Catalogue* and their role in the present-day indexing of medical literature, it is necessary to retrace one's steps to 1879, when the first issue of *Index Medicus* was published. If the format of the *Index-Catalogue* was incapable of coping with the rapid indexing of current literature, it was largely because Billings had not intended it for such a purpose. It was to be the repository catalogue of the Surgeon General's Library, and it was *Index Medicus* which was intended for the role of current indexing. In the prospectus contained in the first issue of *Index Medicus* of 31 January 1879, Billings declared that it would 'record the titles of all new publications in medicine, surgery and the collateral branches received during the preceding month', and that they 'will be followed by the titles of valuable original articles upon the same subject, found, during the like period, in medical journals and transactions of medical societies. The periodicals thus indexed will comprise all current medical journals and transactions of value, so far as they can be obtained.'

The odd fact about *Index Medicus* is that, although it was based on material already prepared for the *Index-Catalogue*, Billings did not seek public funds for its publication. It was a private commercial venture and, as such, was beset by financial difficulties from the start. Three separate publishers undertook responsibility for it at different times during the early years, and in 1899 publication was entirely suspended. In 1903 it was resumed with financial help from the Carnegie Institution of Washington, and publication continued until 1927, when *Index Medicus* was merged with the American Medical Association's *Quarterly Cumulative Index* to *Current Medical Literature* to form the *Quarterly Cumulative Index Medicus*. For some years thereafter, the Army Medical Library's only bibliographical publication was the *Index-Catalogue* and it was not until 1960, under quite new circumstances, that it re-introduced the title *Index Medicus*.

The earlier *Index Medicus* was published in three separate series:

> Series 1: 1879–1899
> Series 2: 1903–1920
> Series 3: 1921–1927

The first two series were issued monthly in classified form, with subject headings that were more general and less subdivided than those in the *Index-Catalogue*. Under each subject, books and theses were listed by authors, followed by an author listing of journal articles. An annual index was provided for both authors and subjects, but in these, as reference was made only to the number of the page on which a particular item occurred, the finding of that item could be a time-consuming business. In the third series (1921–1927), *Index Medicus* became a quarterly instead of a monthly, the subject arrangement became alphabetical instead of classified, and the annual indexes were limited to authors only. The prime importance of *Index Medicus* is that, for the period 1879–1927, it is an author guide to periodical literature, and, as such, is an indispensable supplement to the *Index-Catalogue*.

For the years 1899–1902, when *Index Medicus* was not published, there are two substitute bibliographical aids. *Bibliographia Medica (Index Medicus)*, 1–3, 1900–1902, was published monthly by the Institut de Bibliographie in Paris. As with *Index Medicus,* both books and journal articles were listed under subjects in a classified arrangement; an annual author index was provided, but an abbreviated index to the classification formed the only annual guide to subjects. *Bibliographia Medica* supplies a bridge to the gap in *Index Medicus,* but the literature for late 1899 is not covered and the indexing is neither as comprehensive nor as accurate. *Index Medicus Novus* was published in Vienna between 15 June 1899 and 10–25 February 1900, and is another source of bibliographical information for the missing years of *Index Medicus.* Its classified arrangement and lack of annual indexes, however, make it of very limited value.

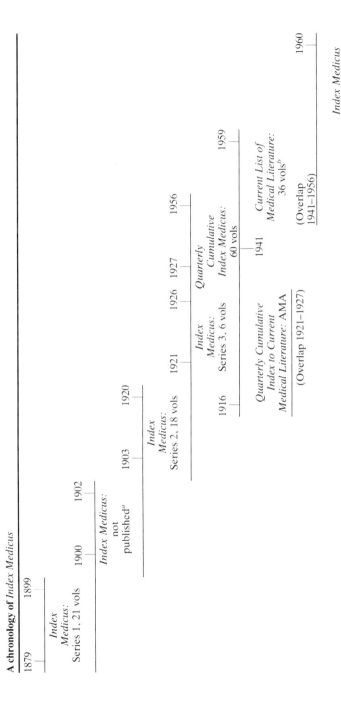

A chronology of *Index Medicus*

1879 1899
Index Medicus:
Series 1, 21 vols

1900 1902
Index Medicus:
not published[a]

1903 1920
Index Medicus:
Series 2, 18 vols

1921 1926 1927 1956
Index Medicus:
Series 3, 6 vols

Quarterly Cumulative Index Medicus:
60 vols

1916
Quarterly Cumulative Index to Current Medical Literature: AMA
(Overlap 1921–1927)

1941 1959
Current List of Medical Literature:
36 vols[b]
(Overlap 1941–1956)

1960
Index Medicus

[a] Partial substitutes were *Bibliographia Medica*, 3 vols, Paris, 1900–1903; *Index Medicus Novus*, Vienna. Nos 1–12, 1899, 1–3, 1900.
[b] From 1957–1959 the only source of references to medical periodical literature.

In the years following 1927, after *Index Medicus* had ceased publication, the main instruments for indexing contemporary medical literature were the *Quarterly Cumulative Index Medicus* and, at a later date, the *Current List of Medical Literature.*

Quarterly Cumulative Index Medicus

In 1916 the American Medical Association had begun publication of a *Quarterly Cumulative Index to Current Medical Literature,* an index which was intended primarily for the general practitioner, and its coverage of the literature was, accordingly, very selective and restricted in the main to the clinical field. In 1926, for example, only 326 periodical titles were indexed. From 1916 to 1925 the quarterly issues were cumulated annually; for 1926 there are two semi-annual cumulations. At the start of each volume are to be found lists of new books arranged by authors, of new books arranged by subject, of book publishers, of US Government publications and of the journal titles indexed in the main text. This main index of journal articles is one of authors and subjects in a single alphabetical sequence, a form that is extremely simple to use. The titles of foreign-language articles are translated into English.

By 1926 this publication had run into financial difficulties, and was merged with *Index Medicus* to form the *Quarterly Cumulative Index Medicus,* which, from 1927 to 1931, was sponsored jointly by the American Medical Association and the Army Medical Library; from 1932 until it ceased publication in 1956 it was the responsibility of the American Medical Association alone.

All the features of the previous *Quarterly Cumulative Index* were maintained, with the exception of the list of US Government publications. Coverage of journal literature was much more complete; in 1956, the final year of publication, 933 biomedical periodicals were indexed. It remained a quarterly publication, with semi-annual cumulations, until 1948; from 1949 to 1956 it was published in the form of semi-annual volumes only. Entries under authors' names in the main index are given in the original language, if that is English, French, German, Spanish, Italian or Portugese; other languages are translated into English. The titles of all subject entries are in English.

The fact that full details of each reference are to be found with every entry, and that those entries are arranged in a self-indexing sequence of authors and subjects makes the *Quarterly Cumulative Index Medicus* the easiest of all medical bibliographies to use. The format, however, was not a suitable one for rapid production. Delays in publication were made worse by the effects of World

War II, with the result that, by the 1950s, volumes were appearing over two years late. For purposes of medical research, this meant that they were of little value, and that radical change was necessary.

Current List of Medical Literature

The imperative need for a more rapid indexing service had first become apparent during the early years of World War II, and in 1941, in response to that need, the *Current List of Medical Literature* was first issued. Although based on cards already prepared for the *Index-Catalogue,* it was initially a private venture and was not formally taken over by the Army Medical Library until 1945. It was intended as a service primarily for US Army medical officers serving overseas by providing them with an up-to-date weekly list of the contents of some of the more important journals in the Army Medical Library. From 1950 onwards it appeared monthly.

The arrangement of each number of the *Current List* constitutes an alphabetical sequence of journal titles, and under each title are to be found the contents of one or more issues of that title. Each entry provides details of author and title of the article, together with a translation of items in foreign languages, and inclusive pagination. Each article is numbered for indexing purposes, and semiannual indexes for both authors and subjects were published.

The strength of the *Current List* was its speed of publication; a survey in 1954 showed that 56 per cent of all material published was less than one year old. Its great weakness is that its format makes it a laborious work to consult; it cannot be used without referring first to an index, and, as entries in that index can refer to several numbered items in the main text, location of a particular item is rarely straightforward. Up to the end of 1956 the *Quarterly Cumulative Index Medicus* and the *Current List* should be used as complementary indexes, as each covered some part of the literature not dealt with by the other; following the demise of the *QCIM* at the end of 1956, the *Current List* is the only guide to medical periodical literature for the years 1957 to 1959. At the end of the latter year it also ceased publication and 1960 saw the introduction of an entirely new look to medical indexing in general.

The new arrangements were based initially on a return to the co-operation between the National Library of Medicine and the American Medical Association, which had existed between 1927 and 1931 for the publication of the *Quarterly Cumulative Index Medicus*. There were two new features in 1960 which must be stressed. In all the principal indexes which have been mentioned up to this time, both book and periodical literature were listed within the same framework to a greater or lesser degree. From 1960 onwards the fundamental difference between the techniques required for indexing the two types of literature is finally recognized, and the published guides to each type, issued by the National Library of Medicine, went their separate ways. Periodical literature is henceforth indexed in *Index Medicus* and *Cumulated Index Medicus*; new books and monographs are listed in the *National Library of Medicine Catalog* and the *National Library of Medicine Current Catalog.*

The second innovation, in 1960, was mechanization. Up to that time, all the published indexes, including the *Quarterly Cumulative Index Medicus* and the *Current List,* had been compiled basically by the manual manipulation of cards. For compiling the new *Index Medicus* of 1960, the National Library of Medicine system involved three elements of mechanization:

(1) Typewriters which operated from punched tape enabling the typing of entries on IBM cards.
(2) IBM sorters and collators for filing entries in alphabetical sequence.
(3) The Eastman-Kodak Listomatic camera, which could photograph text imprinted along the top edge of an IBM card at the rate of 230 cards per minute (Crawford, 1960).

Mechanization was further developed in 1964, when *Index Medicus* was produced for the first time by the National Library of Medicine's automated medical literature analysis and retrieval system (MEDLARS), and was composed for printing, binding and distribution by the Library's Photon 900 graphic arts composing equipment (GRACE) (*see* page 56). These technical developments were timely in the extreme in the face of the mounting volume of medical literature. They made possible, in 1982, the coverage of approximately 2700 journal titles and the publication of more than 250 000 citations to articles; the listing of those articles could appear as little as three months after their original publication; and the *Cumulated Index Medicus* is published about four months after the close of the year which it covers. The system by which journals are evaluated for inclusion in *Index Medicus* has been described by Karel (1967).

Index Medicus and Cumulated Index Medicus

Since January 1960, *Index Medicus* has been published in monthly parts, each part being divided into subject and author sections arranged alphabetically. Citations are given in full in every entry. In the subject section, under each heading, entries are grouped according to the original language of the articles, with the English-language items first, followed by citations for articles in other languages arranged alphabetically by language. Titles in foreign languages are translated into English and shown in square brackets, together with an indication of the language concerned. Since 1972 each citation to a foreign-language article includes the phrase, 'Eng. Abstr.', if the original article is accompanied by an English-language abstract.

Since 1978 all authors' names, however many, have been included in citations in the author section and a cross-reference is given from each author to the first author. The citations in the subject index include only the first author.

In the process of indexing at the National Library of Medicine, each article is given as many subject headings as are necessary to describe adequately its content. Only those subject headings which represent the most important concepts are cited in *Index Medicus*, but all subject headings are stored in MEDLARS, the National Library of Medicine's computer-based file of citations for use in machine retrieval. As a guide to the choice of the correct headings when a search is made, a list of headings currently in use is published annually as Part 2 of the January issue of *Index Medicus* under the title, *Medical Subject Headings (MeSH)*. This includes an alphabetical list of headings with cross-references, categorized lists of headings, and full information on new and altered headings.

Part 1 of the January issue of *Index Medicus* contains a section which lists, by both full and abbreviated titles, the journals which are currently being indexed. This section is also published separately as *List of Journals Indexed in Index Medicus*, in which the journals concerned are given additional listings under subjects and countries. Since March 1965 each issue of *Index Medicus* has contained a section entitled *Bibliography of Medical Reviews*, which is discussed at greater length later in this chapter.

In 1976 *Index Medicus* introduced coverage of selected non-serial monographs containing papers presented at congresses and symposia. In 1981, however, this was discontinued in order to devote the entire capacity of *Index Medicus* to an expanding journal literature.

The monthly issues of *Index Medicus* are cumulated annually into *Cumulated Index Medicus*. This brings together the subject and author sections of *Index Medicus*, *List of Journals Indexed*, *Medical Subject Headings* (since 1966) and *Bibliography of Medical*

Reviews (since 1967). In the early years volumes of *Cumulated Index Medicus* tended to be heavy and unwieldy, but, since 1977, each year has been published in 14 volumes of more reasonable size.

Since January 1970 the National Library of Medicine has also issued a monthly *Abridged Index Medicus* which cites articles from 118 English-language journals, using the same subject headings as in *Index Medicus*. The issues are brought together annually into *Cumulated Abridged Index Medicus*. The low cost of this index makes it an attractive proposition for the individual practitioner or smaller library, but the selection of such a limited number of journals for indexing must inevitably be a matter for some controversy.

The centenary of *Index Medicus* in 1979 was celebrated in the National Library of Medicine by a symposium, the papers at which have been published in Blake (1980).

National Library of Medicine Current Catalog

Index Medicus is a guide only to periodical literature; detailed information on monographs must be sought in the *National Library of Medicine Current Catalog*, which was first published in 1966 as an additional product of MEDLARS. We have seen that the *Index-Catalog*, when it finally ceased publication, had listed monographs published up to 1950. Details of books published between that date and the appearance of the *National Library of Medicine Current Catalog* in 1966 are to be found in the following:

> *Armed Forces Medical Library Catalog*, 1950–1954; 6 vols; 1955
> *National Library of Medicine Catalog*, 1955–1959; 6 vols; 1960
> *National Library of Medicine Catalog*, 1960–1965; 6 vols; 1966

These furnish comprehensive author and subject guides to books of world-wide imprint reflecting, as they do, the international acquisitions policy of the National Library of Medicine.

As from January 1966, the *National Library of Medicine Current Catalog* was computer-generated and was produced by GRACE. It began as a twice-monthly publication, with quarterly and annual cumulations. The bi-weekly parts contained entries for books catalogued by the Library which had been published during the current or two previous years. The cumulations cited all books catalogued by the Library with the exception of those printed before 1801.

Until the end of 1969 each issues of the *Current Catalog* contained:

(1) A subject section in which the headings are taken from MeSH.
(2) A name section listing authors and titles, providing guidance

on subject headings and cross-references, and giving information on prices when available.

(3) A technical reports section listing reports under both subjects and names.

Beginning with January 1970 the bi-weekly issues were replaced by monthly ones, which contained a name section only and listed imprints for the current and two previous years only; there were quarterly and annual cumulations which had both name and subject sections, and which listed all imprints. The monthly issues ceased in December, 1973 and the *Current Catalog* is now published quarterly with an annual cumulation. Proof sheets of the *Catalog* are published weekly by the Medical Library Association in Chicago.

In 1971 Audiovisual Subject and Name Sections were introduced, but after 1977 these were cumulated annually in an entirely separate publication, *National Library of Medicine Audiovisuals Catalog*. In 1973 Serials Subject and Name Sections were brought in and these became permanent features.

A sexennial cumulation of the *Current Catalog*, covering the years 1965 to 1970, has been published, and a further cumulation for the five years 1971 to 1975 were published in 1976. A microfiche version covers 1976 to 1980.

From July 1968 onwards, the *Current Catalog* also includes entries for books owned and catalogued by the Countway Library at Boston and by the Upstate Medical Library of New York State University, Syracuse.

An indication of the comprehensive coverage of monograph material by the *Current Catalog* is the fact that some 16 795 items were catalogued in the year 1971. This information is made available rapidly in the quarterly parts of the *Catalog*, and for retrospective search in the annual and larger cumulations.

Discussion of the indexes to current medical literature has, so far, been confined to those published by the National Library of Medicine. There are, however, a number of guides published elsewhere which deserve attention. Two such, published by the Institute for Scientific Information in Philadelphia, are *Current Contents, Clinical Practice* and *Science Citation Index*.

Current Contents, Clinical Practice

Current Contents, Clinical Practice first appeared in January 1973, and in 1982 it contained the titles of papers and all other substantive material from more than 775 journals which reported advances in the practice of medicine and allied health sciences. This weekly publication contains copies of the contents pages of journals, mainly photographically reproduced, and, in some cases, this information on contents can appear before the original journal is received. Each issue has a subject index and an author address directory which greatly facilitates the acquisition of reprints.

Further series of *Current Contents* are devoted to *Life Sciences, Physical Chemical and Earth Sciences, Agriculture Biology and Environmental Sciences, Social and Behavioral Sciences* and *Engineering Technology and Applied Sciences.*

Science Citation Index

The concepts behind citation indexing have been described by Garfield (1979). Essentially, it consists of a list of references (cited works) in which each reference is followed by a list of the sources (citing works) which quote it. The main purpose behind the index is to lead the searcher from a key article to others which have referred to it on the basic assumption that they will be relevant.

The first issues of *Science Citation Index* were published by the Institute for Scientific Information, Philadelphia, in 1964; since that time, annual volumes have been published covering the period 1961 to 1963, and a cumulation for the years 1955 to 1964 was in production in 1981. *Science Citation Index* is published bimonthly with an annual cumulation; five-year cumulations for 1965 to 1969, 1970 to 1974 and 1975 to 1979 have been published.

Science Citation Index indexes both journals and non-journal items and a list of source material is included in each issue. In 1981 more than 3600 journals and other publications were covered and more than 500 000 articles were indexed in over eight million reference citations. The complete contents of every journal covered are indexed.

Science Citation Index is particularly useful in information retrieval when a key reference, rather than a key word is known. From such a key reference it is possible to trace more easily subsequent developments in a particular field. It can also be claimed, with justification, that it provides a novel link between literatures of different scientific disciplines. *Science Citation Index* consists of a number of separate parts: the Citation Index itself; the Source Index (equivalent to an author index); the Permuterm Subject Index (which acts like a keyword index); and the Corporate Index (which lists authors by institution).

The basic principle of *Science Citation Index* is that a scientific paper cites other articles which are relevant to its own subject content. By the same token a paper will itself be cited by later papers dealing with the same topic. Thus *Science Citation Index* can move the user *forward* in time to relevant references, whereas other indexing and abstracting publications move the user *backwards* to older material. Although useful as a supernumerary tool, *Science Citation Index* cannot provide the coverage in depth of the conventional medical indexes and abstracts.

Bibliographies

Before turning to sources of information on recently published books, mention should be made of an extremely useful compilation of recent references. This is *Problems in Internal Medicine; Selected Topics with Annotated Bibliography* edited by B. M. Greene *et al.* (University Park Press, 1980), an annotated selection of representative references arranged under a wide variety of subject headings. All the references concern specific problems of individual patients and emphasize practical clinical issues. This is a handy, well-organized one-volume guide to the medical literature that every library can afford. It claims to be quicker and easier to use than any other source.

Current-awareness sources for monographs

Current awareness of monograph publications in the medical field can be maintained from a number of sources, apart from the *National Library of Medicine Current Catalog*. Book reviews in medical journals constitute one such source, and they have the great advantage of giving an authoritative assessment of the value of individual books. They may not, however, appear until long after the books themselves have been published, and, except in journals of a very specialized nature, reviews can provide only limited coverage of the total number of books published.

For complete guidance to what is being published there are, in the first instance, the various advertising methods employed by publishing firms, varying from leaflets describing individual books to lists of recent publications or batches of standard catalogue cards giving full bibliographical details. To co-ordinate this ill-assorted material, there are a number of useful book lists, among which can be included the following.

Cumulative Book Index

Published by the H. W. Wilson Co. of New York, this seeks to include the majority of books in the English language wherever published.

Excluded, however, are government documents, most pamphlets, cheap paperbacks and, in general, all material of a local, fugitive and ephemeral nature. Entries are arranged alphabetically by authors, subjects and titles. It is published monthly, except in August, with a bound cumulation each year.

Medical Books and Serials in Print

Medical Books and Serials in Print, published by R. R. Bowker Company of New York and London, is an annual publication which lists current literature in the health and biomedical sciences. The indexes to books contain titles which are in print and which have been, or will be, published or exclusively distributed in the US. The coverage of serial literature is international and includes selected titles of periodicals issued more frequently than once a year and usually published at regular intervals, together with irregular serials and annuals provided the last issue date was not earlier than 1968.

Book titles are indexed by subject, author and title and serials are listed by subject and title. The author and title indexes to books in the 10th edn of 1981 include 46 519 entries for titles available from some 2200 publishers; the subject index to periodicals lists 8553 titles. a useful list of publishers' addresses is included in the work.

British National Bibliography

British National Bibliography is confined to British publications and provides virtually complete coverage in that field, based as it is on new books received by the Copyright Receipt Office of the British Library. Details are also included of forthcoming publications derived from information supplied by publishers. *British National Bibliography* is published weekly with cumulations for the periods January to April, May to August, and September to December.

Entries are arranged by subject according to the 19th edition of the *Dewey Decimal Classification* and the cataloguing is in accordance with the provisions of the 2nd edn of the *Anglo-American Cataloguing Rules.* Each weekly issue has an index for authors, titles and series; the weekly issue at the end of each month has separate author – title and subject indexes for the preceding month and these indexes are cumulated in the annual volume.

British Medicine

British Medicine first appeared in January 1972, when it was published by the Medical Department of the British Council as an expanded version of the former *British Medical Book List*. In May 1980, publication of *British Medicine* was transferred to Pergamon Press Ltd. and, since 1981, the work has been issued with the support of the Royal Society of Medicine. Its aim is to provide a guide to new books and non-book material, pamphlets, official publications, brochures and reports by research institutions and voluntary societies; to list the main contents of current issues of British medical periodicals; and to note forthcoming international congresses. It seeks to provide readers with a comprehensive picture of medical work being done in Britain.

British Book News

British Book News is published monthly by the British Council. Every issue contains about 240 short reviews by specialists in their subjects. There is a separate section devoted to the medical sciences, and the sections on social sciences and pure sciences may also contain material of interest. There is a monthly inset giving details of books due for publication in the forthcoming month with a section for medical sciences.

Books and Periodicals for Medical Libraries in Hospitals

Originally published by the Medical Section of the Library Association, this work constitutes a select list of books and periodicals intended as a guide to those unfamiliar with the literature in particular subject fields. The most recent edition is the fifth (1978). Shortly after that date the Medical Section was merged in the Medical, Health and Welfare Libraries Group of the Library Association, and the book section has since been updated by Howard Hague in *Medical Textbook Review: Books for Medical Libraries* (5th edn, compiled by V. Daniels, 1982). A similar select list suitable for American Libraries is published regularly in the *Bulletin of the Medical Library Association*, the most recent being that by Brandon and Hill (1983).

Catalogue of Lewis's Medical, Scientific and Technical Lending Library

This *Catalogue*, which lists the books available to subscribers to H. K. Lewis's Library, provides an extensive guide to hard-cover books in the English language. The latest edition, published in 1975, includes books published up to 31 December 1972. This is a two-volume work, vol 1 being devoted to authors and titles and vol 2 to a subject index. Three *Supplements to the Catalogue* covering the years 1973 to 1975, 1976 to 1978 and 1979 to 1981 have been published. Details of more recent books can also be found in Lewis's weekly and quarterly lists.

Index of Conference Proceedings (received by the BLLD)

The *Index of Conference Proceedings* is issued monthly, with an annual cumulation, by the British Library Lending Division, and is of considerable assistance in tracing recent conference proceedings; such proceedings can be both valuable and difficult to locate. A ten-year cumulation covering the years 1964 to 1973 was published in 1974 and a five-year cumulation for 1974 to 1978 appeared in 1978. A list of 363 older congress proceedings is to be found in Bishop (1958).

British Reports, Translations and Theses (received by the BLLD)

British Reports, Translations and Theses is a monthly publication of the British Library Lending Division with annual cumulations. It lists 'grey' or semi-published literature, such as reports and translations produced by British government organizations, industry, universities and learned institutions, and most doctoral theses accepted at British universities during and after 1970. It also covers reports and unpublished translations from the Republic of Ireland and selected British official publications of a report nature that are not published by HMSO. Prior to 1981 the work had been entitled the *BLLD Announcement Bulletin*.

Abstracts

Attention must now be turned from publications of the index type, which point solely to the existence of particular medical literature, to abstracting publications which provide greater detail of the content of that literature. Their purpose may be to indicate briefly the importance of the original articles or to give more complete summaries of those articles for the benefit of readers unable to obtain them without difficulty. In their coverage of the literature, abstracting services may seek to be either selective or comprehensive.

Abstracts have been a feature of medical literature since the earliest times, both as separate publications and as an integral part of conventional medical journals. A nineteenth-century example of the former type was *Braithwaite's Retrospect of Practical Medicine and Surgery*, which was published in 123 volumes from 1840 to 1901. From the early years of the twentieth century, the *Berichte* and *Zentralblätter*, published by the firm of Julius Springer, provided German abstracts with the set intention of furnishing complete cover in many areas of medicine and surgery. A typical example of abstracts included in an ordinary medical journal was the *Epitome of Current Medical Literature*, which was a supplement to the *British Medical Journal* from 1892 to 1939. Abstracts sections are a feature, at the present time, of the *Journal of the American Medical Association*.

In the years immediately following World War II, a number of comprehensive abstracting services, covering the field of general medicine, were developed as one means of combating the problems caused by the increasing amount of medical literature, and by the language barrier, which hindered the flow of medical information. Among these was *Abstracts of World Medicine* (British Medical Association, 1947–1977), which scanned 1500 journals and published about 3000 informative abstracts a year.

Excerpta Medica

The Excerpta Medica Foundation, an international non-profit organization, was founded in 1946 with headquarters in Amsterdam and with, as its principal aim, the furthering of 'the progress of medical knowledge by making information available to the medical and related professions on all significant basic research and clinical findings reported in any language, anywhere in the world'. The abstracting publication, *Excerpta Medica*, the main instrument for carrying out this aim, first appeared in 1947. It is divided into different sections, each of which covers a special subject field and may be purchased separately: the number of sections in 1982 totalled 43. The individual issues in each section appear monthly, and the abstracts, all in the English language, are arranged in classified order. Subject and author indexes are provided with each issue and for the annual cumulated volumes. Both the issues and the indexes are computer-produced.

Excerpta Medica publishes a number of user aids to its abstracting service. These include the *Excerpta Medica User Manual*, the *List of Journals Abstracted* and the *Guide to the Excerpta Medica Classification and Indexing System*. The latter title lists alphabetically over 5000 classification and indexing terms (including the most frequently used *MeSH* terms) which direct the user to the most relevant Excerpta Medica abstract journals.

In 1982 more than 3500 journals were being screened by

Excerpta Medica. Compiled by experts in the relevant subject fields, the abstracts are well written but are of the informative rather than the indicative type. They appear with reasonable rapidity, the average time being some 12 months after publication of the original articles.

Bulletin Signalétique

Published in Paris since 1940 by the Centre National de la Recherche Scientifique, *Bulletin Signalétique* provides abstracts of articles in approximately 9000 periodicals. It is published in sections devoted to a wide range of scientific subjects. Theses, congress proceedings and reports are covered. The abstracts, in French, are of the brief, indicative type.

Kongresszentralblatt für die gesamte innere Medizin

The main medical abstracting medium in the German language is the *Kongresszentralblatt für die gesamte innere Medizin* which has been published in Berlin since 1912. It is divided into six sections, each devoted to a special subject field and each comprising six issues a year. The sixth issue includes an author and subject index to the volume. Abstracts are in either German or English and there is some coverage of monograph literature.

Medicinskij Referativnyi Zhurnal

Abstracts in Russian are to be found in *Medicinskij Referativnyi Zhurnal,* which began publication in 1957, and which, since 1982 has been published in 22 sections, each having monthly parts with an annual subject index. Abstracts are in Russian, but authors and titles are given in the language of the original articles and an author index is provided for each issue.

Chemical Abstracts

In view of the increasingly interdisciplinary nature of the study of medicine, brief mention must be made of three important abstracting services in allied subject fields. *Chemical Abstracts,* the first volume of which appeared in 1907, provides as near to complete coverage of chemical literature as could be desired. The literature covered includes journal articles, proceedings of congresses and symposia and edited collections, technical reports, deposited documents, dissertations, new-book announcements and patent literature. The abstracts, which are classified in 80 subject groups or sections, provide brief, informative summaries. A substantial proportion of the material published is of biochemical interest.

Chemical Abstracts is published weekly in two 26-issue volumes per year. Each issue contains keyword, author and patent indexes. Each volume is provided with indexes to authors, general subjects, chemical substances, formulae and patents. Collective indexes are also published at regular intervals; the most recent covers vols 86 to 95, published in the years 1977 to 1981.

The computer-base for the Chemical Abstracts Service is also used to produce a current-awareness service in the form of *Chemical Titles*, a bi-weekly index to approximately 750 journals. A detailed account of *Chemical Abstracts* is given by Bottle (1979).

Biological Abstracts

Biological Abstracts, which has been in existence since 1926 and which is published by BIOSciences Information Service (BIOSIS) of Philadelphia, is important for the medical research worker who is interested in such subjects as genetics, biophysics, biochemistry and nutrition. In 1978, 8580 serials were screened and 262 000 items were added to the BIOSIS Data Base

The abstracts in *Biological Abstracts* are generally well-written and informative. Issues appear semi-monthly and abstracts are arranged in classified order with author, biosystematic, generic, concept and subject indexes, which are cumulated semi-annually. The subject indexes to *Biological Abstracts* have a complicated history, an account of which is to be found in Bottle and Wyatt (1971).

International Abstracts of Biological Sciences

International Abstracts of Biological Sciences, which first appeared in 1954 under the title of *British Abstracts of Medical Sciences*, covers the more important papers in biochemistry, physiology, pharmacology, microbiology, immunology, oncology, cell biology, genetics, anatomy, animal behaviour and experimental zoology. The applications of biology in clinical medicine are covered only in so far as they depend on the development of fundamental research.

In 1980 all papers in approximately 90 specified journals were covered by abstracts, titles or expanded titles. In the case of some 350 additional journals, all papers which fell within the aims and scope of *International Abstracts of Biological Sciences* were covered by titles or expanded titles. In each issue, which appear monthly or bi-monthly, abstracts are arranged in classified order with an author index; there are two volumes to the year.

A number of useful lists of abstracting services are available. Blake and Roos (1967) and the supplements to their work (*see* page 70) give detailed information on a considerable number of current and discontinued medical abstracting journals. The third edition of *World Medical Periodicals,* published by the World Medical Association in 1961, and its *Supplement* published in 1968, list over 100 titles with the publishers' addresses. In 1969 the International Federaton for Documentation published at The Hague a second edition of its *Abstracting Services,* the first volume of which is devoted to 'Science, Technology, Medicine, Agriculture'. In this volume entries are arranged alphabetically by title, and detailed information is given for each service; in two further sections the services are listed by subject and by country.

A very comprehensive guide to current medical abstracting and indexing journals has been provided by Dalby (1975).

Reviews

Reviews are a more sophisticated version of abstracts. They bring together, summarize and critically annotate information on a special subject which has been published over a period of time. If they are compiled with expert knowledge, give adequate coverage of the literature and are well written, with full bibliographical detail, they are of inestimable service, as they can save much time in tracking down and consulting relevant references.

Review articles have always been a feature of scientific journals, and, since the beginning of the nineteenth century, the number of periodicals or serials which confine themselves entirely to reviewing has steadily increased. A detailed account of reviews and yearbooks is included in Chapter 4 and references to those in special subjects are in the appropriate chapters. In the sphere of general medicine the following titles are among the most useful of those currently being published.

Advances in Internal Medicine

Advances in Internal Medicine first appeared in 1942 and is now published annually by Year Book Medical Publishers of Chicago and London. Each volume contains articles of reasonable length which synthesize from the literature 'a wide range of developments that should be important to the practice of all internists'. Substantial bibliographies are appended to the articles. The most recent edition, vol 27 of 1982, includes a cumulative subject index to vols 23 to 27.

Annual Review of Medicine: Selected Topics in Clinical Sciences

Published by Annual Reviews Inc. of Palo Alto, California, the above title seeks to treat in depth topics in internal medicine in which there have been remarkable recent advances. In general, the articles are not as lengthy as those in *Advances in Internal Medicine*, but the bibliographies are more extensive. Each volume contains a subject index and a classified list of chapter titles covering the previous five years.

Medical Annual

Medical Annual has been published continuously by John Wright of Bristol since 1883–1884. It comprises a selection of special articles on topics of current interest and a section devoted to reviews of the past year's work covering the whole field of medicine. There is a subject index to the volume. This is an invaluable work of reference, particularly for practitioners with no ready access to medical literature.

Recent Advances in Medicine (Beaumont and Dodds)

Published by Churchill Livingstone, *Recent Advances* first appeared in 1924, and subsequent volumes have been issued at irregular intervals, the most recent being the eighteenth of 1981 edited by A. M. Dawson *et al.* It seeks to provide readable and critical surveys of subjects in which there have been significant advances since the previous edition; the authors are active workers in the subjects concerned. It is designed for undergraduate and postgraduate students and for specialists with interests outside their field. Each chapter has a good bibliography, and there is a subject index but no name index to the volume (for further information on the *Recent Advances* series, *see* page 73).

Year Book of Medicine

Year Book of Medicine, an annual publication since 1901, is divided into sections covering broad subject headings. Each section contains abstracts of individual articles coupled with critical editorial comment. The complete volume has both author and subject indexes.

Bibliography of Medical Reviews

For tracing up-to-date review articles, workers in the medical field are fortunate in having a comprehensive reference tool in the *Bibliography of Medical Reviews*, which is published in Washington by the National Library of Medicine. The articles included in the *Bibliography* are indexed from the journals covered for *Index Medicus*. It was an annual publication from 1955 to 1966 and a monthly from 1967 to 1977 after which it ceased to appear as a separate publication. It continued as a section within the monthly issues of *Index Medicus*, a practice which was introduced in March 1965. Annual cumulations have been included in *Cumulated Index Medicus* since 1967. Vol 6 of 1960 consolidated the reviews for the period 1955 to 1960 and further cumulations covering 1966 to 1970, 1971 to 1975 and 1976 to 1980 have been published.

The criterion for inclusion in *Bibliography of Medical Reviews* is that articles should be well-documented surveys of recent literature. As with *Index Medicus*, the arrangement of each issue is a dual one of subjects and authors; the subject headings are taken from *MeSH*, but are somewhat broader than those used in *Index Medicus*. A very useful feature is that the number of references cited by each article is given.

Conclusions

Can it be said that indexes, abstracting services and reviews which have evolved since John Shaw Billings launched the *Index-Catalogue* constitute adequate guides to the medical literature of 1983 and of the past hundred years? Despite the prodigious volume of that literature, it can fairly be said that the tools are available for the medical worker to keep up to date with current developments and to retrieve past information in a reasonably comprehensive and efficient way. It cannot be denied, however, that there are some flies in the bibliographical ointment. Subscription rates to the more important reference works are so high that the maintenance of a complete collection is possible only for libraries with substantial financial resources. The haphazard manner in which the various bibliographical aids have been developed to meet particular situations have resulted in the large number of publications which are involved. This is one of the factors responsible for high cost, and has also led to a considerable duplication of effort by the different services. The advent of computerization should have helped to eliminate this overlapping and recent hopeful signs in this connection have been the co-operation between *Chemical Abstracts* and *Index Medicus* in linking their data bases (Baker, 1970) and the efforts of Unesco to develop a world science information system (UNIsist) (Wysocki and Tocatlian, 1971). Of late, however, an opposite and worrying tendency has been manifested in the legal challenge by the private information industry in the US to the bibliographical services operated by the National Library of Medicine (Davies, 1982). The whole subject of medical bibliography is inevitably a complex one and an excellent account of its development and of the external forces that exert an influence upon it is given by Adams (1981).

In the meantime, the medical worker with access to the bibliographies and with the skill to use them is better placed to locate what is required of the literature than many fellow scientists.

References

Adams, S. (1981), *Medical Bibliography in an Age of Discontinuity*, Chicago, Medical Library Association

Baker, D. B. (1970), Communication or chaos? *Science*, **169**, 739

Bishop, W. J. (1958), *Bibliography of International Congresses of Medical Sciences*, Oxford, Blackwell

Blake, J. B. (1980), *Centenary of Index Medicus, 1879–1979. Papers given at a Program held in the National Library of Medicine*, Bethesda, National Library of Medicine

Blake, J. B. and Roos, C. (1967), *Medical Reference Works, 1679–1966; a Selected Bibliography*, Chicago, Medical Library Association

Bottle, R. T. (1979), *Use of Chemical Literature*, 3rd edn, London, Butterworths

Bottle, R. T. and Wyatt, H. V. (1971), *The Use of Biological Literature*, 2nd edn, London, Butterworths

Brandon, A. N. and Hill, D. R. (1983), Selected list of books and journals for the small medical library, *Bull. Med. Libr. Assoc.*, **71**, 147

Crawford, S. (1960), Introduction to: *Cumulated Index Medicus*, vol 1, Part 1

Dalby, A. K. (1975), *Medical Abstracts and Indexes, 1975: a Bibliography of Abstracting, Indexing and Current Awareness Services in Medicine and Related Subjects* (Cambridge University Library, Librarianship Series 2), Cambridge, University Library

Davies, N. E. (1982), The health-sciences information struggle. The private information industry versus the National Library of Medicine, *New Engl. J. Med.*, **307**, 201

Garfield, E. (1979), *Citation Indexing: its Theory and Application in Science, Technology and Humanities*, New York, John Wiley

Karel, L. (1967), Selection of journals for *Index Medicus*: a historical review. *Bull. Med. Libr. Assoc.*, **55**, 259

Marson, J. (1969), John Shaw Billings as a bibliographer, *Bull. Med. Libr. Assoc.*, **57**, 379

Rogers, F. B. and Adams, S. (1950), The Army Medical Library's publication program, *Tex. Rep. Biol. Med.*, **8**, 271

Wysocki, A. and Tocatlian, J. (1971), A world science information system; necessary and feasible, *UNESCO Bull. Libr.*, **25**, 62

4

Standard Reference Sources

J. L. Thornton*; revised by H. R. Hague

It is sometimes assumed that reference librarians have the answer to all possible queries in their heads. This is, of course, far from the truth, but what librarians should have is a good idea of where to start looking for the answer. Experience tells which particular source is likely to produce a good result, and consequently which should be consulted first. To this end even the smallest library should have available a basic stock of reference and bibliographical sources. Even a specialized library is expected to provide the answers to many general questions.

The most comprehensive guide to medical reference material is *Medical Reference Works 1679–1966: a Selected Bibliography* edited by J. B. Blake and C. Roos (Medical Library Association (MLA), 1967), which contains 2700 entries. Arranged alphabetically by sub-divisions of medicine, each section has lists of material under sub-headings such as indexes and abstracts, reviews, bibliographies, dictionaries, lists of periodicals, directories and histories. *Supplement I, 1967–1968* compiled by M. V. Clark (MLA 1970) contains 315 items. *Supplement II, 1969–1972* compiled by J. S. Richmond (MLA, 1973), lists some 500 items, and *Supplement III, 1973–1974* (MLA, 1975) includes 244 annotated entries. No further supplements have been issued. Instead the role of updating Blake and Roos has been taken over by entries in the *National Library of Medicine Current Catalog*, using the subject heading 'Reference Books, Medical'. The *NLM Current Catalog* appears

*Formerly Librarian, St Bartholomew's Hospital Medical College, London

quarterly, with annual cumulations, and the 1981 annual cumulation contained 90 entries under this subject heading, most provided with a brief annotation.

Volume one of the *Guide to Reference Material* edited by A. J. Walford (4th edn, Library Association,, 1980) covers science and technology in general, with 48 pages devoted to medicine and veterinary medicine. It is arranged according to the Universal Decimal Classification. Although Walford's *Guide* is inevitably selective, many important works are listed, and the section devoted to dictionaries is particularly helpful. It is also useful for fringe subjects.

Encyclopaedias

It must be admitted that encyclopaedias are now of little value in the medical field. Even when updated by means of annual supplements, they are unsatisfactory for finding information on particular topics when compared with other sources, such as textbooks, monographs and reviews. Medical encyclopaedias should be regarded mainly as recording the state of knowledge on a particular subject at the time of writing, and are therefore primarily of historical interest.

The *McGraw-Hill Encyclopaedia of Science and Technology* (5th edn, 15 vols, 1982) is of little relevance for clinical medicine, though it may be of some value in the basic sciences and for related fields such as biophysics and computing. With this work extensive use should be made of the analytical index.

A small, but valuable, work is the *Penguin Medical Encyclopaedia* by P. Wingate (3rd edn, 1983). This is aimed at patients or anyone concerned with the care of sick people. Entries range in size from a few lines to over a page, and explain diseases, organs and bodily processes in straightforward, non-technical language.

Handbooks

Before World War II, a number of multi-volumed works were published in Germany as *Handbücher*. These were usually issued in parts, bound or unbound, sometimes out of numerical sequence, so that often several years elapsed before volumes were completed. These *Handbücher* were expensive yet of great importance, because they consisted of authoritative surveys by writers with international reputations, and reviewed the literature historically and bibliographically. Despite a modern tendency to regard any scientific literature more than five to ten years old as obsolete, there is a persistent demand for reliable reviews surveying progress to date and evaluating the material. This is particularly so when theses are being written and prior to research work being undertaken. A surprising number of these handbooks are still being issued today, and an interesting trend in recent years has been the adoption of English as the language of publication for some of them.

Examples include W. von Möllendorff's *Handbuch der mikroskopischen Anatomie des Menschen* (Springer), which was started in 1929 and is still appearing; the *Handbuch der speziellen pathologischen Anatomie und Histologie* (Henke/Lubarsch) in 40 volumes (Springer, 1925–1978); the *Handbook of Experimental Pharmacology* (Springer, 1950–), which from volume 36, 1973, is entirely in English; and the *Handbook of Sensory Physiology* (Springer, 1971–1981) which was completed upon publication of the 23rd part, all volumes being in English. Individual volumes in these series can normally be bought separately, and they can usually be borrowed from the British Library Lending Division.

The *Handbook of Physiology*, published by the American Physiological Society and distributed by Williams and Wilkins, commenced in 1959 and appeared in nine sections. A new edition is now in progress (from 1977), with some changes in the titles of sections, and this will maintain its place as a work of great significance. Equally important is P. J. Vinken and G. W. Bruyn's *Handbook of Clinical Neurology* (North Holland–Elsevier), which started publication in 1969 and is still appearing (vol 43 being published in 1982). Other examples are the *Handbook of Neurochemistry* edited by A. Lajtha (7 vols, Plenum Press, 1969–1972) and the *Handbook of Psychopharmacology* edited by L. L. Iversen *et al.* (14 vols, Plenum Press, 1975–1978).

Year books, annual reviews

Individual items in these series are detailed in other chapters and are many and varied in scope, reliability and coverage. Generally, they survey the literature of the previous year, evaluating it in chapters contributed by experts.

The *Year Book* series is published regularly by Year Book Medical Publishers (Chicago) and currently covers 25 areas of medicine. Recent additions to the series are the volumes devoted to *Family Practice* (1977–), *Sports Medicine* (1979–), *Clinical*

Pharmacy (1981–) and *Emergency Medicine* (1981–). A number of the earlier volumes have changed their titles over the years. Academic Press (New York) publishes *Recent Progress in Hormone Research* and also issues the *Advances* series, of which more than 30 titles are in the biomedical field, including the well known volumes for *Cancer Research, Clinical Chemistry, Immunology* and *Pharmacology and Chemotherapy*. Year Book Medical Publishers produce another *Advances* series covering *Internal Medicine, Nephrology, Pediatrics, Surgery* and a new volume, *Advances in the Management of Cardiovascular Disease* (1980–). Grune and Stratton publish the *Progress* series, which appear irregularly. The subjects covered include *Clinical Immunology, Clinical Pathology, Gastroenterology, Hematology, Liver Diseases*, and a new title, *Progress in Diseases of the Skin* (1981–).

The *Annual Reviews* series (Palo Alto, Annual Reviews Inc.) now contains some 12 titles of medical interest, and recent additions cover *Immunology* (1983–), *Neuroscience* (1978–), *Nutrition* (1981–) and *Public Health* (1980–). The various chapters in all these volumes normally contain extensive lists of references. One British publication which does not always receive the recognition it deserves is the *Medical Annual* (John Wright), published regularly since 1883. Each volume includes one or more special, original articles, and the remainder is devoted to a review of the year's work, arranged under broad headings which are divided into subsections. References to the literature are given at the end of each section. Many libraries treat all these annual volumes as bound periodicals, rather than as books.

Volumes in Churchill Livingstone's *Recent Advances* series are issued irregularly. Some 38 different titles are now available, covering most branches of medicine. Recent additions to the series include the volumes for *Clinical Biochemistry* (No 1, 1978), *Clinical Oncology* (No 1, 1982), *Clinical Pharmacology* (No 1, 1978), *Community Medicine* (No 1, 1978), *Geriatric Medicine* (No 1, 1978), *Infection* (No 1, 1979, *Neuropathology* (No 1 1979), *Occupational Health* (No 1, 1982) and *Perinatal Medicine* (No 1, 1983). These are now numbered serially rather than being designated as editions. Earlier issues provide a guide to the historical development of the subject.

The series of *Clinics* published by W. B. Saunders are issued bound as separate symposia, usually in three, four or six parts each year. Those published in Britain cover *Endocrinology and Metabolism* (1972–), *Gastroenterology* (1972–), *Haematology* (1972–), *Immunology and Allergy* (1981–), *Obstetrics and Gynaecology* (1974–) and *Rheumatic Diseases* (1975–), while those published in

North America are more numerous and include the *Dental Clinics,
Medical Clinics, Orthopedic Clinics, Pediatric Clinics, Radiologic
Clinics, Surgical Clinics* and *Urologic Clinics*, amongst others.

The *Modern Trends* series published by Butterworths covered
many areas of medicine in volumes issued every few years, but gradually ceased publication during the 1970s. There is now, however,
a major new series, *Butterworths International Medical Reviews*,
which covers 16 different specialties. Individual volumes within each
subject are issued annually, but they focus on a single topic or major
theme of current interest rather than attempting to survey the whole
field. The series covers the following subject areas:

Anesthesiology (1983–)
Cardiology (1982–)
Clinical Endocrinology (1981–)
Clinical Immunology (1983–)
Clinical Pharmacology and Therapeutics (1982–)
Gastroenterology (1981–)
Hematology (1983–)
Neurology (1981–)
Obstetrics and Gynecology (1981–)
Ophthalmology (1983–)
Orthopedics (1983–)
Otolaryngology (1982)
Pediatrics (1982–)
Rheumatology (1982–)
Surgery (1981–)
Urology (1983–)

As an example, the first volume of the *Gastroenterology* series was
devoted to 'Foregut', the second to 'The Small Intestine' and
volume three to 'The Large Bowel'. The annual volumes in each
subject area may be purchased on a subscription basis.

Directories

There is available a wide range of directories, national and international, and only a brief selection can be given here. The *Medical
Register* has been published annually since 1859 by the General
Medical Council, and is the official register of doctors qualified to
practice in this country. More detailed information is given in the
Medical Directory (Churchill Livingstone) which has been issued
annually since 1845. This provides names, addresses, telephone
numbers, qualifications, past and present posts held and a list of up
to three publications. Information is also given on hospitals
(including the names of consultants in each department), societies,
medical schools, postgraduate medical centres, geographical listing

of doctors and other topics. Directories for other countries include the *Medical Directory of Australia* (Sydney, 1935–), the *Canadian Medical Directory* (Toronto, 1955–) and the *American Medical Directory* (Chicago, 1906–), published irregularly by the American Medical Association (28th edn, 1982). This also lists the chief medical societies, hospitals and medical journals, while the *Directory of Medical Specialists* (19th edn, 3 vols, Marquis, 1979) includes details of 220 000 American specialists. The *Dentists Register* (London) has been published since 1879 by the General Dental Council, and the American Dental Association has issued the *American Dental Directory* since 1947.

The General Medical Council publishes a *List of Hospitals and House Officer Posts in the United Kingdom which are Approved or Recognised for Pre-Registration Service* (9th edn, 1980). The Council for Postgraduate Medical Education in England and Wales regularly issues a *Directory of Postgraduate Medical Centres*. The *Hospitals and Health Services Yearbook* (Institute of Health Service Administrators, annual) provides a wealth of information on government departments, statutory bodies, health authorities, all types of hospitals, circulars and statutory instruments, important reports and hospital suppliers. Further details of the organization of the National Health Service are found in *Health Care in the United Kingdom* edited by N. W. Chaplin for the Institute of Health Service Administrators (Kluwer Medical, 1982), while the *Directory of Schools of Medicine and Nursing* issued by the International Hospitals Group (Kogan Page, 1983) provides more information about the training and qualifications of the professions supplementary to medicine than is elsewhere available. Brian Watkin's *Documents on Health and Social Services 1834 to the Present Day* (Methuen, 1975) is a very useful source for older official reports and legislation.

The annual *World of Learning* (2 vols, Europa Publications) is arranged alphabetically by country and provides information on universities, colleges, research institutes, museums and libraries. It also has a section listing international organizations. *The Commonwealth Universities Yearbook* (Association of Commonwealth Universities) gives very detailed information about the universities in the countries it covers, including historical background, courses offered and full lists of staff by department. The World Health Organization issues the *World Directory of Medical Schools* (5th edn 1979), and this is updated by regular entries in *WHO Chronicle*. For Great Britain and Ireland, courses are listed in the *Summary of Postgraduate Diplomas and Courses in Medicine*, issued at the start of each year by the Council for Postgraduate Medical Education. Advisory, governmental and semi-official bodies in British public life are listed in *Councils, Committees and Boards* (4th edn, C.B.D. Research, 1980).

Details of research being undertaken is covered by *Research in British Universities, Polytechnics and Colleges* published by the British Library in three vols: vol 1, *Physical Sciences* (2nd edn, 1981); vol 2, *Biological Sciences* (2nd edn, 1981); and vol 3, *Social Sciences* (2nd edn, 1981). This will eventually be available as an online data base via the British Library. The Medical Reseach Council *Handbook* (MRC, annual) provides details of research sponsored by the Council, and the *DHSS Handbook of Research and Development* (HMSO, annual) lists projects sponsored by the Department of Health during the preceding year. Details of research sponsored by the US Government are provided by the National Institute of Health's *Research Grants Index*, which is arranged by subject, grant number and name of investigator.

Information about grants available in this country can be found in the *Grants Register 1981–83* (Macmillan, 1980) and the *Directory of Grant-Making Trusts 1983* (CAF Publications, 1983). On a smaller scale are the *Handbook of British Medical Research Charities* (Association of Medical Research Charities, annual, free) which is restricted to the major trusts and foundations, and the British Medical Association's *Research Funds Guide* (3rd edn, BMA, 1976). The Association of Commonwealth Universities publishes *Awards for Commonwealth University Staff 1981–83* (ACU, 1980), giving details of fellowships, visiting professorships and grants, and *Scholarships Guide for Commonwealth Postgraduate Students 1983–1985* (ACU, 1982), providing information on scholarships, grants, loans and assistantships for postgraduate study outside the home country. More general information about foundations and trusts is found in the *International Foundation Directory* (2nd edn, Europa Publications, 1979).

In addition to the directories listed above, university and medical school calendars and the annual reports of institutions often provide additional information. This section would not be complete, however, without mention of *Whitaker's Almanack*, published annually since 1868, which contains a vast amount of information of all kinds. An up-to-date copy should be available in every library, however small.

Dictionaries

The most comprehensive British medical dictionary is *Butterworths Medical Dictionary* with Macdonald Critchley as editor-in-chief (2nd edn, Butterworths, 1978), first published in 1961 as the *British Medical Dictionary* and edited by Sir Arthur MacNalty. This contains biographical and eponymous material, as well as abbreviations, and includes as an appendix an 80-page anatomical nomenclature. The *Faber Medical Dictionary,* which was originally edited by Sir Cecil Wakeley and is now revised by J. G. Bate (2nd edn, Faber, 1975), is smaller, but may be particularly useful for medical secretaries and others who need English as opposed to American spelling. Another short, but valuable, compilation is the *Concise Medical Dictionary* (Oxford University Press, 1980) which gives good explanations of 9500 terms and contains some illustrations.

There are several large American dictionaries of long standing which are popular in this country. *Dorland's Illustrated Medical Dictionary* (26th edn, Saunders, 1981) has been published since 1900, though successive editions have tended to include fewer illustrations. It contains biographical and eponymous material and, because of its reliability, is included in the bibliography accompanying the list of Medical Subject Headings used by *Index Medicus.* An abridged version is published as *Dorland's Pocket Medical Dictionary* (23rd edn, Saunders, 1982). *Stedman's Medical Dictionary* (24th edn, Williams and Wilkins, 1982) was first issued in 1911 and has some 100 000 entries. It is easy to use and contains a number of additional tables and appendices, including a 30 page section on medical etymology. *Blakiston's Gould Medical Dictionary* (4th edn, McGraw-Hill, 1979), first compiled by G. M. Gould in 1894, has very full coverage of terms and many extra tables. On a smaller scale is *Taber's Cyclopedic Medical Dictionary* now edited by C. L. Thomas (14th edn, F. A. Davis, 1981) with some 47 000 entries and 150 good illustrations.

Three polyglot dictionaries are worth noting, as smaller medical libraries may stock one of these in preference to multiple foreign-language dictionaries: E. Veillon and A. Nobel's *Medical Dictionary* (6th edn, Huber, 1977), which contains over 40 000 numbered terms, the main section being English with references back from German and French words; A. Sliosberg's *Elsevier's Medical Dictionary in Five Languages* (2nd edn, Elsevier, 1975), covering English–American, French, Italian, Spanish and German, with over 20 000 English-base entries; and *Lexicon Medicum: Anglicum, Russicum, Gallicum, Germanicum, Latinum, Polonium* edited by B. Zlotnicki (Polish Medical Publishers, 1971), Part I of which contains some 15 000 English terms with their equivalents in Russian, French, German, Latin and Polish, and Part II being an index in these languages referring back to the numbered terms in Part I.

Foreign-language medical dictionaries are numerous. The following are suggested as examples:

FRENCH

Vocabulary of Medicine and Related Sciences: English–French, French–English by
W. J. Gladstone (Masson, 1971)

English–French Dictionary of Medical Terms by J. Delamare and T. Delamare-Riche (Paris, Maloine, 1971)

Dictionary, French–English/English–French, of Medical and Biological Terms by
P. Lépine and P. R. Peacock, (2nd edn, H. K. Lewis, and Flammarion, 1974)

GERMAN

Medical Dictionary of the English and German Languages by D. W. Unseld (7th edn, Wissenschaftliche Verlagsgesellschaft, 1978), containing English–German and German–English sections in one small volume

Medical and Pharmaceutical Dictionary English–German by W. E. Bunjes (4th edn, Thieme, 1981) with a *Supplement* comprising more than 17 000 new entries

Wörterbuch der Medizin und Pharmazeutik, Deutsch–Englisch by W. E. Bunjes (3rd edn, Thieme, 1981)

RUSSIAN

English–Russian Medical Dictionary by M. P. Multanovsky and A. Y. Ivanova (Collets, 1969)

Russian–English Biological and Medical Dictionary by E. A. Carpovich (2nd edn, Technical Dictionaries Co., 1960) containing over 32 000 entries

S. Jablonski's Russian–English Medical Dictionary edited by B. S. Levine (Academic Press, 1958) with 29 000 entries

Russian–English Medical Dictionary (Russian Language Publishers, 1975), containing 50 000 terms and using American spelling

SPANISH

Spanish–English/English–Spanish
Medical Guide by H. H. Hirschhorn (Bailey Bros, 1968)

Diccionario Inglés–Español y Español–Inglés de Medicina by F. Ruiz Torres (3rd end, Editorial Alhambra, 1965, reprinted 1979) which contains over 50 000 entries, with eponyms and abbreviations

OTHER

Hitti's Medical Dictionary: English–Arabic, with an Arabic–English Vocabulary by
Y. K. Hitti (4th edn, Librairie du Liban, 1982), with some 40 000 English entries and 31 coloured anatomical plates

A Short English–Swahili Medical Dictionary by T. H. White (Churchill Livingstone, 1978)

Dictionaries dealing with a particular subject are referred to in the relevant chapters. A useful and necessary addition to the literature is the *Dictionary of Medical Ethics* edited by A. S. Duncan *et al.* (2nd edn, Longman and Todd, 1981), which contains entries on such important topics as abortion, bereavement, embryo transfer, psychosurgery, etc.

Nomenclature, terminology and abbreviations

Medical terminology is of vital importance, and the clear description of a clinical condition assumes a standard nomenclature. The

Nomenclature of Disease was drawn up by a committee of the Royal College of Physicians (8th and final edition, HMSO, 1960). It has two sections: the first is an aetiological classification which, in the second section, is applied to the body as a whole and to its systems. It is a nomenclature only, concerned with absolute specificity in the description of disease, and cannot be used to code or classify. E. T. Thompson and A. C. Hayden prepared the *Standard Nomenclature of Diseases and Operations* for the American Medical Association (5th edn, McGraw-Hill, 1961). This incorporates a classification and is intended primarily as a diagnostic code for record-keeping and for statistical purposes – as such it is readily adaptable for use in machine-readable data handling systems.

Standardization is particularly necessary for international co-operation and for statistical purposes. The World Health Organization manages the *International Classification of Diseases (ICD)*, the ninth revision of which was published in the *Manual of the International Statistical Classification of Diseases, Injuries and Causes of Death* (2 vols, WHO, 1977–1978). The first volume gives a tabular list of diseases and causes of death, and the second volume is an alphabetical index to the first. The classification is widely used in the recording of pathological conditions and forms the basis of many national mortality and morbidity statistical compilations. The *International Classification of Procedures in Medicine* (2 vols, WHO, 1978) was published for trial purposes following a resolution at the Twenty-Ninth World Health Assembly in May 1976 and is intended to present, in a systematic fashion, the many procedures used in the different branches of medicine. The *International Classification of Impairments, Disabilities and Handicaps* (WHO, 1980) is concerned with the consequences of disease and has also been issued in an experimental first edition. Both these volumes are intended to supplement the *ICD* itself.

The Committee on Nomenclature and Classification of Disease of the College of American Pathologists has produced two important classifications: *Systematized Nomenclature of Pathology (SNOP)* (College of American Pathologists, 1965) and *Systematized Nomenclature of Medicine (SNOMED)* (2nd edn, 2 vols, 1979). Both these publications aim to help pathologists and clinicians organize and utilize their material, and the codings are sufficiently comprehensive and flexible to have many applications in the storage and retrieval of clinical information. Anatomical nomenclature is covered by the International Anatomical Nomenclature Committee's *Nomina Anatomica* (4th edn, Excerpta Medica, 1977); this edition incorporates the *Nomina Histologica* and the *Nomina Embryologica*. Also relevant is T.

Donath's *Anatomical Dictionary with Nomenclatures and Explanatory Notes;* the English edition is by G. N. C. Crawford (Pergamon Press, 1970). This brings together the *Basle Nomina Anatomica* (1895), the *Jena Nomina Anatomica* (1935) and the *Nomina Anatomica Parisiensia* (1955) in a comparative dictionary, and also contains a list of eponymous authors, with dates of birth and death, nationality and subject specialty. First published in Hungarian in 1958, this has also been translated into German (1960) and Russian. The *Enzyme Nomenclature 1978* (Academic Press, 1979) comprises the recommendations of the Nomenclature Committee of the International Union of Biochemistry on the nomenclature and classification of enzymes.

Guides to the derivation, construction and meaning of medical terms include H. A. Skinner's *The Origin of Medical Terms* (2nd edn, Williams and Wilkins, 1961), which contains about 4000 terms; F. Roberts' *Medical Terms: their Origin and Construction,* revised by B. Lennox (6th edn, Heinemann Medical, 1980); P. M. Davies' *Medical Terminology in Hospital Practice* (3rd edn, Heinemann Medical, 1978), which is aimed especially at the professions supplementary to medicine; and D. Anderson and R. Buxton's *A Pocket Etymology of Medical Terms – an Introduction to the Greek and Latin Roots of Medical Terminology* (Bristol Classical Press, 1981), aimed primarily at medical students. M. A. Collins' *Medical Terminology and the Body Systems* (Harper and Row, 1974) is arranged by systems, while *Henderson's Dictionary of Biological Terms,* now edited by S. Holmes (9th edn, Longman, 1979), provides definitions of over 22 000 terms in related fields. J. Parkinson's *Manual of English for the Overseas Doctor* (2nd edn, Churchill Livingstone, 1976) is concerned mainly with language and terminology, but is also one of the few books to contain a sample curriculum vitae.

Medical and scientific abbreviations appear in some of the dictionaries referred to earlier, but two separate compilations are E. B. Steen's *Abbreviations in Medicine* (4th edn, Baillière Tindall, 1978), listing over 13 000 items, and *Medical Abreviations and Acronyms* by P. Roody *et al.* (McGraw-Hill, 1977) with some 14 000 entries and cross-references.

Eponyms, syndromes and quotations

The use of eponyms in medical literature has been criticized because some diseases, syndromes, etc., may have more than one eponymous name associated with them and this can lead to confusion. However they are undoubtedly here to stay, and it can be argued that they do have a mnemonic quality. Several guides to this kind of terminology have been produced and the most comprehensive is the *Dictionary of Medical Syndromes* by S. I. Magalini and E. Scrascia (2nd edn, Lippincott, 1981). This is arranged alphabetically, and under each syndrome are listed synonyms, symptoms, signs, etiology, pathology, diagnostic procedures, therapy, prognosis and bibliography – the way that a doctor might approach a particular medical problem. Several references are given in the bibliography, including the original reference, but where books are quoted page references are seldom given. S. Jablonski's *Illustrated Dictionary of Eponymic Syndromes and Diseases and their Synonyms* (Saunders, 1969) is arranged alphabetically by personal names, with dates of birth and death where appropriate, followed by synonyms, definition and original source. Cross-references and numerous illustrations are included. Two older compilations are R. H. Durham's *Encyclopaedia of Medical Syndromes* (Hoeber–Harper, 1960), which includes a classification of syndromes by system or type, but which does not always refer to the original description, and E. C. Kelly's *Encyclopedia of Medical Sources* (Williams and Wilkins, 1948), which provides full references to the original source and often gives brief biographical information. A useful addition to the literature, and one intended for the laboratory coat pocket, is J. Lourie's *Medical Eponyms: Who Was Coudé?* (Pitman Books, 1982). This short compilation of some 900 entries does not give original sources or a bibliography, but instead aims to provide biographical details about the individual in question, something notably lacking from a number of the earlier guides.

The field of anatomy is adequately served by J. Dobson's *Anatomical Eponyms: being a Biographical Dictionary of those Anatomists whose Names have become Incorporated into Anatomical Nomenclature . . .* (2nd edn, Livingstone, 1962), while *Notable Names in Medicine and Surgery* by H. Bailey and W. J. Bishop (3rd edn, H. K. Lewis, 1959; reprinted 1972) is also useful for eponymous material. C. Allan Birch's *Names We Remember* (Ravenswood Publications, 1979) consists of 56 short eponymous medical biographies. A vital source for tracing original descriptions, as well as sign-posting the development of medicine, is *A Medical Bibliography (Garrison–Morton)* by L. T. Morton (4th edn, Gower 1983). The texts of the various declarations and codes of ethics are often sought, and a useful source for these is *Decision-Making in Medicine: the Practice of its Ethics* edited by G. Scorer and A. Wing (Arnold, 1979, pages 190–201). Amongst others this includes the text of the Declarations of Geneva, Helsinki, Oslo and Tokyo, as well as the Hippocratic Oath.

Medical quotations are frequently requested, as are their sources, and these can be traced in *Familiar Medical Quotations* edited by M. B. Strauss (Little, Brown, 1968). This is arranged by subjects, and dates of birth and death are appended to names, but few of the sources are provided with dates or other bibliographical details, making it difficult to trace original sources (for example, if one wants to place a quotation in its original context). Strauss provides some 7500 quotations, and there are indexes of authors and keywords. More general in coverage, but equally fascinating, is A. L. Mackay's *The Harvest of a Quiet Eye* (Institute of Physics, 1977), a delightful and stimulating collection of scientific quotations.

Medical writing

Most members of the medical profession become involved in formal writing at some stage during their careers, whether for a thesis, a book or a journal article. The following are suggested as general guides: V. Booth's *Writing a Scientific Paper/Speaking at Scientific Meetings* (5th edn, Biochemical Society, 1981) combining two previously separate publications; *Writing Scientific Papers in English* by M. O'Connor and F. P. Woodford (revised edn, Pitman Medical, 1978), which gives a step-by-step approach for authors from first draft to correcting proofs; H. A. F. Dudley's *The Presentation of Original Work in Medicine and Biology (Churchill Livingstone, 1977); Thorne's Better Medical Writing* revised by Stephen Lock (2nd edn, Pitman Medical, 1977); and the King's Fund *Preparing for Publication* (Pitman Medical, 1976), which is a style-manual for authors, editors, compilers and typists.

Technical guidance is provided by the Royal Society of Medicine's *Units, Symbols and Abbreviations* edited by D. N. Baron (3rd edn, RSM, 1977), which is intended for biological and medical editors and authors, and by three British Standards: *BS 1629: 1976, Recommendations for Bibliographical References; BS 4821: 1972, Recommendations for the Presentation of Theses*, and *BS 5261c: 1976, Marks for Copy Preparation and Proof Correction*. The Institute of Medical and Biological Illustration's *Charts and Graphs: Guidelines for the Visual Presentation of Statistical Data in the Life Sciences* edited by D. Simmonds (MTP Press, 1980) is a practical guide for anyone concerned with preparing charts and graphs either for teaching or for publication. Copyright is often another area of concern, and assistance is provided by M. F. Flint's *A User's Guide to Copyright* (Butterworths, 1979).

A number of compilations give advice to authors about the requirements of particular journals, though it should be remembered that instructions are revised from time to time. N. D. Lane and K. L. Kammerer's *Writer's Guide to Medical Journals* (Ballinger, 1975) gives publication data and instructions for over 300 journals, while D. B. Ardell and J. Y. James' *Author's Guide to Journals in the Health Field* (Haworth, 1980) covers 260 titles. Many eminent journals in both Europe and North America have decided to adopt the so-called 'Vancouver Style', which proposes uniform requirements for manuscripts submitted to biomedical journals. Details will be found in the *British Medical Journal* for 12th June 1982, vol 284, pages 1766–1770, including a list of those periodicals currently using the new style. It should be noted that this code requires the titles of journals to be abbreviated according to the *List of Journals Indexed in Index Medicus*, which is published in the January issue of *Index Medicus* each year, and which is also available separately.

In addition to writing, many doctors are also required to address meetings of various kinds. Sound advice is provided by J. Calnan and A. Barabas' *Speaking at Medical Meetings: a Practical Guide* (2nd edn, Heinemann Medical, 1981), which ranges from classroom teaching to giving a paper at an international conference and is very humorously illustrated. Finally, the *British Medical Journal* has issued a most useful compilation entitled *How to do it* (BMJ, 1979), which gives guidance on many topics including writing an MD thesis, planning a research project, giving a lecture, writing a paper, using slides, appearing on television, etc.

Data books

Data books are intended to provide basic scientific data in concise form and they include such information as mathematical, statistical, chemical and physical tables; dosages; toxicities; normal values; etc. Devoted mainly to subjects connected with scientific medicine, they embrace chemistry and biochemistry, biology and allied topics. Organic chemistry boasts a most comprehensive tool in Beilstein's *Handbuch der Organischen Chemie* (4th edn, Springer, 1913), a monumental work listing all known compounds. 'Beilstein' is described in detail in R. T. Bottle's *The Use of Chemical Literature* (3rd edn, Butterworths, 1979, Chapter 11). This also provides extensive information on literature on physicochemical data (Chapter 8), and sources of biological data are indicated in R. T. Bottle and H. V. Wyatt's *The Use of Biological Literature* (2nd edn, Butterworths, 1972, Chapter 8). A few standard reference books are mentioned below.

Geigy Scientific Tables should be available in every medical library. Vol 1–2 of the 8th edition appeared in 1983 (Geigy Pharmaceuticals, Horsham) and the remaining 3 volumes will be issued at yearly intervals. Providing basic scientific information in concise form, it includes sections devoted to mathematical and statistical tables, physics, physical chemistry, biochemistry, nutrition, composition and functions of the body, body fluids, body measurements and hormones. Another popular source is *The Merck Index: An Encyclopedia of Chemicals and Drugs* (9th edn, Merck, 1976), providing information on the chemical and physical properties, dosages and toxicities of about 10 000 compounds, with references to the literature.

The *Biology Data Book* edited by P. L. Altman and D. S. Dittmer and published by the Federation of American Societies for Experimental Biology (2nd edn, 3 vols, 1972–1974) contains evaluated reference data for the life sciences, and is particularly useful because full details of the original sources are given. The FASEB series of *Biological Handbooks* includes *Blood and Other Body Fluids* (1961, reprinted 1971), *Environmental Biology* (1966), *Respiration and Circulation* (1971), *Cell Biology* (1976), *Human Health and Disease* (1977) and *Inbred and Genetically Defined Strains of Laboratory Animals* (2 vols, 1979).

Compounds, reagents and techniques used in biochemistry are described in *Data for Biochemical Research* by R. M. C. Dawson *et al.* (2nd edn, Clarendon Press, 1969). G. D. Fasman has edited the *Handbook of Biochemistry and Molecular Biology* (3rd edn, 8 vols, CRC Press, 1976), while R. C. Weast edits the regularly revised *Handbook of Chemistry and Physics* (63rd edn, CRC Press, 1982). G. W. C. Kaye and T. H. Laby's *Tables of Physical and Chemical Constants* (14th edn, Longman, 1973) covers general physics, chemistry, atomic and nuclear physics, and some mathematical functions. All tabulated volumes are expressed in SI units. Statistical tables are often in demand, and a suitable small compilation is F. C. Powell's *Cambridge Mathematical and Statistical Tables* (Cambridge University Press, 1976), while A. M. Bold and P. Wilding's *Clinical Chemistry Companion* (Blackwell, 1979) is a handy source of information on normal reference values and standard laboratory tests in medicine.

Vital statistics and statistical tables

For further information on this topic, *see* Chapter 8, page 185. Statistical information is often hard to find in the format required. Workers require more up-to-date figures than may be available, or else they need them broken down in different ways from their published form. It may be that a recent journal article, located through *Index Medicus,* is the only source of a certain subject. However, a good starting point for many enquiries is the *Guide to Official Statistics* compiled by the Central Statistical Office (4th edn, HMSO 1982). This is a highly detailed source of reference, not only to published statistical tables, but also to the journal articles and to reports. Also useful is M. Alderson and R. Dowie's *Health Surveys and Related Studies* (Pergamon Press, 1979) which forms vol 9 of that publisher's *Reviews of United Kingdom Statistical Sources* series. A quick source of basic information about the incidence of particular types of illness and disease in this country is J. Fry's *Common Diseases: their Nature, Incidence and Care* (3rd edn, MTP, 1983), which gives figures gathered mainly from general practice. G. M. Howe's *The National Atlas of Disease Mortality in the United Kingdom* (2nd edn, Nelson, 1970) was compiled on behalf of the Royal Geographical Society, and indicates by means of maps the varying pattern of disease mortality in the UK.

On the international level the World Health Organization published *Annual Epidemiological and Vital Statistics* from 1939–1951, which was then succeeded by the *World Health Statistics Annual* (Geneva, 1952–). This is published in three volumes: I *Vital Statistics and Causes of Death;* II *Infectious Diseases: Cases;* and III *Health Personnel and Hospital Establishments.* From 1979, vol 1 appeared annually, but the other topics are only covered periodically. Since 1948 the United Nations has issued the *Demographic Yearbook* (New York), providing statistics from over 220 countries or areas on population, births, mortality, marriage and divorce and international migration. M. Alderson's *International Mortality Statistics* (Macmillan, 1981) is an important source of information, giving serial mortality tables for European and other selected countries by sex, calendar period, and cause of death. It is valuable both for analysing long-term mortality trends within a particular country and for comparing patterns of mortality in different countries during this century.

The Registrar-General's *Statistical Review of England and Wales* came to an end with the three volumes for 1973 (published 1975–1976), and this has been replaced by a series of smaller annual volumes, each dealing with one topic or a number of related topics (HMSO, 1974–). The volumes issued include: *Birth Statistics, Mortality Statistics – Cause; Mortality Statistics – Childhood and Maternity; Mortality Statistics – Accidents and Violence; Mortality Statistics – Area; Cancer Statistics; Communicable Disease Statistics; Hospital In-Patient Enquiry;* and *Abortion Statistics*. This is a selection only, and full details are found in *Sectional List No. 56: Office of Population Censuses and Surveys (OPCS)*, revised every eighteen months or so and available free from HMSO. Each main subject carries a colour and reference code; For example, volumes in the morbidity series are pale blue and carry the reference number MB. The aim is to publish figures more quickly than was possible before. The annual reference volumes are supplemented by a series of OPCS *Monitors*, designed for the quick release of selected information as it becomes available. The *Monitors* are divided into the same colour and reference codes as the annual volumes, and their frequency may be monthly, quarterly or 'occasional'. The Registrar-General's *Weekly Return for England and Wales* is published as one of the *Monitors*, and includes notifications of infectious diseases for each administrative area. It is issued about ten days after the end of the week to which figures relate. The *Monitors* are available free from OPCS, whereas the annual volumes must be bought from HMSO. *Population Trends*, the quarterly journal of OPCS, contains regular and up-to-date tables on vital statistics, births, marriages, divorces, migration, deaths and abortions.

Figures relating to the management of the National Health Service (NHS) are found in *Health and Personal Social Services Statistics for England, with Summary Tables for Great Britain; Scottish Health Statistics;* and *Health and Personal Social Services Statistics for Wales* (all HMSO, annual). The Office of Health Economics' *Compendium of Health Statistics* (3rd edn, OHE, 1979) contains information on the costs of the NHS, staffing, hospital services, family practitioner services, mortality and morbidity. This includes particularly clear tables and graphs. Another important title is the OPCS *Classification of Occupations* (HMSO, 1980), not least for its explanation of social classes and socio-economic groups, while *Social Trends 1983* (No 13, HMSO, 1982) gives a great deal of statistical and other information about British society today.

Texts for research workers in the statistical field include:

Statistical Methods in Medical Research by P. Armitage (2nd edn, Blackwell, 1983)
Statistical Methods in Biology by N. T. J. Bailey (2nd edn, Hodder and Stoughton, 1981)
Statistics at Square One by T. D. V. Swinscow (6th edn, British Medical Journal, 1980)

Survey Methods in Community Medicine by J. H. Abramson (2nd edn, Churchill Livingstone, 1979)

Statistics in Operation by W. M. Castle (Churchill Livingstone, 1979)

Short Textbook of Medical Statistics by A. Bradford Hill (Hodder and Stoughton, 1977)

Interpretation and Uses of Medical Statistics by G. J. Bourke and J. McGilvray (2nd edn, Blackwell, 1975)

Statistics in Medicine by T. Colton (Little, Brown, 1974)

A Guide to Medical Mathematics by D. A. Franklin and G. B. Newman (Blackwell, 1973)

Statistical Tables for Biological, Agricultural and Medical Research by R. A. Fisher and F. Yates (6th edn, Oliver and Boyd, 1963)

Congresses

It is estimated that some 10 000 scientific meetings take place each year and that three-quarters of these result in some kind of published record of the papers given. The proceedings of congresses, conferences and symposia are notoriously difficult to trace, and references to them may appear in many forms. Some proceedings are published separately, though not always by the well-known commercial publishers; some appear as supplements to journals or as reports; and individual papers may appear as articles in journals. The British Library Lending Division at Boston Spa, West Yorkshire, aims to acquire conference proceedings on a comprehensive basis, and issues the monthly *Index to Conference Proceedings Received* (1964–), which is arranged by keywords. This cumulates annually, and the 1981 volume gave details of 19 000 conferences in all subject fields. Cumulations for 1964–1973 and 1974–1978 have been published. This file is also available online as the *Conference Proceedings Index*, via the British Library Automated Information Service (BLAISE). The foregoing titles index only the proceedings of a conference as a whole, while the Institute for Scientific Information's *Index to Scientific and Technical Proceedings* (1978–) indexes the individual papers given. This appears monthly, with semi-annual cumulations, and covers some 3000 published proceedings each year, of which it estimated that 35 per cent are in the field of the life sciences and clinical medicine. Some earlier congresses can be traced in W. J. Bishop's *Bibliography of International Congresses of Medical Sciences* (Blackwell, 1958), listing 363 congresses. *Index Medicus* indexed certain selected conference proceedings between 1976 and 1981.

Future meetings are listed by Aslib's *Forthcoming International Scientific and Technical Conferences*, issued quarterly, and the *International Congress Calendar*, published by the Union of

International Associations (Brussels, 1961–). On the medical side are *British Medicine: a Monthly Guide to the Literature* (Pergamon Press, May 1980–, previously The British Council) which includes a list of forthcoming congresses and meetings up to three years ahead; *World Meetings: Medicine,* published quarterly by the World Meetings Information Centre, Chestnut Hill, Mass., US (1978–), covers more than 1000 meetings a year in considerable detail; and the *Calendar of Congresses of Medical Sciences,* issued annually by The Council for International Organizations of Medical Sciences (CIOMS, Geneva), lists meetings up to five years hence. One of the main tasks of the CIOMS since its establishment in 1949 has, indeed, been to assist with the co-ordination of international medical congresses, and to offer advice on their planning and organization. For the US, forthcoming meetings are listed regularly in the *Journal of the American Medical Association,* monthly in the case of home meetings and quarterly for foreign meetings.

Societies

Information on current medical and scientific societies can be obtained from their own handbooks and annual reports, or from more general reference books. The *Medical Directory* and the *American Medical Directory* both contain lists of medical societies, and the *World of Learning* has broader coverage of this material under the heading 'learned societies'. The *Directory of British Associations and Associations in Ireland* (7th edn, C. B. D. Research, 1982) covers some 8500 organizations and is updated every two to three years. It is arranged alphabetically by the name of the association, with subject and abbreviation indexes. Although general in scope it covers a considerable number of medical and scientific societies. The same firm issues the *Directory of European Associations* in two parts: Part 1 covers industrial, trade and professional associations (3rd edn, 1981) and Part 2 covers learned, scientific and technical societies (2nd edn, 1979).

For the US the most comprehensive work is the *Encyclopedia of Associations* (17th edn, 3 vols, Gale, 1983), which lists 16 500 national organizations in all subject fields in some detail. The names, addresses and chief office-holders of medical societies are also listed quarterly in the *Journal of the American Medical Association.* An older source is *Scientific and Learned Societies of the United States,* published by the National Academy of Sciences (9th edn, Washington, 1971), which covers over 500 organizations and gives details of their history and activities.

Current biographical sources

Information on contemporary medical men and women is difficult to acquire except for the brief details of addresses, posts held, qualifications, etc to be found in the *Medical Directory* and equivalent publications for other countries. A few very eminent people have books and issues of journals dedicated in their honour, and are written about on the occasion of their retirement or when awards are bestowed on them. But these are few, as are those who achieve the pages of *Who's Who,* which inevitably contains only a small percentage of medical people. *Who's Who in Science in Europe: a Reference Guide to European Scientists* (3rd edn, 4 vols, Hodgson, 1978) contains over 44 000 entries for the whole of Europe and includes medicine in its coverage. The *Who's Who of British Scientists 1980–81* (3rd edn, Simon Books, 1980) is a revised edition of a work formerly published by Longman, while the *International Medical Who's Who* (2 vols, Longman, 1980) aims to be a biographical guide to those engaged in medical research.

American Men and Women of Science (15th edn, 7 vols, Bowker, 1982) contains entries for 130 000 active US and Canadian scientists in the physical and biological sciences, and cross-references are provided for those listed in previous editions, but not in the current one. This compilation is available as an online database via the Lockheed Dialog information system from early 1983. Historical biographical sources are described in Chapter 22.

5

Mechanized sources of information retrieval

C. Norris

Online information retrieval has become a large and rapidly changing field, and that part of it which relates to biomedical information is no exception. The problems of knowing what is available, which database to choose, the differences between versions of the same database available on different host systems, and the real costs and value-for-money of searching a particular database on a particular host, grow year by year.

Online versus hand searching

When is it appropriate to search by hand, and when is it better to search by computer? A bibliographic search which requires few headings to be scanned and which is intended to produce a small number of citations may be carried out quickly and effectively in an abstract or index journal. However, many searches of this kind are now being done online because the terminal can quickly produce a typed list of citations to take away and use. For more complex questions where several concepts must be linked together, and searches where a large number of citations is required, a machine search is not only quicker and more efficient than hand-searching, but cheaper as well, taking into account the time and salary of the reader.

The ability to scan large numbers of terms, the facility to enlarge or narrow the search in response to the output produced, and the almost instantaneous nature of online searching give great power and flexibility to the searcher. Most databases are updated with new citations several weeks before the corresponding printed issue of the abstract journal is published, so one receives information sooner. In addition, most databases carry information which is not available in the printed version, but which can be searched by computer.

All lists of citations produced by computer searches are liable to contain some irrelevant citations, called 'false drops' or 'noise'. These citations have been correctly retrieved by the computer in response to its given strategy. The indexing headings or search parameters which qualify the citation for retrieval are all present, but the relationship between them is not that implied by the searcher. For example, if I wished to retrieve citations on the brain in liver disease using the three search words 'brain', 'liver' and 'disease' linked by the operator 'AND', I instruct the computer to search for the occurrence of 'brain AND liver AND disease'. This would retrieve citations on 'the brain in liver disease' as I wished, but would also find articles on 'the liver in brain disease' which I would consider as 'noise'. The amount of 'noise' can be reduced by altering the search strategy in various ways to make it more specific. However, there is a trade-off between precision and recall in every search. Relevant citations may be lost in the attempt to increase specificity and most searches aim to achieve a compromise between these two factors.

Choosing a database

A number of general directories of databases and databanks have been published covering all subject fields, including Cuadra Associates *Directory of Online Databases,* updated quarterly, *Directory of Online Information Resources,* updated annually, both American, the *Eusidic Database Guide,* updated annually, *Databases in Europe 1982* from Euronet Diane, and Hall and Brown (1981). The Online Information Centre, 3 Belgrave Square, London SW1X 8PL (Tel: 01-235 1732) was established by Aslib, with support from the British Library Research and Development Department and the Department of Industry, to give practical advice on all aspects of online searching. The Centre publishes a series of guides, including a *Medical Databases* (1983), a guide to accessing bibliographic databases, which includes information about the costs of equipment and searching as well as the staff implications of online retrieval. It also includes an appendix giving the addresses of the major online vendors and telecommunications network suppliers.

The two major biomedical databases are MEDLINE and EXCERPTA MEDICA. Both databases add around 250 000 citations to their files each year and both claim to give reasonably comprehensive coverage of the literature of biomedicine. Surprisingly, the amount of overlap is only around 40 per cent in most searches due to the particular journals covered and the selection policies of the database producers. EXCERPTA MEDICA scans many journals and adds citations selectively from them, whereas MEDLINE coverage of articles in its journals is comprehensive, although the list itself is smaller. EXCERPTA MEDICA has a bias towards the pharmaceutical and environmental health literature. MEDLINE includes dentistry, nursing and veterinary medicine in its biomedical coverage, whereas those topics are generally excluded by EXCERPTA MEDICA. MEDLINE is cheaper, more widely available and more extensively used than EXCERPTA MEDICA. A more detailed account of each database is given below.

Many smaller databases exist covering specialized subject fields or types of material. Medical ethics is served by BIOETHICS, oncology by CANCERLIT, CANCERPROJ and CLINPROT, health planning and administration by HEALTH, medical history by HISTLINE and toxicology by RTECS, TDB and TOXLINE. EPILEPSYLINE covers epilepsy and NIMH the field of mental health. PSYCINFO covers the literature of psychology, POPLINE the area of population, family planning and contraception, while INTERNATIONAL PHARMACEUTICAL ABSTRACTS, and PHARMACEUTICAL NEWS INDEX provide information about pharmaceuticals.

Special types of material are covered by the files AVLINE (audiovisual materials on health care and medicine) and CATLINE (books on medicine and related areas). These and other files are discussed in more detail below.

MEDLINE (MEDLARS)

The world's first computerized database was MEDLARS (MEDical Literature Analysis and Retrieval System) which was started in mid-1963. The database is derived as a by-product of the compilation of *Index Medicus*, the *Index to Dental Literature* and the *Inter-*

national Nursing Index. The online files of the database are called MEDLINE (MEDlars onLINE). The term MEDLARS is sometimes used to cover the family of databases produced by the US National Library of Medicine (NLM).

Coverage

MEDLARS covers the whole field of biomedicine from 1964 onwards, although most sources offer the files from 1966 onwards only. 3200 journals published in over 70 countries are indexed for the database, amounting to 250 000 citations each year, the total file size being over four million citations. The *List of Serials and Monographs Indexed for Online Users,* published annually, gives bibliographic information about journals indexed for MEDLINE, HEALTH and POPLINE and indicates those which are selectively indexed to include only articles of medical interest – for example, *Nature.*

Substantive editorials, letters, biographies and obituaries are indexed in addition to articles. Short abstracts of society proceedings are no longer taken, although full length papers of proceedings continue to be indexed.

Major clinical journals receive priority treatment and are indexed with an average of eight to ten descriptors per article. Experimental and preclinical journals are indexed in similar detail, but articles from the more practical clinical and paramedical journals are indexed in less depth with an average of four to five descriptors. However, each article is treated on its merits, and up to 25 descriptors are permitted. Of the descriptors used for indexing, only three on average are used as headings to cite the article in *Index Medicus.* These correspond to the main point of the article. The remaining descriptors covering minor points and experimental details are available only on the MEDLARS files. Since 1975 author abstracts have been added to the records of the MEDLARS files and these are available for direct textword searching. Over 40 per cent of records now have abstracts added, with an upper limit of 250 words per abstract.

MeSH

The descriptors used in indexing are taken from *MeSH (Medical Subject Headings),* which is published in revised form each year. *Medical Subject Headings – Annotated Alphabetic List (Annotated MeSH)* is a thesaurus of the 14 500 descriptors used in indexing with individual terms annotated with information and instructions for indexing and searching. The alphabetical listing includes many cross-references from synonyms and related headings. *MeSH Tree Structures* is an arrangement of the headings into subject categories, A – anatomical terms, B – organisms, C – diseases, and so on, each category being subdivided and having an hierarchical arrangement of the headings into 'trees'. *Figure 5.1* gives part of the tree for category C4 – diseases–neoplasms. Up to seven levels of specificity of headings are available in the trees.

Individual headings can be in more than one category, and can have different relations and arrangements in different categories. Since indexing is done using the most specific term available for a concept, with no posting-on of entries to higher levels, the trees are important in tracing the relationships of headings and are used extensively in searching for groups of related headings in MEDLARS.

Permuted MeSH is a keyword out-of-context index to *MeSH*, often found useful by searchers.

Annotated MeSH contains minor descriptors, geographical headings and check tags. Check tags include such concepts as age groups of patients, common experimental animals, types of study such as case reports and *in vitro* experiments, and types of article, for example, historical articles. These are minor concepts looked for routinely in indexing, preprinted on the indexing data form and checked automatically. These three types of headings are available only for searching on the MEDLARS files and never appear in *Index Medicus*.

Qualifiers

A total of 76 qualifiers or subheadings are available to modify *MeSH* headings and minor descriptors. *Annotated MeSH* lists the qualifiers with definitions of their usage and indicates the subject categories of headings to which, broadly speaking, each can be applied. Individual headings in *MeSH* are annotated with specific limitations to the use of qualifiers. The qualifiers were introduced to break up the list of citations under each main heading in *Index Medicus* into convenient groups for reading. They can also be used in searching, either tied to descriptors for specificity or used free floating to give blanket retrieval of all headings modified by the particular qualifier.

Co-ordination of headings

The most common form of co-ordination in MEDLARS is the

combination of a *MeSH* heading with a qualifier. For example 'X-ray diagnosis of osteoporosis' indexed as OSTEOPOROSIS/radiography, and 'metabolism of iron' by IRON/metabolism. The combination is physically linked when co-ordinated in this way. Sometimes no suitable qualifier is available to modify the heading, and two separate headings are used; for example, 'biophysics of the hip joint' indexed by BIOPHYSICS and HIP JOINT. Qualifiers are restricted to particular categories of headings and it may not be possible to use a combination. For example, PREGNANCY is in category G8, but the qualifier 'blood' is available only to categories B2, C, D, and F3, so 'serum levels of iron in pregnancy' is indexed as PREGNANCY (no qualifier) and IRON/blood.

MeSH contains a very large number of pre-co-ordinated headings, which are always used in preference to other forms of co-ordination. For example, LIVER DISEASES is used in preference to LIVER and DISEASE; LEAD POISONING in preference to LEAD and POISONING or LEAD/poisoning. The annotations in *Annotated MeSH* indicate forbidden combinations of headings and qualifiers and give directions to the appropriate pre-co-ordinated headings.

Missing concepts

Although *MeSH* headings are available for the majority of required concepts, it is sometimes necessary to use combinations of headings when the exact required term is not available, or to use the next most general heading to cover a specific. For example, the bacterium *Moraxella liquefaciens* is indexed by the broader heading MORAXELLA. The specific bacterium can, of course, be retrieved by searching a combination of the *MeSH* heading MORAXELLA with the textword 'liquefaciens' if this is required.

Drugs and chemicals pose a particular problem due to the sheer number of compounds mentioned in the literature. The *Supplementary Chemical Records* file maintained by the National Library of Medicine has entries for all chemicals that have appeared in the literature indexed for MEDLARS, with indexing and mapping instructions. The file is maintained online for internal use and a new edition of the printed version became available to outside users in 1983.

MEDLARS in the UK

From 1966, when the UK MEDLARS Service began, until 1974

C4 – DISEASES–NEOPLASMS

NEOPLASMS	C4		
APUDOMA	C4.70		
CHORISTOMA	C4.131		
CYSTS	C4.182		
BONE CYSTS	C4.182.89	C4.557.499.	C5116.70
JAW CYSTS	C4.182.89.530	C5.500.470.	
NONODONTOGENIC CYSTS	C4.182.89.530.660	C5.500.470.	
ODONTOGENIC CYSTS	C4.182.89.530.690	C5.500.470.	
BASAL CELL NEVUS SYNDROME*	C4.182.89.530.690.150	C4.557.117.	C16.131.77.
DENTIGEROUS CYST	C4.182.89.530.690.310	C5.500.470.	
PERIODONTAL CYST	C4.182.89.530.690.790	C7.465.714.	
RADICULAR CYST	C4.182.89.530.690.790.820	C7.465.690.	
BRANCHIOMA	C4.182.117		
DERMOID CYST	C4.182.201	C4.557.537.	
EPIDERMAL CYST	C4.182.254		
ESOPHAGEAL CYST	C4.182.281	C6.306.316	
FIBROCYSTIC DISEASE OF BREAST*	C4.182.289	C19.146.378	
KIDNEY, CYSTIC	C4.182.394	C12.777.419.	
KIDNEY, POLYCYSTIC	C4.182.394.420	C12.777.419.	
KIDNEY, SPONGE	C4.182.394.586	C12.777.419.	
MEDIASTINAL CYST	C4.182.444	C23.304.612.	
MESENTERIC CYST	C4.182.473	C6.772.420	
MUCOCELE	C4.182.511		
OVARIAN CYSTS	C4.182.612		C16.131.939.
CORPUS LUTEUM CYST	C4.182.612.278	C13.371.56.	
STEIN–LEVENTHAL SYNDROME	C4.182.612.765	C13.371.56.	
PANCREATIC CYST	C4.182.640	C6.689.500	
PANCREATIC PSEUDOCYST*	C4.182.640.692	C6.689.500.	
PAROVARIAN CYST	C4.182.668	C13.371.56.	
PILONIDAL CYST	C4.182.710		
RANULA	C4.182.766	C7.465.780	
SEBACEOUS CYST	C4.182.811	C17.805.711.	
SYNOVIAL CYST	C4.182.867		
THYROGLOSSAL CYST	C4.182.902		

URACHAL CYST	C4.182.946			
NEOPLASM REGRESSION, SPONTANEOUS	C4.495			
NEOPLASMS BY HISTOLOGIC TYPE (NON MESH)	C4.557	C4.805.670		
CARCINOID TUMOR	C4.557.112			
MALIGNANT CARCINOID SYNDROME	C4.557.112.524			
CARCINOID HEART DISEASE*	C4.557.112.524.329	C14.280.129		
CARCINOMA	C4.557.117			
CARCINOMA 256, WALKER	C4.557.117.45			
CARCINOMA, BASAL CELL	C4.557.117.110	C4.619.45		
BASAL CELL NEVUS SYNDROME*	C4.557.117.110.150	C4.182.89	C5.500.470	C16.131.77
CARCINOMA, BASOSQUAMOUS	C4.557.117.141			
CARCINOMA, BROWN–PEARCE	C4.557.117.172			
CARCINOMA, DUCTAL	C4.557.117.234	C4.619.124		
PAGET'S DISEASE, EXTRA-MAMMARY	C4.557.117.234.500			
PAGET'S DISEASE OF BREAST*	C4.557.117.234.666			
CARCINOMA, EHRLICH TUMOR	C4.557.117.265			
CARCINOMA IN SITU	C4.557.117.327	C4.619.169		
CARCINOMA, KREBS 2	C4.557.117.358			
CARCINOMA, MUCINOUS	C4.557.117.390			
KRUKENBERG'S TUMOR	C4.557.117.390.500	C4.619.214	C4.557.576.	C4.588.322.
CARCINOMA, OAT CELL	C4.557.117.421	C4.557.576.	C13.371.56.	C4.588.945.
CARCINOMA, PAPILLARY	C4.557.117.452			
CARCINOMA, SCIRRHOUS	C4.557.117.483			
LINITIS PLASTICA*	C4.557.117.483.515			
CARCINOMA, SQUAMOUS CELL	C4.557.117.490			
BOWEN'S DISEASE*	C4.557.117.490.318			
CARCINOMA, TRANSITIONAL CELL	C4.557.117.514			
LEUKEMIA	C4.557.337	C4.619.531		
LEUKEMIA, EXPERIMENTAL	C4.557.372			

Figure 5.1 Part of the MeSH tree structure. * Indicates minor descriptor

MEDLARS searches in the UK were processed offline in weekly batches. The first experimental online system, AIM-TWX *(Abridged Index Medicus* via the Teletypewriter Exchange Network) was developed by the NLM in the US and was inaugurated in June 1970. The system developed from AIM-TWX was MEDLINE, which became operational in October 1971 to a limited number of users in the US. The system was greatly enlarged by the use of the Tymshare Inc. network of data transmission lines from over 50 'node' cities in the US and Europe. MEDLINE via the Tymshare network was used by a limited number of British users from 1974 until BLAISE (The British Library Automated Information Service) became operational in April 1977. BLAISE was the first UK-based online retrieval service of any size and used the Elhill software developed specifically for MEDLINE. A number of other databases from the MEDLARS family were gradually added to BLAISE, as well as UK MARC, LC MARC and other files.

Up until January 1982, BLAISE had enjoyed monopoly rights to provide MEDLARS services within the UK free from outside competition, similar to the rights enjoyed by other national MEDLARS Centres in Europe and elsewhere. When the monopoly was ended in January 1982, MEDLINE became available from a choice of vendors. The MEDLARS files were dismounted and replaced by the BLAISE-LINK service which provides access to the NLM databases in Washington, US, via the telecommunication networks. BLAISE-LINK came into operation in July 1982.

Users now have a choice of vendors of MEDLINE and some other services. Unfortunately, the command languages of different vendors and the software used for retrieval are not identical.

Online searching

Online searches take place in the form of an interactive dialogue between the searcher and the computer program. However, it is wise to consider what kind of citations one wishes to retrieve, and to do preparatory work and planning before going online. Time spent in preparation can save frustration and anxiety at the terminal as well as expensive online time. *Figure 5.2* shows part of a MEDLINE search on 'mental disorders due to surgery' performed on Elhill software. Depending on experience, new or experienced user format may be used for searching. New user format gives explanations of the facilities available and the meanings of commands. For the sake of brevity, the example is given in experienced user format, with annotations.

Figure 5.2 Part of a MEDLINE search

HELLO FROM ELHILL AT NLM.
YOU ARE NOW CONNECTED TO THE MEDLINE FILE.

SS 1 /C?   (Program: Give search statement 1 or
                                  command)

USER: (User: Pre-explosion of surgery,
SURGERY, OPERATIVE (PX)   operative (all subsidiary terms) and the
AND AE   qualifier 'adverse effects')

PROG: (Program: SS1 has postings for 7121
SS (1) PSTG (7121)   citations)

SS 2 /C?

USER:
EXP C23.814   (User: Explode 'postoperative
                                  complications' C23.814)

PROG: (Program: SS2 has 11570 postings)
SS (2) PSTG (11570)

SS 3 /C?

USER: (User: Adverse effects of surgery or
1 OR 2   postoperative complications)

PROG: (Program: Total postings 17293)
SS (3) PSTG (17293)

SS4 /C?

USER: (User: Pre-explosion of mental
MENTAL DISORDERS (PX) AND   disorders with the qualifier 'etiology')
ET

PROG:
SS (4) PSTG (3695)

SS 5 /C?

USER: (User: Surgery causing mental
3 AND 4   disorders)

PROG: (Program: 162 postings)
SS (5) PSTG (162)

(cont.)

SS 6 /C?

USER: TS (LA) ENG	(User: Stringsearch for citations in English)
PROG: (148) SCHD (108) QUAL;CONT? (Y/N)	(Program: 148 of the citations have been scanned so far, 108 qualify: – shall I continue?)
USER: Y	
PROG: SS (6) PSTG (116)	(Program: 116 citations found)

SS 7 /C?

| USER: PRT 5 | (User: Print 5 citations in standard format) |

| PROG:
1
AU – McGuinness BW
TI – The health of sterilized women.
SO – Practitioner 1982 May;
      226 (1367):925–8
2
AU – Gath D
AU – Cooper P
AU – Bond A
AU – Edmonds G
TI – Hysterectomy and psychiatric disorder: II Demographic psychiatric and physical factors in relation to psychiatric outcome.
SO – Br J Psychiatry 1982 Apr; 140:343–50 | (The citations are listed showing authors, title and source) |

SS 7 /C?

| USER:
SUBS APPLY PX | (In the light of these citations the user decides to look at a related area: psychological aspects of gynaecological surgery)
(apply the qualifier 'psychology' to all subsequent headings) |

PROG:
SUBHEADINGS ACCEPTED

(*cont.*)

SS 7 /C?

USER:	(User: psychological aspects of these
MASTECTOMY OR HYSTEREC-	headings)
TOMY OR STERILIZATION, TUBAL	

PROG:
SS (7) PSTG (150)

SS 8 /C?

USER: (User lists ten citations by title only)
PRT TI 10

PROG:
1
TI   – The role of support in relation to recovery from breast surgery.
2
TI   – Differences in crisis reactions among cancer and surgery patients.
3
TI   – [Subjective feelings during the stress provoked by hysterectomy (author's
         transl)].
etc

Textwords from the titles and abstracts of citations may be used for retrieval in MEDLARS as well as *MeSH* headings, categories and sub-categories of headings from the trees. The text of titles and abstracts is held in inverted form, so that text searching is independent of the *MeSH* headings.

Sources for MEDLINE

BLAISE-LINK

Five online files give access to all records from 1966 to date. MEDLINE covers the years 1980 to the present; B77 (MED77), 1977–1979; B75 (MED75), 1975–1976; B71 (MED71), 1971–1974; and B66 (MED66), 1966–1970. The current month is also available as a separate online file SDILINE. BLAISE-LINK provides access to the NLM computer in the US and is not available to users outside the UK and Eire.

BRS

The database is called MEDLARS on BRS. 1975 to the present is available as online files and 1966–1974 as offline files.

DATA-STAR

Four online files are available covering the years 1979 to date, 1975–1978, 1971–1974 and 1966–1970. The latest month is also available as a separate file.

DIALOG

Three online files give access to all records from 1966. File 152 (1966–1974), File 153 (1975–1979) and File 154 (1980 to date, updated monthly).

DIMDI

The database is referred to as MEDLARS. Access back to 1964 is available. 1978 to date is available online, 1966–1977 is processed offline, and Backfile 64–65 is searchable online at particular times.

MIC-KIBIC

1977 to the present is available online and 1966–1976 as offline files.

NLM

For NLM services in the UK and Eire, *see* BLAISE-LINK. File details are as given there.

MeSH VOCABULARY FILE

MeSH Vocabulary File is available as a separate online file on BLAISE-LINK and DIMDI.

EXCERPTA MEDICA (EMBASE)

The computer database which is used for the production of the Excerpta Medica's 43 English-language abstract journals and two drug-related literature indexes covers the whole field of biomedicine apart from nursing, psychology, dentistry, veterinary medicine and the paramedical fields.

Coverage

A total of 3500 biomedical journals are screened for the abstract journals. In addition, 1500 journals are screened for the Environmental Health Section by abstracters in the Royal Netherlands Academy of Arts and Sciences, the Agricultural Institute, Wageningen, and the Technological University, Delft. From this material, approximately 250 000 articles each year are selected for indexing, and of these some 150 000 are abstracted for the individual abstract bulletins. Around 60 000 indexed citations a year are listed in the *Drug Literature Index*, which is a published partial version of the file available as the DRUGDOC service.

As well as original articles, Excerpta Medica also covers editorials, conference proceedings and letters to the editor, where these are substantive. The indexing and abstracting is undertaken by around 100 specialist physicians. A series of editorial boards consisting of some 400 leading scientists and physicians from 43 countries advise on editorial policy.

EMCLASS

Each abstract journal covers a particular subject field. The abstracts in each journal are arranged by a detailed classification scheme designed to give roughly equal numbers of citations under each subdivision. The classifications can go to a depth of four decimal subdivisions, and are often based on anatomical aspects of the subject, or, in the case of the Drug Literature Service, on pharmacological activities. The combined classification of all the abstract journals is known as the Excerpta Medica CLASSification System (EMCLASS) and consists of 3500 polyhierarchical categories which cover the whole medical literature. The classification is flexible in that new categories may be added at any time. Part of the classification scheme for the abstract journal covering Anatomy, Anthropology, Embryology and Histology is given in *Figure 5.3*.

Up to ten different classification numbers can be assigned to each article within each abstract journal. Articles overlapping into more than one subject field are included in all the appropriate abstract journals. The classification numbers may be used as search parameters and are highly effective for searches where the classification scheme corresponds to some aspect of the search.

Indexing

Indexing is done at two levels. The more important concepts are put into the computer using a controlled thesaurus of terms, called MALIMET (MAster LIst of MEdical indexing Terms). On

Anatomy, Anthropology, Embryology and Histology

1. GENERAL ASPECTS
   1.1. History, philosophy
   1.2. Biometrics
2. ANATOMY
   2.1. Descriptive anatomy
      2.1.1. Technique and apparatus
      2.2.2. Osteology
      2.1.3. Syndesmology
      2.1.4. Myology
      2.1.5. Digestive system
      2.1.6. Respiratory system
      2.1.7. Urogenital system
      2.1.8. Peritoneum
      2.1.9. Endocrine system
      2.1.10. Cardiovascular system
      2.1.11. Nervous system
      2.1.12. Sense organs
      2.1.13. Integument
      2.1.14. Lymphatic system
   2.2 Functional and experimental anatomy
      2.2.1. Skeleton
      2.2.2. Locomotion
      2.2.3. Digestion and excretion
      2.2.4. Circulation and respiration
      2.2.5. Nervous system and sense organs
3. ANTHROPOLOGY
   3.1. Technique and apparatus
   3.2. Phylogeny, paleontology
   3.3. Evolution
   3.4. Variability
   3.5. Heredity of normal features
   3.6. Body build and body composition
   3.7. Ecologic factors and adaption
4. HISTOLOGY
   4.1. Technique and apparatus
      4.1.1. Fixation
      4.1.2. . . . . . .

5. MICROSCOPIC STRUCTURE OF VERTEBRATES
   5.1. Sense organs
      5.1.1. Eye
      5.1.2. Ear
      5.1.3. Lateral line system
      5.1.4. Olfactory organ
      5.1.5. Taste buds
   5.2. Peripheral nervous system
      5.2.1. Nerves and ganglia
      5.2.2. Nerve terminations
   5.3. Central nervous system
      5.3.1. Brain
      5.3.2. Spinal cord
      5.3.3. Tracts
      5.3.4. Meninges
   5.4. Neuroendocrine system
   5.5. Endocrine glands
      5.5.1. Adenohypophysis
      5.5.2. Thyroid
      5.5.3. Parathyroid
      5.5.4. Endocrine pancreas
      5.5.5. Adrenal cortex
      5.5.6. Adrenal medulla
      5.5.7. Paraganglia
   5.6. Digestive system
      5.6.1. Teeth
      5.6.2. Tongue and oral mucosa
      5.6.3. Pharynx
      5.6.4. Alimentary canal
      5.6.5. Salivary glands
      5.6.6. Liver, biliary system
      5.6.7. Exocrine pancreas
      5.6.8. Mesentery, peritoneum
   5.7. Respiratory system
      5.7.1. Nasal cavity, nasopharynx
      5.7.2. Larynx
      5.7.3. Trachea, bronchi
      5.7.4. Lung
      5.7.5. . . . . . .

Figure 5.3 Part of EMCLASS

average, eight primary terms are assigned to each article and a maximum of 50 are allowed for each record. A number of secondary indexing terms are also added without the use of the thesaurus, including the species of experimental animal and detailed descriptors. A third group of concepts, EMTAGS, is available only on the computer tapes. This is used for recording 200 routine concepts such as sex, age, different types of studies, common experimental animals and routes of drug administration. Up to 25 item index numbers may be used for each article.

MALIMET

The thesaurus MALIMET is a computer file that forms part of the database. The indexer is free to assign concepts from each article in the form in which they appear. The terms and phrases are fed into the computer in their original form, where they are checked against MALIMET. The entry vocabulary consists of 200 000 primary terms, including more than 40 000 drugs and chemicals together with 275 000 synonyms. Synonyms are automatically converted into the preferred term by the MALIMET program. There are also some limited cross- references between related terms and from broad terms to more specific terms, but the thesaurus has no further hierarchical structure built into it.

If the MALIMET program does not recognize an indexing term, it is printed on an 'error list' which is examined by the thesaurus committee of the editorial department. After correcting typographical errors, the terms on the error list are entered into MALIMET either as valid, new preferred terms or as new synonyms of existing preferred terms. At present few terms other than drug names are being added as preferred terms. Synonyms are added at a much more significant rate.

MALIMET is published in microfiche form, a new version being produced several times each year as *MALIMET, EMCLASS and EMTAGS on Microfiche*.

Sources for EXCERPTA MEDICA (EMBASE)

BRS

A service providing the most recent three years' records online is planned for the early part of 1983.

DATA-STAR

Files containing records from 1977 to date are available online.

DIALOG

Excerpta Medica records are held on three online files. File 172 contains 1 200 000 records entered from June 1974 to December

1979; File 72 contains records entered from 1980 to date and is updated every two months. File 73 is an in-process file, updated monthly. Both File 72 and File 73 should be accessed for current information.

DIMDI

The files are known as EMBASE on DIMDI. Records are held from 1973 onwards, with the current file updated monthly. All records placed on the current file are updated there, if necessary, as processing is completed by Excerpta Medica.

Databases for special areas

ALCOHOL USE/ABUSE

See DRUGINFO/ALCOHOL USE/ABUSE

ARZ-DB

Arzneimittel und Wirkstoffe databank covers drugs and active ingredients of drugs. Access is planned to be available through DIMDI.

AVLINE

AVLINE contains bibliographic records of all types of audiovisual materials in the field of medicine and health care, including dentistry and nursing. The file is produced by the National Library of Medicine and covers the period 1976 to date. It is updated weekly, and the present file size approaches 11 000 records. Reviews and critical assessments (abstracts) are given on most records. The file may be searched for type of media or for specific running time, as well as the more usual bibliographic features. Both textwords and *MeSH* headings are available for subject searching.

AVLINE is available online through BLAISE-LINK (UK and Eire only) and NLM (US).

BIOETHICS

The BIOETHICS file contains bibliographic information on medical ethics and public policy in the areas of health care and biomedical research, including abortion, euthanasia, genetic intervention and organ transplantation. The file is produced from a variety of sources, including MEDLINE and CATLINE, by the National

Library of Medicine and the Kennedy Institute of Ethics. It includes newspaper articles, US Court decisions and legislation. Abstracts are not available. The file contains 11 000 records from 1973 to date and is updated every four months. Subject searching using textwords, *MeSH* headings and a special Bioethics thesaurus is available.

BIOETHICS is available online through BLAISE-LINK (UK and Eire only) and NLM (US).

CANCERLINE

See the individual files: CANCERLIT, CANCERPROJ and CLINPROT.

CANCERLIT

CANCER LITerature is a bibliographic file produced by the US National Cancer Institute. It covers all aspects of cancer research from 3000 journals together with reports, monographs, conference proceedings and theses from 1963 onwards. The file contains over 250 000 records and is updated monthly. All records carry abstracts, and from 1980 onwards all records have been indexed with *MeSH* headings. Earlier years must be searched by means of textwords. *Figure 5.4* gives an example of a CANCERLIT search.

CANCERLIT is available online through BLAISE-LINK (UK and Eire only), DIMDI, MIC-KIBIC and NLM (US).

Figure 5.4 A CANCERLIT search using textwords

FILE CANCERLIT

PROG:
YOU ARE NOW CONNECTED TO THE CANCERLINE FILE.

SS 1 /C?

USER:
ALL NITRATE: (TW) AND ALL FERTILIZER: (TW) OR AMMONIUM (TW) AND NITRATE (TW)

PROG:
SS (1) PSTG (39)

SS 2 /C?

USER:
PRT COMPR   *(cont.)*

PROG:
1
AU – Armijo R; Detels R; Coulson AH; Medina E; Orellana M; Gonzales A
TI – EPIDEMIOLOGY OF GASTRIC CANCER IN CHILE.
SI – ICDB/81/28532
SO – Rev Med Chil; 109(6): 551–556 1981
2
AU – Zaldivar R
TI – A NOTE ON THE USE OF NITRATE FERTILIZERS IN A HIGH-
       RISK GEOGRAPHICAL AREA FOR STOMACH CANCER.
SI – CARC/79/00065
SO – Z Krebsforsch; 92(2): 215–216 1978
etc.

CANCERNET

Literature on cancer and related medical research in biochemistry, virology and immunology from 1968 to date, and updated monthly. The system is in the French language and is available through Telesystemes-Questel.

CANCERPROJ

CANCER Research PROJects (CANCERPROJ) is a file of research projects in progress and from the two preceding years, provided by researchers from over fifty countries through the Smithsonian Science Information Exchange (SSIE). The file is compiled by the National Cancer Institute and contains over

Figure 5.5 A CANCERPROJ record

1
TI – GASTRIC CANCER AND NITRATE INGESTION – nitrate in drinking
       water
IR – Fraser PM
IR – Chilvers CE
IR – Hill MJ
AD – London School of Hygiene and Tropical Medicine; Dept. of Medical
       Statistics and Epidemiology; Keppel St., Gower St., London WC1E 7HT,
       United Kingdom (principal investigator's preferred address)
AB – Evidence is accumulating that populations ingesting large amounts of nitrate
       have a high mortality from cancer, particularly of the stomach, due to the
       formation *in vivo* of carcinogenic nitrosamines. Nitrate levels in some water
       sources in the eastern regions of England are rising steadily due to increasing
       use of fertilizer and changes in farming practice. Mortality from gastric
       cancer within these regions in 1969–1978 is being examined in relation to the
       nitrate concentration in drinking water 15 to 20 years previously, to establish
       whether there is an increase risk of gastric cancer in populations exposed to
       moderately high levels.
ID – 01106
YI – 7700
Y2 – 8100

20 000 entries. It is updated quarterly. Subject searching is by means of textwords and by subject captions and hierarchical subject codes from the SSIE thesaurus. Part of a CANCERPROJ record is shown in *Figure 5.5*.

CANCERPROJ is available online through BLAISE-LINK (UK and Eire only), DIMDI and NLM (US).

CATLINE

The National Library of Medicine CATalogue onLINE (CAT-LINE) contains records of almost 400 000 monographs and first issues of periodicals published since 1801. The file covers medicine, health care, nursing and dentistry in all languages. Coverage from 1965 onwards is comprehensive and records of earlier material are at present being converted and added to the online catalogue. Subject searching of the file may be carried out by means of textwords, keywords, *MeSH* headings or NLM classmarks. The records are updated weekly.

CATLINE can be accessed online through BLAISE-LINK (UK and Eire only) and NLM (US).

CHEMLINE

CHEMLINE is the National Library of Medicine chemical dictionary file often used in conjunction with RTECS and TOXLINE. It contains records for over 526 000 compounds with more than one million synonyms.

Access is through BLAISE-LINK (UK and Eire only), DIMDI and NLM (US).

CHILD ABUSE AND NEGLECT

CHILD ABUSE AND NEGLECT covers the period 1965 to date for English-language material only. Three subfiles cover ongoing research project descriptions and preventive programs in the US as well as bibliographic references. The file contains over 10 000 records and is updated half-yearly.

The file is produced by the US National Center for Child Abuse and Neglect and is available through DIALOG (File 64).

CIS-BIT

The Safety and Occupational Health database produced by the Centre International d'Informations de Securité et d'Hygiène du Travail (International Labour Organization) covers literature from 1974 to date. It is updated seven times per year and French and English-language versions are available. The English version has translated titles, indexing terms and abstracts. CIS-BIT is available through SPIDEL.

CLINPROT

CLINical PROTocols contains summaries of current clinical investigations of new anti-cancer agents and treatment protocols. Summaries of over 2000 current investigations are available, including data on clinical trials, patient entry criteria, therapeutic regimens and areas of special study. Investigators' names, addresses and supporting agencies are included together with a detailed abstract. The file is produced by the National Cancer Institute and is updated quarterly.

Online access is available through BLAISE-LINK (UK and Eire only), DIMDI, MIC-KIBIC and NLM (US).

DRUGINFO/ALCOHOL USE/ABUSE

This file covers psychological and educational aspects of drug and alcohol abuse from 1969 to date and contains 17 000 bibliographical records with abstracts and keywords. It is updated quarterly and is available through BRS.

DZF

The DZF database covers the field of biomedical engineering, engineering and optics from 1977 to date. German and English versions are available, and the file is updated monthly. The host is Fiz-Technic.

EMBASE

See EXCERPTA MEDICA.

EPILEPSYLINE

EPILEPSY onLINE contains 36 000 references and abstracts to articles on epilepsy that have been abstracted by Excerpta Medica under the sponsorship of the US National Institute of Neurological and Communicative Disorders and Stroke. The file contains references from 1945 to date.

EPILEPSYLINE is available through BRS.

HEALTH

Non-clinical aspects of health care are the field of HEALTH (Health Planning and Administration) including health facilities, health insurance, financial management and personnel administration. The file includes over 200 000 citations from 1975 to date derived from MEDLINE and 300 selectively indexed health administration journals. The file is produced by NLM in co-operation with the American Hospital Association and the Health Resources Administration, and has a structure and search capabilities similar to MEDLINE.

HEALTH is available online through BLAISE-LINK (UK and Eire only), BRS, DIALOG, MIC-KIBIC, DIMDI and NLM (US).

HISTLINE

HISTLINE (HISTory of medicine onLINE) contains over 50 000 citations to articles, monographs and symposia on the history of medicine from 1970 to date. The database is the source of *Bibliography of the History of Medicine*, published annually by NLM. The file is updated quarterly. Subject searching is available by textwords or keywords (75 per cent of keywords are *MeSH* headings), and searches can be limited to particular historical periods or geographic areas.

HISTLINE is available through BLAISE-LINK (UK and Eire only) and NLM (US).

HSELINE

The bibliographic database compiled by the Health and Safety Executive of the Department of Employment, UK, is called HSE-LINE. It covers articles, conference papers, legislation and patents relating to occupational health and safety.

HSELINE is available through ESA-IRS.

INTERNATIONAL PHARMACEUTICAL ABSTRACTS (IPA)

IPA contains over 62 000 citations from more than 500 pharmaceutical, medical and related journals from 1970 to date. The file contains information on all phases of the development of drugs and their clinical use. Abstracts of clinical studies include detailed information on the design, patients and dosage parameters of the studies. The file is updated every two months.

IPA is available through DIALOG (File 74).

ISI/BIOMED

The Institute for Scientific Information file of biomedical information (ISI/BIOMED) contains citations indexed from 1300 biomedical journals from 1979 to date. Searches are available using words from article titles, source journals, cited papers and by 2700 research front specialty codes.

ISI/BIOMED is available through ISI and DIMDI.

MEDIC

The Central Medical Library, Helsinki, Finland mounts a file of around 7500 citations to approximately 100 Finnish medical publications not included in the international databases. Searching can be done using *MeSH* headings. The file covers the period 1978 to date and is updated quarterly. Access is direct to the Central Medical Library via SCANNET.

MEDOC

MEdical DOCuments (MEDOC) covers US government documents in the field of health sciences from 1975 to date and contains over 8000 records. The file is updated quarterly and is produced by the Eccles Health Sciences Library, University of Utah, using *MeSH* headings as descriptors.

MEDOC is available through BRS.

MENTAL HEALTH ABSTRACTS

See NIMH.

MeSH

MeSH Vocabulary File is available through BLAISE-LINK (UK and Eire), DIMDI and NLM. *See* MEDLINE for fuller details.

NARIC

Rehabilitation literature from 1956 to date is covered by NARIC. The file contains over 7000 citations, and is produced by the US National Rehabilitation Information Center. The file is available through BRS.

NIMH

NIMH (MENTAL HEALTH ABSTRACTS) is compiled by the US National Institute of Mental Health from 12 000 journals, as well as books, technical reports and conference proceedings, on mental health and psychology. The file covers from 1969 to date and contains over 400 000 citations. It is updated monthly.

NIMH is available through BRS, DATA-STAR and DIALOG (File 86).

PDQ

PDQ (Protocol Data Query) contains descriptions of approximately 700 cancer therapy research protocols, listing the institutions where the protocol is in use for treatment of patients. The database is closely related to the CLINPROT file and was developed by the National Cancer Institute. At present use of the file is limited to users in the US through NLM, although it may become more widely available later.

PHARMACEUTICAL NEWS INDEX

PHARMACEUTICAL NEWS INDEX, produced by Data Courier, Inc., provides current news about pharmaceuticals, cosmetics and medical devices from *SCRIP World Pharmaceutical News, FDC Reports, Drug Research Reports, Medical Devices, Diagnostics and Instrumentation Reports, Weekly Pharmacy Reports* and *Quality Control Reports*. Business information, legislation, regulations and court decisions are included as well as research grant applications and news items. The file includes information from December 1975 to date.

PHARMACEUTICAL NEWS INDEX is available through DIALOG (File 42).

POPLINE

POPulation information onLINE (POPLINE) is a bibliographic file covering population, family planning, fertility and contraception and is produced by NLM in co-operation with the Population Information Program of John Hopkins University and the Centre for Population and Family Health of Columbia University. It includes family planning programs and related legislation and policy issues. Types of material covered include journal and newspaper articles, books, technical reports and unpublished reports. Of the citations 90 per cent have abstracts and the file has comprehensive coverage of the period from 1970 to date. Some earlier material is also included. The file contains 100 000 citations and is updated monthly. Keywords taken from the POPLINE thesaurus may be used for subject searching, as well as *MeSH* headings without qualifiers.

POPLINE is available through BLAISE-LINK (UK and Eire only) and NLM (US).

PRE-MED

PRE-MED covers current clinical literature from 108 core journals and includes nursing, psychiatry and hospital literature. The file is available through BRS and DATA-STAR.

PSYCINFO

PSYCINFO, formerly PSYCHOLOGICAL ABSTRACTS, covers the field of psychology. Over 900 journals, as well as conference proceedings, books and technical reports, are scanned. The file covers the period 1967 to date and contains over 334 000 citations. It is produced by the American Psychological Association and is updated monthly.

PSYCINFO is available through BRS, DIALOG (File 11), DATA-STAR (as PSYCHOLOGICAL ABSTRACTS), DIMDI and SDC.

RTECS

The Registry of Toxic Effects of Chemical Substances (RTECS) is a databank of toxicity data for over 40 000 substances compiled by the US National Institute for Occupational Safety and Health. Records include threshold limit values, recommended standards and toxicity data, as well as bibliographic details of the source of the data. The file is updated quarterly.

RTECS is available through BLAISE-LINK (UK and Eire only), DIMDI, MIC-KIBIC and NLM (US).

SDILINE

Selective Dissemination of Information onLINE (SDILINE) is the current month of the MEDLINE file and contains about 20 000 citations, which are replaced by new citations at each monthly update. Users may store searches and have them run automatically each time the file is updated.

SDILINE is available through BLAISE-LINK (UK and Eire only), DIMDI, MIC-KIBIC and NLM (US).

SERLINE

SERials onLINE is the NLM file of serial titles. Approximately 38 000 titles in the field of biomedicine, including nursing and dentistry, have records in the file.

Access is through BLAISE-LINK (UK and Eire only) and NLM.

TDB

The Toxicology Data Bank (TDB) is an online file, prepared by

NLM, which contains chemical, pharmacological and toxicological data for over 3000 substances. The records contain 60 different data elements giving chemical, physical, biological, pharmacological, toxicological and environmental properties and information.

TDB is available online through BLAISE-LINK (UK and Eire only), NLM (US) and is planned for DIMDI.

TOXLINE

TOXicology information onLINE (TOXLINE) is the NLM bibliographic file of toxicology information, including human and animal toxicity, environmental effects of chemicals and teratology. Eleven subfiles derived from various sources exist within the database which can be searched simultaneously or individually. These include *Chemical–Biological Activities* (a subset of *Chemical Abstracts*), *Abstracts on Health Effects of Environmental Pollutants* (from BIOSIS), *International Pharmaceutical Abstracts* and *Toxicity Bibliography*. Most records on TOXLINE have abstracts. There is some duplication of records derived from the different sources.

The file contains references from 1974 to date online (800,000 records) with older material from 1940 onwards (400 000 records) on TOXBACK and available offline. Searches can utilize textword searching for words from titles, index term fields and abstracts. CAS Registry numbers for chemical substances may also be used as search parameters. CAS Registry numbers may be traced by means of CHEMLINE, an online chemical dictionary.

TOXLINE and TOXBACK are available through BLAISE-LINK (UK and Eire only), DIMDI and NLM (US).

OTHER DATABASES

A number of major databases whose primary subject coverage is in other fields have some areas of overlap with biomedicine, and are discussed below. BIOSIS PREVIEWS contains citations from *Biological Abstracts* and *Biological Abstracts/Reports, Reviews, Meetings*, the major English language abstracting services in the biological sciences. The files cover 8000 journals and other material from 1969 to date, amounting to over 3 000 000 records. Experimental medicine, immunology, microbiology, nutrition, physiology and public health are some of the areas included. BIOSIS PREVIEWS is available through BRS, DATA-STAR, DIALOG (Files 5 and 55), DIMDI, ESA-IRS and SDC.

CA SEARCH is the online files of *Chemical Abstracts* covering the period from 1967 to date, containing over 5 000 000 citations. The files have extensive information from areas such as biochemistry pharmacology, analytical techniques and environmental pollution. CA SEARCH is available through DIALOG (Files 2, 3, 4 and 104).

INSPEC, the online files of *Physics Abstracts, Electrical and Electronics Abstracts* and *Computer and Control Abstracts,* contain over 1 600 000 citations from 1969 to date. Areas of interest include computer applications in biomedicine, electrophysiology, biomechanics and biomedical effects of radiation. INSPEC is available through BRS, DATA-STAR, DIALOG (Files 12 and 13) ESA-IRS and SDC. In addition, the INSPEC Topics Service provides a series of weekly computer searches on fixed topics of general interest, including the areas listed above: for example, T001 on *Electrophysiology* and T006 on *Nuclear medicine and radio-isotopes.* Topics are available from Marketing Department, Institution of Electrical Engineers, Station House, Nightingale Road, Hitchin, Herts. SG5 1RJ, England.

LIFE SCIENCES COLLECTION corresponds to the 15 abstract journals of Information Retrieval Ltd, covering animal behaviour, biochemistry, genetics, immunology, microbiology, toxicology and virology and other subject areas. The online file contains over 330 000 records from 1978 to date and is updated monthly. LIFE SCIENCES COLLECTION is available on DIALOG (File 76).

SCISEARCH is a multidisciplinary file of over 3 000 000 citations from 1974 to date. The service provides a novel approach to the literature searching problem, a citation index, which allows retrieval of newly published articles which quote an existing citation as an authority. When a scientist cites an earlier work in this way it implies a subject relationship in the content of the two papers. *Science Citation Index* and SCISEARCH, the online file, permit use of the inverted relationship, allowing one to list all papers in which the authority is currently quoted. As well as citation searching, SCISEARCH allows the use of the more usual forms of subject retrieval by textwords or phrases in titles etc. Medicine is one of the subject areas covered by the files, which are available through DIMDI and DIALOG (Files 34 and 94).

SOCIAL SCISEARCH, also produced by the Institute for Scientific Information, is a multidisciplinary database for the social and behavioural sciences, including these aspects of medicine. It covers the period from 1972 to date and contains 1 000 000 records. Like its sister file SCISEARCH, it permits citation searching as well as the conventional forms of retrieval. SOCIAL SCISEARCH is available through BRS, DIALOG (File 7) and DIMDI. Access through DATA-STAR is planned.

Online ordering of documents

Once a search has been run and citations retrieved, a user will wish to read at least some of the cited documents. Several host systems provide automatic document ordering facilities which can be used to obtain the cited documents. These include the Automatic Document Request Service (ADRS) of BLAISE, DIALOG Dialorder and the SDC Orbit Maildrop.

Sources of education and training

A useful general introduction to the field of online searching is given by Henry *et al.* (1980). This goes into some detail about many aspects of searching using a variety of host systems. The book also covers the equipment required for searching, the use of telecommunication networks and education and training.

Database producers and the host system suppliers are active in providing training courses relating to the use of their search systems in general and to individual databases. Information about the dates and venues is given in the house journals of the different hosts; for example, *BLAISE Newsletter, Chronolog* (DIALOG) and the *NLM Technical Bulletin.* This information is collated and included in *Online Notes* from the Online Information Centre for British online users. *Online Notes* also provides news of changes to files, announcements of new databases, conferences and meetings and a book review column.

A number of training databases are available online, for example, MEDLEARN available on BLAISE-LINE and NLM. MEDLEARN is a computer-assisted instruction programme in the use of MEDLINE, which teaches how to perform simple searches on the database. A number of simulations of searches on different hosts and databases have been developed by library schools and academic institutions using microcomputers and Mediatrons.

To keep up to date with developments and to improve their expertise as searchers, online searchers have organized themselves into national and local Online User Groups. The Online User Groups have regular meetings which often feature talks by experts from database producers and host systems. They also provide a useful forum for the exchange of views, experience and problems. A list of UK online user groups is included as an appendix in *Going Online* (Online Information Centre). The UK Online User Group publishes a *Newsletter* which summarizes its own and other major meetings and provides commentary on developments in the field of online retrieval.

A number of independent professional journals have appeared in order to cater for the needs of the online searcher. These include *Database, Online* and *Online Review,* which are all published quarterly.

Future developments

The electronic journal has been under development for a number of years. Authors submit papers through their online terminals directly to a central computer. Editing and refereeing are also carried out online before the paper is released into general availability on the network. An experimental electronic journal on the subject of *Computer Human Factors* (the study of people interacting with computers from either a computing or human science point of view) is being financed by the British Library, and other electronic journals are in operation in the US

It has recently been announced that the full text of 20 medical journals will be made available online by Elsevier in 1983. If these trends continue, then perhaps we really are entering the age of the paperless society!

References

Hall, H. L. and Brown, M. J. (1981), *Online Bibliographic Databases: An International Directory,* 2nd edn, Aslib
Henry, W. M., Leigh, J. A., Tedd, L. A. and Williams, P. W. (1980) *Online Searching: An Introduction,* Butterworths

Appendix: Database host addresses

BLAISE
BLAISE Marketing Office, Bibliographic Services Division, The British Library, 2 Sheraton Street, London W1V 4BH, England
Tel: 01-636 1544

BRS
Bibliographic Retrieval Services, Corporation Park, Bldg. 702, Scotia, New York 12302, USA
Tel: 800/833-4707 or 518/374-5011

DATA-STAR
Data-Star, 199 High Street, Orpington, Kent, BR6 0PF, England
Tel: 0689–38488

DIALOG

DIALOG Information Retrieval Service, P.O. Box 8, Abingdon, Oxford, OX13 6EG, England
Tel: 0865-730969

DIMDI

DIMDI, Weisshausstrasse 27, Postfach 42 05 80, Cologne 41, Federal Republic of Germany
Tel: (0221) 44 20 81–83

ESA-IRS

ESA Information Retrieval Service, ESRIN, Via Galileo Galilei, CP 64, I-00044 Frascati (Roma), Italy
Tel: (+39) 694 011

FIZ-TECHNIC

Fachinformationszentrum Technik e.V., Ostbahnhofstrasse 13, D-6000 Frankfurt am Main 1, Federal Republic of Germany
Tel: (611) 430 82 39

ISI

ISI European Branch, 132 High Street, Uxbridge, Middlesex, England
Tel: 0895–30085

MIC-KIBIC

Medical Information Centre, Karolinska Institute, PO Box 60201, S-104 01 Stockholm, Sweden
Tel: 46 8-23 22 70

NLM

MEDLARS Management Section, National Library of Medicine, 8600 Rockville Pike, Bethesda, Maryland 20209, USA
Tel: 301-496-6193

SDC

Derwent–SDC Search Service, Stuart House, 47 Crown Street, Reading, Berks RG1 2SG, England
Tel: 0734-866811

SPIDEL

Société pour l'Informatique, 98 Bd. Victor Hugo, 92115 Clichy, France
Tel: (+33) 1 731 11 91

TELESYSTEMES-QUESTEL

Telesystemes-Questel, 40 Rue du Cherche-Midi, 75006 Paris, France
Tel: (+33) 1 544 38 13

6

Anatomy and physiology

C. F. A. Marmoy*; revised by S. Gove

If any evidence was needed to demonstrate how greatly the scope
of the anatomical and physiological sciences has been extended,
examination of the last edition of *Research in British Universities,
Polytechnics and Colleges, Vol 2, Biological Sciences* (2nd edn, British Library, 1981) would suffice. Widespread use is being made of
electronic apparatus – in particular, the electron microscope,
micro-electrodes and the digital computer; developments in
biochemistry have also extended the fields of embryology and histology. With instrumentation and various physical techniques also
continuing to advance, progress in the preclinical sciences has
accelerated, and with increasing contact between previously separated disciplines, the resulting literature has also undergone
changes. Consideration of the literature of anatomy must take into
account the modern approach which, in regarding the body as a
living object, also gives more attention to the beginning and end of
existence – developmental biology and ageing – as well as investigating in particular the organization of the nervous system. Such a
shift in emphasis is reflected in teaching, as was acknowledged in
the *Royal Commission on Medical Education Report, 1965–1968.*
  One would like to be able to say that bibliographical control of
the relevant literature had kept pace with scientific progress, but
while the computer has helped considerably in indexing the periodical literature, the coverage of other forms, especially sympo-

* Formerly Assistant Librarian in Charge, Thane Library of Medical Sciences,
University College, London

sia, is still imperfect. This may or may not be serious, according to the needs of the enquirer; tracking down literature on a given subject must be related to the degree of coverage required, and on whether it is for a limited period of research or for regular, continuing scrutiny. In some cases it may be necessary to consult retrospective bibliographies, but more generally only recent literature is required: while some prefer to scan current-awareness publications and go straight to the material gleaned, others may use abstracts to avoid unnecessary reading.

Primary sources of information

Periodicals

Although original work appears principally in periodicals, other forms must be kept in mind: the many symposia produced by conferences of all kinds, research reports and theses. Because of the lack of an organized bibliographical service, these forms have often been missed. *BioResearch Index* gives a comprehensive coverage citing articles from symposia, reviews, preliminary reports, semi-popular journals, selected institutional and government reports, research communications and other secondary sources (*see* Indexing services, page 124).

It should not be necessary to stress that many relevant papers in anatomy and physiology appear in journals of general scientific or of clinical interest. Preliminary communications are found in *Nature, Federation Proceedings* and the *Proceedings of the Society for Experimental Biology and Medicine;* important full papers may be included in the *Proceedings of the Royal Society of London, Series B* or the *Proceedings of the National Academy of Sciences.* Medical periodicals which often contain articles bearing on the normal subject are many, e.g. *Gut, Thorax, Gastroenterology* and the *Journal of Experimental Medicine.* Thus many other periodicals are likely to be needed in research in these two basic medical sciences. A *List of Journals Indexed in Index Medicus* is published each year in the January issue of *Index Medicus* (*see* page 124), and also separately; in the latter form it includes subject and geographical listings. A check of the subject lists under the headings Anatomy (which includes histology and morphology), Cytology (which includes microscopy), Embryology (which includes developmental biology and teratology), Genetics (which includes biochemical genetics, eugenics and heredity), Histocytochemistry and Physiology, shows that over two hundred other periodicals are likely to be needed. Even then, these headings do not include still more specialized journals, e.g. *Circulation Research*. Incidentally, the subject and geographical sections of the *List* enable one to ascertain quickly the titles of journals in any particular field or country, so that it is not necessary to give here more than a representative selection of the most important titles in these basic sciences. Naturally, each country has its leading journals – in Britain the *Journal of Anatomy* and the *Journal of Physiology*, in the US the *American Journal of Anatomy* and the *American Journal of Physiology*. Obviously these four could not possibly publish the leading work in every field and some periodicals have gained equal repute in their more circumscribed spheres, such as the *Journal of Neurophysiology*, which attracts the best from the English-speaking world.

The following list is confined to the more important journals published in English; those in other languages may, of course, be traced through the subject and country listings in the *List of Journals Indexed in Index Medicus*.

Acta Anatomica
American Journal of Anatomy
Anatomical Record
Anatomy and Embryology
Journal of Anatomy

Cell
Cell and Tissue Research
Experimental Cell Research
Journal of Cell Biology
Journal of Cell Science
Journal of Histochemistry and
*   Cytochemistry*
Journal of Ultrastructure Research
Tissue and Cell
*Zeitschrift für Zellforschung und
*   mikroskopische Anatomie*

Annals of Human Genetics
Developmental Biology
Journal of Embryology and
*   Experimental Morphology*
Acta Physiologica Scandinavica
American Journal of Physiology
Biophysics of Structure and Mechansim
Comparative Biochemistry and
*   Physiology*

Journal of Applied Physiology
Journal of Cellular Physiology
Journal of General Physiology
Journal of Physiology
*Pflugers Archiv: European Journal of
*   Physiology*
Physiology and Behaviour
Quarterly Journal of Experimental
*   Physiology*

Cardiovascular Research
Circulation Research
Respiration Physiology

Endocrinology
Journal of Endocrinology
Journal of Reproduction and Fertility
Developmental Neuroscience
Journal of the Autonomic Nervous
*   System*
Journal of Neuroscience
Journal of Comparative Neurology
Journal of Neurophysiology
Brain Research
Experimental Brain Research
Experimental Eye Research
Pain

*These journals are now very largely in English.

For those who wish to keep abreast of the latest developments there is the choice of either regularly scanning the new issues of journals in a library or following a current-awareness service. The former may not be sufficient unless the library has a very good coverage of relevant periodicals; an alternative is to see the weekly issues of *Current Contents, Life Sciences* (Institute for Scientific Information), which gives the contents of over 1100 journals. Each issue has an author index, including addresses, and since January 1972 an edition with a subject index is available, this index having entries for all significant words in every article title. As copies of this service are flown over from the US, they often give contents of journals from overseas still on their way to Britain.

Abstracting services

Though abstracting services are discussed in Chapter 3, some account of those serving these basic medical sciences is necessary here. Currently there are two main agencies providing extensive informative abstracts, *Excerpta Medica* and *Biological Abstracts*. *Excerpta Medica* has, since 1968, provided a keyword subject index in each issue, and the cumulated annual indexes appear two to three months after completion of the volume; the abstracts are reasonably informative. *Biological Abstracts* vies with *Chemical Abstracts* in its massive sophisticated structure and extensive coverage; dealing with 8000 primary journal and monograph titles, it serves all the life sciences. Each issue has a classified arrangement with a CROSS index (subject specialties) and a BASIC (keyword in context) index.

Of the various sections of *Excerpta Medica*, the following are relevant here:

1. Anatomy, anthropology, embryology and histology
2. Physiology
3. Endocrinology
8. Neurology and neurosurgery
21. Developmental biology and teratology
22. Human genetics
27. Biophysics, bio-engineering and medical instrumentation

Other relevant abstracting services confined to certain fields include the following:

Calcified Tissue Abstracts (monthly, classified; monthly author indexes only)
Chemoreception Abstracts (quarterly, each containing an author and subject index, annual author and subject indexes)
Genetics Abstracts (monthly, classified with author index; annual author and subject indexes)
Muscular Dystrophy Abstracts (fortnightly; annual author and subject indexes)
Nutrition Abstracts and Reviews (quarterly, classified with author index; annual author and subject indexes)

Indexing services

For most anatomists and physiologists the *Index Medicus* is indispensable, although new users should study the introduction (printed in each issue) and the annual subject headings list (*MeSH*). The latter, in particular, needs scrutiny as it still lacks a number of terms, rendering searches in these topics a matter of sifting through much irrelevant material. Thus, headings for 'cell membranes' and 'synaptic membranes' can be found but not for 'nerve membranes', and for 'myofibrils' but not 'muscle fibres'; 'smooth muscle' has a separate heading but papers on striated muscle and skeletal muscle are under the general heading 'muscles'. Otherwise the methodical arrangement of entries under each heading makes selection reasonably straightforward.

The development in 1967 of *BioResearch Index* as an adjunct to *Biological Abstracts* has greatly assisted in tracing papers in symposia, preliminary reports, letters, notes, etc. Each year this index reports '100 000 research papers in addition to and different from' the more than 140 000 reports in *Biological Abstracts.* The index appears monthly and is provided with a complete list of publications covered and the same types of author and subject indexes as its parent publication. Hitherto the only source of information on symposia has been the invaluable *Index of Conference Proceedings received by the BL,* which cannot, however, list the contents of the thousands of such proceedings it receives annually. The *Index to Scientific and Technical Proceedings,* published by ISI, was started in 1978 and includes biomedical material. It is now available online.

In addition to these general indexes, there are two or three smaller ones which serve limited areas. The *Bibliography of Reproduction,* begun in 1963, is a classified monthly index to books and periodical articles on all aspects of reproduction in vertebrates, including man. A bibliographical service is run by the producing body, Reproduction Research Information Service, Cambridge. Each monthly issue has an author index as well as a co-ordinated subject index – these are cumulated half-yearly – and also a separate bibliography on a selected topic.

Another field having its own index was histochemistry, although its appearance was irregular. From 1959 *Acta Histochemica* devoted certain volumes to *Bibliographia Histochemica,* the last being Bd. 40, 1971. This became an exhaustive index including books and papers in symposia and other composite works; it can be found in the following volumes of the journal: 7, 11, 14, 16, 24, 29 and 40; over 34 000 items were listed in classified order, with author and subject indexes. A more limited source of information in this field is the citation index published monthly in the *Journal of Histochemistry and Cytochemistry*, compiled from the Automatic Subject Citation Alert (ASCA) of the Institute for Scientific Information: this is however, confined to papers in that journal during the previous three to five years.

Tissue culture has been well indexed in retrospect, as is shown in the next section. It is currently served by the *Index of Tissue Culture* edited by H. E. Cesvet, sponsored by the Tissue Culture Association co-operating with the National Library of Medicine. This index is derived from the tapes of the *Index Medicus*, and so far volumes covering 1966–1974 have appeared.

Researches on the nervous system represent many forms of approach and different kinds of indexes have resulted, both current and retrospective. Of the former, one example is *Bibliographia Neuroendocrinologica*, a quarterly publication also containing abstracts; each issue contains about 500 items arranged by authors with a subject index. Electroencephalography also has its own indexes: an *Index to Current Literature* appears quarterly from the publishers of *Electroencephalography and Clinical Neurophysiology*, prepared by the Brain Information Service, UCLA. There is a classified arrangement beginning with a general selection including reviews and books.

Retrospective bibliographies

Continuing with the field of electroencephalography, the excellent series of KWIC indexes begun by R. G. Bickford continued regularly. The first volume appeared in 1965 and has over 10 000 items published up to the end of 1963: this was the *KWIC Index of EEG Literature (and Society Proceedings)* (Elsevier, 1965). Two further volumes covering 1964 to 1969 have since appeared as *Supplements 29–30* to *Electroencephalography and Clinical Neurophysiology* (Elsevier, 1970–1971). Earlier supplements to the same journal were No 1, *Bibliography of Electroencephalography 1875–1948* (1950), compiled by M. Brazier, and No 23, *A Selected Bibliography of Electroencephalography in Human Psychopharmacology 1951–62* (1964) by M. Fink.

Tissue culture is another field which has received much attention in bibliography. The *Bibliography of the Research in Tissue Culture 1884 to 1950* edited by M. R. Murray and G. Kopech (Academic Press, 1950), is concerned with the living cell cultivated *in vitro* and excludes bacteria unless cultivated along with tissue cells. It is in 'dictionary' form, authors and subjects in one alphabet, covering all forms of literature as well as films and even unpublished cinemicrographs. It was supplemented by an author index of literature 1950–1953, and an annual volume with the same editors was planned, but only vol 5 for 1965 appeared. Since then the *Index of Tissue Culture* mentioned earlier has taken over.

Other bibliographies of potential value are:

(1) Ageing: *A Classified Bibliography of Gerontology and Geriatrics* by N. W. Shock, with two supplements (Stanford University Press, 1951–1963). This is classified with indexes of authors and subjects, and includes books and chapters of books, also abstracts. It was continued in each quarterly issue of the *Journal of Gerontology* until 1980.

(2) Bone: *The Structure, Composition and Growth of Bone, 1930–53* compiled by M. C. Spencer and K. Uhler (US Armed Forces Medical Library, 1955).

(3) Electron microscopy: *The International Bibliography of Electron Microscopy (1950–1961)* (2 vols, New York Society of Electron Microscopists, 1959–62).

(4) Genetics: *Bibliographia Biotheoretica (Section VII)*, compiled at the University of Leiden, covers the field in volumes each of five years. *Bibliographia genetica* began in 1925, and was a series of reviews or monographs, each with a bibliography, e.g. vol 15, 1952, which was the second edition of *The Genetics of the Mouse* by H. Grüneberg, but unfortunately this ceased publication in 1970.

(5) Hearing: *Bibliography on Hearing* by S. S. Stevens *et al.* (Harvard University Press, 1955), has over 10000 items including books and theses.

(6) Muscle receptors: *Bibliography on Muscle Receptors, their Morphology, Pathology and Physiology* by E. Edred *et al.* (Academic Press, 1967), appeared as supplement to *Experimental Neurology*, and includes articles up to 1966.

(7) Taste: *Bibliography on the Sense of Taste 1566–1966* compiled by R. M. Pangborn and I. M. Trabue is appended to *The Chemical Senses and Nutrition* edited by M. R. Kare and O. Maller (Johns Hopkins, 1967). A second volume published by Academic Press appeared in 1977, but the bibliography was not updated.

Secondary sources

While it may be convenient to speak of primary and secondary sources, one cannot forget that periodicals contain material that is not necessarily original, while new information may first appear in a symposium or some other non-periodical publication. There are also periodicals which are in any case secondary source material since they are devoted to the review type of article.

The following section deals with those forms of literature which present an ordered statement of knowledge on a given subject, though of varying scope and depth, i.e. handbooks, treatises, textbooks, monographs and symposia. As an intermediate step, however, consideration must first be given to reviews, mostly collected in serial publications, though occasionally found in isolated surveys of progress. Authorship may be collective, and some symposia offer the best exposition available on certain topics. Other methods of presenting facts may be pictorial (atlases), documentary (data handbooks) or simply explanatory (dictionaries, terminology), and these are treated in succeeding sections.

The changing approach to the study and teaching of the medical sciences has resulted, as already noted, in a new literature. Some of these works concern individual subjects and are mentioned in those contexts, but four publications of a general interdisciplinary nature may be cited here. The first is intended for both teachers and students: *The Biological Basis of Medicine* edited by E. E. and N. Bitter (6 vols, Academic Press, 1968–1969), which uses cellular biology as the key to explaining normal and pathological processes. This is the work of over 100 investigators and is well documented and indexed. The second is also well produced, though designed for undergraduates: *A Companion to Medical Studies* edited by R. Passmore and J. S. Robson (3 vols, 2nd edn, Blackwell Scientific 1976,1980), the first two volumes covering the preclinical medical sciences, structure and function being co-ordinated. The other two publications are shorter but also based on the wider approach to the study of human structure and function: *Introduction to the Study of Man* by J. Z. Young (2nd edn, Oxford University Press, 1974), and *Human Biology: An Introduction to Human Evolution, Variation and Growth* edited by G. A. Harrison (2nd edn, Oxford University Press, 1977).

Reviews

The value of this type of secondary source material is perhaps best underlined by the existence of the *Bibliography of Medical Reviews* as a prominent feature of *Index Medicus*. While the majority of such articles are contained in serials entirely devoted to this form of literature, there are still many reviews to be found in periodicals intended primarily for original papers; in addition, reports of the review type may be found in the annual volumes of symposia of various societies, e.g. the Society for Experimental Biology. Discovering such articles is facilitated by the *Bibliography of Medical Reviews.*

The following list may be of use in searching for reviews in the fields concerned:

Advances in Anatomy, Embryology and Cell Biology
Advances in Cell Biology
Advances in Comparative Physiology and Biochemistry
Advances in Gerontological Research
Advances in Human Genetics
Advances in Morphogenesis
Advances in Oral Biology
Advances in Reproductive Physiology
Annual Review of Neuroscience
Annual Review of Physiology
Biological Reviews
British Medical Bulletin
Cold Spring Harbor Symposia on Quantitative Biology
Contributions to Sensory Physiology
Currents in Modern Biology
Current Topics in Bioenergetics
Current Topics in Developmental Biology
Endocrine Reviews
Harvey Lectures
International Review of Connective Tissue Research
International Review of Cytology
Nutrition Abstracts and Reviews
Physiological Reviews
Progress in Biophysics and Molecular Biology
Progress in Brain Research
Progress in Histochemistry and Cytochemistry
Quarterly Review of Biology
Quarterly Reviews of Biophysics
Reviews of Physiology, Biochemistry and Pharmacology
Scientific Basis of Medicine Annual Reviews
Symposia of the Society for Developmental Biology (formerly The Society for the Study of Development and Growth)
Symposia of the Society for Experimental Biology
Topics in Developmental Biology
Trends in Neurological Sciences (TINS)

Systematic works, textbooks, monographs

Anatomy, histology, embryology

The old anatomical handbooks in this field have become dated and with changes in terminology often difficult to use: Bardeleben's *Handbuch der Anatomie des Menschen* (8 vols in 19, Jena, 1896–1934) and Quain's *Elements of Anatomy* (11th edn, 4 vols in 8, Longmans, 1908–1929) are without successors. For general works with the most detail there is still *Gray's Anatomy* by P. L. Williams and R. Warwick (36th edn, Churchill Livingstone, 1980) and *Cunningham's Textbook of Anatomy* by G. J. Romanes (12th edn Oxford University Press, 1981), both of which successfully resist the passage of time. For students there are Grant's *Method of Anatomy* by J. V. Basmajian (10th edn Williams and Wilkins, 1980), *Clinically Orientated Anatomy* by K. L. Moore (Williams and Wilkins, 1980), and *Clinical Anatomy for Medical Students* by R. S. Snell (2nd edn, Little, Brown, 1981). The regional approach is used in *Anatomy, Regional and Applied* by R. J. Last (6th edn, Churchill Livingstone, 1978), and in *Anatomy: a Regional Study of Human Structure* by E. Gardner (4th edn, Saunders, 1975). For guides in dissecting there are *Cunningham's Manual of Practical Anatomy* (14th edn, vol 1–, Oxford University Press, 1976–), and the *Manual of Human Anatomy* by J. T. Aitken *et al.* (3rd edn, 3 vols, Churchill Livingstone, 1975). The various techniques in the preparation of anatomical specimens are ably described in *Anatomical Techniques* by D. H. Tompsett (2nd edn, Livingstone, 1970).

Histology is one subject still comprehensively covered by one of the great German treatises: the *Handbuch der mikroskopischen Anatomie des Menschen* founded by W. von Möllendorff and now edited by W. Bargmann (7 Bde, in 38 parts to date, Springer, 1927–). The latest volume (1982) is on the *Paraganglia* and each volume is finely illustrated and exhaustively documented and indexed. Thus, the latest volume has a bibliography of 50 pages and indexes of 36 pages.

There is no lack of textbooks of histology, of which the most important include those by W. Bloom and D. W. Fawcett (10th edn, Saunders, 1975), *Histology* by A. W. Ham and D. H. Cormack (8th edn, Lippincott, 1979), L. C. Junqueira (3rd edn, Lange, 1980) and P. R. Wheater *et al.* (Livingstone, 1979). Researches on ultrastructure have led to more specialized works: *Cell and Molecular Biology* by E. D. De Robertis (CBS Company, 1980), *Ultrastructure of the Mammalian Cell* by R. V. Kristic (Springer, 1979), *Human Microscopic Anatomy* by S. S. Han and J. O. V. Holmstedt (McGraw-Hill, 1981) and *Biological Membranes* by D. S. Parsons, (Clarendon, 1975). There are also numerous works on techniques, e.g. H. M. Carleton's *Histological Technique* (5th edn, Oxford University Press, 1980), *Principles of Biological*

Microtechnique by J. R. Baker (Wiley, 1958), *Handbook of Histopathological Technique* by C. F. A. Culling (3rd edn, Butterworths, 1974), and *Histological Techniques for Electron Microscopy* by D. C. Pease (2nd edn, Academic Press, 1964). More specialized works of value are the *Physical Techniques in Biological Research* edited by A. W. Pollister, Vol 3, Parts A–C (2nd edn, Academic Press, 1966–1969), *Biological Stains* by H. J. Conn (9th edn, Williams and Wilkins, 1977), the Academic Press series on *Biological Techniques* and *Three Dimensional Reconstruction in Biology* by P. N. and W. A. Gaunt (Pitman Medical, 1978). Histochemical methods are ever growing in number: guides to their use include *Histochemistry* by R. W. Horobin (Butterworths, 1982), *Histochemistry, Theoretical and Applied* by A. G. E. Pearse (4th edn, vol 1–, Churchill Livingstone, 1980–), and *Histopathologic Technic and Practical Histochemistry* by R. D. Lillie and H. M. Fullmer (4th edn, McGraw-Hill, 1976).

For the techniques of autoradiography there is *Autoradiography* by A. W. Rogers (3rd edn, Elsevier, 1979); and *Physical Techniques in Biological Research* edited by A. W. Pollister, of which vol 3, Part B, is on *Autoradiography at the Cellular Level* (Academic Press, 2nd edn, 1969).

In the field of embryology useful textbooks for medical studies are *Human Embryology* by M. J. T. Fitzgerald (Harper and Row, 1978) and *Medical Embryology* by J. Langman (4th edn, Williams and Wilkins, 1981), *The Developing Human* by K. L. Moore (2nd edn, Saunders, 1977) and *Essentials of Human Embryology* by F. D. Allan (2nd edn, Oxford University Press, 1969), while the scientific worker has *An Introduction to Embryology* by B. I. Balinsky (5th edn, Saunders, 1981). Monographs of note are *Interacting Systems in Development* by J. D. Ebert and I. M. Sussex (2nd edn, Holt Rinehart, 1970), *Developmental Processes in Higher Vertebrates* by M. R. Bellairs (Logos Press, 1971, *Introductory Concepts in Developmental Biology* by A. Monroy and A. A. Moscona (University of Chicago Press, 1979) and *Tissue Interactions and Development* by N. K. Wessells (Benjamin, 1977). Experimental methods may be found in *Methods in Developmental Biology* edited by F. H. Wilt and N. K. Wessells (Crowell, 1967), *Methods in Mammalian Reproduction* edited by J. C. Daniel (Academic Press, 1978), *Culture of Vertebrate Embryos by D. A. T. New (Logos Press, 1966), and Methods in Experimental Embryology of the Mouse* by K. A. Rafferty (Johns Hopkins, 1970). Among works of reference for embryologists are the 'normal tables', containing descriptions of embryos at successive stages of development; at best not only external details are given, but also an account of the various organs. The existence of these standard descriptions obviates the need for repeating them and also assists identification of which stage another author is discussing, if this should be in doubt. The basic series of these works was the *Normentafeln zur Entwicklungsgeschichte der Wirbeltiere* edited by F. Keibel (16 vols, G. Fischer, 1897–1938). Many others have since been published and a detailed list is given in Bellairs' *Developmental Processes in Higher Vertebrates*, cited above (page 130). *See also* vol 1, Section III, of the *Biology Data Book* edited by P. L. Altman and D. S. Dittmer (2nd edn, FASEB Biological Handbooks, 1972).

The culture of cells and tissues has applications in other branches of medical research, and the bibliographies already mentioned indicate what may be relevant here. A basic text on the subject is *Cell and Tissue Culture* by J. Paul (5th edn, Churchill Livingstone, 1975), while *Cells and Tissues in Culture* edited by E. N. Willmer (3 vols, Academic Press, 1966), is an extensive treatise.

Research in human genetics continues to increase; the Fifth International Congress was held in 1976 and proceedings published (Excerpta Medica, 1977). General works to note in this field are *Human Genetics* by V. A. McKusick (2nd edn, Prentice-Hall, 1969), *Human Genetics* by E. Novitski (MacMillan, 1977), *Principles of Human Genetics* by C. Stern (3rd edn, Freeman, 1973), *Introduction to Medical Genetics* by J. A. F. Roberts (7th edn, Oxford University Press, 1978), and *Principles of Human Biochemical Genetics* by H. Harris (3rd edn, North-Holland, 1980); while *Elements of Medical Genetics* by A. E. H. Emery (5th edn, Churchill Livingstone, 1979) provides a useful introduction to the subject.

To end this section one may refer to the study of ageing. A number of conferences have been held in this field; the proceedings of one of the latest (held in Vichy) were published in 1981 in 3 vols as *Aging: a Challenge to Science and Society* (Oxford Medical Publications). For a comprehensive review of the subject there is *The Biology of Senescence* by A. Comfort (3rd edn, Churchill, 1979).

Physiology

The *Handbook of Physiology* (Williams and Wilkins, 1959–1978) is the creation of the American Physiological Society, with contributions by physiologists in many other countries as well. Its aim is 'the comprehensive but critical presentation of the state of knowledge in the various fields of functional biology. It is intended to cover physiological sciences in their entirety once in about ten or twelve years and to supplement them thereafter.' The following volumes appeared in the 1st edn: I *Neurophysiology* (3 vols 1959–1960); II *Circulation* (3 vols, 1962–1965); III *Respiration (2 vols, 1964–1965); IV Adaptation to the environment* (1964); V *Adipose tissue* (1965); VI *Alimentary canal* (5 vols 1967–1968); VII *Endocrinology* (7 vols in 9, 1969–1976); VIII *Renal Physiology (1973)*; and *IX Reactions to Environmental Agents* (1977). So far three volumes have appeared in the revised edition on the nervous and cardiovascular systems. One other recent work of this kind should be cited, since it is to some extent complementary: the *Handbook of Sensory Physiology* with various editors (Springer, 1971–1979). The series is updated by *Progress in Sensory Physiology,* of which three volumes have so far appeared.

General physiology has produced some notable textbooks, e.g. Bayliss' *Principles of General Physiology* (5th edn, 2 vols, Longmans, 1959–1960) and H. Davson's *Textbook of General Physiology* (4th edn, 2 vols, Churchill, 1970). Established texts in human physiology are *An Introduction to Human Physiology* by A. H. Green (4th edn, Oxford University Press, 1976), *Physiology and Biophysics* edited by T. C. Ruch and H. D. Patton (20th edn, 4 vols, Saunders, 1973–1982), *Introduction to Physiology* by H. Davson and M. B. Segal (5 vols, Academic Press, 1975–), *Textbook of Physiology* by G. H. Bell *et al.* (10th edn, Churchill Livingstone, 1980), *Physiology* by E. E. Selkurt (4th edn, Little Brown, 1976).

Medically slanted texts are *The Physiological Basis of Medical Practice* by C. H. Best and N. B. Taylor (10th edn, Williams and Wilkins, 1979), *Samson Wright's Applied Physiology* by C. A. Keele and E. Neil (13th edn, Oxford University Press, 1982) and *Textbook of Medical Physiology* by A. C. Guyton (6th edn, Saunders, 1982), among others.

Experimental Physiology by B. L. Andrew (9th edn, Livingstone, 1973) and *Experiments in Cell Physiology* by L. Packer (Academic Press, 1967) are useful for students. For the research worker there is the series *Experiments in Physiology and Biochemistry* edited by G. A. Kerkut (6 vols, Academic Press, 1968–1975); for the cell biologist *Methods in Cell Biology* originally edited by D. M. Prescott (25 vols, Academic Press, 1964–). Electrophysiological techniques, including the use of microelectrodes, are covered by vols 5 and 6 of *Physical Techniques in Biological Research* edited by G. Oster and A. W. Pollister (Academic Press, 1963–1964) and *Principles of Applied Biomedical Instrumentation* by L. A. Geddes and L. E. Baker (2nd edn, Wiley, 1975).

Basic concepts in understanding the functions of the body include homeostasis and physiological regulations, and, in association with engineering theory, the study of control mechanisms has been developed from various angles. Works on these subjects include *Origins of Physiological Regulations* by E. F. Adolph (Academic Press, 1968); two Ciba Foundation symposia, *Homeostatic Regulators* edited by G. E. W. Wolstenholme and J. Knight (Churchill, 1969), and *Control Processes in Multicellular Organisms* with the same editors (Churchill, 1970); and a monograph, *Control Theory and Physiological Feedback Mechanisms* by D. S. Riggs (Williams and Wilkins, 1970). Other topics of general physiological interest are dealt with in *Membrane Transport in Biology* edited by G. Giebisch *et al.*, (5 vols, Springer, 1978–), *Fluids and Electrolytes* by K. Smith (Churchill Livingstone, 1980), *Ion Transport and Membranes* by A. B. Hope (Butterworths, 1971), and the series *Studies in Biology* produced by the Institute of Biology. Adaptation to the environment, to which one volume of the *Handbook of Physiology* is devoted, has also been covered by 3 volumes in the series *International Review of Physiology* published by University Park Press.

Systems of the body

The nervous system more than any other has seen a widespread increase in all forms of the relevant literature; at the same time older material may still be needed, such as the *Histologie du Système Nerveux de l'Homme et des Vertébrés* by S. Ramón y Cajal (2 vols, Paris, 1909–1911; reprint Madrid Instituto Ramón y Cajal, 1952–1955). Also, some forms are confused, e.g. *Progress in Brain Research* (1–, Elsevier, 1963–), the scope of which is wider than the title indicates, and which includes symposia, monographs and reviews of progress; work of basic importance may be found in *Publications of the Association for Research in Nervous and Mental Diseases* (vol 1–, Williams and Wilkins, 1920–). The integrated approach to the study of the nervous system is found in a multi-volume treatise, *Structure and Function of Nervous Tissue* edited by G. H. Bourne (vols 1–6, Academic Press, 1968–1972); as well as in single volume works, e.g. *Medical Neurobiology* by W. D. Willis and R. G. Grossman (3rd edn, Mosby, 1981) and *Neurological Anatomy in Relation to Clinical Medicine* by A. Brodal (3rd edn, Oxford University Press, 1981). Useful textbooks include *Functional Neuroanatomy* by N. B. Everett (6th edn, Lea and Febiger, 1971) and *Human Neuroanatomy* by M. B. Carpenter (7th edn, Williams and Wilkins, 1976).

The embryology and histology of the nervous system are treated in various works: *Developmental Neurobiology* edited by W. A. Himwich (Thomas, 1970), from the research angle, and *Developmental Neurobiology*, a monograph by M. Jacobson (2nd edn, Plenum, 1978) and *Fine Structure of the Nervous System* by A. Peters *et al.* (2nd edn, Saunders, 1976). The only recent textbooks on neurophysiology are *The Neurophysiology of the Cerebral Cortex* by L. Bindman and O. Lippold (Arnold, 1981), *Fundamentals of Neurophysiology* by R. T. Schmidt (Springer, 1978) and *Structure and Function of the Nervous System* by A. C. Guyton (2nd edn, Saunders, 1976).

Monographs and other works on special topics of importance are:

The Conduction of the Nervous Impulse by A. L. Hodgkin (University of Liverpool Press, 1964)
Nerve, Muscle and Synapse by B. Katz (McGraw-Hill, 1966)
Synapses by G. A. Cottrell and P. N. R. Usherwood (Blackie, 1977)
Neuronal Plasticity by C. W. Cotman (Raven Press, 1978)
Structure and Function of Synapses edited by G. D. Pappas and D. P. Purpura (North Holland, 1972)
Intracellular Functions and Synapses edited by J. Feldman *et al.*, (Chapman and Hall, 1978)
The Physiology of Excitable Cells by D. J. Aidley (2nd edn, Cambridge University Press, 1978)
Nerve–muscle interaction by G. Vrbova (Chapman and Hall, 1978)
Adrenergic Neurons by G. Burnstock and M. Costa (Chapman and Hall, 1975)
Limbic System edited by R. L. Isaacson (Plenum, 1974)
Cerebellar Cortex by S. L. Palay and V. Chan-Palay (Springer, 1973)
The Hippocampus by R. L. Isaacson and K. H. Pribram (2 vols, Plenum, 1975)
Structure of the Autonomic Nervous System by G. Gabella (Chapman and Hall, 1976)
Nerve and Muscle Excitation by D. Junge (Sinauer, 1981)

Lastly, by way of aiding research, there is *Tissue Culture in Neurobiology* edited by E. Giacobinini *et al.* (Raven Press, 1980).

The literature on the brain has grown to such volume that it has its own history, *The Human Brain and Spinal Cord: A Historical Study . . . from Antiquity to the Twentieth Century* by E. Clarke and C. D. O'Malley (University of California Press, 1968). It is not possible here to cover all aspects of research on the structure and function of the brain: some current studies still refer to classic works such as *Histological Studies on the Localisation of Cerebral Function* by A. W. Campbell (Cambridge University Press, 1905), *The Integrative Action of the Nervous System* by C. S. Sherrington (Yale University Press, 1906) and *The Cytoarchitectonics of the Human Cerebral Cortex* by C. von Economo (Oxford University Press, 1929). Many have worked in this field since, and the following is a select list in chronological order of some major works still in use:

Brain Mechanisms and Intelligence by K. S. Lashley (Chicago University Press, 1929; Dover, 1963)
The Primate Thalamus by A. E. Walker (Chicago University Press, 1938)
The Hypothalamus by W. E. Le Gros Clark *et al.* (Oliver and Boyd, 1938)
The Cerebral Cortex of Man by W. Penfield and T. Rasmussen (Macmillan, 1950)
Aspects of Cerebella Anatomy by J. Jansen and A. Brodal (Tanum, Oslo, 1954)
Organization of the Cerebral Cortex by D. A. Sholl (Methuen, 1956)
Reticular Formation of the Brain Stem by A. Brodal (Oliver and Boyd, 1957)
Excitable Cortex in Conscious Man by W. Penfield (Liverpool University Press, 1958)
Model of the Brain by J. Z. Young (Oxford University Press, 1964)
From Neuron to Brain by S. W. Kuffler and J. B. Nicholls (Sinauer, 1976)
Molecular Neurobiology of the Mammalian Brain by P. L. McGeer *et al.* (Plenum, 1978)

The series *Progress in Brain Research,* already cited, informs on the various aspects of current research. The special sense organs are treated in the *Handbook of Sensory Physiology* mentioned above. Two introductions to the subject are *Fundamentals of Sensory Physiology* by R. T. Schmidt (Springer, 1978) and *The Senses* by A. B. Barlow (Cambridge University Press, 1982). For individual organs the following works are important:

(1) Vision: the two works by S. Polyak, *The Retina* (Chicago University Press, 1941) and *The Vertebrate Visual System* (Chicago University Press, 1957); supplemented by two volumes on *The Structure of the Eye,* the first edited by G. K. Smelser (Academic Press, 1961), the second by J. W. Rohen (Schattauer, Stuttgart, 1965); and also *The Eye* edited by H. Davson (2nd edn, 6 vols, Academic Press, 1967–1974), *Vision* by D. Marr (Freeman, 1982) and *Physiology of the Retina and Visual Pathway* by G. S. Brindley (2nd edn, Arnold, 1970).
(2) Hearing: *An Introduction to the Anatomy and Physiology of Speech and Hearing* by J. F. Jarvis (Juta, 1978) and *An Introduction to the Physiology of Hearing* by J. O. Pickles (Academic Press, 1982).
(3) Taste and smell: This is the subject of a series of international symposia, *Olfaction and Taste,* of which the latest is the 7th, (IRL Press, 1980).
(4) Touch: *Mechanisms of Cutaneous Sensation* by D. Sinclair (Oxford University Press, 1981).

With respect to other systems of the body, the secondary literature is smaller and sometimes out of date. Where no recent treatise or monograph exists, reference should be made to the appropriate section of the *Handbook of Physiology* or to one of the larger general textbooks. For physiology the valuable monograph series of the Physiological Society should be remembered; this began in 1953, and so far 25 volumes have been published by Arnold and, more recently, by Cambridge University Press and Academic Press; recent volumes include *Local Mechanisms Controlling Blood Vessels* by W. R. Keatinge and M. C. Harman (Academic Press, 1980), *The Electrophysiology of Gland Cells* by O. H. Petersen (Academic Press, 1980) and *The Physiology of Thirst and Sodium Appetite* by J. T. Fitzsimons (Cambridge University Press, 1979).

The following list is of titles likely to be of use for other systems:

(1) Locomotor system: *Biochemistry and Physiology of Bone* edited by G. H. Bourne (2nd edn, vols 1–4, Academic Press, 1972); *Physiology and Pathophysiology of the Skin* edited by A. Jarrett (7 vols, Academic Press, 1973–); *Structure and Function of Muscle* edited by G. H. Bourne (2nd edn, 4 vols, Academic Press, 1972–1973).

(2) Circulatory system: *Cardiovascular Physiology* edited by A. C. Guyton and C. E. Jones (3 vols in the series *International Review of Physiology* previously mentioned on page 133); *Circulatory Physiology* edited by A. C. Guyton and C. E. Jones (Butterworths, 1973); *Cardiovascular Dynamics* by R. F. Rushmer (4th edn, Saunders, 1976); and *The Human Cardiovascular System* by J. T. Shepherd and P. M. Vanhoutte (Raven Press, 1979).

(3) Respiratory system: *Physiology of Respiration* by J. T. Comroe (2nd edn, Year Book Medical Publishers, 1974) and *Regulation of Breathing* by R. Hornbein (2 vols, Dekker, 1981).

(4) Digestive system: *Physiology of the Digestive Tract* by H. W. Davenport (5th edn, Year Book Medical Publishers, 1982); *Digestive System Physiology* by P. A. Sanford (E. Arnold, 1982) and, for a short introduction, *A Digest of Digestion* by H. W. Davenport (2nd edn, Year Book Medical Publishers, 1978).

(5) Urinary system: *The Kidney* by B. M. Brenner and F. C. Rector (2nd edn, 2 vols, Saunders, 1981); *Physiology of the Kidney and Body Fluids* by R. F. Pitts (3rd edn, Year Book Medical Publishers, 1974); and *Principles of Renal Physiology* by C. J. Lote (Croom Helm, 1982)

(6) Lymphatic system, body fluids: *Lymphatics, Lymph and the Lymphomyeloid Complex* edited by J. M. Yoffey and F. C.

Courtice (Academic Press, 1970); and *Physiology of the Cerebrospinal Fluid* by H. Davson (Churchill, 1967).

(7) Endocrine system: *Textbook of Endocrinology* edited by R. D. Williams (6th edn, Saunders 1981); *Endocrine Physiology* by R. N. Hardy (Arnold, 1981); *Endocrinology* by L. J. Degroot *et al.* (3 vols, Grune and Stratton, 1979); *Essential Endocrinology* by J. Laycock and P. Wise (2nd edn, Oxford University Press, 1983).

(8) Reproductive system: F. H. A. Marshall's *Physiology of Reproduction* by A. S. Parkes (3rd edn, 3 vols in 4, Longmans, 1952–1966); M. H. Johnson and B. Everett's *Essential Reproduction* (Blackwell, 1980); *Human Reproduction and Developmental Biology* by D. J. Begley *et al. (Macmillan, 1980)*; *The Ovary* edited by S. Zuckerman (2nd edn, 3 vols, Academic Press, 1977–1978); *Milk: the Mammary Gland and its Secretion* edited by S. K. Kon and A. T. Cowie (2 vols, Academic Press, 1961); *Lactation: A Comprehensive Treatise* edited by B. L. Larson and V. R. Smith (4 vols, Academic Press, 1974–).

(9) Nutrition: *Human Nutrition and Dietetics* by S. Davidson *et al.* (7th edn, Churchill Livingstone, 1979); *Human Nutrition: a Comprehensive Treatise* by R. B. Alfin-Slater and D. Kritchevsky (3 vols in 4, Plenum, 1979–).

Atlases

While the older type of anatomical atlas continues, newer works resulting from the use of the electron microscope and of the stereotaxic instrument are multiplying. J. C. B. Grant's *Atlas of Anatomy* (7th edn, Williams and Wilkins, 1978), R. M. H. McMinn and R. T. Hutchings *A Colour Atlas of Human Anatomy* (Wolfe Medical Publications, 1977) and *Atlas of Clinical Anatomy* by R. S. Snell (Little, Brown, 1978) are all popular; the first two also include descriptive text. To microscopic anatomy is added ultrastructure: an example of the combined approach is *Cells and Tissues by Light and Electron Microscopy* by E. G. Sandborn (2 vols, Academic Press, 1970; other atlases of micrographs with accompanying descriptions are *Atlas of Descriptive Histology* by E. J. Reith and M. H. Ross (3rd edn, Harper and Row, 1977), *Ultrastructural Pathology of the Cell and Matrix* by F. N. Ghadially (2nd edn, Butterworths, 1981) and *Fine Structure of the Cells and Tissues* by K. R. Porter and M. A. Bonneville (4th edn, Lea and Febiger, 1974).

For the study of embryology there are W. W. Matthe's *Atlas of Descriptive Embryology* (2nd edn, Macmillan, 1976), and the three volumes of H. Tuchmann-Duplessis *et al.*, *Illustrated Human Embryology* (Chapman and Hall, 1972–1974). Of those atlases with more specialized objectives, the following are available: for general studies on the brain the *Atlas of the Human Brain* by D. H. Ford *et al.*, (3rd edn, Elsevier, 1975), while for dissecting *Human Brain* by N. Gluhbegovic and T. H. Williams (Harper and Row, 1980) is valuable: for dental studies there are *A Colour Atlas and Textbook of Oral Anatomy* by B. K. B. Berkovitz *et al.* (Wolfe Medical Publications, 1978); *A Colour Atlas of the Head and Neck* by R. M. H. McMinn (Wolfe Medical Publications, 1981). In the field of comparative anatomy there are the *Atlas of Cat Anatomy* by H. E. Field and M. E. Taylor (2nd edn, Chicago University Press, 1969), and – with atlases incorporated in the text – the *Anatomy of the Dog* by M. E. Miller *et al.* (Saunders, 1964), and the *Anatomy of the Rat* by E. C. Greene (1935; reprinted, Hafner, 1968).

The stereotaxic instrument for the three-dimensional investigation of the brain was invented by R. H. Clarke some years before World War I. However, it is only during the past two decades that it has been widely used and atlases of the deep structures of the brain of man and of various animal species published as a result. The *Introduction to Stereotaxis with an Atlas of the Human Brain* by G. Schaltenbrand and P. Bailey (3 vols, Thieme, 1959), and *Stereotaxic Atlas of the Human Thalamus and Adjacent Structures* by J. Andrew and E. S. Watkins (Williams and Wilkins, 1969), relate to man. For comparative studies the following stereotaxic atlases may be noted: for the baboon by R. Davis and R. D. Huffman (University of Texas Press, 1968); the chimpanzee by M. R. DeLucchi *et al.* (University of California Press, 1966); the rhesus monkey *Macaca mulatta*, by R. S. Snider and J. C. Lee (Chicago University Press, 1961); the Java monkey, *Macaca irus*, by T. R. Shantha *et al.* (Karger, 1968); the Cebus monkey by S. L. Manocha *et al.* (Clarendon, 1968); the squirrel monkey, *Saimiri sciureus*, by R. Emmers and K. Akert (University of Wisconsin Press, 1963). For the cat there are atlases by R. S. Snider and W. T. Niemer (Chicago University Press, 1961), of the brain stem by A. L. Berman (University of Wisconsin Press, 1968) and of the hypothalaums by R. Bleir (Johns Hopkins Press, 1961). For the dog there are atlases by S. Dua-Sharma *et al.* (MIT Press, 1970) and by R. K. S. Lim *et al.* (L. C. Thomas, 1960). For the rat there is a general atlas by R. J. and J. R. Olds (Wolfe Medical Publications, 1977), and one for the developing rat brain by N. M. Sherwood and P. S. Timiras (University of California Press, 1970), for the rat diencephalon by D. Albe-Fessard *et al.* (CNRS, Paris, 1971), and for the forebrain and lower brain stem by J. F. R. König and R. A. Knippel (Williams and Wilkins, 1963).

Reference works

Data handbooks

The great volume of data established in anatomical and physiological research has been digested and made available in several publications. Probably the biggest compilation of this kind is the series *Tabulae Biologicae* (22 vols, W. Junk, 1925–1963): the last four volumes are vol 19 '*The Cell*' (1939–1951), vol 20 '*Growth of Man*' (1941), vol 21 '*Digestion*' (1954) and vol 22 '*The Eye*' 1947–1963). This work contains a mass of fully documented data not always accessible elsewhere.

More recently an excellent series edited by P. L. Altman and D. S. Dittmer for the Federation of American Societies for Experimental Biology, called the *FASEB Biological Handbooks*, has appeared. So far the following volumes have been issued: *Blood and Other Body Fluids* (1961, re-issued 1971), *Growth, Including Reproduction and Morphological Development* (1962), *Environmental Biology* (1966), *Metabolism* (1968), *Respiration and Circulation* (1971), *Biology Data Book* (3 vols, 1972–1974), *Cell Biology* (1976), *Human Health and Disease* (1977), and *Inbred and Genetically Defined Strains of Laboratory Animals* (2 vols, 1979).

The application of mathematics and physics to pre-clinical medical sciences may involve both theory and practice. The encyclopaedic *Medical Physics* edited by O. Glasser. (3 vols, Year Book Medical Publishers, 1944–1960), may still be of use in the physical and mathematical aspects of biomedical research. *Biomathematics: the Principles of Mathematics for Students of Biological and General Science* by C. A. B. Smith (4th edn, 2 vols, Griffin, 1966–1969), is very useful; methodology is covered by *Statistical Methods for Research Workers* by R. A. Fisher (15th edn, Hafner, 1973), and data by the *Statistical Tables for Biological, Agricultural and Medical Research* by R. A. Fisher and F. Yates (6th edn, Longman, 1974). For the student there are *Statistical Exercises in Medical Research* by J. F. Osborn (Blackwell, 1979), and *Statistics at Square One* by T. D. V. Swinscow (7th edn, British Medical Association, 1980).

Dictionaries

While the major medical dictionaries are described in Chapter 4, mention may be made of the *Dictionary of Biological Terms* edited by I. F. and W. D. Henderson (9th edn, Longmans, 1979); a useful specialized work is the *Glossary of Genetics and Cytogenetics*,

Classical and Molecular by R. Rieger *et al.* (4th edn, Springer, 1976), which includes a bibliography giving the citations for many of the entries.

   Modern anatomical nomenclature is based on the *Basle Nomina Anatomica* (BNA) of 1895, which was revised in Britain in 1933 by the Anatomical Society at Birmingham (BR) and in Germany in 1935 by the German Anatomical Society at Jena (JNA or INA). The Fifth International Congress of Anatomists at Oxford in 1950 agreed to produce a new standard revision, which was ready for the Paris Congress in 1955 (PNA); the next two congresses approved minor corrections and the current authority is found in the *Nomina Anatomica* (3rd edn, Excerpta Medica, 1966). A comparative study of three systems – BNA, JNA and PNA – has been made by T. Donath in his *Anatomical Dictionary* (Pergamon, 1969), which presents the three systems with an explanatory dictionary and a list of authors named in eponyms, with biographical data. For a straightforward equation of PNA and BR nomenclatures Appendix I of *Butterworths Medical Dictionary* edited by MacDonald Critchley (Butterworths, 1978), is useful. A guide for students is *Anatomical Terms: Their Origin and Derivation* by E. J. Field and R. J. Harrison (3rd edn, Heffer, 1968).

Historical sources

Anatomy

Charles Singer's *Evolution of Anatomy* (Paul Kegan, 1925), an invaluable reference work, was reprinted as *A Short History of Anatomy from the Greeks to Harvey* (Dover, 1957). Two other useful works are G. W. Corner's *Anatomy* (Hoeber, 1930) and R. H. Hunter's *A Short History of Anatomy* (2nd edn, Bale, 1931). J. L. Choulant traced the evolution of anatomical illustration in *Geschichte und Bibliographie der anatomischen Abbildung* (Weigel, 1852); an English translation was published in 1920 (Chicago University Press) and reprinted with additional material in 1945. Jessie Dobson's *Anatomical Eponyms* (2nd edn, Livingstone, 1962) is a biographical dictionary of anatomists whose names are perpetuated in the nomenclature; it includes definitions of the structures eponyms and references to the works in which they are described.

Embryology

Joseph Needham's *History of Embryology* (2nd edn, Cambridge

University Press, 1934) is an exhaustive account with good illustrations and a valuable bibliography. *The Rise of Embryology* by A. W. Meyer (California University Press, 1939) includes a good bibliography, and vols 2–5 of H. B. Adelmann's *Marcello Malpighi and the Evolution of Embryology* (Cornell University Press, 1966) provide an extensive account of the development of embryology.

Physiology

J. F. Fulton's *Selected Readings in the History of Physiology* (2nd edn, C. C. Thomas, 1966) is an excellent introduction to the subject. The readings extend from Aristotle to twentieth-century writers and give access to many classical accounts otherwise difficult to come by. Other languages are translated into English. Michael Foster's *Lectures on the History of Physiology* (Cambridge University Press, 1901; reprinted 1924), although lacking in modern material, is worth reading. K. J. Franklin's *Short History of Physiology* (2nd edn, Staples, 1949) and Fulton's *Physiology* (Hoeber, 1931) though small, are useful. The best systematic account is probably K. E. Rothschuh's *Geschichte der Physiologie* (Springer, 1953) of which there is a revised and expanded English translation by G. B. Risse (Krieger, 1973). This includes a new English bibliography. A more recent account of the development of physiology is to be found in *The Pursuit of Nature – Informal Essays on the History of Physiology* by A. L. Hodgkin *et al.* (Cambridge University Press, 1977).

7

Biochemistry, biophysics and molecular biology

J. F. B. Rowland

Biochemistry is the study of the molecular changes that occur within living tissues. Biophysics is the study of living organisms by the techniques and concepts of physics. Out of the two subjects has grown Molecular Biology, which has so greatly enhanced man's understanding of the fundamental processes of life. The boundaries between these three disciplines are arbitrary. Biochemistry has traditionally concerned itself with the elucidation of metabolic reaction pathways, the study of the enzymes that catalyse the steps in those pathways and the mechanisms of control of the pathways. Molecular biology is taken to mean the study of the processes whereby an organism reproduces itself: the replication of DNA, the synthesis of RNA, the synthesis of protein and the relationships between the structure and the function of nucleic acids and of proteins. Biophysics has concentrated on the study of systems, such as membranes, biological fluids and muscle, where physical models are most applicable.

The field covered by these three subjects is itself interdisciplinary. They draw most heavily upon the fundamental concepts of chemistry, physics and mathematics – which may explain their relative unpopularity among medical students! Basic biological knowledge is necessary for the biochemist (this word, here and later, is taken to encompass the biophysicist and the molecular biologist), and this becomes the more true the closer to the molecular level the biological knowledge draws. So cell biology physiology and microbiology are disciplines closely related to biochemistry. Pharmacy, medicinal chemistry and agricultural chemistry are sciences where biochemical knowledge is extensively used. As is conventional, I have omitted 'the chemistry of natural products' from my definition of biochemistry. This area – the study, by purely chemical methods, of materials of organic origin, without any intention of elucidating the reactions that occur *in vivo* – is normally considered part of organic chemistry. However, chemical or physical studies of model systems are included in the subject matter of this chapter; an example might be the physical study of a model membrane.

There is a tendency for scientists to read, and to contribute to, the literature of the subject in which they originally trained. As biochemical techniques and concepts have achieved wider and wider usage, this has meant that essentially biochemical work has been reported in the literature of adjoining disciplines, because the authors regard themselves as 'chemists', say, or 'pharmacists', rather than 'biochemists'.

One other important point must be borne in mind about biochemistry. It is an essentially bipartite profession. On the one hand, the research biochemist has a general responsibility to broaden human knowledge and is therefore a very heavy user of the literature, and a prolific contributor to it. He or she may well work in a medical research laboratory, but has no responsibility, directly or indirectly, to specific patients. Clinical biochemists on the other hand, belong to one of the professions ancillary to medicine. They are primarily practitioners rather than researchers and are responsible to physicians and through them to patients. Their responsibility is to assist in diagnosis and treatment by the application of biochemical techniques and so they write rather less in the literature, and probably read it rather less, than research biochemists. Further, there is a separate literature of clinical biochemistry in which they write and read. When one reads of the spectacular growth of biochemistry and its literature over recent decades, it is mainly research biochemistry that is meant. Clinical biochemistry has grown in both volume and importance, and is an essential department in every hospital, but its growth has not been of such a spectacular kind.

That all of science has grown at a remarkable rate in recent years is well known. But biochemistry has grown even faster than most sciences. A measure of this is the biochemical sections of *Chemical Abstracts*. As is discussed later, there are some biochemical papers in other sections of *Chemical Abstracts,* but the biochemical sections do give an indication of the size and growth of the subject. A third of the abstracts in *Chemical Abstracts* are now in the biochemical sections, in spite of the youth of biochemistry compared with other branches of chemistry.

The actual numbers of papers in the biochemical sections for 1968–1977 are shown in *Table 7.1.*

TABLE 7.1 Number of abstracts appearing in the biochemical sections of *Chemical Abstracts,* **1968–1977**

Year	Number of abstracts in biochemical sections	Total number of abstracts in Chemical Abstracts	Biochemical sections as % of whole
1968	59 484	229 755	25.9
1969	70 472	252 320	27.9
1970	81 587	277 124	29.4
1971	94 027	308 976	30.4
1972	103 627	334 007	31.0
1973	100 748	321 005	31.4
1974	103 288	333 624	31.0
1975	132 278	392 234	33.7
1976	129 646	390 905	33.2
1977	138 351	410 137	33.7

* The figures for 1968–1970 were provided by Dr. J. T. Dickman, Chemical Abstracts Service; those for 1971–1977 were calculated by the author.

The very rapid growth of biochemical research in recent years is thought, by some biochemists, to stem from the development of new laboratory techniques. It is certainly true that biochemical research has always faced formidable difficulties of practical technique, attempting as it does to elucidate the chemical changes that occur within living cells. The major sources of this difficulty are:

(1) The chemical changes involve very small quantities of reactants.
(2) The biological samples under investigation are, by chemical standards, very complex mixtures.
(3) It is desirable to study the reactions while the cell continues to live.

It is also certainly true that certain modern techniques have rapidly become the standard methods of the biochemical research laboratory. Among these, the various chromatographic and electrophoretic separation methods are of primary importance: gas–liquid, thin-layer, paper, ion-exchange and molecular-sieve chromatography, and paper, thin-layer and gel electrophoresis are examples of the many different techniques now in use. Another important technique is the use of radioactively and other isotopically labelled compounds; these assist in solving both the problem of small quantities and the problem of studies *in vivo*; radioautography is especially useful with the latter problem. Thus, the literature of methods and techniques is of high importance to the biochemist; with the usual indexes it is often harder to track down a method that one needs than to find a general discussion of results in an area of the subject.

Primary journals

Research biochemists are rather more likely than some other types of scientist (chemists, for example) to work in universities, colleges, medical schools, medical research institutes or hospitals, and rather less likely to work in commercial or industrial employment. This is another factor that contributes to their very large production of literature; their work is not so likely to be written in the form of confidential internal reports. Patent literature is also of correspondingly limited importance in pure biochemistry – a contrast to its very great importance in the literature of the adjoining field of pharmaceutical chemistry. Furthermore, the very rapid development of techniques, concepts and factual knowledge in biochemistry means that the delays inherent in book publication are not often tolerable to the research biochemist. Consequently, publication in the scientific journals is of the highest importance. There is a large and increasing number of major journals covering the whole breadth of biochemistry, biophysics or both. The most important of these (with year of foundation and country of publication) are:

Journal of Biological Chemistry (1905) (US) is a journal of very high standards, well respected in the field; it is produced by the American Society of Biological Chemists.

Biochemistry (1962) (US) is published by the American Chemical Society and carries the biochemical papers that previously would have appeared in *Journal of the American Chemical Society*; as this origin suggests, it has a slight stress on the more chemical side of biochemistry. It is a journal of very high standards.

Biochemical Journal (1906) (UK) is the oldest established British journal in the field, and is published by the Biochemical Society. It is the preferred channel of publication for most British biochemists, but also carries a considerable amount of overseas matter; its standards are high, although it is sometimes criticized for its stress on the more classical areas of the subject; more modern material tends to find its way into the *Journal of Molecular Biology*. Since January 1973, it has been published in two series, *Molecular Aspects* and *Cellular Aspects*. At the same time, papers delivered at meetings of the Society, formerly carried at the back of the journal in a Proceedings section, were transferred to a separate journal called *Biochemical Society Transactions* (1973).

Biochimica et Biophysica Acta (1947) (Netherlands) accepts papers in English, French or German and is, perhaps, the journal of choice for most continental biochemists. It is also the most voluminous of the leading biochemical journals and appears in several simultaneous volumes, divided by subject matter (*Lipids and Lipid Metabolism; Nucleic Acids and Protein Synthesis; Biomembranes; Gene Structure and Expression; Protein Structure and Molecular Enzymology; Molecular Cell Research; Bioenergetics; General Subjects*). Review volumes are now also included, among them *Reviews on Cancer*, *Reviews on Biomembranes*, and *Reviews on Bioenergetics*.

Journal of Biochemistry (1922) (Japan) is published in English, and is the preferred journal of Japanese authors. Biochemically based industries, especially those based on fermentation processes for chemical and pharmaceutical production, are prominent in Japan and consequently much biochemical research of a high calibre is performed there.

Biokhimiya (1936) (USSR) is the leading Russian journal in this field. The Soviet Union is less renowned for life sciences than for engineering and physical sciences; however, the life sciences have been catching up in recent years. A cover-to-cover translation of *Biokhimiya*, entitled *Biochemistry: Biokhimiya*, is published in the US.

Hoppe-Seyler's Zeitschrift für physiologische Chemie (1877) (Germany) was the first journal devoted to the biochemical field, but, with the relative decline of Germany from its former position as the predominant scientific nation, it is less pre-eminent than it once was.

Biochemische Zeitschrift (1906) (Germany) was a similar publication to *Hoppe-Seyler;* however, when in 1967 the Federation of European Biochemical Societies started to publish the new *European Journal of Biochemistry* (1967) (Germany), it replaced the *Zeitschrift*, which had been entirely in German. The new *European Journal* accepts papers in English, French or German.

Journal of Molecular Biology (1959) (UK) has rapidly established itself as one of the most respected scientific journals in the world. It is edited from the Laboratory of Molecular Biology in Cambridge, a laboratory of exceptional renown, and its subject field is the most rapidly developing and exciting part of the whole biochemical area. These factors combine to make publication in this journal unusually prestigious, and consequently its editorial standards are particularly high.

Biochemical and Biophysical Research Communications (1959) (US) is a fast-publication organ. Urgent papers are published very quickly by photographic reproduction of the author's original typescript.

FEBS Letters (1968) (Germany) is a similar fast-publication journal produced by the Federation of European Biochemical Societies.

Archives of Biochemistry and Biophysics (1942) (US), *International Journal of Biochemistry* (1970) (UK) and *Bioscience Reports (Short Papers and Reviews in Molecular and Cellular Biology)* (1981) (UK) complete the list of the major journals that tend to contain papers from a variety of countries.

In addition, there are an increasing number of essentially 'national' biochemical journals, and some of these are:

Acta Biochimica et Biophysica Academiae Scientiarum Hungaricae (1966) (Hungary)
Acta Biochimica Polonica (1954) (Poland)
Biochimica e Biologia Sperimentale (1961) (Italy)
Canadian Journal of Biochemistry (1923) (Canada)
Indian Journal of Biochemistry (1964) (India)
Physiological Chemistry and Physics (1969) (US)
Studii si Cercetari de Biochimie (1959) (Romania)

In addition to these, there are also several purely biophysical journals, of which the best known is *Biophysical Journal* (1960) (US). Others are:

Biofizika (1956) (USSR)
Biophysik (1963) (Germany)
Bulletin of Mathematical Biophysics (1939) (US)
Studia Biophysica (1966) (Germany)

As one might expect in an interdisciplinary field that is growing rapidly, biochemistry has spilled out of its own journals and a large proportion of the important papers appear in more general periodicals. A large amount of biochemistry, biophysics and molecular biology appears in *Nature* (1868) (UK), for example.

The *Proceedings of the National Academy of Sciences of the*

United States of America (1915) has been the journal chosen for the announcement of many major biochemical discoveries, and doubtless will continue to be so in the future. Other general journals that regularly carry biochemical papers are:

Annals of the New York Academy of Sciences (1823) (US)
Comptes Rendus Hebdomadaires des Séances de L'Académie des Sciences, Série C: Sciences Chimiques et Série D: Sciences Naturelles (1835) (France)
Doklady Akademii Nauk SSSR (1828) (USSR)
Endeavour (1942) (UK)
Experientia (1945) (Switzerland)
Life Sciences (1962) (UK)
Naturwissenschaften (1913) (Germany)
Proceedings of the Royal Society, Series B (1800) (UK)
Proceedings of the Society for Experimental Biology and Medicine (1903) (US)
Science (1883) (US)

In recent years, the growth in biochemistry and the increasing specialization of biochemists have led to the appearance of a number of journals covering specific areas of biochemistry. These include:

Biochemical Genetics (1967) (US)
Biochemical Pharmacology (1951) (UK)
Biochemical Systematics and Ecology (1973) (UK)
Biopolymers (1963) (US)
Biorheology (1962) (US)
Carbohydrate Research (1965) (Netherlands)
Cereal Chemistry (1924) (USA)
Chemistry and Physics of Lipids (1966) (Netherlands)
Comparative Biochemistry and Physiology (1960) (US)
Enzymologia Biologica et Chimica (1961) (Switzerland)
Histochemical Journal (1968) (UK)
Histochemistry (1958) (Germany)
Immunochemistry (1964) (UK)
Insect Biochemistry (1971) (UK)
Journal of Bioenergetics and Biomembranes (1970) (US)
Journal of Histochemistry and Cytochemistry (1953) (US)
Journal of Lipid Research (1959) (US)
Journal of Neurochemistry (1957) (US)
Journal of Steroid Biochemistry (1969) (UK)
Journal of Supramolecular Structure (1972) (US)
Journal of Vitaminology (1954) (Japan)
Lipids (1966) (US)
Molecular and Cellular Biochemistry (1973) (Netherlands)
Molecular and Cellular Biology (1981) (US)
Molecular Immunology (1964) (US)
Molecular Pharmacology (1965) (US)
Nucleic Acids Research (1974) (UK)
Photochemistry and Photobiology (1962) (UK)
Phytochemistry (1961) (UK)
Process Biochemistry (1966) (UK)
Soil Biology and Biochemistry (1969) (UK)
Steroids (1963) (US)

A great deal of biochemical research is reported in the journals of adjoining fields of science. It is clearly not possible to mention all of these, and many are covered in other chapters of this book. Some of the more important that often contain biochemical work are listed below:

CHEMISTRY

Acta Chemica Scandinavica (1947) (Denmark)
Journal of the American Chemical Society (1879) (US)
Journal of the Chemical Society (various sections) (1849) (UK)

PHYSIOLOGY

American Journal of Physiology (1898) (US)
Journal of Cell Physiology (1932) (US)
Journal of General Physiology (1918) (US)
Journal of Physiology (1878) (UK)
Pflügers Archiv: European Journal of Physiology (1868) (Germany)

PHARMACY AND PHARMACOLOGY

British Journal of Pharmacology (1947) (UK)
Journal of Pharmacology and Experimental Therapeutics (1909) (US)
Journal of Pharmacy and Pharmacology (1919) (UK)
Journal of Pharmaceutical Sciences (1911) (US)

MEDICINAL CHEMISTRY AND BIOCHEMISTRY

Arzneimittelforschung (1951) (Germany)
Biochemical Medicine (1967) (US)
Journal of Experimental Medicine (1896) (US)
Journal of Medicinal Chemistry (1959) (US)

MICROBIOLOGY

Archiv für Mikrobiologie (1930) (Germany)
Japanese Journal of Microbiology (1957) (Japan)
Journal of Applied Bacteriology (1945) (US)
Journal of Bacteriology (1916) (US)
Journal of General Microbiology (1947) (UK)
Journal of General Virology (1967) (UK)

AGRICULTURAL AND FOOD CHEMISTRY

Journal of the Agricultural Chemical Society of Japan (1924) (Japan)
Journal of Agricultural and Food Chemistry (1950) (US)
Journal of Food Science (1936) (US)
Journal of the Science of Food and Agriculture (1953) (UK)

MEDICAL PHYSICS

Physics in Medicine and Biology (1956) (UK)

CANCER RESEARCH

British Journal of Cancer (1947) (UK)
Cancer (1948) (US)
Cancer Research (1944) (UK)
European Journal of Cancer and Clinical Oncology (1965) (UK)
International Journal of Cancer (1966) (Switzerland)
Journal of the National Cancer Institute (1940) (US)

NUTRITION
British Journal of Nutrition (1947) (UK)
Journal of Nutrition (1928) (US)

BIOENGINEERING
Biotechnology and Bioengineering (1962) (US)
Journal of Biochemical and Microbiological Technology and Engineering (1959) (UK)
Journal of Medical Engineering and Technology (1977) (UK)
Medical and Biological Engineering and Computing (1963) (UK)

CELL SCIENCE
Journal of Cell Biology (1955) (US)
Journal of Cell Science (1966) (UK)

In addition to these, there are the specialized journals for the clinical biochemist, such as:

Clinica Chimica Acta (1956) (Netherlands)
Clinical Chemistry (1955) (US)
Clinical and Experimental Pharmacology and Physiology (1974) (UK)
Clinical Pharmacology and Therapeutics (1960) (US)
Clinical Science and Molecular Medicine (1933) (UK)
European Journal of Clinical Pharmacology (1968) (Germany)
Journal of Clinical Pathology (1947) (UK)
Journal of Laboratory and Clinical Medicine (1915) (US)
Laboratory Investigation (1952) (US)
Medical Laboratory Sciences (1944) (UK)
Metabolism (Clinical and Experimental) (1952) (US)
Scandinavian Journal of Clinical Laboratory Investigation (1949) (Norway)

And also, there are the very useful journals devoted to techniques, of which the most significant are:

Chromatographia (1968) (Germany)
Journal of Chromatographic Science (1969) (US)
Journal of Chromatography (1958) (Netherlands)
Journal of Electron Microscopy (1953) (Japan)
Journal of Labelled Compounds (1968) (Belgium)
Laboratory Practice (1952) (UK)
Medical Laboratory Technology (1915) (US)
Organic Mass Spectrometry (1968) (UK)
Science Tools – The LKB Instrument Journal (1953) (Sweden)
Separation Science (1966) (US)

And, most important of all the methodological journals, there is *Analytical Biochemistry* (1960) (US).

As the amount of biochemical research undertaken and the number of practising biochemists have increased, so the pressure on space in the established journals has caused them to increase in size, and has brought new ones into being. Further, the rapid development of the subject has brought impatience with the slow and gentlemanly publishing methods that once prevailed. The

'Letter to *Nature*' has long been popular with authors as a vehicle for brief and urgent communications of important discoveries; work can appear in print within a month of being written. The popularity of this method of publication led to the establishment of *Biochemical and Biophysical Research Communications*, which photographically reproduces the author's typescript to achieve very rapid publication of short reports. *FEBS Letters*, produced by the Federation of European Biochemical Societies, now provides a European counterpart. Established journals carrying full-length papers now often contain a section of short communications, receiving accelerated treatment; *Biochimica et Biophysica Acta* and *Biochemical Journal* now both do this. None of these fast-publishing media, however, dispenses with strict editorial control of the quality of the papers; the short papers, like full-length papers in all the reputable primary journals, are published only after being approved by acknowledged scientific experts acting as editors and referees. It was intended that these fast-publishing media should carry preliminary reports of work that would ultimately appear as a full-length archival paper, and consequently the editing of the short papers is less stringent than that of full-length ones. Unfortunately it often happens that the fuller paper never appears, and the short communication remains the only report in the literature of that particular piece of work. Another recently launched rapid-publication journal for short papers is *Bioscience Reports*.

The Elsevier–North Holland group of publishers have also launched a series of rapid publication journals called '*Trends in . . .*', in newspaper format. *Trends in Biochemical Sciences*, known as *TIBS*, is probably the most successful of these chatty news journals.

Abstracts, title-lists and indexes

It is impossible for a hard-working research scientist to look at all the journals that might contain articles of interest, and for many years scientists have depended on abstracts journals. The first twenty sections of *Chemical Abstracts* cover biochemistry very fully. These sections are listed in *Table 7.2*; they appear fortnightly in the odd-numbered issues. Certain biochemical papers – notably those on biochemical macromolecules – can appear in other sections of *Chemical Abstracts*. The biochemical sections can be purchased as a separate publication if required. *Chemical Abstracts* covers conference proceedings, books and patents as well as journal articles. *Biological Abstracts* also covers this field in its sections entitled '*Biochemistry*', '*Metabolism*', '*Enzymes*' and '*Biophysics*'. Biochemical papers in other sections (such as Chemotherapy, Medical and Clinical Microbiology, Muscle, Immunology, or Plant Physiology, Biochemistry and Biophysics) can be traced by use of the CROSS index. The publishers of *Biological Abstracts* also publish *BioResearch Index*, a Keyword-in-Context index of papers and conference proceedings that are *not* included in *Biological Abstracts*. Another abstracts journal in this field is *Excerpta Medica*; Section 29: '*Biochemistry*', contains relevant abstracts in this field, but Section 3: '*Endocrinology*', Section 4: '*Microbiology*' and Section 26: '*Immunology, serology and transplantation*' may contain items of biochemical interest as well. The biochemical sections of two famous general abstracts journals – the French *Bulletin Signalétique* and the Russian *Referativnyi Zhurnal* – are also very valuable, especially for their coverage of foreign-language material.

TABLE 7.2. Biochemical Sections of *Chemical Abstracts*, 1972

Section number	Section title
1	Pharmacodynamics
2	Hormone pharmacology
3	Biochemical interactions
4	Toxicology
5	Agrochemicals
6	General biochemistry
7	Enzymes
8	Radiation biochemistry
9	Biochemical methods
10	Microbial biochemistry
11	Plant biochemistry
12	Non-mammalian biochemistry
13	Mammalian biochemistry
14	Mammalian pathological biochemistry
15	Immunochemistry
16	Fermentations
17	Foods
18	Animal nutrition
19	Fertilizers, soils, and plant nutrition
20	History, education and documentation

Each of these journals gives full bibliographical references to papers, a summary of their contents, and author and subject indexes. A somewhat different type of abstract is provided by *Current Abstracts of Chemistry and Index Chemicus*. Here the abstracts are mostly in the form of structural diagrams of chemical compounds, with little text; however, it is a rather specialized abstracts journal covering organic and pharmaceutical chemistry, and biochemistry is rather on the fringe of its coverage. Numerous other specialized abstracts journals exist; relevant titles worth mentioning here are *Analytical Abstracts,* useful for methodological information, and some of those produced by Information Retrieval Ltd: *Genetics Abstracts, Virology Abstracts, Nucleic Acids Abstracts* and *Microbiology Abstracts.*

Clinical biochemistry has, since 1969, had its own abstracts journal, entitled *Clinical Biochemistry.*

There are other journals which give only the titles and bibliographic references of papers, without any abstract. The most widely used of these is *Current Contents,* which consists of photographic reproductions of the contents pages of the original journals. There are several editions in different subject areas, each appearing weekly; *Current Contents, Life Sciences* covers biochemistry and chemistry. It also contains an author index to the title pages. Another title-list journal is the computer-produced *Chemical Titles;* the main body of the journal consists of a Keyword-in-Context (KWIC) index of the titles; each index entry gives an abstract number, and this refers to a list of the full bibliographic citations in the back of the issue. Biochemistry is towards the margin of the coverage of *Chemical Titles,* however. *Index Medicus* is another title-list journal; in this case the entries are given under index headings, chosen from a standard list of terms ('Medical Subject Headings'). Many of the more medical biochemical papers appear in it.

Reviews

While the abstracts and the title-list journals help the scientist to keep up with the flood of new papers appearing, they do not offer any critical appraisal of the research. In most fields of science, there are now regular series of publications entitled *Annual Review of . . ., Advances in . . ., Progress in . . .,* or some similar title. In these volumes, which are usually annual and in hard covers, acknowledged authorities review the year's progress in various fields, sifting the work and criticizing it, and providing bibliographies. Usually the book contains a number of such review articles, so as to cover the whole range of the subject given in the book's title. These volumes are of great value to research workers, especially, perhaps, in keeping up to date in fields a little way removed from their central interest. Numerous such series exist in biochemistry and biophysics, of which the most important is probably *Annual Review of Biochemistry*, published by Annual Reviews Inc., founded in 1932.

Other more specialized publications are:

Advances in Carbohydrate Chemistry and Biochemistry (Academic Press)
Advances in Comparative Physiology and Biochemistry (Academic Press)
Advances in Enzyme Regulation (Pergamon Press)
Advances in Enzymology (Interscience)
Advances in Lipid Research (Academic Press)
Advances in Microbial Physiology (Academic Press)
Advances in Protein Chemistry (Academic Press)
Advances in Steroid Biochemistry and Pharmacology (Academic Press)
Progress in Biochemical Pharmacology (Karger)
Progress in Nucleic Acid Research and Molecular Biology (Academic Press)
Progress in Phytochemistry (Interscience)
Recent Progress in Hormone Research (Academic Press)
Subcellular Biochemistry (Plenum)

For the biophysicist there is also *Advances in Biophysics* (University of Tokyo Press), and for the clinical biochemist there are *Advances in Clinical Chemistry* (Academic Press), *Progress in Clinical Pathology* (Grune and Stratton) and *Year Book of Pathology and Clinical Pathology* (Year Book Medical Publishers).

Series in adjoining fields often contain reviews relevant to biochemists; among these are:

Advances in Applied Microbiology (Academic Press)
Advances in Biomedical Engineering (Academic Press)
Advances in Cancer Research (Academic Press)
Advances in Drug Research (Academic Press)
Advances in Immunology (Academic Press)
Advances in Metabolic Disorders (Academic Press)
Advances in Pharmaceutical Sciences (Academic Press)
Advances in Pharmacology and Chemotherapy (Academic Press)
Annual Reports on the Progress of Chemistry (The Royal Society of Chemistry)
Annual Review of Microbiology (Annual Reviews Inc.)
Annual Review of Pharmacology and Toxicology (Annual Reviews Inc.)
Annual Review of Physiology (Annual Reviews Inc.)
Annual Review of Plant Physiology (Annual Reviews Inc.)
Current Topics in Membranes and Transport (Academic Press)
Progress in Industrial Microbiology (Churchill Livingstone)
Progress in Medical Genetics (Grune and Stratton)
Progress in Medicinal Chemistry (North Holland)
Progress in Medicinal Chemistry (Butterworths)
Year Book of Cancer (Year Book Medical Publishers)

All these series are annual and in hard covers. There are also review journals that appear more frequently, commonly quarterly, in soft covers; they do not attempt to cover the whole of their field in each issue. No such journal exists in biochemistry, but in biophysics there are *Quarterly Review of Biophysics* and *Progress in Biophysics and Molecular Biology* – the latter was formerly one of the annual volumes, but has been converted into a review journal. In adjoining fields there are:

Bacteriological Reviews
Biological Reviews
British Medical Bulletin
Chemical Reviews
Chemical Society Reviews (a merger of *Quarterly Reviews of the Chemical Society* and *Royal Institute of Chemistry Reviews*)
Physiological Reviews

In biochemistry there exists also *Essays in Biochemistry*; this appears annually in soft covers and contains a number of specialized reviews, but not a comprehensive coverage every year. The value of this publication is that it is aimed at undergraduates reading biochemistry, and therefore assumes rather less prior knowledge than most scientific journals. It is published by Academic Press for the Biochemical Society. The same idea has now been extended to clinical biochemistry. The Biochemical Society and the Association of Clinical Biochemists jointly publish *Essays in Medical Biochemistry,* the first issue of which appeared in 1975. In a similar context, mention should be made of *Scientific American;* articles in this journal often give excellent coverage of a topic for a newcomer.

Some journals mostly concerned with primary scientific papers include review articles from time to time. Among journals that do this are *Journal of Lipid Research* and *Physics in Medicine and Biology*. The journal *Progress in Histochemistry and Cytochemistry* (Gustav Fischer Verlag) appears in soft covers and consists of just one review per issue.

Finally, among these various types of review, come the less frequent type of review series that attempt to take a longer term view of progress, no easy task in such a rapidly evolving subject, but one that needs to be undertaken by some leading researchers if the subject is to have a sense of direction. Unfortunately, the three main series that exist have all been allowed to fall seriously behind events; it is to be hoped that at least one of them will appear again in a new edition. They are:

Currents in Biochemical Research, edited by D. E. Green (2nd edn, Interscience, 1956)
Progress in Biochemistry since 1949, edited by F. Haurowitz (5th edn, Interscience, 1959)
Recent Advances in Biochemistry, edited by T. W. Goodwin (4th edn, Churchill, 1960)

To assist in keeping track of the review literature, a third tier of 'indexes to reviews' now exists. Relevant to the problem in bio-chemistry are:

Bibliographic Index, edited by M. Frank (Wilson, 1958–)
Index to Reviews, Symposia, Volumes and Monographs in Organic Chemistry (Pergamon, 1962–)

Each of these is a continuing series, updated annually.

Conferences and symposia

Another source of information that is extensively used in many fast-progressing areas of science is the scientific meeting, conference or symposium. These can be divided into two types: the regular general meetings of scientific societies, and specialized meetings to discuss a particular topic, though there are, of course, borderline cases. The general meetings – international, or more local – provide opportunities for scientists to deliver a large number of short papers describing their current work. The information that emerges from them is therefore up to date, but it is usually subject to far less quality control than is applied to journal articles. Some of the work subsequently appears in such articles, in a fuller form; other pieces of work do not reach a conclusive enough state for publication and are never heard of again. In the biochemical field the most important such meetings are the International Congresses of Biochemistry, of which a number have now been held. The publication of their proceedings has taken rather variable forms; for example, the fourth congress (Vienna, 1958) ran to 15 volumes because full texts of all the papers were given, whereas the sixth (New York, 1964) appeared in only two volumes. In the latter case, only abstracts of the ordinary papers were issued, and they occupied one volume; the plenary lectures, which are of a more review-like nature, were given in full in the other volume.

The meetings of the Federation of European Biochemical Societies are of similar importance; their proceedings are, however, published as a regular series, *Proceedings of the Federation of European Biochemical Societies*. In the US a number of societies publish their proceedings in a joint journal called *Federation Proceedings*, the joint body being called the Federation of American Societies for Experimental Biology. Closer to home, the papers given at the regular meetings of the (British) Biochemical Society are published as *Biochemical Society Transactions;* again, however, it must be stressed that they are not subject to the editorial control that is applied to the *Biochemical Journal*. The Biochemical Society also holds more specialized symposia from time to time, and these are published as a separate series entitled *Biochemical Society Symposia.*

The information value of the large general meetings is, however, probably greater for those who attend the meetings than for those who read the proceedings afterwards. The specialized symposia, on the other hand, often provide, in their published proceedings, reviews of specialized topics that remain authoritative and valuable for years. Important series of symposia regularly covering biochemical topics are:

Biochemical Society Symposia
Brookhaven Symposia in Biology
Ciba Foundation Symposia
Cold Spring Harbor Symposia on Quantitative Biology
Colloquia on Protides of the Biological Fluids
Federation Proceedings, Symposia
Symposia of the International Society for Cell Biology
Symposia of the Society for Experimental Biology
Symposia of the Society for General Microbiology

Each of these series is published regularly, on a different topic on each occasion, in book form except for the last mentioned. If a recent volume in one of these series covers a topic of interest, it will be of great value.

There are, of course, also many 'one-off' symposia and ones in lesser series, whose proceedings subsequently appear. These can be difficult to track down, though they are covered by *Chemical Abstracts.* Some examples are:

Regulation of Macromolecular Synthesis by Low Molecular Weight Mediators edited by G. Koch and D. Richter (Academic Press, 1979)
Biochemical Aspects of Prostaglandins and Thromboxanes edited by N. Kharasch and J. Fried (Academic Press, 1977)
Nonsense Mutations and tRNA Suppressors edited by J. E. Celis and D. Smith (Academic Press, 1979)
Phosphatidylcholine edited by H. Peeters (Springer-Verlag, 1976)
Natural Sulfur Compounds edited by D. Cavallini, G. E. Gaull and V. Zappia (Plenum, 1980)
Biotechnological Applications of Proteins and Enzymes edited by Z. Bohak and N. Sharon (Academic Press, 1977)
Biomolecular Structure and Function edited by P. Agris (Academic Press, 1978)

Various lists of forthcoming and past conferences exist to help a searcher to locate an appropriate volume of proceedings. Probably the most useful is *Interdok – Directory of Published Proceedings* (Interdok Corp.). This appears monthly and gives a list of conferences, arranged chronologically by the date of the conference, each entry giving the title, editor, publisher and price of the proceedings. At the back there are indexes of subjects, sponsors, and editors of the proceedings. A similar service is provided by the

Index to Conference Proceedings Received, published by the British Library Lending Division (Boston Spa, West Yorkshire, UK).

There are also series of invited lectures, whose published texts subsequently serve as reviews of the field. Among those that appear as independent publications are:

Ciba Lectures in Microbial Chemistry
The Harvey Lectures
E. R. Squibb Lectures on the Chemistry of Microbial Products

Other similar lectures are given in response to the award of a medal or prize to a distinguished scientist by a scientific society, and are subsequently published in the society's journal. Journals which contain such lectures from time to time include the *Biochemical Journal, Journal of General Microbiology* and *European Journal of Biochemistry.*

Metabolic Maps

A form of 'review' which is peculiar to biochemistry is the metabolic map. This is a chart showing diagrammatically the metabolic pathways that have been demonstrated to exist. These are often supplied by the manufacturers or distributors of biochemical laboratory materials. Koch-Light Laboratories, for example, distribute a large chart entitled *Metabolic Pathways* by D. E. Nicholson, which is updated annually. It is in four colours and covers all the main areas of metabolism. It is accompanied by an explanatory booklet containing an index and notes on the reactions. The same author, with S. Dagley, has also produced a more detailed book entitled *An Introduction to Metabolic Pathways* (Blackwell, 1970) in which the evidence for the pathways is presented. Two other manufacturers who produce charts are Boehringer *(Biochemical Pathways,* two charts, 1965) and Gilson Medical Electronics *(Intermediary Metabolism* by H. J. Sallech and R. W. McGilvery four charts, 1963). The famous biochemist W. W. Umbreit produced a set of charts bound into book form, entitled *Metabolic Maps* (two volumes, Burgess, 1952–1960), but this publication is now out of date. The textbook *Introduction to Modern Biochemistry* by P. Karlson (4th edn, Academic Press, 1974) contains several large pull-out charts of metabolic pathways. Another book *Graphic Biochemistry: Metabolism of Biological Molecules* by T. B. Bennett (Macmillan, 1968), contains many reactions laid out in diagrammatic form.

Any of the large charts can be used very profitably as a rapid *aide mémoire*; it is a good idea to have one of them up on the laboratory wall so that one can consult it to refresh one's memory when reading something else.

Books

It is more true in biochemistry than in most subjects that a book is bound to be out of date before it is published, but this does not deter biochemists from writing and reading them. The books may be classified into several types:

(1) Large multi-volume treatises covering an area of the subject in great depth.
(2) Monographs covering a very specialized area – these may be published as part of a monograph series, of which *Methuen's Monographs on Biochemical Subjects* is probably the best-known, or as an isolated event.
(3) Textbooks for students at various levels.
(4) Encyclopaedias and dictionaries.
(5) Handbooks and other compilations of data.

The leading multi-volume treatises are:

Comparative Biochemistry edited by M. Florkin and H. S. Mason (7 vols, Academic Press, 1960–1964)

The Enzymes edited by P. D. Boyer (12 vols, 3rd edn, Academic Press, 1970–)

The Carbohydrates by W. Pigman and D. Horton (3 vols, 2nd edn, Academic Press, 1972)

The Proteins edited by H. Neurath (5 vols, 3rd edn, Academic Press, 1977)

The Hormones edited by G. Pincus, K. V. Thimann and E. B. Astwood (5 vols, Academic Press, 1948–1964)

The Vitamins edited by W. W. Sebrell and R. S. Harris (vols 1–5) and P. Gyorgy and W. N. Pearson (vols. 6–7) (7 vols, 2nd edn, Academic Press, 1967–)

Enzymes and Metabolic Inhibitors edited by J. L. Webb (5 vols, Academic Press, 1963–)

Metabolic Pathways edited by D. M. Greenberg (6 vols, 3rd edn, Academic Press, 1967–1972)

Biochemistry of Animal Development edited by R. Weber (2 vols, Academic Press, 1965–1967)

Handbuch der Pflanzenphysiologie edited by W. Ruhland (18 vols, Springer, 1955–)

Mammalian Protein Metabolism edited by H. N. Munro and J. B. Allison (4 vols, Academic Press, 1964–1970)

Molecular Biology of Human Proteins, with Special Reference to Plasma Proteins by H. E. Schultze and J. F. Heremans (Elsevier, 1966–)

Chemistry of the Amino Acids by J. B. Greenstein and M. Winitz (3 vols, Wiley, 1961)

Biochemistry of the Amino Acids by A. Meister (2 vols, 2nd edn, Academic Press, 1965)

The Amino Sugars edited by R. W. Jeanloz and E. A. Balazs (Academic Press, 1965–)

Metabolic Inhibitors: A Comprehensive Treatise edited by R. M. Hochester, M.
   Kates and J. H. Quastel (3 vols, Academic Press, 1972)
Bio-organic Chemistry by E. E. van Tamelen (4 vols, Academic Press, 1978)
Isozymes: Genetics and Evolution by C. L. Markert (4 vols, Academic Press, 1975)

The most ambitious of these publications, however, is *Comprehensive Biochemistry* edited by M. Florkin and E. H. Stotz (31 vols,
Elsevier, 1961–). This treatise covers the entire subject, each
volume being devoted to a specialized area. One drawback of these
treatises, especially the larger ones, is the fact that the different
volumes are always out of date to different extents at any one time.
   Monographs appear in large numbers every year. In addition to
the Methuen series already mentioned, there are also three relevant series from Academic Press (*Molecular Biology, Advanced
Biochemistry,* and *Medicinal Chemistry*), and also Elsevier's '*BBA
Library*' (linked with the journal *Biochimica et Biophysica Acta*).
Springer-Verlag produces a series called *Molecular Biology,
Biochemistry and Biophysics.* In Butterworths *MTP International
Review of Science* there is a Biochemistry Series. Any list of recent
significant titles will soon be overtaken by time, but some recent
monographs are nevertheless mentioned:

Fundamentals of Enzymology by N. C. Price and L. Steven (Oxford University
   Press, 1982)
Collagen: The Anatomy of a Protein by J. Woodhead-Galloway (Arnold, 1980)
Energy and the Living Cell by W. M. Becker (Lippincott, 1977)
Prostaglandin Synthesis by J. S. Bindra and R. Bindra (Academic Press, 1977)
Prostaglandins in Reproduction by N. L. Poyser (Research Studies Press, 1981)
Fundamentals of Enzyme Kinetics by A. Cornish-Bowden (Butterworths, 1978)
Molecular Biology and Biochemistry: Problems and Applications by D. Freifelder
   (Freeman, 1978)
Enzymatic Reaction Mechanims by C. Walsh (Freeman, 1979)
Molecular Biophysics by M. V. Volkenshtein (Academic Press, 1977)

Over the years many leading biochemists have set out to produce textbooks of the subject for students at various levels. Many
of the ones now in use are of American origin, and have been written in response to the trend in the US for basic college courses in
biology to have a considerable biochemical emphasis. Others are
larger works, intended to cover the whole of the subject for the
student specializing in it. They rarely succeed, since an undergraduate specializing in biochemistry will, by the time the latter part
of the course is reached, need to be more up to date than a textbook can be. Nonetheless, every student needs to have one of the
large texts within easy reach for continual reference, and these can
be of similar use to non-students. Not all the major textbooks have
been regularly up-dated, and the appended list includes only those
that have appeared in a new edition relatively recently:

Introduction to Physiological and Pathological Chemistry by L. E. Arnow (9th edn, Mosby, 1976)

The Biochemistry of the Tissues by W. Bartley and L. M. Birt (2nd edn, Wiley, 1976)

Biochemistry: A Comprehensive Review by N. V. Bhagavan (2nd edn, Lippincott, 1978)

Companion to Biochemistry: Selected Topics for Further Study by A. T. Bull, J. R. Lagnado, J. O. Thomas and K. F. Tipton (Longmans, vol 1, 1974, and vol 2, 1979).

Biochemistry Illustrated by P. N. Campbell and A. D. Smith (Churchill Livingstone, 1982)

Outlines of Biochemistry by E. E. Conn and P. K. Stumpf (4th edn, Wiley, 1976)

Biochemistry by S. P. Datta and J. H. Ottaway (3rd edn, Baillière Tindall, 1976)

Biochemistry for Medical Sciences by I. Danishefsky (Little Brown, 1980)

Review of Physiological Chemistry by H. A. Harper (18th edn, Lange Medical, 1981)

Biochemistry by A. L. Lehninger (2nd edn, Worth Publishers Inc., 1975)

Biochemistry – A Case-Oriented Approach by R. Montgomery, K. L. Dryer, T. W. Conway and A. A. Spector (3rd edn, Mosby, 1980)

Introduction to Human Biochemistry by C. A. Pasternak (Oxford University Press, 1979)

The Chemistry of Life by S. Rose (2nd edn, Pelican, 1979)

Biochemistry by L. Stryer (2nd edn, Freeman, 1981)

Introduction to Biochemistry by J. W. Suttie (Holt Saunders, 1977)

Principles of Biochemistry by A. White, P. Handler, E. L. Smith, R. L. Hill and I. R. Lehman (6th edn, McGraw-Hill, 1978)

Comprehensible Biochemistry by M. Yudkin and R. Offord (Longmans, 1973)

Textbooks on the clinical side are *Fundamentals of Clinical Chemistry* by N. W. Tietz (Saunders, 1970), *Clinical Biochemistry (Cantarow and Trumper)* edited by A. L. Latner (7th edn, Saunders, 1975) and *The Biochemistry of Clinical Medicine* by W. S. Hoffman (4th edn, Year Book Medical Publishers, 1970).

A recent development is the appearance of programmed texts for the biochemistry student. Unlike more orthodox textbooks, these cannot be used as reference books, but only as learning aids. As such, therefore, they are perhaps of less interest to the average reader of this book; a few are, however, mentioned, in case the reader should happen to be a complete newcomer to biochemistry:

Concepts in Biochemistry by W. K. Stephenson (Wiley, 1967)

Enzyme Kinetics by H. N. Christensen and G. A. Palmer (Saunders, 1967)

Chemistry of Amino Acids, Peptides and Proteins by T. C. Myers and J. S. Allender (Harper and Row, 1968)

Guide to Cellular Energetics by L. C. Carter (W. H. Freeman, 1973)

Multiple-Choice Questions in Biochemistry by D. G. O'Sullivan and W. R. D. Smith (Arnold, 1980)

Life's Basis: Macromolecules by G. E. Parker and T. B. Mertens (Wiley, 1973)

Biochemistry – A Functional Approach by R. W. McGilvery (2nd edn, Saunders, 1980)

Also aimed at the student reader are books of quantitative

problems for use as exercises, such as *Quantitative Problems in Biochemistry* by E. A. Dawes (6th edn, Longmans, 1980) and *Quantitative Problems in Biochemical Science* by R. Montgomery and C. A. Swenson (2nd edn, Freeman, 1976).

There have been very few attempts to produce alphabetically arranged dictionaries or encyclopaedias in this field, possibly because of the frequent updatings that would be necessary. An attempt is *The Encylopaedia of Biochemistry* edited by R. J. Williams and E. M. Lansford, Jr (Van Nostrand Reinhold, 1967), which is very useful as a quick reference tool for information outside one's own special area of knowledge. It is to be hoped that it will be revised from time to time. *The Merck Index of Chemicals and Drugs* (9th edn, 1976), though confined to information about individual compounds, is another very useful tool. Two other alphabetical books, both edited by P. Gray, that are also of value in the biochemical field are *Encylopaedia of Biological Sciences* (2nd edn, Van Nostrand Reinhold, 1969) and *Dictionary of the Biological Sciences* (1967). Further alphabetical dictionaries have recently appeared: *Dictionary of Biochemistry* by J. Stenesh (Wiley-Interscience, 1975), *Glossary of Molecular Biology* by A. Evans (Butterworths, 1974) and, on the clinical side, *Glossary of Clinical Chemical Terms* by P. Haisman and B. Muller (Butterworths, 1974).

A number of handbooks exist for use when one needs not so much a full discussion or a definition, but more a single piece of reliable data. The 'Rubber Bible', *Handbook of Chemistry and Physics* (62nd edn, 1981), is as indispensable to biochemists or biophysicists as it is to their non-biological colleagues. The same publishers (Chemical Rubber Publishing Co.) have now also produced another handbook more specifically for biochemists: *Handbook of Biochemistry: Selected Data for Molecular Biology* (2nd edn, 1971). Apart from this, the most important purely biochemical handbook is probably *Data for Biochemical Research* edited by R. M. C. Dawson, D. C. Elliott, W. H. Elliott and K. M. Jones (2nd edn, 1969); it is designed specifically to be useful in the laboratory and has therefore been kept compact. For more exhaustive coverage, one might turn to *The Biochemist's Handbook* edited by C. Long (1961), which contains over 300 tables of data on all aspects of biochemistry – for example, enzymes, chemical composition of biological tissues, nutritional data and metabolic pathways. It is now out-of-date and a new edition would be welcome. Another compilation that, like the *Merck Index*, concentrates on compound data is *Specifications and Criteria of Biochemical Compounds* (Committee on Biological Chemistry and Chemical Technology, US National Academy of Sciences; this is loose-leaf so that supplements can be added to it. It first appeared in 1960 and supplements have appeared since. It gives full information on each compound: structure, sources, method of preparation, physical criteria (melting point, specific rotation, chromatographic mobilities and extinction coefficients), methods of assay, stability, and methods of storage. Another handbook of considerable value is *Biochemisches Taschenbuch* edited by H. M. Rauen (2 vols, 2nd edn, 1964), and another is *Handbook of Biochemistry and Biophysics,* edited by H. C. Ramm (1966). Several handbooks that cover parts of the subject exist; these include *The Enzyme Handbook* edited by T. E. Barman (1969, 2 vols; *Supplement I,* 1974) and *The Pfizer Handbook of Microbial Metabolites. Atlas of Protein Structure and Sequence* edited by M. O. Dayhoff, attempts to give the amino acid sequence of every protein for which the sequence has been determined, and by 1978 had reached the third supplementary volume to volume 5. A competitor to Dayhoff is *Handbook of Protein Sequence Analysis* by L. R. Croft (2nd edn, Wiley, 1980), and an equivalent volume in a specialized area of protein chemistry is *Variable Regions of Immunoglobulin Chains* by E. A. Kabat, T. T. Wu and H. Bilofsky (National Institutes of Health, 1976). An indispensable volume for the serious biochemist is *Enzyme Nomenclature: Recommendations 1972 of the International Union of Pure and Applied Chemistry and the International Union of Biochemistry* (Elsevier, 1973); this gives not only the rules for the classification and nomenclature of enzymes, but also coverage of enzyme kinetics; it also contains 2743 references and is thus an important bibliography of enzymology.

There are also two handbooks designed for the clinical biochemist. The older one is another of the Chemical Rubber Publishing Co.'s publications, *Handbook of Clinical Chemistry Data* (2nd edn, 1968), and the newer is *Biochemical Values in Clinical Medicine* by R. D. Eastham (6th edn, John Wright, 1978).

Methods and techniques

The importance of technical information has already been stressed and some specifically 'methods' journals have been mentioned. However, many of the most important techniques were originally described in the 'experimental' section of a paper in a general biochemical journal. The most celebrated example is a paper by O. H. Lowry (*Journal of Biological Chemistry,* vol 193, page 265, 1951). This paper describes the standard method of measuring the concentration of protein in a solution and is reckoned to be the most frequently cited reference in the whole of science. How would one find a similar, but less famous, reference to a method, if one did not know where to look?

There fortunately exist numerous handbooks of laboratory methods for biochemists. Some of these appear as serial publications, often annually:

Methods of Biochemical Analysis edited by D. Glick (Interscience, 1954–). Volumes appear annually, and both chemical and biological assays of materials of biochemical importance are described in full laboratory detail.

Biochemical Preparations (Wiley, 1949–) appears less frequently (about once every 1–2 years) and gives details of methods for the preparation or isolation of compounds and enzymes, independently checked.

Methods in Medical Research (Year Book Medical Publishers, 1955–) is more general but usually includes methods of interest to the biochemist.

Chromatography Reviews edited by M. Lederer (Elsevier, 1959–), which covers electrophoretic as well as chromatographic methods, is an important aid to the biochemist, these separation methods being so central in biochemical research.

Advances in Tracer Methodology edited by S. Rothschild (Plenum, 1962–), covers this important area of isotopic tracer methods.

Methods in Enzymology previously edited by S. P. Colowick and N. O. Kaplan, but now with various editors (Academic Press, 1955–), was originally a multi-volume treatise, but since 1966 has been converted into a serial publication, volumes appearing two or three times a year. It is probably the most authoritative of these series, the scope of the work being far broader than the title suggests. Methods for the preparation and for the assay of a large number of enzymes are indeed given, but so are the preparation of enzyme substrates, methods for the handling of biological materials, protein purification techniques, metabolic studies and isotopic methods. Sufficient detail is given for the methods to be used without further reading.

Advances in Chromatography is edited by J. C. Giddings and R. A. Keller (Arnold, 1966–).

Laboratory Techniques in Biochemistry and Molecular Biology edited by T. S. Work and R. H. Burdon (North Holland, 1969–) is one of the major series of this type.

Methods in Molecular Biology edited by J. A. Last and A. I. Laskin (Marcel Dekker, 1972–) covers the important molecular biology area.

Clinical biochemistry is also served by one of the series, *Standard Methods of Clinical Chemistry* edited by D. Seligson (Academic Press, 1953–).

Several large treatises exist on the methodological side of biochemistry. Amongst these are:

Methods in Hormone Research edited by R. I. Dorfmann (2nd edn, Academic Press, 1968–)

Physical Techniques in Biological Research edited by G. Oster and A. W. Pollister (6 vols, 2nd edn, Academic Press, 1968)

Techniques in Protein Biosynthesis edited by P. N. Campbell and J. R. Sargent (3 vols, Academic Press, 1967–1973)

Newer Methods of Nutritional Biochemistry by A. A. Albanese (Academic Press, 1964–)

Methods in Carbohydrate Chemistry edited by R. L. Whistler and M. L. Wolfrom (5 vols, Academic Press, 1962–1965)

Moderne Methoden der Pflanzenanalyse edited by K. Paech and M. V. Tracey (vols 1–4), H. F. Liskens and M. V. Tracey (Vols 5–) (Springer, 1956–). This book is mostly in English

Experimental Biochemistry by J. M. Clark and R. L. Switzer (Freeman, 1977)

Electron Microscopy of Enzymes edited by M. A. Hayat (4 vols, Van Nostrand Reinhold, 1975)

A Laboratory Manual of Analytical Methods in Protein Chemistry edited by P. Alexander and R. J. Block (5 vols to date, Pergamon, 1960–)

Monographs on methods are legion, but some are in such constant use in biochemical laboratories that they must be singled out. I. Smith's *Chromatographic and Electrophoretic Techniques* (vol 1: *Chromatography;* vol 2: *Electrophoresis*) (4th edn, Heinemann, 1976) is an essential book of this kind. Other important works on separation methods are:

Separation Methods in Biochemistry by C. J. O. R. Morris and P. Morris (Pitman, 1964)

New Biochemical Separations by A. T. James and L. J. Morris (Van Nostrand, 1963)

Separation Techniques in Chemistry and Biochemistry by R. A. Keller (Dekker, 1967)

Laboratory Handbook of Chromatographic Methods edited by O. Mikes (Van Nostrand, 1966)

Separation Methods in Organic Chemistry and Biochemistry by F. J. Wolf (Academic Press, 1969)

There are also numerous more specialized works on different separation methods. A representative selection is given:

Thin-Layer Chromatography: A Laboratory Handbook by J. S. Kirshner (Interscience, 1967)

Quantitative Paper and Thin-Layer Chromatography edited by E. J. Shellard (Academic Press, 1968)
Techniques of Thin-Layer Chromatography in Amino Acid and Peptide Chemistry by G. Pataki (2nd edn, Ann Arbor Science Publishers, 1968)
The Practice of Gas Chromatography by L. S. Ettre and A. Zlatkis (Interscience, 1967)
A Programmed Introduction to Gas Chromatography by J. B. Pattison (Heyden, 1969)
Gas-Phase Chromatography of Steroids by K. B. Eik-Nes and E. C. Horning (Springer, 1968)
Quantitative Gas–Liquid Chromatography of Amino Acids in Proteins and Biological Substances by C. W. Gehrke (Analytical Biochemistry Laboratories, 1969)
Gas Chromatography by H. Determan (Springer, 1968)
Electrophoresis by D. J. Shaw (Academic Press, 1969)
Electrophoresis and Immunoelectrophoresis by L. Cawley (Little, Brown, 1969)
Methods in Zone Electrophoresis by J. R. Sargent (BDH Publications, 1969)

As mentioned earlier, the use of radioactive tracers in elucidating biological reactions has been very great and, not surprisingly, a large number of books on these techniques have also appeared. Some of these are mentioned below:

Principles of Radioisotope Methodology by G. D. Chase and J. L. Rabinowitz (2nd edn, Burgess, 1966)
Radiotracer Techniques in Biological Sciences by C. H. Wang and D. L. Willis (Prentice-Hall, 1965)
Tritium-Labelled Molecules in Biology and Medicine by L. E. Feinendegen (Academic Press, 1967)
Isotopes in Biology by G. Wolf (Academic Press, 1964)
Radioactive Isotopes in Biochemistry by E. Broda (Elsevier, 1960)
Labelled Nucleotides in Biochemistry by R. Monks, K. G. Oldham and K. C. Tovey (Radiochemical Centre, 1971)

The spectroscopic techniques that have revolutionized organic chemistry in recent years have, with the exception of ultraviolet spectroscopy, been rather slower to be adopted in the biochemical laboratory. This is probably because the complexity of the chemical systems within living organisms makes the spectra very hard to interpret. Nevertheless, most of these methods have now come into use in the biochemical laboratory, often with the aid of the computer for interpretation. Books describing the particular application of these methods to biological systems are listed; there are, of course, also large numbers of books describing the techniques themselves without special reference to biological use:

Nuclear Magnetic Resonance in Biochemistry by T. L. James (Academic Press, 1975)
Interpretation of the Ultraviolet Spectra of Natural Products by A. I. Scott (Pergamon, 1964)
Structure Elucidation of Natural Products by Mass Spectrometry by H. Budzikiewicz, C. Djerassi and D. H. Williams (2 vols, Holden-Day, 1964)
Magnetic Resonance in Biological Systems edited by A. Ehrenberg, B. G. Malstrom and T. Vanngard (Pergamon, 1967)

The Biological and Biochemical Applications of Electron Spin Resonance by D. J. E. Ingram (Hilger, 1969)

Fluorescence Assay in Biology and Medicine by S. Udenfreund (1st vol, 3rd printing, Academic Press, 1965; 2nd vol, Academic Press, 1969)

One technique very specific to biochemistry is ultracentrifugation, for the separation of sub-cellular particles and biological macromolecules, and the measurement of their molecular weights. The authoritative work on this technique is *The Ultracentrifuge in Biochemistry* by H. K. Schachman (Academic Press, 1959), and a very useful book for the newcomer to the subject is *An Introduction to Ultracentrifugation* by T. J. Bowen (Wiley, 1970). Other works on the subject are:

Mathematical Theory of Sedimentation Analysis by H. Fujita (Academic Press, 1962)

Ultracentrifugal Analysis in Theory and Experiment edited by J. W. Williams (Academic Press, 1963)

Ultracentrifugation by J. S. McCall and B. J. Potter (Baillière Tindall, 1973)

Some of the less modern, but still important, classic methods are provided with major works that are essentials of the biochemical laboratory. One of these is H. U. Bergmeyer's *Methods of Enzymatic Analysis* (Verlag-Chemie and Academic Press, 1963), which describes the use of enzymes as analytical tools, often for the assay of other enzymes – a technique which has been responsible for many of the most elegant determinations of metabolic pathways, and one that also finds use in clinical biochemistry. H. U. Bergmeyer has now produced a more up-to-date book entitled *Principles of Enzymatic Analysis* (Verlag-Chemie, 1978). Another classic is *Manometric Techniques* by W. W. Umbreit, R. H. Burris and J. F. Stauffer (Burgess, 1963). Manometric techniques were one of the earliest major tools of the biochemist, and are still very useful today in the study of any enzymic reaction that involves the evolution or absorption of a gas. The book is much more general than the title suggests and could, indeed, serve as an introductory text to practical biochemistry in general.

In the specialized but important area of protein chemistry, *Techniques in Protein Chemistry* by J. Leggett Bailey (2nd edn, Elsevier, 1969) is the authoritative work; it describes all the major methods used in elucidating the amino acid sequence of proteins. A number of other recent books on methods in particular areas of the subject are also mentioned herein, although, as with monographs in biochemistry generally, the list given is only a selection of recent publications from an enormous number:

Biochemistry and Methodology of Lipids edited by A. R. Johnson and J. B. Davenport (Wiley-Interscience, 1971)

Amino Acid Determination – Methods and Techniques by S. Blackburn (Arnold, 1968)
Procedures in Nucleic Acid Research edited by G. L. Cantoni and D. R. Davies (Harper and Row, 1967)
Protein Sequence Determination edited by S. B. Needleman (Chapman and Hall, and Springer, 1970)
An Introduction to Isozyme Techniques by G. J. Brewer and C. F. Sing (Academic Press, 1970)
Analysis of Triglycerides by C. Litchfield (Academic Press, 1972)
A Flexible System of Enzymatic Analysis by O. H. Lowry and J. V. Passoneau (Academic Press, 1972)
Handbook of Micromethods for the Biological Sciences by G. Keleti and W. H. Lederer (Van Nostrand Reinhold, 1974)
Introduction to Protein Sequence Analysis by L. R. Croft (Wiley, 1980)

And, on the clinical side, there are *Clinical Chemistry and Automation: A Study in Laboratory Proficiency* by R. Robinson (Griffin, 1972) and *Automation of a Biochemistry Laboratory* by G. E. Sims (Butterworths, 1972).

History of biochemistry

The serious student of biochemistry ought to spend at least a little time learning about the history and development of the subject; indeed, I have found that the historical method of approach improves one's understanding of some of the more complex areas of the subject, such as molecular biology. One follows the train of thought of the pioneers and thus better appreciates the reasons why currently held theories have evolved.

No journals are devoted specifically to the history of biochemistry, but papers on the history of biochemistry can be found in the more general *Journal of the History of Medicine and Allied Sciences* (1946–) (US), *Medical History* (1957–) (UK), *Koroth* (1953–) (Israel), etc. Papers in *Perspectives in Biology and Medicine* (1957–) (US) are often written in a more personal and biographical style than those in most journals. A valuable source for biographical data is *Selected Bibliography of Biographical Data for the History of Biochemistry since 1800* by J. S. Fruton (2nd edn, American Philosophical Society, 1977).

The treatise *Comprehensive Biochemistry* edited by Florkin and Stotz, mentioned earlier, devotes vols 30 to 33 to the history of the subject. The most recent editions of these volumes date from 1979. Other important works on the subject are:

The Biochemical Approach to Life by F. R. Jevons (2nd edn, Allen and Unwin, 1968)
Reflections on Biochemistry edited by A. Kornberg, B. L. Horecker, L. Cornudella and J. Oro (Pergamon, 1977)

Search and Discovery edited by B. Kaminer (Academic Press, 1977)
The Chemistry of Life edited by J. Needham (Cambridge University Press, 1970)
Molecules and Life edited by J. S. Fruton (Wiley-Interscience, 1972)
Development of Biochemical Concepts from Ancient to Modern Times by H. M. Leicester (Harvard University Press, 1974)
Wanderings of a Biochemist by F. Lipmann (Wiley-Interscience, 1971)
Machina Carnis: The Biochemistry of Muscular Contraction and its Historical Development by D. M. Needham (Cambridge University Press, 1971)

And perhaps the most famous book yet written describing biochemical history in the making is *The Double Helix* by James Watson (Weidenfeld and Nicholson, 1968).

Current awareness: aid from mechanized services

A large proportion of biochemists – especially those in academic institutions – obtain help in keeping up to date from an 'invisible college' of associates, former colleagues and friends working in different laboratories around the world. The members of such informal groups correspond with one another, visit one another's laboratories, and meet at various international congresses, meetings, symposia and like events. In considering the flow of information in any science, it is important to remember the 'invisible college' and to consider both its merits and its drawbacks. Its greatest merit is its timeliness; its second is probably the ease with which one can keep up to date by this method – indeed, research scientists tend to mingle their personal and working lives to such an extent that it may become virtually a leisure activity. Perhaps because of this, its drawbacks tend to be overlooked. First, this form of communication is rather exclusive; information reaches only those who belong to the 'college', and this tends both to intensify specialization and to undervalue work done by outsiders or written in an unfamiliar language. Secondly, the information that passes is informal, and thus research workers' enthusiasm for their current project may lead them to describe it in a biased way; also, verbal communications are unlikely to be filed properly for future reference, and the recipients of the information have to depend on their fallible memory of what was said. The 'invisible college' is probably most important at the frontiers of knowledge, where only a small number of groups of high-powered specialists are working on the same problem. Once the number of interested parties becomes large, then the formal communication system has to be used. Biochemistry, biophysics and, especially, molecular biology are rapidly-developing subjects and thus a fair proportion of their practitioners are working on the frontiers. However, one must not forget the large groups of workers who do not belong to the international 'jet-set' of scientists – the university teachers in the lesser research schools with a large teaching load; the research workers in industrial laboratories; the practising physicians; the students. Their need for keeping up to date is for a quick method of sorting through the large weekly output of papers to establish the few that they need to read.

Many maintain that it is sufficient to scan a few leading journals – typically 6 to 10 – and that 'everything important' is in these. Many studies have demonstrated that this argument is false, relevant papers in almost any specialization being scattered over a surprisingly large number of journals. Further, this attitude tends to devalue any work not published in English. A wiser approach is regularly to scan *Current Contents* or (less effectively for biochemistry) *Chemical Titles* or *Index Medicus* for relevant-looking titles. A fair number of scientists, however, use *Chemical Abstracts, Biological Abstracts* or *Excerpta Medica* directly for their current awareness, despite the large number of abstracts that each now includes and the consequent tedium of scanning them.

The magnitude of the task of keeping up to date with the flood of literature has produced its own specialists, the information scientists. To date they have been more active in industrial than in academic laboratories, possibly because industry is more ready to direct the way in which research workers should use their precious time. Thus, biochemistry being an essentially academic subject, biochemists are perhaps less aware than, say, chemists of recent activities in the field of information handling.

Computer-based 'selective-dissemination-of-information' services are now publicly available in a number of disciplines. These result as by-products from the computerized typesetting now used by the major abstracts journals. The magnetic tapes used for the typesetting are themselves sold by the abstracts journals' publishers, and these can be searched by computer for topics of interest to the individual user. Large industrial concerns buy the tapes and search them in-house for their own scientists. But services are available publicly as well.

ASCA (the magnetic-tape version of *Science Citation Index*, which is mentioned later) is searched by the tape's producers, the Institute for Scientific Information, whose British office is in Uxbridge, Middlesex; and the machine-readable versions of *Chemical Abstracts* and *Biological Abstracts* are both searched by the Royal Society of Chemistry at Nottingham. One can also do current-awareness searches on the interactive online search systems mentioned below.

Each of these services searches regular issues of the tapes for the user's interests, and sends a print-out of the relevant references. It is important to realize, however, that the potential users must be prepared to put some work initially into compiling their search formulation; the computer looks only for those words it is told to look for, and thus a poorly thought-out search formulation gives poor results.

The subject area in which scientists need to keep absolutely up to date is probably fairly specific. They will, however, need to keep more generally abreast of developments in a wider area. The scientific news magazines, such as *New Scientist* and *Nature,* are helpful here. But for more regular, if less frequent, background coverage, the *Annual Reviews, Advances* and *Progress* series described earlier are probably paramount. Though a few months out of date when they appear, they do give authoritative descriptions of the previous year's progress in their specific fields. As the sheer quantity of scientific research increases, these reviews are likely to become more and more important – provided always that sufficiently eminent scientists are prepared to write them.

Exhaustive retrospective searches

There are a number of occasions when an exhaustive search of the past literature of a subject is needed; for example, when a completely new research project is due to commence. This is commonly when a new research student is starting work, when an industrial researcher is required to change to a new topic, or when an academic researcher moves to a different establishment with a different research emphasis. Another occasion is when some unexpected result alters the course of research, and reveals that the research team lacks knowledge of the new area. Again, results may suggest a new hypothesis, and this has to be tested by checking on past work that might refute or confirm the new theory. In all these cases one wants to find every publication that has ever had a bearing on the subject.

Such a search is usually an iterative process; the area of information required is first defined, and a first search reveals too much information or (less likely) too little. The area is then redefined and the search continued.

Probably the place to start in such a search is in the indexes of the appropriate review serials, or the 'Interdok' index of conferences. This leads to reviews of different ages that are relevant to the topic and yield some references to the primary literature. For the period since the latest relevant review, one needs to resort to the indexes of the appropriate abstracts journal. *Chemical Abstracts* is probably the first choice. It has decennial or (more recently) quinquennial indexes; for the period since the last quinquennial index, one has to use the volume (six-month) indexes. All of these indexes can be used to search for topics or for authors, but if the subject indexes are used, it must be remembered that one is confined to the index headings which the indexer thought appropriate for the paper; titles, as such, are not indexed. For the period since the last six-month index, the Keyword-In-Context (KWIC) index of the titles that appears at the back of each weekly issue must be used. If this last procedure seems too tedious, one could try looking through the reproduced contents pages in the recent issues of *Current Contents* instead.

Another method of covering the recent literature is to use *Science Citation Index*. This tool is quite widely available in libraries, but is probably badly understood by many scientists. It is essentially a list of papers (arranged alphabetically by first authors) with, appended to each paper, a list of those *subsequent* papers that have cited the first paper in their bibliographies. Thus, if a particularly important paper is known, central to the subject of the search, but published some years ago, e.g. 'A. Scientist, *Journal of Speculative Biochemistry*, vol 2, page 103, 1965', say, one looks up Scientist, A. in the *Science Citation Index* for 1971 and scans down the various writings until one comes to '*J. Spec. Biochem.*, **2**, 103, 1965'. Under this is found a list of all the 1971 papers that cited Scientist's 1965 paper in their reference lists. One year's *Science Citation Index* does not replace the previous year's; each covers the citations of one year, and if we also wanted the 1970 papers that cited Scientist's 1965 paper, we would need to look it up again in the 1970 *Science Citation Index*. This is the only method that enables one to move forward in time from a known relevant paper to more recent papers on the same topic. It is not, of course, perfect; it depends on authors' compiling their reference lists rationally and conscientiously, neither including references capriciously nor omitting others carelessly.

Thus, a list of relevant (hopefully) references has been found from various sources; a note of the methods used to find them should be kept. The papers are then checked, in the original journal if possible, or failing that in an abstracts journal; in the original journals, one checks these papers' own reference lists for references not previously encountered. By such means one proceeds until there seem to be no more relevant references to be found.

A recent development is the availability of the major scientific databases for online searching at a terminal in the scientist's own laboratory. Most computer terminals that the laboratory may possess can be used; the public telephone lines are used for access to a network which links the searcher to a distant computer. Public telecommunications networks, such as the International Packet-Switching System or Euronet, are used to provide connection to the host, the distant computer on which the databases are available online. There are now a number of such hosts, among them Lockheed DIALOG, Derwent-Systems Development Corporation, European Space Agency, Pergamon-Infoline and DATA-STAR. The databases available are generally the machine-readable versions of the major abstracts and indexes journals mentioned above, such as *Chemical Abstracts* and *Biological Abstracts*. The data bases corresponding to *Index Medicus* are accessed from the UK by means of BLAISE-LINK, a service of the British Library connecting to computers at the National Library of Medicine in the US.

Acknowledgement

In writing this chapter, I have referred constantly to the corresponding chapter in *The Use of Biological Literature* edited by R. T. Bottle and H. V. Wyatt (Butterworths, 2nd edn, 1971). I am very grateful to the author of that chapter, Dr J. M. Turner, for having saved me a great deal of work in compiling lists of publications. The opinions expressed in this chapter and any errors and omissions, however, are entirely my own.

8

Public health

V. J. Glanville

The present-day concept of public health or community health embraces such a wide range and diversity of interests that it is necessary to begin this chapter with a statement of intent. Important subjects which would have ordinarily been included, but which are dealt with elsewhere in this book, are those of child health, geriatrics and nutrition. Food hygiene and food poisoning, water supplies and sanitation, pollution and other aspects of environmental hygiene are largely the concern either of microbiologists, whose needs are covered elsewhere, or of engineers. These subjects, therefore, are excluded. It is the intention to deal herein with those other subjects with which the State is concerned in its promotion of health, to take account of the rapidly growing fields of social medicine and medical sociology and, in a less specific way, to include epidemiology and vital statistics which are the bases of all health programmes.

Many publications mentioned below deal also with some of the subjects excluded from specific consideration, but this emphasizes that there is almost no aspect of our lives which does not involve, in some way, the health of the community. An attempt is made here merely to give a guide to some of the more important sources of information in the fields selected, and if some of these sources provide a wider view, then so much the better. The sources are considered under the following headings: firstly, primary sources – that is text books, journals and official publications; secondly, abstracting and indexing services and other bibliographies.

Textbooks and monographs

These are important sources of information. Only a limited and highly selective number are given below as the field is expanding and changing so rapidly.

Comprehensive reviews included in encyclopaedic works make a useful beginning to any search – such as *A Textbook of Public Health* edited by W. W. Holland *et al.* (Oxford University Press, 1983) and *The Theory and Practice of Public Health* edited by W. Hobson (5th edn, Oxford University Press, 1979). A short work on British practice is J. B. M. Davies' *Community Health, Preventive Medicine and Social Services* (4th edn, Baillière Tindall, 1979) and A. J. Essex-Cater's *A Manual of Public Health and Community Medicine* (Wright, 1979) which again relates to Britain and is synoptic in style but encyclopaedic in content. An excellent guide to the organization of British medical services is provided in *Health Care in the United Kingdom: Its Organisation and Management* edited by N. W. Chaplin (Kluwer, 1982). *Public Health and Preventive Medicine* edited by J. M. Last (11th edn, Appleton-Century-Crofts, 1980) is a comprehensive and authoritative American text.

A small volume, *World Health* by F. Brockington (3rd edn, Churchill Livingstone, 1975), synthesizes the basic principles of administration and practice in a permanent public health structure; international aspects of public health are further dealt with in the monumental *Health Handbook: An International Reference on Care and Cure* edited by G. K. Chacko (North Holland, 1979) and *Health Care: an International Study. Report of the World Health Organization/International Collaborative Study of Medical Care Utilization* edited by R. Kohn and K. L. White (Oxford University Press, 1976). A European conspectus is provided by *The Planning of Health Services. Studies in Eight European Countries* edited by G. McLachlan (WHO, 1980). There is a review series, of which the latest is *Recent Advances in Community Medicine – 2*, edited by A. Smith (Churchill Livingstone, 1982).

Important works in occupational health are *Industrial Hygiene and Toxicology* edited by F. A. Patty (4 vols, 3rd edn, Wiley, 1978–1981) which covers the American scene, and *Occupational Health Practice* edited by R. S. F. Schilling (2nd edn, Butterworths, 1981) which describes the international scene. A standard reference is *The Diseases of Occupations* by D. Hunter (6th edn, Hodder and Stoughton, 1978) and more specialized, but equally indispensable, is W. R. Parkes' *Occupational Lung Disorders* (2nd edn, Butterworths, 1982). Recently begun is a review series *Recent*

Advances in Occupational Health – 1, edited by J. C. McDonald (Churchill Livingstone, 1982).

A comprehensive treatise on epidemology is A. M. and D. E. Lilienfeld's *Foundations of Epidemiology* (2nd edn, Oxford University Press, 1980) and J. H. Abramson's *Survey Methods in Community Medicine* (2nd edn, Churchill Livingstone, 1979) provides an introduction to the design and conduct of investigations in health and disease. Also important are *A World Geography of Human Disease* edited by G. M. Howe (Academic Press, 1977) and *The Epidemiology of Diseases* by D. L. Miller and R. D. T. Farmer (Blackwell, 1982).

Useful introductions to the growing literature on medical sociology are *Basic Readings in Medical Sociology* edited by D. Tuckett and J. M. Kaufert (Tavistock, 1978) and *Sociology as Applied to Medicine* edited by D. L. Patrick and G. Scambler (Baillière Tindall, 1982). The American scene is dealt with in *Medical Sociology* edited by W. C. Cockerham (2nd edn, Prentice Hall, 1982).

Journals

Such is the nature of 'public health', with its close interdependence of many facets, that any attempt at classification must, to some extent, be misleading, but some broad groupings of subjects have been made to try to meet the needs of particular groups of readers. Many papers of public health and epidemiological interest appear not in 'public health literature', but in general medical journals, such as *The Lancet* and the *British Medical Journal*, and in their equivalents in other countries. These are important sources which should not be overlooked.

Journals aimed more specifically at those whose concern is the public health in its widest sense may be grouped roughly into those dealing with the subject in general, and with epidemiology; journals of occupational and environmental health; journals of social medicine and medical sociology; those which cover medical care and its planning and utilization; and those concerned with studies on population and its control.

Public health

Public health, in the widest sense, is well served by a new series, *Annual Review of Public Health* (Palo Alto, 1980–). Other journals include *Public Health* (London), *Journal of Hygiene* (Cambridge), *Community Medicine* (Bristol) (formerly *Medical Officer*) and *American Journal of Public Health* (Washington, DC). *The Journal of Infectious Diseases* (Chicago) is far more than its title might indicate, and is a major source of information on the clinical, microbiological, epidemiological and public health aspects of the subject.

Among publications with more emphasis on epidemiology are *American Journal of Epidemiology* (Baltimore), *Epidemiologic Reviews* (Baltimore), *Journal of Chronic Diseases* (Oxford) and *International Journal of Epidemiology* (Oxford). The *Journal of Epidemiology and Community Health* (London) publishes important papers over the wide field indicated in its title, and the *Bulletin of the World Health Organization* (Geneva) includes many papers of epidemiological and public health interest. *Preventive Medicine* (New York) aims at covering the preventive aspects of medicine in the widest sense, from the epidemiology of causes of death and disability, to population control, and the influence of social factors. Those who seek information on the epidemiology of specific diseases or groups of diseases should also consult the specialist journals, such as *Tubercle* (Edinburgh), *British Journal of Cancer* (London) and *British Journal of Venereal Diseases* (London). These are only examples – there are many published in other countries and in other fields.

Occupational and environmental health

With regard to occupational and environmental health, the following are among the leading journals in the English language: *British Journal of Industrial Medicine* (London), *Journal of the Society of Occupational Medicine* (Bristol), *Archives of Environmental Health* (Washington, DC) and *Journal of Occupational Medicine* (Chicago). *Environmental Research* (New York) includes not only epidemiological and clinical papers on, for example, the dust diseases, but also articles on air and other environmental pollution.

Social medicine and medical sociology

Publications in the field of social medicine and medical sociology are many and so a short list of some of the more useful must suffice. These include *Social Science and Medicine* (Oxford), *Psychological Medicine* (London) and *Social Biology* (Madison). Although published in Berlin, most papers in *Social Psychiatry* are in English, some in German or French. *Social Policy and Administration* (Oxford) and the *Journal of Health and Social Behaviour* (Albany) provide a link between the more purely sociological aspects of community health and the planning and use of health services. The *Scandinavian Journal of Social Medicine* (Stockholm) is also in this category and includes many papers of significance, not only in the Scandinavian countries.

Addiction

Addiction, in particular to drugs and alcohol, is now a major medico-social problem. Many papers on the subject appear in the general medical literature, but *Alcoholism* (New York), *British Journal of Addiction* (London) and *Bulletin on Narcotics* (Geneva) are major publications.

Organization and use of health services

One of the journals concerned with the organization and use of health services is the *International Journal of Health Services* (New York); its subtitle – planning, administration, evaluation – well illustrates its scope. Another publication devoted to medical services and their use is *Medical Care* (Philadelphia), although this is largely, but not entirely, concerned with the situation in the US. The *Milbank Memorial Fund Quarterly* (New York) publishes symposia, many of which deal with various aspects of medical care.

Populations and their control

There is a wealth of literature on a subject of growing concern – the study of populations and their control, including family planning. Those who wish to do more than maintain a general awareness such as can be gained from the ordinary medical and public health literature, should seek the help of bodies such as the Population Council (New York) or the International Planned Parenthood Federation. The former has published *Reports on Population/Family Planning* and *Studies in Family Planning*, which include 'Current Publications' and 'Abstracts' sections in each issue; the *IPPF Medical Bulletin* and *IPPF Cooperative Information Service* are also valuable sources. *Population Studies* (London) is a specialized journal of interest to the demographer and statistician, as also is *Demography* (Chicago). *Population Trends* and *Social Trends* are useful occasional publications of the UK Government.

Foreign-language journals

For present purposes only those serials with a wider significance for comparative or international studies can be included. However, *Revue d'Epidémiologie, Médecine Sociale et Santé Publique* (Paris) gives much factual and statistical information on public health and health services in France, and *Boletín de la Oficina Sanitaria Panamericana* (Washington) is of interest to those concerned with Central and South America. Valuable national sources of information for this area are journals such as *Revista Venezolana de Sanidad y Asistencia Social* (Caracas, suspended 1977) and *Salud Pública de México* (Mexico). *Gigiena i Sanitariya* (Moscow) is an important source of information; English summaries are included after some papers and an English translation was published for 1964 to 1971 by the Israel Program for Scientific Translation. No one whose interest is in occupational health can neglect *Archives des Maladies Professionelles, de Médecine du Travail et de Securité Sociale* (Paris), *International Archives of Occupational and Environmental Health* (Heidelberg) or *Medicina del Lavoro* (Milan).

Official publications of international agencies, government departments and other organizations

The publications of the World Health Organization (Geneva) are of great value. Those in the series *Public Health Papers* and *Public Health in Europe* range widely and are intended to stimulate discussion and planning on topics such as mental health, perinatal mortality, health services, water supplies and community waste disposal. Those in the *Technical Report Series* usually embody the findings of a special or expert committee set up to study a particular problem. Among recent reports have been those on personal health care and social security, the organization of health administration, food additives, occupational exposure, the selection of essential drugs, and the safe use of pesticides.

The World Health Organization also publishes much useful epidemiological and statistical information in the *Weekly Epidemiological Record*, the *World Health Statistics Quarterly* and the *World Health Statistics Annual*. To these should be added *Morbidity and Mortality Weekly Report* by the US Department of Health, Education and Welfare Centre for Disease Control. The same US Department publishes *Public Health Reports* (Atlanta) as well as numerous papers and reports on subjects of public health concern, and the British Department of Health and Social Security publishes *Health Trends*.

For information on the vital statistics and health status of individual countries, census reports and the annual medical reports provide detail not available elsewhere. For England and Wales the Office of Population Censuses and Surveys (OPCS) publishes an annual reference series, including the following subjects: Family statistics, Deaths, Morbidity, Population estimates and projections, Abortions, etc. This is supplemented by a series of *OPCS Monitors,* designed for the quick release of selected information. OPCS publications are listed in HMSO *Sectional List 56,* last revised February 1982. These supersede the *Registrar General's Statistical Review of England and Wales,* published over many years. There are also the annual reports of the Chief medical Officer of the Department of Health and Social Security (*On the State of the Public Health*), and equivalent reports of the Welsh Office and the Scottish Home and Health Department. Both have also published reports on special subjects from time to time, e.g. on services for the mentally handicapped in England and Wales, on the misuse of drugs, and on health education in relation to alcoholism in Scotland.

Similar annual and other reports are published for other countries. Those who seek information of this sort on a particular country probably do best by applying direct to the country concerned, or through the embassy or consulate, although some of the larger or special libraries carry a selection of such reports. The *Eurohealth Handbook* (5th edn, Robert S. First, Inc., 1978) includes reviews of the health care systems, morbidity, mortality, etc of 18 European countries; and it also provides a section on 'sources of information' for statistics and government agencies in each country. Similarly, *Health Statistics: a Guide to Information Sources* by F. D. Weise (Gale, 1980) provides a review of sources for the US with some coverage of world health statistics.

Abstracts, indexes and other bibliographies

Personal health and health education

Personal health and health education are intermingled, bibliographically speaking, but distinct sources of information are few. *Health Education Abstracts* (New York, 1966–1968) was a publication of promise and of reasonable coverage of the literature.

While both *Health Education Journal* (1943–) and *International Journal of Health Education* (1968–) provide book reviews related to their subject, one must turn to the appropriate section of *Excerpta Medica* or to *Index Medicus* for current awareness of new papers on health education and personal health. Useful bibliographies of recent literature can be found in texts such as *Health Education in Practice* edited by D. C. Anderson (Croom Helm, 1979) or *Health Education Perspectives and Choices* edited by I. Sutherland (Allen and Unwin, 1979).

Occupational health

Turning to occupational health as a specialty, one finds a wider bibliographical field. The International Labour Office (ILO) has, befittingly, for many years actively disseminated information about progress in this field; and its International Occupational Safety and Health Information Centre is currently issuing abstracts of the literature of the world as *CIS Abstracts* (1974– formerly *Occupational Safety and Health Abstracts*). This series is now used as a database for an ILO information service. Earlier series published by the ILO, with less wide coverage, were *Bibliography of Industrial Hygiene* (1924–1941), *Bibliography of Occupational Medicine* (1948–1950) and *Occupational Safety and Health* (1951–1959).

Excerpta Medica also abstracts the important world literature of occupational health and hygiene in its *Section 35: Occupational Health and Industrial Medicine* (1971–), and *Industrial Hygiene Digest* (1937–) has fairly wide, though not comprehensive, coverage of papers relating to the causation and prevention of industrial disease. From commercial publishers, the *Journal of Industrial Hygiene and Toxicology* (1919–1949) carried an abstract section in each issue which had good coverage, with informative abstracts, of the important literature of the period.

In a still more specialized aspect of industrial health, the influence of the National Library of Medicine in dissemination of knowledge is also seen in *Toxicity Bibliography* (1968–1977), which covered all types of poisonous substances, including industrial ones; the database is now included in *Index Medicus* and MEDLARS. The study of work itself is well covered by *Ergonomics Abstracts* (1969–), which has a very useful coverage of the literature, with informative, readable abstracts. Similarly, abstracts of the literature of dust diseases are collected in *Pneumoconiosis Abstracts* (Bureau of Hygiene and Tropical Diseases, London), in three volumes collected from the *Bulletin of Hygiene* for the years 1926 to 1955 inclusive. The *Kettering Abstracts . . . on . . . Lead* (1965–) are published by the laboratory of the same name with wide coverage and good abstracts. Other bibliographies, which can be found through library catalogues such as those included in the Public Health section below, are available and are extremely valuable in collating the literature on particular substances hazardous to man. Good examples are those on fluorine compounds, on carbon monoxide and on sulphur dioxide.

Occupational Health: a Guide to Sources of Information by S. Gauvain (Heinemann Medical, 1974) is a comprehensive review of all types of information sources, including bibliographical, for the industrial medical officer or hygienist. Another excellent review of current knowledge is the *Encyclopaedia of Occupational Health and Safety* (ILO, Geneva, 3rd edn, 1983). *Handbook of Occupational Hygiene* by B. Harvey (Brentford, 1980) is a compendium of current knowledge in loose-leaf format for easy up-dating which includes a chapter on information sources and organizations. The US National Institute for Occupational Safety and Health has also published *NIOSH Publications Catalog, 1970–1977* (Cincinnati, 1977) as a guide to availability of an important series of publications. *Literature Sources in Toxicology: a Survey* by J. M. Hargreaves (British Library Research and Development Report No 5542, 1980) provides a useful conspectus of 'manual' and database sources. *The Barbour Health and Safety Library* is a microfiche compilation, regularly up-dated, of all relevant literature and codes of practice.

Public health – the state and health of the people

Public health – the state and the health of the people – is bibliographically fragmentary: and a number of sources are needed to gain a conspectus of the literature of any particular topic. Library catalogues are an obvious prime source; and here the various series of the catalogue of the National Library of Medicine, Washington (*see* Chapter 3) and its *Current Catalog* must have priority. *The Dictionary Catalogue of the London School of Hygiene and Tropical Medicine* (7 vols, G. K. Hall 1965, and *Supplement*, 1970) forms a wide-ranging bibliography of the literature of preventive as well as tropical medicine. The *John Crerar Library (Chicago) Classified Subject Catalog* (vols 18 and 19, G. K. Hall, 1967) is part of the catalogue of a great scientific library which shows its holdings in hygiene and public health. The library of the World Health Organization at Geneva lists current books, reports, etc, that relate to public health in all parts of the world as *Recent Acquisitions*. A useful guide to publications and sources, mainly in Britain, is *Health Care Administration: an Information Sourcebook* by A. J. Bunch (Capital Planning Information, 1979); and the library of the Royal Institute of Public Administration (RIPA) has produced *Health Services in Britain: a Short Bibliogra-*

phy (4th edn, RIPA, 1979). *Health Planning and Health Services Research* (Springfield, 1979–) abstracts US federal literature; and *An Introduction to the Primary Health Care Approach in Developing Countries: a Review with Selected Annotated References* by G. Walt and P. Vaughan (Ross Institute of Tropical Hygiene, 1981) provides an excellent introduction to its subject.

Three major abstract journals cover the literature of public health, though not exhaustively. *Excerpta Medica*, Section 17: *Public Health, Social Medicine and Hygiene* (1947–), with Section 46: *Environmental Health and Pollution Control* (1971–), abstracts a wide range of the world's literature. *Abstracts on Hygiene and Communicable Diseases* (formerly *Bulletin of Hygiene*) (1926–) abstracts, only selectively, literature which shows advances in knowledge or provides 'state of the art' reviews. This title is now being published within the Commonwealth Agricultural Bureaux computer system and abstracts will be available from that database. In this group, three other publications should be included for their value. The *World Bibliography of Social Security* (1960–) largely achieves the object denoted by its title; and *Abstracts of Health Care Management Studies* (Ann Arbor, 1979–), formerly published as *Abstracts of Hospital Management Studies*, now achieves wide coverage of both published and unpublished information. Finally, the *International Digest of Health Legislation* (1948–), though not strictly an abstract journal, is a valuable survey and digest of the public health legislation of the world.

Bibliographies of public health are generally national rather than cosmopolitan. Examples can be found through the library catalogues mentioned above. The USSR, China and Sweden are amongst the countries which are surveyed bibliographically in the Geographic Health Studies project of the Fogarty International Center, USDHEW National Institute of Health.

For the older literature of public health, recourse is necessary to works such as the *Surgeon General's Index-Catalogue* (*see* Chapter 3) or to the following excellent German works: *Zentralblatt für die gesamte Hygiene* (1922–1944), *Hygienische Rundschau* (1891–1922), *Jahresbericht über die Fortschritte und Leistungen auf dem Gebiete der Hygiene* (1833–1913) and *Bibliographischer Jahresbericht über soziale Hygiene, Demographie und Medizinalstatistik* (1900–1921).

Hospitals

Hospitals – their finance, administration and efficiency – are an important part of any state health system. *Hospital Abstracts*

(1961–) is published by the UK Department of Health and Social Security library, and achieves a wide and up-to-date coverage of the world's literature. *Hospital Literature Index* (1945–), a publication of the American Hospital Association, has a wider coverage of the literature, but with index entries only. *Abstracts of Hospital Management Studies* (1964–1978) was more restricted in scope, but included good abstracts in its field. For the historical bibliography of hospitals *Medical Reference Works, 1679–1966* edited by J. B. Blake and C. Roos (Medical Library Association, 1967; *Supplements,* 1970, 1973, 1975), has a useful source list.

Social medicine and medical sociology

Social medicine and medical sociology, as comparatively new extensions of long-standing sciences, have less bibliographical support and control than is available for some other subjects, but those works available are good. Apart from those library catalogues which have already been quoted in earlier sections of this chapter, another source of respectable seniority and of considerable bibliographical authority must be included here. This is the *London Bibliography of the Social Sciences* (LSE, later Mansell, London, 1931–), which is effectively the catalogue of the library of the London School of Economics and Political Science, although additional material found in other University of London libraries was included in the earlier series. The wide subject coverage of this great library makes its catalogue a prime source for monographic material. The *International Bibliography of the Social Sciences* (Sociology, Anthropology sections; Paris, 1957–) is a useful adjunct of this, covering the whole range of related sociological subjects in periodical and other literature.

Focusing more closely, the area of interrelationship of sociology and medicine has three useful guides to current literature. The *Medical Care Review* (Ann Arbor, 1944–) began under the title *Public Health Economics.* It has a strong bias to US sources, but includes a wide variety of excerpts and abstracts from different forms of literature. Two non-periodical bibliographies are also useful basic tools: *Medical Behavioral Science: a Selected Bibliography of Cultural Anthropology, Social Psychology and Sociology in Medicine* (University of Kentucky, 1963) is by M. Pearsall and provides a basic reading list in these subject areas of over 3000 references to various types of mainly English language literature; and an earlier bibliography, published in *Current Sociology* (1962–, vols 10/11, No 3), has a wider geographic spread. This latter was entitled *The Sociology of Medicine: a Trend Report and Bibliography.*

Others which may be of particular value in development programmes are *Housing, the Housing Environment, and Health: An Annotated Bibliography* by A. E. Martin *et al.* (World Health Organization, Geneva, 1976), and *SALUS: Low-cost Rural Health Care and Health Manpower Training: An Annotated Bibliography with Special Emphasis on Developing Countries* by various editors (International Development Research Centre, Ottawa, 1975–).

Vital statistics and epidemiological bibliographies

Vital statistics and epidemiological bibliographies are not common, but those available are good. The more general library catalogues and bibliographies already mentioned are a first source; so also must be international and government publications lists. The *United Nations Documents Index* (New York, 1950–) includes all the publicly available papers and books of all the different agencies set up under the UN; but it does not include, for example, the publications or the mimeographed working papers of the World Health Organization, which are so often cited in the literature, but which are not published or generally available. British Government publications are listed daily and monthly and cumulate in the *HMSO Annual Catalogue*. The now quinquennial *Consolidated Index to Government Publications* has listed publications of the British government since the nineteenth century; and included are such departmental reports as those of the General Register Office, now the Office of Population Censuses and Surveys, and those of the Department of Health and Social Security and its predecessors. Similarly, the *Monthly Catalog of United States Government Publications* lists the more numerous reports and papers of the various Federal agencies and departments, including the Department of Health, Education and Welfare, the National Institutes of Health and the Bureau of the Census. Similar lists are available for tracing demographic publications of other countries.

Bibliographies of health and disease statistics can save a great deal of research. Examples of merit are: *Reviews of United Kingdom Statistical Sources, vol. IX. Health Surveys and Related Studies* by M. Alderson and R. Dowie (Pergamon, 1979), with earlier volumes in this series, of which the general editor is W. F. Maunder; *A Guide to Health and Social Services Statistics* (G. B. Department of Health and Social Security, 1974); *Health Statistics: a Guide to Information Sources* by F. O. Weise (Gale, 1980), *US Public Health Service: Clearing House on Current Morbidity Statistics Projects, Sources of Morbidity Data* (vols 1–11, Washington, 1953–1963); and *Sanitarnaia Statistica – Bibliografiya Sovetski*

Literatury, 1918–1960 gg by A. M. Merkov (Moskva, Medgiz, 1963). A valuable compendium is M. Alderson's *International Mortality Statistics* (Macmillan, 1981).

Bibliographies of diseases are too numerous to mention, but should not be ignored. Collective works of value which are basic tools for any chronological epidemiological study are, among others, *Handbook of Geographical and Historical Pathology* by A. Hirsch translated from the German 2nd edn by C. Creighton (New Sydenham Society, London 1883–1886), *Welt-Seuchen-Atlas . . . World Atlas of Epidemic Diseases* by E. Rodenwalt (Hamburg, 1952–1957) and G. M. Howe's unique *National Atlas of Disease Mortality in the United Kingdom* (2nd edn, Nelson, 1970). These are particularly valuable examples in their class; and also histories of diseases and of epidemiology are of equal use as sources.

The study of population growth and control is becoming more urgent and increasingly significant in the field of vital statistics. The United Nations plays a leading role in this advance and its *Documents Index*, already quoted, is a guide to a significant proportion of the literature. The *Population Index* (Princeton, 1935–) has a good coverage of the literature of demography generally, including morbidity and mortality, and many of the references include abstracts. A review of bibliographical value is *Demographie: Tendences Actuelles et Organisation de la Recherche, 1955–1965* by L. Tabah and J. Viet (Mouton, 1966). In this field there are many good bibliographies of particular geographical areas; and these can be traced through *Population Index* or library catalogues.

Lastly, but of great importance, should be included the *Current Bibliography of Epidemiology* (1969–1977), which covers the major literature of not only epidemiology, but also preventive medicine. As a derivative from the MEDLARS computer tapes, it had a greater depth of indexing than *Index Medicus*, and the division into two sequences (i.e. into topics such as accident prevention and into diseases such as hookworm infection and occurrence) was valuable. The references are now only available in *Index Medicus;* and the more detailed indexing may be accessed through the MEDLARS service.

History

The origins and development of the public health movement are succinctly described in the first chapter by S. P. W. Chave of vol 1 of *A Textbook of Public Health*, edited by W. W. Holland *et al.*

(Oxford University Press, 1983). C. F. Brockington's *A Short History of Public Health* (2nd edn, Churchill, 1966), G. Rosen's *A History of Public Health* (MD Publications, 1958), and W. M. Frazer's *A History of English Public Health 1834–1919* (Baillière Tindall, 1950) provide modern accounts. Sir John Simon's *English Sanitary Institutions* (Cassell, 1890), recently reprinted by William Dawson, records the development of public health in England in the nineteeth century

N. M. Goodman has given a systematic account of international health work from its beginnings to modern times in his *International Health Organizations and their Work* (2nd edn, Churchill Livingstone, 1971), and N. Howard-Jones has published a detailed study of one aspect of international health work in *The Scientific Background of the International Sanitary Conferences 1851–1938* (History of International Public Health series, No 1, WHO, 1975), pointing out that 'The history of the International Sanitary Conferences is largely the history of public health in international perspective. It is more particularly a history of the first gropings towards what is now the World Health Organization.'

An account of the development of medical statistics is provided by M. Greenwood's *Medical Statistics from Graunt to Farr* (Cambridge University Press, 1938).

Recent accounts of the history of the National Health Service are to be found in B. Abel-Smith's *The NHS: the First Thirty Years* (DHSS, 1978) and J. E. Pater's *The Making of the National Health Service* (King Edward's Hospital Fund for London, 1981). Finally, H. E. Sigerist in *On The Sociology of Medicine,* edited by M. I. Roemer (New York, MD Publications, 1960), provides fascinating historical glimpses.

9

Pharmacology and therapeutics

D. H. Calam

The information sources considered in this chapter have been selected to cover not only the fields of pharmacology and therapeutics in the strict sense, but also areas of pharmaceutical science concerned particularly with drugs, their development and control. This wider coverage has been chosen advisedly, since such areas are not considered elsewhere in the volume. Although the flow of new drugs, in the sense of new chemical entities, has slowed during the past few years, our understanding of drug action and the importance of pharmacodynamics and pharmacokinetics has increased. This knowledge, together with mounting legislative control, has had a significant influence on the range of medicines available. Although the traditional and jealously guarded right of physicians to prescribe whatever they believe appropriate for their patients remains, many little-used preparations or those whose efficacy has been questioned have disappeared. Nevertheless, the next few years may bring further changes with the introduction of sophisticated drug delivery systems permitting continuous, controlled release of the active principles, and with new products resulting from advances in genetic manipulation.

Information sources play a crucial role in meeting the challenge of maintaining awareness of these developments. Rapid progress in the field of communications and computers will have a striking effect on these sources. The time has already arrived when the doctor in the hospital ward can call up a patient's records on a local terminal and check information on individual drugs and their interactions and when physicians can, through their home computer and telephone links, monitor from home the laboratory results as they are produced for their patients. Data in a compendium like *Martindale* can now be studied online as they are updated and the time cannot be far off when pharmacopoeial requirements can be examined in the same way.

History

Although historical sources are considered in Chapter 22 the reader's attention is drawn to a few sources of particular relevance. Early works are annotated in L. T. Morton's *A Medical Bibliography* (4th edn, Gower, 1983), which includes original publications up to about 1950 (for example, the original descriptions of the isolation of antibiotics) together with later histories. The special supplement to the *Journal of Pharmacy and Pharmacology* in April 1976 entitled *Frontiers in Pharmacology* consists of a collection of papers to mark the fiftieth anniversary of the founding of the pharmacological laboratories of the Pharmaceutical Society of Great Britain and includes several entertaining accounts of the early activities of those laboratories. A further source of historical information is the lectures given on the occasion of award of the Nobel Prizes. These are collected into volumes, but also appear in *Science* within a few months of delivery.

Many standard textbooks acquire historical value over the years because, apart from their rarity, they provide an insight into the scientific development of a field. R. T. Williams' *Detoxication Mechanisms* (1st edn, Chapman and Hall, 1947) is an example from the area of metabolism. The acquisition and study of such books can be an interesting and enlightening pastime.

Indexing services and abstracts

These have been dealt with comprehensively in Chapters 3 and 5. This section only summarizes briefly the main sources which contain information relevant to the subjects of this chapter. *Current Contents* (*see* page 57) is one of the most timely indexing systems. For those who prefer their literature sifted to a greater extent, a number of computerized systems are available. *Index Chemicus,* *Chemical Titles* and *Index Medicus* all appear in periodical form, but their contents are also held on magnetic tape and can be searched by the appropriate keyword method. The *Index Medicus* entries are much more extensive than those in the hard copy. These searches (MEDLINE, CT (*Chemical Titles*), CBAC (*Chemical–Biological Activities*)) are relatively inexpensive and permit research workers and others to keep abreast of current literature in a relatively confined area. Their value becomes lost if the search becomes too broad, since the material retrieved has, essentially, to be re-sorted. These searches are discussed at length in Chapter 5. However, the power of online information retrieval systems should not be underestimated. The Lockheed Dialog system, for example, provides access to over 10 million references in medical, pharmaceutical and biochemical sciences in the MEDLINE, *Excerpta Medica, BIOSIS (Biological Abstracts), International Pharmaceutical Abstracts, Life Science Collection* and *SciSearch* databases.

A drawback of many abstracting periodicals is the inevitable delay between appearance of the primary literature and appearance in abstracted form. This drawback is particularly acute with *Chemical Abstracts*, where production of indexes lags behind the individual volumes and a search of volumes since the last five-year index is a major undertaking. Some of the *Excerpta Medica* series, such as that on *Pharmacology and Toxicology*, are more useful for this purpose. *International Pharmaceutical Abstracts* is a semi-monthly publication (American Society of Hospital Pharmacists) in 25 sections, all concerned with various aspects of pharmacy, and *Abstracts on Drug Interactions* (1971 onwards) is a computer-based compilation of this. For those who need to know about new adverse reactions as quickly as possible after being reported, *Clin-Alert* (Science Editors Inc., US) published about 30 times per year, is of value.

A manual search of recent literature can be carried out efficiently using the *Science Citation Index (SCI) (see* Chapter 3). Given a key article or review, *SCI* permits direct entry to the literature in which such an item has been cited and enables the construction of citation trees from which the major contributors to a field can be identified and a fresh search developed.

Primary sources

Over the years it has become more and more difficult to read widely and in depth in any discipline because of the steady increase in size and number of journals. The individual reader must decide which are core journals of prime interest and which are of less importance. This is probably done most easily by studying issues of *Current Contents, Life Sciences* (Institute for Scientific Information) over a period of several weeks. The contents pages, taken as a whole, of journals published frequently (at least monthly) provide an excellent insight to the subject matter and degree of specialization of the journal. Review publications produced quarterly or annually can be located by reference to the cumulated journal index, which appears tri-annually, and to the lists of journal coverage.

The following list includes a selection of primary journals, arranged roughly by discipline. The list is intended to provide a range within which, for a variety of needs, a source journal for original research papers may be found. The classification of some titles is arbitrary since they span several areas.

Pharmacology and therapeutics

Acta Pharmacologica et Toxicologica
Agents and Action*
Archives Internationales de Pharmacodynamie et de Thérapie
Archives of Toxicology
Biochemical Pharmacology
British Journal of Pharmacology
European Journal of Pharmacology
Farmakologiya i Toksikologiya
General Pharmacology*
Journal of Pharmacokinetics and Biopharmaceutics
Journal de Pharmacologie
Journal of Pharmacology and Experimental Therapeutics
Molecular Pharmacology
Naunyn-Schmiedeberg's Archives of Pharmacology
Pharmacological Research Communications*
Pharmacology and Therapeutics
Teratology
Toxicology and Applied Pharmacology

Clinical pharmacology sources

British Journal of Clinical Pharmacology
Clinical Pharmacology and Therapeutics
Drugs
European Journal of Clinical Pharmacology
International Journal of Clinical Pharmacology
Therapy and Toxicology
Thérapie

together with core medical journals, e.g.: *The Lancet, British Medical Journal, Journal of the American Medical Association*

Pharmaceutical and chemical sciences

Acta Pharmaceutica Suecica

Annales Pharmaceutiques Françaises
Antimicrobial Agents and Chemotherapy
Archiv der Pharmazie
Arzneimittel-Forschung
Chemical and Pharmaceutical Bulletin
Chemico-Biological Interactions
Die Pharmazie
European Journal of Medicinal Chemistry – Chimica Therapeutica
Il Farmaco Edizione Scientifica
Journal of Antibiotics
Journal of Antimicrobial Chemotherapy *
Journal of Medicinal Chemistry
Journal of Pharmaceutical Sciences *
Journal of Pharmacy and Pharmacology *
Khimiko-Farmatseuticheskii Zhurnal
Pharmaceutica Acta Helvetiae

Some primary information on the development of drugs appears in core chemical journals, such as *Helvetica Chimica Acta, Journal of the American Chemical Society, Journal of the Chemical Society (Perkin Transactions), Bulletin de la Société Chimique de France, Chemische Berichte.*

Reviews

Some of the journals listed above, indicated by an asterisk, frequently contain brief reviews and annotations that cover a wide range of topics. Similar brief reports may also be found in periodicals such as *Pharmaceutical Journal, Deutsche* and *Schweizerische Medizinische Wochenschrift,* and longer articles in those such as *Pharmacological Reviews.* The annual review issue of *Analytical Chemistry* includes a literature review on pharmaceutical chemistry. Articles on 'Today's Treatment' appear in the *British Medical Journal* and are cumulated in useful little volumes published by the British Medical Association under the same title. A valuable interdisciplinary journal is *Trends in the Pharmaceutical Sciences.*

There are, of course, several series publications of the 'Advances' type. Among the more important of these are *Annual Review of Pharmacology* and . . . *of Medicine* (Annual Reviews Inc.), *Advances in Drug Research* edited by Harper and Simmonds (Academic Press) and published since 1964, which consists of long articles on specific topics; *Advances in Pharmacology and Chemotherapy* (Academic Press), published from 1969 (vol 7) as a continuation of the two previously separate series; *Progress in Drug Research* edited by E. Jucker (Birkhauser Verlag), provides survey articles of pharmaceutical research; *Progress in Medicinal Chemistry* (Butterworths) contains reviews by specialists in different disciplines concerned with development and study of new drugs; *Annual Reports in Medicinal Chemistry* (Academic Press) has similar aims. Both these last-mentioned publications are available in soft covers. The sphere of drug metabolism is specifically covered by two series: *Drug Metabolism Reviews* edited by F. J. Di Carlo (Dekker) beginning in 1973, and *Progress in Drug Metabolism* edited by J. W. Bridges and L. F. Chasseaud (Wiley), an annual series, the first volume of which appeared in 1976.

Three other periodicals which contain short articles rather than reviews and which attempt to provide unbiased and critical information need to be mentioned. All are produced by non-profit organizations. The first is the *Drug and Therapeutics Bulletin* edited by A. Herxheimer and published for doctors by the Consumers Association (London). It consists of four pages every fortnight and contains general articles (e.g. drugs to prevent relapse after myocardial infarction), as well as others, that reassess old drugs and critically discuss new ones, particularly in comparison with existing methods of treatment. The second of this type is the *Adverse Drug Reaction Bulletin* edited by D. M. Davies, published every two months by the Northern Regional Hospital Authority and sent free with the *Drug and Therapeutics Bulletin*. It has the same four-page format and is similar in style. The editors have prepared a *Textbook of Adverse Drug Reactions* (2nd edn, Oxford University Press, 1981) and are associated with the new quarterly *Adverse Drug Reactions and Acute Poisoning Reviews*. The third short-article periodical is an American counterpart: the *Medical Letter on Drugs and Therapeutics* (editorial chairman, H. Aaron), published fortnightly by The Medical Letter Inc. (New York). This has similar aims and format to the others and was formerly known as *Drugs and Therapeutic Information*.

Side-effects to drugs are known to account for a significant proportion of hospital admissions. The importance of this subject is clear from the number of information sources available. As well as the indexes and bulletins, an annual series *Side Effects of Drugs* (Excerpta Medica) has been published since 1977 as a supplement to *Meyler's Side Effects of Drugs* edited by M. N. G. Dukes (9th edn, Excerpta Medica, 1980), which is a comprehensive and authoritative guide. A helpful feature of the annual series is the provision of indexes cumulated for about four years.

Information on topics of current importance to practitioners is also circulated from official sources. In Britain the Committee on Safety of Medicines produces, as an occasional series, *Current Problems,* which draws attention to problems under consideration and seeks reports from doctors. The *FDA Bulletin* is a similar American publication.

Monographs

The selection of significant books and monographs is a difficult task because few are read from cover to cover, and in any rapidly changing field they have an inherent tendency to date rather quickly. This short list is not exhaustive.

The Pharmacological Basis of Therapeutics edited by A. G. Gilman, L. S. Goodman and A. Gilman (6th edn, Macmillan, 1980), is a classic work which provides a bridge between basic medical science and clinical usage of drugs. The 70 chapters, in 17 main sections, have been prepared by many distinguished contributors. A minor disadvantage is the emphasis on American trade names. Other major reference monographs include the Springer-Verlag series of *Handbooks of Experimental Pharmacology;* the constituent volumes of the *International Encyclopedia of Pharmacology and Therapeutics* (Pergamon), many of the most recent of which have been published as supplements to the review journal *Pharmacology and Therapeutics;* and the massive compendium *Hager's Handbuch der Pharmazeutische Praxis* (also Springer-Verlag) edited by P. H. List and L. Hörhammer (began in 1967, and the most recent volume of which appeared in 1980), which deals with all aspects of pharmaceutical chemistry and manufacture. *Remington's Pharmaceutical Sciences* edited by A. Osol *et al.* (16th edn, Mack Publishing, 1980) is a massive volume (108 chapters, about 300 contributors) intended as a 'treatise on theory and practice of pharmaceutical sciences and essential information about pharmaceutical and medicinal agents.' The reader should judge how far this intention is met.

The following provide a guide to some books on pharmacology and therapeutics which may be of value. *An Introduction to Human Pharmacology* by J. D. P. Graham (Oxford University Press, 1979), *Textbook of Pharmacology* by W. C. Bowman and M. J. Rand (2nd edn, Blackwell, 1980), *Essentials of Pharmacology: Introduction to the Principles of Drug Action* by J. A. Bevan and 32 others (2nd edn, Harper and Row, 1976), are introductory volumes which vary in their depths of coverage. *Clinical Pharmacology* by P. Turner and A. Richens (4th edn, Churchill Livingstone, 1982) and *Poisoning Diagnosis and Treatment* edited by J. A. Vale and T. J. Meredith (Update Books, 1981) cover more specific areas. The *Pharmaceutical Handbook* (19th edn, Pharmaceutical Press, 1980) is a handy guide.

Drugs of Choice 1980–81 edited by W. Modell (Mosby, 1980) is the latest in a series of practical guides to the selection of drugs for therapeutic use. It is a multi-author volume with chapters on specific groups of drugs and a drug index. Two similar volumes are the *Year Book of Drug Therapy* edited by D. G. Friend (Year Book Medical Publishers) and *Current Therapy 1982* edited by H. F. Conn, with about 30 contributors (Saunders). For British readers more timely and pertinent advice, not without some controversy, is given in the rearranged *British National Formulary* (page 203). The *Merck Manual of Diagnosis and Treatment* editor-in-chief R. Berkow (14th edn, 1982) is a well-established American handbook for physicians, giving information about the aetiology, investigation and treatment of a wide range of conditions, both common and rare. American names for drugs are, of course, used and many US trade names are given.

Adverse drug reactions and interactions are discussed in *Evaluations of Drug Interactions* (2nd edn, American Pharmaceutical Association), *A Manual of Adverse Drug Interactions* by J. P. Griffin and P. F. D'Arcy (2nd edn, Wright, 1979), the soft-covered *Adverse Reactions to Drugs* by O. L. Wade and L. Beeley (2nd edn, Heinemann, 1976), and *Adverse Reactions to Intravenous Drugs* by J. Watkins and A. M. Ward (Academic Press, 1978), the proceedings of a meeting.

Pharmacopoeias

The object of a pharmacopoeia is to lay down specifications for the quality of important and widely used drugs. These specifications are 'official' and are intended to ensure that all marketed versions of such drugs are of high quality. This activity long pre-dates, and is complementary to, control of quality through national licensing systems where information is confidential to the producer and the licensing authority. Further, pharmacopoeial requirements apply throughout the life of a product and may differ from those applied at the time of manufacture. Many countries produce their own pharmacopoeias which are revised periodically by committees of experts. The escalating cost of developing new drugs means that a world market is sought for their sale and one consequence is an increasing tendency to apply uniform criteria of drug quality through multi-national use and production of pharmacopoeias.

The duty to publish a *British Pharmacopoeia (BP)* was laid upon the General Medical Council by the Medical Act of 1858, and the first edition was published six years later. In recent times, revisions here appeared every five or seven years with addenda to the main volume in between. Under the provisions of the Medicines Act 1968, responsibility for the *BP* was transferred to the Health

Ministers, who authorize publication after the edition has been prepared on behalf of the Medicines Commission. The 1973 edition was the first to appear under these arrangements. The *BP*, like others, declares a date from which its contents become 'official' and supersede those of previous volumes. The current *BP 1980* is in two volumes with a companion volume of *Infra-red Reference Spectra*. The first volume contains monographs on drug substances, including definitions, descriptions, tests for identity, purity and properties, assays and information about action and use, dosages and labelling. The second volume consists of specifications for preparations (such as tablets and injections), blood and immunological products, and surgical materials, together with a series of appendices with information about reagents, procedures and general requirements. At present the *BP* is the only pharmacopoeia to provide a compilation of infrared reference spectra for identification, instead of reference materials with which analysts prepare their own spectra. Unlike certain other pharmacopoeias (for example, the French), the tests are advisory not mandatory, but in the event of disputes there is an obligation to justify any departure from them. Addenda containing new material are published between the main editions. The *Addendum 1982* became effective in December 1982 and is cumulative, including all material from the *Addendum 1981*. Complementary supplements of infra-red spectra have also been published. Because the proportion of reprinted matter will increase, it is possible that future Addenda may include only new material. The considerable increase in size of the *BP 1980* compared with *BP 1973* is largely due to incorporation of requirements from the *European Pharmacopoeia* and of material previously published in the *British Pharmaceutical Codex*. This latter was a second book of drug standards and information published by the Pharmaceutical Society (*see* page 203). After the introduction of the Medicines Act responsibility for official specifications was transferred to the *BP*. However, until new standards are set for materials in the *British Pharmaceutical Codex 1973* and its *Supplement 1976*, the requirements therein continue to have legal status. The requirements of the *British Pharmacopoeia* are enforced legally in the Commonwealth and are accepted by many other countries as their own standards. Medicines specifically for veterinary use feature in a separate volume, the *British Pharmacopoeia (Veterinary) 1977*.

The *European Pharmacopoeia (EP)* is prepared under the auspices of the Council of Europe by the terms of a Convention of 1964. The events leading up to this are described in the preface to vol 1 of the first edition, published in 1969. Eight countries were involved at the outset: Britain, Belgium, France, Italy, Luxembourg, The Netherlands, West Germany and Switzerland, but the number has increased to 15 with the addition of Austria, Cyprus, Denmark, Iceland, Ireland, Norway and Sweden. At present Finland and Portugal send observers but are not full members. The *EP* is drafted by groups of experts, not necessarily drawn from all the countries, and the draft is approved by a main Commission representative of the national authorities. Thus, the requirements of the *EP* represent the agreed views of most countries in western Europe. However, since the various national pharmacopoeias are used in yet other countries, the influence of the *EP* extends beyond Europe. Under the terms of the Convention, it is agreed that the monographs should become official in each country from a specified date and that, in so far as they are binding, they are included in and supersede existing monographs in the national pharmacopoeias. There is no obligation to include a particular monograph, but if included it must not be changed and no alternative is permitted. The first edition of the *EP* consisted of three main volumes (I, 1969; II, 1971; III 1975) and two supplements (1973 and 1976), produced in two official languages, English and French. Translations into other languages, for example, German, are official only if authorized or if appearing as part of the national pharmacopoeia of a country signatory to the Convention. Publication of the second edition commenced in 1980 in a loose-leaf format. The reasons for adopting this, and the system for publication, are explained in the Preface. In essence, advances in methods and the complexity of drug substances demand frequent revision of monographs. The loose-leaf presentation should facilitate incorporation of monographs in the correct sequence as they are revised and also replacement of sections as required. New pages are issued in fascicules about twice yearly. Because of national variations in prescribing and the large range of excipients that may be incorporated in drug dosage forms, the monographs of the *European Pharmacopoeia* are almost exclusively for parent substances. The few exceptions concern complex biological products.

Before the *EP* convention was signed, the Scandinavian countries had reached a similar agreement to produce a *Nordic Pharmacopoeia*, produced in several languages. The main volumes were produced in 1963 and have been updated by means of loose-leaf addenda. With the accession of the Nordic countries to the *EP* Convention, it is unlikely that further volumes of the *Nordic Pharmacopoeia* will appear.

Following a precedent set by the League of Nations, the World Health Organization supports the production of the *International*

Pharmacopoeia. The third edition is in the course of publication. Unlike earlier editions which employed material from some national pharmacopoeias, this edition is intended to meet the specific needs of developing countries. Volume 1, published in 1979, contains general methods of analysis, and volume 2 (1981) contains quality specifications. The aim is to provide specifications for the drugs appearing on the 'essential' list recommended by WHO, together with common excipients and dosage forms, at a level to ensure their safety and efficacy without recourse to complex methods or imposing unduly stringent criteria. A further aim is to provide general methods which can form the basis for control of other products. The *International Pharmacopoeia*, which is produced by an international group of experts and has no legal force in itself, is available for official adoption by any member state of WHO.

Main editions of the *United States Pharmacopoeia (USP)* (XXth edition, 1980) appear every five years. Although produced by the US Pharmacopoeia Convention, independent of government, the *USP* has official status. Each edition has a preface describing the history of the *USP* and the changes since the previous edition. As in Britain, a second book of drug standards, the *National Formulary (NF)*, was previously published in America, but the *USP* and *NF* merged in 1975. The *National Formulary* now appears as a separate section in the *USP* and deals with pharmaceutical ingredients, whereas the main body of the book concerns drug substances and dosage forms. Regulations for antibiotics, which under American law are the responsibility of the Food and Drug Administration, are included as an Appendix in the pharmacopoeia. Annual supplements are produced between editions, and have previously been cumulative. However, it has been announced that from *Supplement 3* (1982) cumulation will cease because of the large amount of information that has to be reprinted. An interesting insight into pharmacopoeial revision is provided by *Pharmacopoeial Forum*, published every two months. This gives details of in-process revision of monographs for the *USP* with discussion and explanation, and proposes policy changes; comments are sought. Each issue contains a cumulative index.

Although the pharmacopoeias described above are the most important for English readers, a number of others are interesting for comparison of their approach and content. The *Pharmacopoeia Helvetica* (6th edn, 1971), with supplements, is published in loose-leaf form and in three languages (French, German, Italian). The 7th edn will not appear before 1985. An interesting feature is a colour chart for pH indicators, resembling a household paint guide, to be used for matching. The monographs are similar to those of the *BP*, but include cautions (e.g. incompatibility), guidance on possible changes such as sensitivity to light, reference to official preparations (which also appear in the *Pharmacopoeia)* that contain the drug as a main component, and trade names. The supplements bear evidence of the increasing role of the *EP*, as do recent editions of pharmacopoeias in other European countries.

The *Deutsches Arzneibuch (DAB)* is published in two distinct and separate editions, one each for West and East Germany. In the former, the current 8th edn was published in 1978, with a supplement in 1980. It includes a statement permitting the use of non-pharmacopoeial methods if they give the same result as the official one – in accord with the policy of the *BP*. A *Kommentar* (commentary) on *DAB8* is available (by H. Böhme and K. Hartke). This is an annotated version which reproduces the official sections with a black line in the margin and follows each with descriptive and explanatory notes. For example, the monograph on quinine sulphate occupies three pages in the main volume and six pages in the *Kommentar*. The increase comes from details of the synthesis and properties, a detailed explanation of identity and purity tests, an assay, and details of uses and trade names, complete with literature references, as well as notes on differences from other pharmacopoeial tests.

The most recent *Pharmacopée Française* is the 10th edn in loose-leaf format. The monographs follow the *EP* style and, as with the *EP*, the individual pages are dated. The previous edition included information for pharmacists, similar to that in data sheets (*see* below, page 204), and indexes of active ingredients with trade names of products and vice versa. The *Formulaire National* is a complementary volume containing details of preparations such as ointments and tablets. Certain foreign pharmacopoeias are published in English translation and are therefore more readily accessible than might appear at first sight; for example, the *State Pharmacopoeia of the USSR X,* undated, but about 1973, and the *10th Japanese Pharmacopoeia* (1981).

A *British Herbal Pharmacopoeia* (British Herbal Medical Association) is available in three volumes. It represents a revision of earlier herbal materia medica in the light of current knowledge. The monographs include detailed descriptions and therapeutic information.

Drug indexes and compendia

Reference volumes in which are collected details of all drugs currently available fall into two groups: those that merely provide details of proprietary preparations and their manufacturers, and those that provide greater detail about the individual active substances, their indications and adverse reactions, and the preparations containing them. The former group are, of course, essential to pharmacists and are produced in many countries, usually annually. The library of the Pharmaceutical Society of Great Britain, in London, holds a wide range of them. From a practical point of view, the most useful publications are those relating to this country. The *Monthly Index of Medical Specialities (MIMS)* is indeed produced monthly and widely circulated to doctors (free) and to others with a professional interest. Each issue contains details of new products in the form of a data sheet, lists of drugs in a pharmacological classification with presentation, composition and contra-indications, together with a therapeutic index, an alphabetical index and a non-proprietary name index. The *Pharmaceutical Journal* also provides regular information about new products and product changes. The *Chemist and Druggist Directory* (Benn Brothers) is a trade directory and buyers' guide. It contains information about products, a tablet and capsule guide, a résumé of the Medicines Acts and a section providing details of companies with interests in pharmacy and pharmaceuticals. There are other similar publications as well as several which provide more comparative information (described below).

An analogous American volume is the *Drug Topics Red Book* (Medical Economics Co.), an annual which provides product information not only about proprietaries, but also other drug store merchandise, such as cameras, as well as a colour guide for product identification and a section on drug intereactions. An interesting feature of the drug entries is the National Drug Code system. This consists of a four- or five-figure code allotted to each manufacturer by the Food and Drugs Administration. Each product is then further coded with a four-figure code and finally a two-character package code. The identity and package size of each product is thus uniquely defined. There are other similar American publications such as the *American Drug Index* (Lippincott), which gives details of composition, presentation and use of products in alphabetical order with cross-indexing for generic, brand, chemical and *USP/NF* names. Thus, it is relatively simple to find a drug or combination even if only one major constituent is known. There is also a manufacturer/distributor index. Another American book, the *Merck Index* (9th edn, 1976, Merck), is rather more an organic or pharmaceutical chemistry reference work. It includes details of nearly 10 000 substances with a strong medical bias. Each entry contains references to the original literature or reviews and very brief details of therapeutic use where appropriate. There is an extensive cross-index of names.

The indexes for other countries are prepared on similar lines to those described above. The German *Rote Liste* (Editio Cantor, Aulendorf/Württtenberg) is an annual similar to the *American Drug Index*, but contains in addition information about contra-indications and dosages. The French *Dictionnaire Vidal* (OVP) is also an annual, but is brought up to date 10 times during the year by the *Cahiers de Bibliographie Thérapeutique Française*. The *Dictionnaire* is divided into five parts: Part 1, a compound name index with the trade/product name; Part 2, products arranged by pharmacological classification giving the trade names in each group; Part 3, details of therapeutic products with composition, properties, indications, tolerance, dosage, presentation, manufacturer; Part 4, a similar section on other products, such as dietary ones, and mineral waters; Part 5, manufacturers and producers with their product lists.

L'Informatore Farmaceutico (Organizzazione Editoriale Medico-Farmaceutica, Milan), the Italian directory of drugs and manufacturers, is in two volumes. Volume 1 lists all products by trade name with composition, presentation and code, together with over-the-counter preparations (e.g. baby products, diabetic foods) and has a section on prime manufacturers of pharmaceuticals. Volume 2 contains a list of drug substances, a therapeutic classification, a list of dietetic and other products and information about manufacturers and concessionaires. The whole is kept up to date by the *Notiziario Medico Farmaceutico*.

Among many other such indexes, the following are given to provide some indication of geographical coverage: *Prescription Proprietaries Guide* (Australia and New Zealand); *Compendium of Pharmaceuticals and Specialities* (Canada); *Catalogo de Especialidades Farmaceuticos* (Spain); *Vademecum Internacional* (covering Central and South America); *Felleskaterlog* (Norway); *Japanese Drug Directory* (JAPTA list); *Indian Pharmaceutical Guide* and the regional editions of *MIMS*.

The Pharmaceutical Society library holds a comprehensive proprietary drug index on cards listed by trade name with details of composition, action and use, manufacturer and country. This has been compiled from data such as new product indexes and also from the literature. It includes drugs which have not been marketed commercially as well as proprietaries. Many of the entries have been compiled from the journal *Unlisted Drugs* (Pharmaceutical Section, Special Libraries Association, Box 401,

Chatham, New Jersey). This is issued monthly and provides current-awareness coverage of all newly reported drugs which are not yet listed by name, composition and manufacturer in a basic drug compendium such as *Martindale* (*see* below). It also contains reviews of new books on drugs and certain other data. Information about each drug is given under the following headings: name, composition, equivalent preparation, manufacturer, pharmacological or clinical activity, reference. Information may also be provided by a structural diagram, dosage, synonyms and any earlier references in the journal. An interim index of numbers and names appears in July and an annual index after December. There is also a cumulative index. A valuable service is provided in the alternative supply of the data on cards each month.

The second group of drug compendia comprises those which provide more descriptive information than the group dealt with above. Some of these are annual volumes but many appear less frequently. Foremost among the English volumes is *Martindale's Extra Pharmacopoeia* edited by J. E. F. Reynolds (28th edn, Pharmaceutical Press, 1983). The aim of this is to provide practising physicians and pharmacists with up-to-date information on all substances in current use, whether official, unofficial or proprietary. It is compiled from the literature and draws on 28 pharmacopoeias and national formularies. Large numbers of references and abstracts are included. Part 1 contains more than 3990 monographs arranged broadly alphabetically but grouped into chapters covering drugs with similar action and use. Each monograph includes some or all of the following information: name of the drug together with official name and synonyms; molecular formula and molecular weight; list of foreign pharmacopoeias in which the drug may be found; dose, including information as to division and time, and paediatric dose; description and brief details of physical and pharmaceutical properties; dependence; adverse effects; antidotes; precautions, absorption and fate; uses. Brief abstracts may be provided under these headings, compiled from the literature. Finally, details are given of official preparations and of proprietary preparations available in the UK and proprietary names in use elsewhere. Part 2 contains short monographs on 1120 miscellaneous (new, obsolescent) drugs and Part 3 details (including composition but excluding information about claimed actions) of 900 medicines available over the counter and which may be advertised to the public in Great Britain.

Martindale was first published in 1883 and has appeared variously in one or two volumes at intervals since. Formerly, vol 2 included analytical and other data but this is now published as a series of companion volumes. *Martindale* is probably the key book for the bookshelf of anyone whose main interest is covered by the subject matter of this chapter. Certainly it should be readily available. It contains a mass of detailed information and provides direct access to original literature. The individual 'chapters', read as a whole, provide a succinct review of current therapeutics and clearly indicate those areas in which more effective and specific drugs are needed. Like all the best reference books, once opened it tempts one to digress into other pages. This edition has been compiled from a computer-based databank and the data will eventually be available online. Not surprisingly, *Martindale* is often used as the yardstick by which similar volumes are measured in reviews. Few measure up to it.

The format of the *British National Formulary (BNF)* (British Medical Association and the Pharmaceutical Press) underwent complete revision in 1981. Its aim is to promote effective prescribing and it is prepared for the benefit of professional staff in the National Health Service. It contains a main section of chapters dealing with the drugs and preparations used for treatment of disease of particular body systems, such as the respiratory system, or for a particular purpose, such as vaccines. Guidance is given about relative costs, and the preference of the panel of experts who compile the *Formulary* for particular preparations is indicated. In addition, there are sections on drug interactions, advice on prescribing in renal impairment and similar features. A *Dental Practioners' Formulary* is included, as is an extensive index. In its new style, the *BNF* is revised and published every six months. Although the current policy of the *BNF* has been subjected to some criticism, the widespread distribution of the book to doctors, pharmacists and students completing their courses for these professions ensures that its opinions and recommendations have considerable impact.

A further source is provided by the *Pharmaceutical Codex* (11th edn, Pharmaceutical Press, 1979) the greatly revised successor to the *British Pharmaceutical Codex* (*see* page 196). In its new format it is intended to serve as an encyclopaedia of drug information for pharmacists and others concerned with the preparation and use of medicines. The entries on drug substances include trade names, description, metabolism, action and uses, side effects, preparations available and whether British or European pharmacopoeial standards exist. There is additional information for the pharmacist about containers, storage and advice to patients. Other sections of the *Codex* deal with diseases, clinical pharmacy and surgical dressings.

One of the American volumes similar to *Martindale* is *AMA*

Drug Evaluations. The latest edition is that for 1980 (American Medical Association). This provides details of pharmaceutical preparations for those prescribing, dispensing and administering drugs. The chapters are arranged in groups by therapeutic use, with a short introductory section. Each drug has a monograph which includes dose, route of administration and proprietary names. Although there are similarities with *Martindale,* the coverage is in some respects narrower. One area in which confusion may arise is with regard to proprietary names. Those given here are largely confined to those of North America, whereas *Martindale* provides names used in several countries. Although this may be considered a minor point, the immediate relevance of some of the information in the *AMA* volume is lost as a result.

The growing demand for information about products to be available in a defined style for physicians and, particularly in America, for patients, has resulted in publication of compendia in several countries.

The Medicines Act 1968 (*see* page 206) requires that data sheets for medicinal products, to a format prescribed by regulation, be circulated to practitioners by the manufacturer. To simplify the system, the Association of the British Pharmaceutical Industry produces the *ABPI Data Sheet Compendium.* This combines data sheets from most companies, listed in alphabetical order, together with a product (trade mark) index, an index of non-proprietary names and a list of participating companies. Each sheet contains entries under the headings: presentation, uses, dosage and administration, contra-indications, etc., pharmaceutical precautions, legal category, package quantities, further information and product licence number.

The *USP* compiles an annual *USP Dispensing Information* in two volumes. Volume 1 is for the 'health care provider' and contains data similar to the *ABPI* compendium. Each entry comprises official name, dose form, category, pharmacology, precautions, side and adverse effects, patient consultation, dosages and storage. Volume 2 is particularly interesting being intended for use by the patient and for display in a pharmacy or hospital. The entries are written in less technical language and consist of name, explanation of use, information about proper use, precautions and side effects. It is suggested that copies of the relevant entries are made for the patient to take home. The *Physicians' Desk Reference* (Medical Economics) is another American annual, with supplements, whose purpose is clear from its title. The volume contains indexes for manufacturers' and product names, and products by category and generic name. There is a product identification colour guide and information is grouped by manufacturer. An uncommon feature is the section on diagnostic products.

Other similar compendia include the *MIMS Annual*, for Australia, which incorporates the *Australian Drug Compendium* and has entries of the data sheet format; the *Repertorio Terapeutico*, from the publishers of *L'Informatore Terapeutico*, which contains entries for about 5000 drugs and mixtures in both Italian and English; and *FASS (Farmacevtiska Specialiteter i Sverige)*.

A distillation of information from 12 main sources is available in the *Index Guide to Rational Drug Therapy* by H. Fukushima, T. Okazaki and M. Noguchi (Excerpta Medica, 1982) arranged in sections which are classifications of drugs by indication, of drug effects, of drugs by side effect and a main drug index. The information is so designed that drugs can be traced from the name of a disease or symptoms with drug-induced diseases. Entries consist of reference to the sources, which include *Martindale*, *Pharmacological Basis of Therapeutics* by Gilman, Goodman and Gilman (Macmillan, 1975), *Side-effects of Drugs*, *Year Book of Drug Therapy*, *Clin-Alert* and the *Physicians' Desk Reference*, all of which are mentioned above. The drawback of such a volume is the speed with which it dates unless it is frequently revised.

It may be apparent that one problem associated with the study of drugs in current use is the plethora of names which may be used for one substance in several countries. There are three reference volumes which are of importance with regard to the assignment of officially accepted names for drugs. WHO proposed *International Nonproprietary Names (INN)* for drugs in international use. The 20th report of the Expert Committee involved, published as *Nonproprietary Names for Pharmaceutical Substances* (Technical Report Series No 581, WHO, 1975), is a valuable guide to the system. Lists of new names are published every six months in *WHO Chronicle*. The latest cumulative list (International Nonproprietary Names for Pharmaceutical Substances No 6) appeared in 1982 and is a computer print-out of *INN* in Latin, English, French, Russian and Spanish. It includes national names where these differ significantly from the *INN*. Chemical names and graphic formulae are not included and must be found in the separate published lists. *British Approved Names 1981* (HMSO, 1981) is the most recent complete list of official names prepared by the British Pharmacopoeia Commission. The entries give official and chemical names, trade names, *Chemical Abstracts* registry number, manufacturer(s), code numbers and claimed therapeutic activity. The existence of pharmacopoeial monographs is indicated. Guiding principles for selection of names are given, together with guidance on systematic chemical nomenclature of some groups of compounds, and a proprietary name/Approved Name cross-index.

Valuable compilations of synonyms are available: the most extensive is probably *Organisch-chemische Arzneimittel und ihre Synonyma* by M. Negwer in 3 vols (5th edn, Akademie-Verlag, 1978). In German, with an English preface, this lists over 6000 drugs and more than 60 000 synonyms. Entries are included by incremental molecular formulae. The following are given for each drug: structural and empirical formulae; *Chemical Abstracts* registry number; systematic names; salts which may be in use; synonyms, including official names; and therapeutic use. Volume 3 contains a group index for identification of drugs related chemically or pharmacologically.

The *Index Nominum 1982* (Société Suisse de Pharmacie, 1982) is the 11th edn of a volume revised at about two-year intervals. The main language is French, with instructions for use in English and German as well. It is a compilation of synonyms for therapeutic substances on an international basis and consists of an alphabetical list of drug names, including extensive cross-references. The key entries take the *International Nonproprietary Name* or another national approved name and give the chemical name, structural formula, therapeutic class, trade names and sources, and monograph titles in internationally important pharmacopoeias. If one name for a drug is known, any others can be traced very easily. The complete data base is now held on computer for eventual access online.

The corresponding English language volume is *Pharmacological and Chemical Synonyms* by E. E. J. Marler (7th edn, Excerpta Medica, 1983) which lists names only, with no structural formulae or indication of therapeutic use.

Legal requirements

At a time when statutory control over the introduction of new drugs and the safety and efficacy of older ones is steadily increasing in many countries, it is pertinent to add a brief note on legal requirements.

A major piece of legislation in this country is the Medicines Act 1968, which exerts control over all aspects of manufacture, wholesaling, retailing and import of 'medicinal products', a class of substance which is defined very widely. This Act has had far-reaching effects on the pattern of drug development and use, and amplifies earlier controls, which were much less extensive. It is implemented by a series of Statutory Instruments. Editorials on and a survey of the first ten years of the Act are in *Brit. J. Clin. Pharmacol.*, **12,** 447–463, 1981. The *Annual Reports of the Medicines Commission* and of the major committees established under the Act are published collectively by HMSO and provide details of their various activities and terms of reference. The Department of Health and Social Security (Medicines Division) issue *MAIL: Medicines Act Information Letter* several times per year. Although intended primarily for holders of licences issued under the Act, the contents are often of more general interest. The Department also issues booklets giving notes for guidance, including a concise outline of the Control of Medicines in the United Kingdom (MAL99).

The *Medicines and Poisons Guide* prepared by M. E. Pearce (3rd edn, Pharmaceutical Press, 1982) is a guide to, and annotated list of, medicines and poisons the supply of which is restricted by law. Cumulated amendments appear monthly in the *Pharmaceutical Journal*.

Britain's membership of the European Economic Community has resulted in legislative changes in the pharmaceutical field and, of course, many others, under the provisions of EEC Directives. These are published in the *Official Journal of the European Communities*, both when first proposed and when adopted. They are reprinted in the *Pharmaceutical Journal*. Since they have considerable bearing on attempts to remove trading barriers, through harmonization of licencing requirements for example, their importance should not be underestimated.

The major statutory control in America is exercised under the Federal Food, Drug and Cosmetic Act 1938 as subsequently amended. One particularly significant group of amendments (the Kefauver–Harris amendments) were enacted in 1962 and, among other things, place all responsibility for antibiotic specifications on the FDA.

Similar legislation is in force or being introduced in many other countries, and is one field included in the quarterly *International Digest of Health Legislation*, collated and published by WHO. With a greater awareness of the risks as well as the benefits of drug treatment, it is inevitable that such legislation will increase rather than diminish.

10

Tropical medicine

V. J. Glanville

At one time tropical medicine was considered to be the concern only of specialists or of doctors resident in the tropics, but the vast increase in and the greater speed of travel in recent years have meant that the diseases largely peculiar to the tropics are no longer the exotic rarities in temperate climates that they once were. Even today, however, tropical medicine still receives too little recognition in formal medical education, with the result that many of those who may need to seek information on some aspect of the subject are unfamiliar with the literature.

The sources of information are considered under the following headings:

(1) Primary sources – (a) journals, (b) official publications, and (c) catalogues and guides to periodicals.
(2) Principal abstracting and indexing services – other bibliographies.
(3) Review publications.
(4) Monographs and major textbooks.

Journals

General: English language

There are several major periodicals in the English language devoted largely or entirely to general tropical medicine and to associated subjects, such as parasitology and entomology. Among the most important of these are the *Transactions of the Royal Society of Tropical Medicine and Hygiene* (the official journal of the Society), the *Annals of Tropical Medicine and Parasitology* (a publication of the Liverpool School of Tropical Medicine) and the *American Journal of Tropical Medicine and Hygiene* (the official journal of the American Society of this name). To these must be added the *Journal of Tropical Medicine and Hygiene* which, after a long and distinguished history of independent publication since 1898, is now sponsored by the London School of Hygiene and Tropical Medicine. The *Bulletin of the World Health Organization* ranks among the first in order of importance; a high proportion of the papers in most issues being of tropical interest (most of the papers are in English, a few in French. A complete, translation in Russian is available). *Tropical and Geographical Medicine*, published in the Netherlands, has an international authorship. All these journals publish a wide variety of papers, including those of a mainly clinical nature, those of a more scientific and parasitological interest, and descriptions of field surveys and conditions. A rather different periodical is *Tropical Doctor,* which is designed to meet the needs of medical workers, particularly those in remote places, for practical guidance on the conditions and problems they meet. Unlike the other journals mentioned, it does not publish the results of original research. The *Journal of Tropical Paediatrics* is a useful specialized publication.

The increasing frequency with which 'tropical' diseases are seen in temperate climates is reflected in the number of papers on these diseases which now appear in general medical journals, such as *The Lancet,* the *British Medical Journal,* the *Journal of the American Medical Association,* and equivalent publications in other countries as well as general scientific journals. These can be traced through the use of an indexing or abstracting service, a particularly valuable one being the *Tropical Diseases Bulletin.* A separate section on such services is included below.

Regional, national and local: English language

The proportion of papers on tropical medicine and on general or 'non-tropical' medicine in national or local journals largely reflects climatic conditions or levels of development. Thus, the general medical journals of South Africa and Australia (the *South African Medical Journal* and the *Medical Journal of Australia*) often publish papers of tropical interest, and in journals published in regions or countries nearer to or in the tropics the proportion of such papers is naturally higher. The *Indian Journal of Medical Research*, first published in 1913, is among those with the longest history, but no longer is it comprised almost entirely of papers on malaria, plague and dysentery, and among the most important tropical medical journals of the world is the *Southeast Asian Journal of Tropical Medicine and Public Health*, published under the auspices of the Southeast Asia Region Co-operative Project. Other regional and national journals include the *Medical Journal of Malaysia*, the *Journal of the Formosan Medical Association*, the *Journal of the Egyptian Medical Association*, the *East African Medical Journal*, the *Central African Journal of Medicine*, the *Medical Journal of Zambia*, the *Ethiopian Medical Journal*, the *Saudi Medical Journal* and many others.

Special diseases: English language

Virtually the only disease in the Tropics to which English language periodicals are now specially devoted is leprosy, and this is well served by two such journals: the *International Journal of Leprosy*, published in New York, and *Leprosy Review,* published in London for the British Leprosy Relief Association.

Foreign language

There are many periodicals which could be isolated under this heading. A short selection of the most relevant is shown below by title under the principal language of publication.

French

Annales de la Société Belge de Médecine Tropicale (Brussels)
Bulletin de la Société de Pathologie Exotique (Paris)
Dakar Médical (Dakar)
Médecine d'Afrique Noir (Dakar)
Médecine Tropicale (Marseilles)
Revue Internationale du Trachome (Paris)

German

Acta Tropica (Basle; mostly in German, some in English)
Tropenmedizin und Parasitologie (Stuttgart; many important papers in English)

Portuguese

Revista Brasileira de Malariologia e Doenças Tropicais (Rio de Janeiro)
Revista do Instituto de Medicina Tropical de São Paulo (São Paulo)

Revista Medica de Moçambique (Maputo)
Revista de Patologia Tropical (Goiana)

Spanish

Boletín Chileno de Parasitologia (Santiago, Chile)
Boletín de la Oficina Sanitaria Pan-americana (Washington, DC)
Revista Cubana de Medicina Tropical (La Habana)
Salud Pública de México (México)

Associated subjects: parasitology, helminthology, entomology

These and similar fields are, in the main, the preserve of the expert, who will know where to find information, but parasites or insects play a part in so many tropical diseases that any treatment of the subject would be incomplete without at least some mention of some of the more important periodicals. Among these are;

Annales de Parasitologie Humaine et Comparée (Paris)
Annals of the Entomological Society of America (Baltimore)
Bulletin of Entomological Research (London)
Experimental Parasitology (New York)
International Journal for Parasitology (Oxford)
Japanese Journal of Parasitology (Tokyo; many papers in English)
Journal of Economic Entomology (Monasha, Wisconsin)
Journal of Helminthology (London)
Journal of Medical Entomology (Honolulu)
Journal of Parasitology (Lancaster, Pennsylvania)
Journal of Protozoology (New York)
Meditsinskaya Parazitologiya i Parazitarnye Bolezni (Moscow; Russian with short
    English summaries)
Mosquito News (Albany)
Parasitology (Cambridge)
Revista di Parassitologia (Rome)

Official publications of international agencies, government departments and other organizations

The reports of the World Health Organization, especially those in the *Technical Report Series,* are of great value. These reports usually embody the findings of a special or expert committee convened to study a particular problem; and, in general, they provide useful summaries of the recent position, often with recommendations for action and for future research. Reports cover almost the whole spectrum of tropical medicine; and major diseases, such as malaria, African trypanosomiasis, filariasis, cholera and tuberculosis are the subject of regular discussion and report.

Another publication of the World Health Organization, *Public Health Papers,* includes collective studies on control programmes, on health personnel and on management in health services. The *Weekly Epidemiological Record* (WHO) provides up-to-date information on the incidence and epidemiology of many diseases. Other publications of the World Health Organization, such as the *World Health Statistics Annual* and also of the US Department of Health, Education and Welfare, are referred to in Chapter 8. These are especially valuable in the study of the epidemiology of tropical diseases.

The reports of the many research institutions throughout the world concerned with the study of various aspects of tropical disease (and of grant-giving bodies such as the Rockefeller Foundation or the Wellcome Trust) are of interest mainly to the specialist, but some countries still publish regular annual medical reports which give valuable indications of their particular problems.

Catalogues and guides to periodicals

Sources of information concerning books and other monographic publications in tropical medicine are principally the catalogues of libraries; but there are relatively few in this field. The catalogue of publications of the World Health Organization has great value as a guide to the technical reports, monographs, public health papers and other publications of this body. But equally the list *Recent Acquisitions,* which has been published by the World Health Organization library under various titles since 1947, provides a survey of books, reports, symposia, etc., relating to tropical medicine, public health and a wide coverage of the medical and biological sciences. It is arranged in classified subject order (according to the Barnard Classification Scheme) and is available free to appropriate libraries. The *Dictionary Catalogue of the London School of Hygiene and Tropical Medicine* (G. K. Hall) was published in 1965. It is a catalogue, under authors and under subjects, of material in one of the world's largest libraries of tropical medicine and public health. A five-year supplement was added in 1970, and a seventh volume of the main work covers the complete periodical and report series holdings. The list of current periodicals is updated by the publication from time to time, as a supplement to *Tropical Diseases Bulletin* and *Abstracts on Hygiene* of a list of publications examined by the Bureau of Hygiene and Tropical Diseases. Similarly, library accessions lists are issued by other medical libraries such as the *Institut de Médecine Tropicale Prince Leopold, Antwerp, Bibliotheca Brodeniania Bulletin* and the *East African Medical Bibliography*, published by Makerere University. Publication of *PAHODOC: A Computerized Index to Pan American Health Organization and World Health Organization Documents* commenced in 1980.

The firm of G. K. Hall has published many other library catalogues. Included in their list are the following which, among others, are valuable source material for historical and current literature of tropical medicine and related subjects:

Great Britain. Commonwealth Relations Office. India Office. Library. *Catalogue of European Printed Books*, 10 vols, 1964
Great Britain. Colonial Office. *Catalogue of the . . . Library*. 15 vols, 1964; also first supplement, 1967; second supplement 1972
Royal Commonwealth Society [formerly Royal Empire Society]. *Subject Catalogue . . .* 11 vols, 1930–1971

Although these catalogues are large and expensive, access to them in a library can be a fruitful source of references to sociological, geographical or historical literature which is needed in tropical epidemiological studies.

Principal abstracting and indexing services: other bibliographies

The only service exclusively devoted to tropical medicine, the *Tropical Diseases Bulletin*, was started in 1908 as an intergovernmental information service under the titles of *Sleeping Sickness Bureau Bulletin* and *Kala-Azar Bulletin*. It is now published monthly by the Bureau of Hygiene and Tropical Diseases with assistance from the British and some Commonwealth governments. The Bulletin is deliberately selective and abstracts only papers which describe advances in knowledge or treatment of tropical diseases or which provide good reviews of the current state of knowledge. There are also articles on, and summaries of, the literature of important topics, such as malaria or leprosy; and book reviews appear in each issue. Annual author, subject and geographical indexes are provided. It is important to remember that *Abstracts on Hygiene and Communicable Diseases*, published by the Bureau, is complementary and the two publications cover most aspects of health and disease throughout the world. These two abstract bulletins are now published within the Commonwealth Agricultural Bureaux (CAB) computer system; and abstracts will be available as part of the CAB database, as well as those on entomological, mycological, helminthic, protozoal and nutritional subjects from the CAB journals listed below.

There are many other abstracting services that provide a conspectus of the literature of particular sections of the practice of tropical medicine. First, it is worth emphasizing the value of the comprehensive services (which are discussed in Chapter 3) such as *Biological Abstracts,* which reviews the world's literature on the agents and vectors of disease, for example, and *Chemical Abstracts,* with its world-wide coverage of nutritional, biochemical and physiological papers. Second, the computerization of these large and costly services has led to the production of specialized publications for the individual worker. One such important newcomer is the *Quarterly Bibliography of Major Tropical Diseases* (1978–) which is produced from the *Index Medicus* input and which lists papers, with abstracts included in the author section, under the following headings: Filariasis, Leishmaniasis, Leprosy, Malaria, Schistosomiasis, and Trypanosomiasis. The *Bibliography* is prepared and circulated to participating institutions and workers as part of the UNDP/WORLD BANK/WHO Special Programme for Research and Training in Tropical Diseases.

More specialized is *Nutrition Abstracts and Reviews* (CAB, 1931–), perhaps the best example in this group of completeness of coverage, currency of indexes and value of abstracts. It covers both human and animal nutrition in two series and most quarterly issues begin with a review article. As a guide to the literature relating to the vectors of tropical disease, we have two useful periodicals, the *Bulletin Signalétique. Part 364. Protozoaires et Invertébrés,* and the *Review of Applied Entomology, Series B: Medical and Veterinary.* Coverage by these two periodicals appears comparable, although the *Bulletin,* of course, has a higher proportion of entries from French-language journals. Each of these provides input to a major database – the Commonwealth Agricultural Bureaux system and the French Centre de Documentation Scientifique et Technique.

Three other specialized periodicals have especial importance as sources of information in tropical medicine. *Courrier: Revue Médico-Sociale de l'Enfance* (1950–) is a useful guide to the literature of tropical as well as temperate paediatrics and related topics. Each issue contains both review articles and a bibliographical section with abstracts in both English and French. *Helminthological Abstracts, Series A: Animal and Human Helminthology* has a very good coverage, with abstracts, of the world's literature on helminthic agents of disease such as schistosomes or filariae; and a companion series, *Protozoological Abstracts* (CAB, 1977–) is also now produced from the Commonwealth Institute of Parasitology. Similarly, the quarterly *Review of Medical and Veterinary Mycology* (CAB) has covered tropical mycological conditions since 1943.

Again it is necessary to draw attention to those serials which are a valuable source for the bibliography of tropical medicine. The *Bulletin de l'Institut Pasteur* (Paris) was, from 1903 to 1970, first an abstract journal, then an index to the literature of infectious diseases, microbiology, hygiene and related topics. It is a useful source for references to papers by French speaking writers, as well as giving a good coverage of the rest of the world. Similarly, the *Zentralblatt für Bakteriologie, Mikrobiologie und Hygiene. I. Abt. Referate*, has been published separately since 1902 with a wider scope than just tropical medicine, but has much value for the literature of this subject, especially for that emanating from Germany, Eastern Europe and the USSR. Some of the sections of *Excerpta Medica* (for example, *No 25 – Hematology; No 17 – Public Health, Social Medicine and Hygiene;* and *No 4 – Microbiology*) are important sources of reference, with good abstracts.

Other bibliographies

Perhaps the most important survey of epidemic diseases which has been published is the *Welt-Seuchen-Atlas . . . World Atlas of Epidemic Diseases* (3 vols, Falk-Verlag, 1952–1961). This has an excellent coverage of tropical conditions and each map is accompanied by a review of the subject and a bibliography of the source literature. A similar series of maps was begun by the American Geographical Society, *The Atlas of Diseases*, plates 1–17, 1950–1955, but the project was abandoned. In this series, text and bibliography are printed on the back of each map. The World Health Organization continues to record the changing incidence of disease in its various publications (*see* above). Other publications of this type, of value for the epidemiologist or historian, are: *A World Geography of Human Diseases* edited by G. M. Howe (Academic Press, 1977); *A Demographic Survey of the British Colonial Empire* by R. R. Kuczynski (3 vols, Oxford University Press, 1948–1953); the *Bibliographie Géographique Internationale* (Paris, 1915–), which is useful for background material in epidemiology and demography; the series *Studies in Medical Geography* edited by J. M. May and D. M. McLellan (Hafner, 1958–), which includes masterly studies of the ecology of disease and of malnutrition in particular areas; and the series *Geomedical Monographs* edited by H. J. Jusatz (Springer, 1967–), which includes country by country studies of medical geography, e.g. of Libya, Kuwait, Afghanistan and Ethiopia.

There are many important bibliographies of the medical literature of tropical countries. Examples are: *Bibliografia Brasileira de Medicina* (Rio de Janeiro: Instituto Brasileiro de Bibliografia e Documentação) which has been published since 1941, but the earlier parts cover the State of São Paulo only; *Bibliography of the Distribution of Diseases in East Africa* by B. W. Langlands (Makerere University College, 1965) and a continuation, *East African Medical Bibliography* (1970–); *Medicine in British West Africa, 1880–1956 – an Annotated Bibliography* by C. Tettey (Negro University Press, 1971); and *Global Epidemiology* by J. S. Simmons and others (3 vols, Heinemann (later Lippincott), 1944–1954). The last has a world coverage, but there are a number of others devoted to particular countries.

Similarly, there have been many bibliographies of specific tropical diseases and it is necessary to consult a good library catalogue, such as that of the World Health Organization or of the London School of Hygiene and Tropical Medicine, in order to find whether a bibliography of a particular disease has already been compiled. Some international or national organizations have been prominent in recognition of the value of such bibliographies, such as the World Health Organization (e.g. hookworm, yaws) or the South Pacific Commission (filariasis). Bibliographies of special interest, among others, are *Indice Bibliografico da Lepra* by L. Keffer (3 vols, Bibliotca do Departmento de Profilaxia da Lepra, São Paulo, 1944–1948); *Schistosomiasis: a Bibliography of the World Literature from 1852 to 1962* by K. S. Warren and V. A. Newill (Press of Western Reserve University, 1967) and three further works by K. S. Warren and D. B. Hoffman, Jr., in 1973, 1976 and 1978, provide additional citations, abstracts and condensations of significant papers; the bibliography of schistosomiasis, with selected abstracts, is continued in two publications of the Edna McConnell Clark Foundation, New York, namely *Schisto Packet* (2 vols, 1977) and *Schisto Update* (1978–); *Bibliography of Leishmania and Leishmanial Diseases* by D. Heynemann *et al.* (2 vols, Cairo, 1980); *Bibliography of Ticks and Tickborne Diseases from . . . 800 BC to . . . 1973* by H. Hoogstraal (5 vols., USNAMRU, Cairo, 1970–1974, *Chagas's Disease (South American Trypanosomiasis): a Bibliography* by M. A. Miles and J. E. Rouse (Bureau of Hygiene and Tropical Diseases, London, 1970); *Doença de Chagas: Bibliographia Brasileira* (Instituto Brasileiro de Bibliografia e Documentação, Rio de Janeiro, 1958); trypanosomiases are also surveyed in *Trypanosomiasis Current References* (Salford,

1971–1974), which is a continuation of the bibliography in the monograph *The African Trypanosomiases* by H. W. Mulligan (1971), and also *Tsetse and Trypanosomiasis Information Quarterly* (1978–), which includes abstracts but covers African trypanosomiasis only; *Bibliography of Kuru* by M. P. Alpers *et al.* (US National Institutes of Health, Bethesda, 1975). The African Studies Association (Massachusetts) has published *Health and Society in Africa: a Working Bibliography* by S. Feierman (1979) and *Infectious Diseases in Africa: a Bibliography of their Distribution and Consequences* by K. D. Patterson (1979).

Lastly, in this same category of bibliographies and indexes it is essential to notice the value of a more general work. The *Index-Catalogue of Medical and Veterinary Zoology* (Stiles and Hassall; 2nd edn by A. Hassall *et al.*, US Government Printing Office, 1932–1952), is primarily a comprehensive author catalogue of the literature of the world on vectors and agents of disease. It is kept up to date by irregular supplements (published by the Oryx Press) and these supplements are now being enriched by a further series indexed by zoological genera and species (*see also* Chapter 12).

Review publications

The importance of review series in medical bibliography has been discussed elsewhere. Pertaining to tropical medicine as a specialty, there is only one series, the *International Review of Tropical Medicine* (1961–). It is not annual, only four volumes having been published to date; but the reviews of particular topics and diseases are of high standard, as are their supporting bibliographies. The *Tropical Diseases Bulletin* provides regular reviews of the recent literature on specific diseases or groups of diseases. *Nutrition Reviews* (1942–), *Nutrition Abstracts and Reviews* (1931–) and *Revue du Paludisme* (1939–1953) are all useful sources for a conspectus of the literature within their appropriate fields. Finally, the dominance of the microbiological aspects of tropical diseases demands that the reviews in series such as *Advances in Parasitology* (1963–) and the *Annual Review of Microbiology* (1947–) should not be overlooked.

Monographs and major textbooks

For a comprehensive list of recent British books on tropical medicine (102 titles) *see* V. J. Glanville, *British Book News,* November 1980, pages 645–649.

General tropical medicine

The standard textbook on tropical medicine in the English language is *Manson's Tropical Diseases* edited by P. E. C. Manson-Bahr and F. I. C. Apted (18th edn, Baillière Tindall, 1982). This is a comprehensive work, which not only provides full descriptions of all the major diseases, but also includes many minor and obscure conditions, and there are adequate sections on parasitology and medical zoology. The first edition was published in 1898 and it is pleasing to see the continuity of the family tradition of service to tropical medicine, from Sir Patrick Manson, the 'Father of the Science of Tropical Medicine', through Sir Philip Manson–Bahr, who edited all the later editions until his death in 1966, to his son Dr P. E. C. Manson–Bahr.

Another good textbook, which might be regarded as the standard American work, is *Tropical Medicine* by G. W. Hunter, J. C. Swartzwelder and D. F. Clyde (5th edn, Saunders, 1976). Not a textbook, but a book for physicians by authors of wide clinical and research experience is *Adams and Maegraith: Clinical Tropical Diseases* edited by B. G. Maegraith (7th edn, Blackwell Scientific, 1980). *Medicine in the Tropics* edited by A. Woodruff (Churchill Livingstone, 1974) is a collection of authoritative reviews of the whole subject by 36 contributors. A *Textbook of Imported Diseases* by E. Nnochiri (Oxford University Press, 1979) and *Geographic Medicine for the Practitioner* edited by K. S. Warren and A. A. F. Mahmoud (Wiley, 1977) are written for the physician in temperate climates. Other very good textbooks for students and practitioners have been published recently, and there is an excellent comprehensive series entitled *Medicine in the Tropics* published by Churchill Livingstone.

A Colour Atlas of Tropical Medicine and Parasitology by W. Peters and H. M. Gilles (2nd edn, Wolfe Medical, 1981) is an excellent supplement to any textbook of tropical medicine; and epidemiology and control of disease are well covered in *The Control of Disease in the Tropics. A Handbook for Medical Practitioners* by Davey and Lightbody (4th edn, revised by T. H. Davey and T. Wilson, Lewis, 1971) and *Epidemiology and Community Health in Warm Climate Countries* by R. Cruickshank, K. Standard and H. B. L. Russell (Churchill Livingstone, 1976).

Finally, of the books in the English language, two that were major standard works of their time, but now long outdated from the practical viewpoint, should be mentioned because of their valuable early references and for the picture which they give of the state of knowledge some fifty years ago. These are *Manual of Tropical Medicine* by A. Castellani and A. J. Chalmers (3rd edn, Baillière Tindall, 1919) and *The Practice of Medicine in the Tropics, by Many Authorities* edited by W. Byam and R. G. Archibald (3 vols, Oxford Medical Publications, H. Frowde and Hodder and Stoughton, 1921–1923).

General tropical pathology: laboratory medicine

A long-standing need for a good book on this subject was met by the publication of *Pathology in the Tropics* by G. M. Edington and H. M. Gilles (2nd edn, Arnold, 1976) which has a good bibliography and over 2000 references. A much longer and very much more expensive book is *Protozoal and Helminthic Diseases, with Clinical Correlation* edited by R. A. Marcial–Rojas (Williams and Wilkins, and Churchill Livingstone, 1971). This also provides many references. Another excellent and readable, but also expensive, book is *Tropical Pathology*, by H. Spencer *et al.* (Springer, 1973). There is also *Pathology of Tropical and Extraordinary Diseases: an Atlas* edited by C. H. Binford and D. H. Connor (vols 1–2, Castle House, 1979). *Tropical Medicine and Parasitology: Classic Investigations* edited by B. H. Kean, K. Mott and A. J. Russell (2 vols, Cornell University Press, 1978) is a useful source of early texts which may not be easily available. *Toxicology in the Tropics* edited by R. L. Smith and E. A. Bababunmi (Taylor and Francis, 1980), *Clinical Radiology in the Tropics* by W. P. Cockshott and H. Middlemiss (Churchill Livingstone, 1979), *Radiology of Tropical Diseases* by M. M. Reeder and P. S. Palmer (Williams and Wilkins, 1981) and *A Medical Biochemistry for the Tropics* by J. K. Candlish (Baillière Tindall, 1977) are valuable supplementary texts.

Diseases

LEPROSY

Leprosy, an ancient disease which still affects so many millions, is the subject of a number of works. *Leprosy in Theory and Practice* edited by R. G. Cochrane and T. F. Davey (2nd edn, John Wright, 1964) with many contributors is still a valuable account of all aspects of the disease. *The Handbook of Leprosy* by W. H. Jopling (2nd edn, Heinemann Medical, 1978) and *Leprosy* by A. Bryceson and R. E. Pfaltzgraff (2nd edn, Churchill Livingstone, 1979) provide modern accounts of recognition and treatment.

CHOLERA

There is no recent encyclopaediac work on the major scourge of cholera, but publications of the World Health Organization and of the International Centre for Diarrhoeal Diseases Research, Dacca, collect much valuable information on current knowledge and research in progress.

MALARIA

As is to be expected, there is a large volume of literature on malaria, and only a few of the most important works can be considered here. *Malaria* by J. P. Kreier (3 vols, Academic Press, 1980) is a valuable compilation of information on all aspects of the disease. *Essential Malariology* by L. J. Bruce-Chwatt (Heinemann Medical, 1980) combines essential knowledge of the parasite and its vector with basic information on the disease and its control. A book devoted to all aspects of the problems is a *Textbook of Malaria Eradication* by E. Pampana (2nd edn, Oxford University Press, 1969). This has a list of about 650 references. *Chemotherapy of Malaria* edited by L. J. Bruce-Chwatt *et al.* (2nd edn, WHO, 1981) brings this important aspect up to date, with 300 selected references. *Chemotherapy and Drug Resistance in Malaria* by W. Peters (Academic Press, 1970) is not a book for the clinician, but is a valuable collation and analysis of the vast amount of experimental work on this subject, with particular reference to the increasingly important aspect of drug resistance. There are over 2200 references. Finally, with regard to the parasites which cause all the trouble and to many others which do not affect man, P. C. C. Garnham has written a 1000 page monograph, *Malaria Parasites and other Haemosporidia* (Blackwell Scientific, 1966), which is certain to remain the standard work of reference for many years. A very important monograph with more emphasis on the disease process is *The Primate Malarias* by G. R. Coatney, W. E. Collins, McW. Warren and P. G. Contacos (US Government Printing Office, 1971). *Rodent Malaria*, by R. Killick-Kendrick and W. Peters (Academic Press, 1978) is another valuable source of information on related forms of the disease. Amoebiasis, another major protozoal disease, is surveyed in *Pathogenic and Non-Pathogenic Amoebae*, by B. N. Singh (Macmillan, 1975).

TRYPANOSOMIASIS (AFRICAN)

This disease of man and animals in Africa has a literature which must rival that of malaria, but little of it is in the form of books or monographs. Fortunately, the long experience of British workers has recently been brought together in *The African Trypanosomiases* edited by H. W. Mulligan (Allen and Unwin, 1970) which covers this vast subject from the history of sleeping sickness, through all aspects of the infection in man and animals, to the tsetse fly and its control. There are over 1700 reference. The *Role of the Trypanosomiases in African Ecology. A Study of the Tsetse Fly Problem* by J. Ford (Clarendon Press and Oxford University Press, 1971), considers the problem of trypanosomiasis in relation to the ecology of tropical Africa as a whole and to the impact of European civilization. This is fascinating and essential reading for anyone who would attempt a fuller understanding, but its value also lies in its wealth of references, many to little-known historical and ethnographical works.

The natural history of this group of diseases is surveyed in the following titles. *The Trypanosomes of Mammals. A Zoological Monograph* by C. A. Hoare (Blackwell Scientific, 1972) is the first monograph on the trypanosomes to be published since 1912 and ranks with Garnham's book on the malaria parasites. Although zoological in its approach, subjects such as epidemiology and the host–parasite relationships are fully considered. There are over 1700 references. *Biology of the Kinetoplastida* by W. H. R. Lumsden and D. A. Evans (2 vols, Academic Press, 1976–1979) is an exhaustive review of this group. Buxton's monograph *The Natural History of Tsetse Flies. An Account of the Biology of the Genus Glossina (Diptera)* by P. A. Buxton (H. K. Lewis, 1955) is, and will remain, a standard work of reference even though much has been added to knowledge since it was written.

MISCELLANEOUS

Child health is the major problem in the tropical world and there is an extensive literature dealing with all aspects of development, health and disease. Three works which provide a review and also bibliographies are *Paediatrics in the Tropics: Current Review* edited by R. G. Hendrickse (Oxford University Press, 1981), *Paediatric Practice in Developing Countries* by G. J. Ebrahim (Macmillan, 1981) and *Diseases of Children in the Subtropics and Tropics* edited by D. B. Jelliffe and J. P. Stanfield (3rd edn, Arnold, 1978). Burkitt's tumour, of interest to those engaged in virology and cancer research as well as to pathologists and clinicians, has a book devoted to it – *Burkitt's Lymphoma* edited by D. . Burkitt and D. H. Wright (Livingstone, 1970).

In recent years there has been a notable increase in works on basic and primary health care; for example, *Community Diagnosis and Health Action: A Manual for Tropical and Rural Areas* edited by F. J. Bennett (Macmillan, 1980), *Laboratory Manual for Rural Tropical Hospitals: A Basis for Training Courses* by M. Cheesbrough and J. McArthur (Churchill Livingstone, 1975), *Diagnostic Pathways in Clinical Medicine: An Epidemiological Approach to Clinical Problems* by B. J. Essex (2nd edn, Churchill Livingstone 1980) and *Poliomyelitis: A Guide for Developing Countries* by B. J. Huckstep (Churchill Livingstone, 1975).

Snake bites and poisoning by other venomous animals are of concern, not only to people in the tropics, but also to those who keep these creatures in captivity. There are many books, but comprehensive works and key sources of references are *Venomous Animals and their Venoms* edited by W. Bucherl, E. E. Buckley and V. Deulofeu (3 vols, Academic Press, 1968–1972) and *Vol 48, Arthropod Venoms* and *Vol 52, Snake Venoms* in the *Handbook of Experimental Pharmacology* edited by G. V. R. Born (Springer Verlag, 1978, 1979). Much of medical mycology is of tropical interest and a standard work with many references is *Medical Mycology* by C. W. Emmons *et al.* (3rd edn, Henry Kimpton, 1977). Similarly, a recognized standard work on medical entomology is *A Handbook for the Identification of Insects and other Arthropods of Medical Importance* by K. G. V. Smith (British Museum (Natural History), 1973) and *Insects and Hygiene: The Biology and Control of Insect Pests of Medical and Domestic Importance* by J. R. Busvine (3rd edn, Chapman and Hall, 1980). Another work of reference and also a student text is *Entomology in Human and Animal Health* by R. F. Harwood and M. T. James (7th edn, Baillière Tindall, 1980). Probably the most used book on general parasitology is *Craig and Faust's Clinical Parasitology* by E. C. Faust, P. F. Russell and R. C. Jung (9th edn, Lea and Febiger, in preparation). Another very good book is *Textbook of Parasitology* by D. L. Belding (3rd edn, Appleton-Century-Crofts, 1965). A number of other recent textbooks of medical parasitology can be found which all provide a review of current knowledge. But no mention of this subject would be complete without reference to two major classic works of the past: the sixth edition of *Précis de Parasitologie* by E. Brumpt (Masson et Cie), was published in 1949, and Professor Garnham referred to it as 'the testimony of the greatest master living or dead, of the subject'. Another master in his field, indeed he is regarded as the father of protozoology, was C. M. Wenyon and his *Protozoology. A Manual for Medical Men, Veterinarian and Zoologists* (2 vols, Baillière Tindall and Cox, 1926) is unsurpassed. Both these works, apart from their intrinsic interest, are

aluable sources of early references. Helminthic diseases have
)een well surveyed, both clinically and bibliographically, in
Vorms and Disease by R. L. Muller (Heinemann Medical, 1975).

An interesting and most useful development has been the publi-
ation in English of books on the work of Japanese parasitologists;
nuch of it is of great value but hitherto available only in that lan-
,uage. Examples are *Progress of Medical Parasitology in Japan*
dited by K. Morishita *et al.* (5 vols to date, Meguro Parasitologi-
al Museum, Tokyo, 1964–) and *Recent Advances in Researches on
filariasis and Schistosomiasis in Japan* (University of Tokyo Press,
970).

History

1. H. Scott's *A History of Tropical Medicine* (Arnold, 1939) is an
xhaustive study of the subject. Parasitology is well covered by W.
). Foster's *History of Parasitology* (Livingstone, 1965), and R. T.
.eiper's paper 'Landmarks in medical helminthology' in the *Jour-
al of Helminthology*, **7**, 101–110, 1929, is a useful contribution.
V. H. S. Jones's *Malaria and Greek Society* (Manchester Univer-
ity Press, 1909) is a classic in its field. Two works on leprosy
vorthy of note are D. A. Zambaco's *La Lèpre à Travers les Siè-
les et les Contrées* (Masson, 1914) and A. Weymouth's *Through
he Leper Squint: A Study of Leprosy from Pre-Christian Times to
he Present Day* (Selwyn and Blount, 1938). *A History of Bubonic
'lague in the British Isles* by J. F. D. Shrewsbury (Cambridge Uni-
ersity Press, 1970) is an extensive study with 76 pages of refer-
nces and 27 of bibliography. *Health in Tropical Africa during the
'olonial Period* edited by E. E. Sabben-Clare *et al.* (Oxford Uni-
ersity press, 1980) is based on the proceedings of a symposium
eld in Oxford in 1977.

Tropical Medicine and Parasitology: Classic Investigations com-
iled by B. H. Kean *et al.* (2 vols, Cornell University Press, 1978),
rovides a valuable collection of texts not easily available other-
vise. Finally, not a history but a perspective of strategies for the
uture is found in the proceedings of a 1977 conference, *Tropical
Medicine from Romance to Reality* edited by C. Wood (Academic
'ress, 1979).

11

Morbid anatomy: clinical and experimental

D. C. Roberts

Morbid anatomy is that branch of pathology concerned with structural changes in organisms, tissues and cells associated with disease processes. Because morbid anatomy is not concerned with the totality of specific diseases, much of its literature is scattered to be found within the literature of the individual disease. The reader must not believe, therefore, that this chapter will inform adequately: he must be prepared to consult, in addition, that chapter elsewhere in this book which deals with the literature of the ailment in which he is interested.

Somatic disease is normally associated with somatic change. To attempt exhaustively to review sources of information even in the relatively restricted field of clinical morbid anatomy, let alone the much wider field of experimental pathology, is unrealistic. This chapter is intended only to be a guide to those who require access to a particular part of the specialized literature, and is very selective in its coverage. The almost total lack of reference to texts in languages other than English is deliberate, and omission of a particular work does not imply adverse judgement upon it. It is hoped, however, that sufficient sources are included to enable the reader to gain access to that part of the literature relevant to his problem.

Indexes and abstract journals

Indexes and abstract journals are considered in depth in Chapter

3. The morbid anatomist will, however, find most of his needs catered for by *Index Medicus* and its forerunners, and by *Excerpta Medica* and *Current Contents, Life Sciences.*

Index Medicus is, without doubt, a remarkably comprehensive index of the medical sciences, but the reader will not be able to realize its potential unless he is prepared to spend a little time learning how to use it. *Index Medicus* is prepared with the help of a thesaurus containing a list of headings which may be used for indexing. Everything to be indexed must be under one (or more than one) of these index terms; no others may be used. The thesaurus (which is revised annually) is published as *Medical Subject Headings (MeSH)* with the January number each year, and separate copies may be purchased from the Superintendent of Documents, US Government Printing Office, Washington DC 20402, USA. By consulting *MeSH* before starting a search, it is possible to determine the terms which have been used to index the concept of the search, and will be found to be time very well spent. To take an example: it will be found that *mammary gland* is not an index term, but that *breast* and *mammae* are. Reference to these terms in a copy of *Index Medicus* will show that references to the human mammary gland are indexed under *breast*, while those to the non-human mammary gland are indexed under *mammae*.

Excerpta Medica is published in a number of sections, those of most use to the pathologist being *Section 5, General Pathology and Pathological Anatomy; Section 21, Developmental Biology and Teratology;* and *Section 26, Immunology, Serology and Transplantation.* There is a wide journal coverage in this series, and the abstracts are of high quality.

Current Contents, Life Sciences contains facsimile sheets of contents of a wide variety of journals in the life sciences, with excellent coverage of the medical literature. The subject index is arranged by significant words in titles and, at first sight, seems difficult to use, since it is necessary to consider all possible synonyms of the required concept. In practice, familiarity is soon gained, and its use becomes relatively simple. In addition to its immediate use, familiarization is valuable training for future use of computer-driven bibliographic data bases such as MEDLINE and CANCERLINE (*see* Chapter 5) since, although searching by index terms is the norm, textword searching is also permitted, and is often very useful. *Current Contents, Life Sciences* also contains an author index with abbreviated addresses. These addresses, as printed, are very useful to determine the affiliation of the authors, but the reader is advised to use the full postal address when writing for a reprint. Authors are, in general, only too pleased to provide reprints to those they believe have read their papers and to those they believe do not have funds to subscribe to the original journal. Some are less sympathetic on receiving a request from a well-funded organization in a developed country if they believe that the request originates by the reading of a title in an indexing journal. In this context, the reader is urged not to write for reprints unless he really needs them: remember that the cost of reprints, and the postage, has to come out of the author's research budget.

Anatomy and histology

The morbid anatomist will, at all times, require information on his baselines, anatomy and normal histology. These are dealt with fully in Chapter 6, but a few suggestions may not be out of place here. One of the classical texts of anatomy will certainly be required, such as *Gray's Anatomy* edited by P. L. Williams and R. Warwick (36th edn, Churchill Livingstone, 1980) or *Grant's Method of Anatomy* by J. V. Basmajian (10th edn, Williams and Wilkins, 1980), and will probably be the most recent edition of the book the individual used as a student. The choice of textbooks of histology is also often a matter of imprinting as a student: there are many texts, differing in style, and the choice must be, in some degree at least, a matter of individual inclination. *Histology* by A. W. Ham and D. H. Cormack (8th edn, Lippincott, 1979) is a modern classic, graphic in style, and profusely illustrated. Maximow and Bloom's *Textbook of Histology* is one for which many pathologists have a special affection, and those who have a copy of the first edition (Saunders, 1930) still tend to turn to it for advice. The book has gone through many editions since then, and the latest, modern in style and layout, and excellent in content, is *A Textbook of Histology* by W. Bloom and D. W. Fawcett (10th edn, Saunders, 1975). Other texts include *Human Histology* by D. L. Gardner and T. C. Dodds (3rd edn, Churchill Livingstone, 1976), *Histology* by L. Weiss and R. O. Greep (4th edn, McGraw-Hill, 1977), the shorter *Concise Textbook of Histology* by W. J. Krause and J. H. Cutts (Williams and Wilkins, 1981), *Human Histology, Cytology and Microanatomy* by H. Leonhardt (Year Book Medical Publishers, 1976) and *Functional Histology: a Text and Colour Atlas* by P. R. Wheater *et al.* (Churchill Livingstone, 1979). Other examples of atlases are a *Colour Atlas of Histology* by M. B. L. Craigmyle (4th impression, Wolfe Medical, 1980), *An Atlas of Human Histology* by M. S. H. Di Fiore (5th edn, Lea and Febiger, 1982) and *Atlas of Descriptive*

Histology by E. J. Reith and M. H. Ross (3rd edn, Harper and Row, 1977). A book on comparative histology is *Histology of the Vertebrates: a Comparative Text* by W. Andrew and C. P. Hickman (Mosby, 1974).

General textbooks and atlases

Selection of a general textbook of pathology can only be satisfactorily carried out by the individual. There are many excellent, modern texts available, and final choice will probably depend upon presentation in terms of layout and the literary style of the author rather than a judgement of the accuracy of the information. Some dislike double columns of print, some have strong views on the relative merits of one- and two-volume works, while that which to one is an excellent literary style may be pedantry to another. The following is a selection of modern texts which should cater for most tastes:

Pathology edited by W. A. D. Anderson and J. M. Kissane (2 vols, 7th edn, Mosby, 1977)
Muir's Textbook of Pathology edited by J. R. Anderson (11th edn, Arnold, 1980)
A Textbook of Pathology by W. Boyd (8th edn, Kimpton, 1970)
Pathology Illustrated by A. T. Govan and P. S. Macfarlane (Churchill Livingstone, 1981)
Systemic Pathology edited by W. St C. Symmers (6 vols, Churchill Livingstone, 1976–1980)

Books on surgical pathology include

A Textbook of Surgical Pathology by C. Illingworth and B. M. Dick (12th edn, Churchill Livingstone, 1979)
Boyd's Pathology for the Surgeon edited by W. Anderson (8th edn, Saunders, 1967)
Ackerman's Surgical Pathology by J. Rosai (2 vols, 6th edn, Mosby, 1981)
Principles of Pathology in Surgical Practice by K. A. Myers *et al.* (1980)
Surgical Pathology edited by W. F. Coulson (2 vols, Lippincott, 1978)
Introduction to Biopsy Interpretation and Surgical Pathology by J. C. E. Underwood (Springer-Verlag, 1981)

General pathology is catered for by

General Pathology by J. B. Walter and M. S. Israel (5th edn, Churchill Livingstone, 1979)
Processes in Pathology by M. J. Taussig (Blackwell, 1979)
An Introduction to General Pathology by W. G. Spector (2nd edn, Churchill Livingstone, 1980)
Pathologic Basis of Disease by S. L. Robbins and R. S. Cotran (2nd edn, Saunders, 1979)
The Principles of Pathology by A. J. M. Reese (2nd edn, Wright, 1981)
Introduction to the Study of Disease by W. Boyd and H. Sheldon (8th edn, Lea and Febiger, 1980)

Atlases are both popular and useful and include:

A Colour Atlas and Textbook of Histopathology by W. Sandritter and C. Thomas (Year Book Medical Publishers, 1979)

Color Atlas of Pathology by C. F. Geschickter and A. Cannon (Lippincott, 1963)

Colour Atlas of Histopathology by R. C. Curran (2nd edn, Oxford University Press, 1972)

A Colour Atlas of Surgical Pathology by W. Guthrie and R. Fawkes (Wolfe Medical, 1981)

A Colour Atlas of General Pathology by G. A. Gresham (Wolfe Medical, 1979)

Atlas of Ultrastructure: Ultrastructural Features in Pathology edited by C. H. Tseng (Appleton-Century Crofts, 1980), which consists of full-page pictures with short captions on the opposite page

Journals

General journals

Many papers appearing in clinical medical journals contain material relevant to the morbid anatomist. The major weeklies, the *British Medical Journal* and *The Lancet,* must be mentioned, as must the equivalent American journals, such as the *American Journal of Medicine* and *Surgery, Gynecology and Obstetrics,* as well as the journals published by the various State medical societies. The *Journal of the Royal Society of Medicine* publishes accounts of meetings of its various sections: those of interest to the pathologist include the Sections of Pathology, Oncology and Comparative Medicine.

Specialist journals of pathology

Modern pathology is usually considered to date from the publication by Rudolph Virchow of his famous book *Die Cellularpathologie in ihrer Begründung auf physiologische und pathologische Gewebelehre* (Hirschwald, 1858). Some specialist journals of pathology, still in publication, precede this book, as does Virchow's own *Virchow's Archiv für pathologische Anatomie und Physiologie.* By the end of the century, *Zentralblatt für allgemeine Pathologie und pathologische Anatomie* (1892) and the *Journal of Pathology and Bacteriology* (1892) were in publication, and still thrive, the latter (since 1969) being named the *Journal of Pathology* and now being published, regrettably, without either book reviews or obituaries. There are many other journals of pathology, often published by national medical or pathological societies. Examples are *American Journal of Pathology, American Journal of Surgical Pathology, Archives of Pathology and Labor-*

atory Medicine and *Human Pathology*, all from the United States; the Scandinavian *Acta Pathologica et Microbiologica Scandinavica Section A, Pathology, Histopathology* (UK); *Pathology* (Australia); while from Asia there are the *Indian Journal of Pathology and Microbiology* and the *Malaysian Journal of Pathology*.

More specialized and, perhaps, of more interest to the experimentalist are:

British Journal of Experimental Pathology
Experimental Pathology (Jena)
Japanese Journal of Experimental Medicine
Experimental and Molecular Pathology
Journal of Cellular Physiology
Laboratory Investigation
Journal of Comparative Pathology and Therapeutics
Veterinary Pathology
Journal of Invertebrate Pathology (previously the *Journal of Insect Pathology*)

Review series

There are many serial publications of interest to the morbid anatomist. The *International Review of Cytology* (Academic Press) has been edited since its inception in 1952 by Bourne and Danielli. It reached vol 74 in 1982, while vol 24 of *Methods in Cell Biology* edited by L. Wilson (Academic Press) was published in 1982. Publications on general pathology include *Recent Advances in Histopathology, vol 11* edited by P. P. Anthony and N. M. MacSween (Churchill Livingstone, 1981), the *Pathology Annual 1982, vol 17, part 1,* series editors S.C. Sommers and P. P. Rosen (Prentice-Hall, 1982), *Pathobiology Annual* edited by H. L. Oachim since its inception in 1972, the *Year Book of Pathology and Clinical Pathology* (Year Book Medical Publishers), *Pathology Decennials 1966–75* edited by S. C. Sommers, which has seven volumes on various subjects, and *Progress in Surgical Pathology* edited by C. M. Fenoglio and M. Wolff (three vols, Masson, 1980–1981).

Experimental pathology is served by the *International Review of Experimental Pathology* edited by G. W. Richter and M. A. Epstein (Academic Press), which reached vol 23 in 1982, and *Methods and Achievements in Experimental Pathology* series editors G. Jasmin and M. Cantin (Karger, 10 vols to 1981).

The literature of cancer research has its own serial publications. *Advances in Cancer Research* was first published in 1953 and vol 23 is edited by G. Klein and S. Weinhouse (Academic Press, 1982). *Recent Results in Cancer Research* (Springer-Verlag) reached vol 83 in 1982, *Progress in Experimental Tumor Research*, series editor

F. Homberger (Karger) reached vol 25 in 1980, and *Methods of Cancer Research* edited by H. Busch and L. C. Yeoman (Academic Press) reached vol 19 in 1982. The *National Cancer Institute Monographs,* of which there have been 56 to 1981, may be either proceedings of symposia or specially written monographs, while the *Year Book of Cancer* relates significant findings in the literature, both clinical and experimental.

More specialized serials include:

Recent Advances in Haematology–2 by A. V. Hoffbrand *et al.* (Churchill Livingstone, 1977)
Progress in Hematology edited by E. B. Brown, (vol 12, Grune and Stratton, 1981)
Recent Advances in Neuropathology–2 edited by W. T. Smith and J. B. Cavanagh (Churchill Livingstone, 1982)
Progress in Neuropathology edited by H. M. Zimmerman (4 vols Grune and Stratton, 1971–1979)
Perspectives in Pediatric Pathology (4 vols, Year Book Medical Publications, 1973–1978).

Methods

Necropsy

While the pathologist usually has to rely on his surgical colleagues for macroscopic descriptions of lesions *in vivo*, he has at the time of the necropsy, an opportunity to see and to describe the macroscopic appearance of lesions for himself. The quality of his reports will depend, primarily, upon the practical skills and knowledge he has attained by attendance at post-mortem examinations and pathological museums and by conducting necropsies personally whenever this is possible.

He will, however, not be able to do without books. *Color Atlas and Textbook of Macropathology* by W. Sandritter *et al.* (3rd edn, Year Book Medical Publishers, 1979), *Post-Mortem Procedures: an Illustrated Textbook* by G. A. Gresham and A. F. Turner (Year Book Medical Publishers, 1979), *Current Methods of Autopsy Practice* by J. Ludwig (Holt Saunders, 1979), *Autopsy* by J. R. Adams and R. D. Mader (Year Book Medical Publishers, 1976), and *Manual of Surgical Pathology Gross Room Procedures* by J. Rosai (1981), are examples. More specialized is *Medico-Legal Autopsy: the Investigation of Non-criminal Deaths* by B Knight (Churchill Livingstone, 1982), while that excellent book *Pathology of Congenital Heart Disease* by A. E. Becker and R. H. Anderson (Butterworths, 1981) will help with a difficult subject. Atlases are also useful, such as *Gross Pathology: a Colour Atlas* by R. C. Curran and E. L. Jones (Harvey Miller, 1974) and *Atlas of Gross Neurosurgical Pathology* by K. J. Zulch (Springer-Verlag, 1975). Finally, *The Disposal of the Dead* by C. J. Polson and T. K. Marshall (3rd edn, Hodder and Stoughton, 1975) covers all aspects of English practice.

Histological methods

Two journals devoted to histological methods are the *Journal of Histochemistry and Cytochemistry* and the *Histochemical Journal*. A recent book on histological techniques is *Theory and Practice of Histological Techniques* edited by J. D. Bancroft and A. Stevens (Churchill Livingstone, 1982). Dyes and stains, and their use in histology, are described in *Synthetic Dyes in Biology, Medicine and Chemistry* by E. Gurr (Academic Press, 1971) *Conn's Biological Stains* edited by R. D. Lillie (9th edn, Williams and Wilkins, 1977), *Staining Procedures* edited by G. Clark (4th edn, 1981), *Histopathological Stains and their Diagnostic Uses* by J. D. Bancroft and A. Stevens (Churchill Livingstone, 1975) and *Color Atlas of Histological Staining Techniques* by A. Smith and J. W. Bruton (Year Book Medical Publishers, 1978).

In histochemistry, *Histopathological Technic and Practical Histochemistry* by R. D. Lillie and H. M. Fulmer (4th edn, McGraw-Hill, 1976) and *Histochemistry, Theoretical and Applied* by A. G. E. Pearse (4th edn, vol 1, Churchill Livingstone, 1980) are major texts. Pearse's book is to be in three volumes, and 2 and 3 are still to be published at the time of writing. Other texts include:

Histological and Histochemical Methods by K. A. Kiernan (Pergamon, 1980)
Selected Histochemical and Histopathological Methods by S. W. Thompson and L. G. Luna (2nd printing, C. C. Thomas, 1974)
Histochemical Techniques by J. D. Bancroft (2nd edn, Churchill Livingstone, 1975)
Histochemistry: the Widening Horizons of its Applications in the Biomedical Sciences edited by P. J. Stoward and J. M. Polak (Wiley, 1981)
Color Atlas and Manual for Applied Histochemistry by L. W. Chang (C. C. Thomas, 1979).

More specialized are:

Immunocytochemistry by L. A. Sternberger (2nd edn, Wiley, 1979)
Frozen sections in Surgical Diagnosis by A. A. Shivas and S. G. Frazer (Churchill Livingstone, 1971)
Thin is In: Plastic Embedding Tissue for Light Microscopy by W. A. Burns and A. Bretschneider (Raven, 1982)

Finally, the realists among the readers will appreciate *An Atlas of Artefacts Encountered in the Preparation of Microscopic Tissue*

Sections by S. W. Thompson and L. G. Luna (C. C. Thomas, 1978).

Microscopy

Journals concerned with microscopy include the *Journal of Microscopy* (Oxford) and *Scanning Electron Microscopy.* The *Journal of Microscopy* was, before 1969, named the *Journal of the Royal Microscopical Society,* and first appeared in 1878.

It is very sad that there are still many pathologists who use the optical microscope daily, who never realize the potential of their instruments. If all those who have been badly instructed, or have forgotten what they were taught, would buy and read Peter Healey's excellent little paperback *Microscopes and Microscopic Life* (Hamyln, 1969) they would be surprised at the improvements they could make to the performance of their microscopes. Other texts on microscopy include *The Microscope and How to Use It* by P. B. Carona (Gulf Publications, 1970), *Microscope Techniques* by W. Burrells (Halsted Press, 1977), and *The Microscope and How to Use It* by G. Stehli (Dover, 1970). More advanced is the irregular series *Advances in Optical and Electron Microscopy* edited by R. Barer and V. E. Coslett, the most recent being volume 6 (Academic Press, 1979).

Photomicrography is an important skill in microscopy. *The Practical Use of the Microscope* by G. H. Needham (2nd printing, C. C. Thomas, 1977) includes advice on the subject. Other texts are *Microscopy and Photomicrography: a Practical Guide* by R. F. Smith (Prentice-Hall, 1982) and *Photomicrography* by D. Lawson (Academic Press, 1972), while anyone taking up the demanding discipline of time-lapse cinemicrography will find first-class, practical advice in *Time Lapse Cinemicroscopy* by P. N. Riddle (Academic Press, 1979).

Texts on electron microscopy include *Introduction to Electron Microscopy* by C. E. Hall (2nd edn, McGraw-Hill, 1966) and the two series *Principles and Techniques of Electron Microscopy* by M. A. Hayat (9 vols to 1978, Van Nostrand Reinhold) and *Practical Methods in Electron Microscopy* edited by A. M. Glauert (7 vols, 1972–1978, North-Holland). For scanning electron microscopy, there are *Scanning Electron Microscopy* by O. G. Wells (McGraw-Hill, 1974) and *Scanning Electron Microscopy 1978* and *Scanning Electron Microscopy 1979*, both edited by O. Johari and R. P. Becker, while recent texts on applied electron microscopy are *Diagnostic Electron Microscopy* by J. V. Johannessen (McGraw-Hill, 1981), *Introduction to Diagnostic Electron Microscopy* by B.

MacKay (Prentice-Hall, 1981) and *Electron Microscopy in Human Medicine* edited by J. V. Johannessen (10 vols, McGraw-Hill, 1979–1982). More specialized is *Electron Microscopy of Enzymes* by M. A. Hayat (Van Nostrand Reinhold, 5 vols to 1977). Scanning microscopy is catered for by *Introduction to Biological Scanning Electron Microscopy* by M. A. Hayat (University Park, 1978).

Experimental animals

So long as research in pathology was restricted to observation of the human subject, it was impossible effectively to investigate the many problems which arose. This was due, on the one hand, to the lack of reproducible test systems and, on the other, to the ethical impossibility, for many purposes, of subjecting human patients to the conditions of controlled experiments. The proper use of animals permits a wide, but by no means unlimited, range of hypotheses to be tested critically, and it is proper that some mention of the literature on the experimental animal should be made in this chapter.

There are a number of journals devoted to experimental animals, including *Laboratory Animals, Laboratory Animal Science* and the *Journal of the Institute of Animal Technicians*. General textbooks include the *UFAW Handbook on the Care and Management of Laboratory Animals* (5th edn, Churchill Livingstone, 1976), which no laboratory using animals should be without. Other texts include the *Manual of Laboratory Animal Practice and Techniques* by D. J. Short and D. P. Woodnott (2nd edn, Crosby Lockwood, 1969) and *The Laboratory Animal – Principles and Practice* by W. Lane-Petter and A. G. E. Pearson (Academic Press, 1963). A most useful index is the *International Index of Laboratory Animals* edited by M. F. W. Festing (4th edn, MRC Laboratory Animals Centre, 1980) which details holdings of species and strains throughout the world, as is *Standardized Nomenclature for Inbred Strains of Mice: Seventh Listing for the International Committee on Standardized Genetic Nomenclature for Mice* by J. Staats. This is really a journal article (*Cancer Research* **40**, 2083–2128, 1980), but is available from Dr M. F. Lyon, Radiobiological Research Unit, Harwell, Didcot, Berkshire, England or Dr J. Staats, The Jackson Laboratory, Bar Harbor, Maine 04609, USA. This paper lists inbred strains of mice, details holdings and gives much genetic and historical information. *Mouse News Letter,* together with its companion issues *Inbred Strains of Mice* and its bibliographical supplements similarly gives valuable and detailed information on the laboratory mouse. Two textbooks on the subject are *Inbred and Genetically Defined Strains of Laboratory Animals* edited by P. L. Altman and D. D. Katz. *Part 1, Mouse and Rat; part 2, Hamster, Guinea Pig, Rabbit and Chicken* (Federation of American Societies for Experimental Biology, 1979) and *Inbred Strains in Biomedical Research* by M. F. W. Festing (Macmillan, 1979). Books on the application of laboratory animals to research include:

Methods of Animal Experimentation edited by W. I. Gay (vols 1 to 5, Academic Press, 1965–1974)

A Handbook: Animal Models of Human Disease (Armed Forces Institute of Pathology, Washington DC, 1973)

Spontaneous Animal Models of Human Disease edited by E. J. Andrews *et al.* (2 vols, Academic Press, 1979)

Animal Models for Biomedical Research (National Academy of Sciences, 4 vols to 1971)

Immunodeficient Animals in Cancer Research edited by S. Sparrow (Macmillan, 1980)

Reports of symposia include those of the International Committee on Laboratory Animals, while the collected papers of the Laboratory Animals Centre and the *Collected Papers of Carworth, Europe* are useful series on a variety of subjects. Also useful is the irregular publication *Laboratory Animal Handbooks* published by the journal *Laboratory Animals*. Examples are *Laboratory Animals Handbooks 5. Safety in the Animal House* by J. H. Seamer and M. Wood and *Laboratory Animals Handbooks 7. Control of the Animal House Environment* edited by T. McSheehy.

Examples of books on anatomy and cytology are *Histology of the Vertebrates: a Comparative Text* by W. Andrew and C. P. Hickman (Mosby, 1974), *Comparative Animal Cytology and Histology* by U. Welsch and V. Storch (University of Washington Press, 1976) and, more specialized, *An Atlas of Laboratory Animal Haematology* by J. H. Sanderson and C. E. Phillips (Clarendon Press, 1981).

Books on pathology include *Pathology of Laboratory Animals* edited by K. Benirschke *et al.* (2 vols, Springer-Verlag, 1978), *The Pathology of Laboratory Animals* by W. E. Ribelin and J. R. McCoy (2nd printing, C. C. Thomas, 1971), the more general *Pathology of Domestic Animals* by K. V. F. Jubb and P. C. Kennedy (2 vols, 2nd edn, Academic Press, 1970), and, for tumours, *Neoplasms of Domesticated Animals: A Review* by E. Cotchin (Commonwealth Agricultural Bureaux, 1956), *Tumors of Domestic Animals* by J. E. Moulton (University of California Press, 1961), the classic, much sought after *Neoplasms of Domesticated Animals* by W. H. Feldman (Saunders, 1932) and *Animal*

Tumours of the Female Reproductive Tract by E. Cotchin and J. Marchant (Springer-Verlag, 1977).

Further information on the laboratory rat will be found in:

The Anatomy of the Rat by E. C. Greene (Hafner, 1935, reprinted 1971)
Colour Atlas of the Rat: a Dissector's Guide by R. J. Olds (Halsted Press, 1979)
The Microscopic Anatomy of the White Rat by E. M. Smith and M. L. Calhoun (Iowa State University Press, 1968)
The Laboratory Rat, vol 1, Biology and Diseases; vol 2, Research Applications edited by H. J. Baker *et al.* (Academic Press, 1979 and 1980)
The Rat in Laboratory Investigation by E. J. Farris and J. Q. Griffith (2nd edn, 1949, reprinted, Hafner, 1963)
Pathology of Laboratory Rats and Mice edited by E. Cotchin and F. J. C. Roe (Blackwell, 1967)
The Pathology of Aging Rats by J. D. Burek (CRC Press, 1978)
Pathology of Tumours of Laboratory Animals, vol 1, parts 1 and 2: Tumours of the Rat edited by V. S. Turusov *et al.* (International Agency for Research on Cancer, 1972 and 1976), a comprehensive volume

The laboratory mouse is catered for by:

Biology of the Laboratory Mouse by the staff of the Jackson Laboratory and edited by E. L. Green (2nd edn, McGraw-Hill, 1966; reprinted, Dover, 1975)
Handbook on the Laboratory Mouse by C. G. Crispens, Jr, (C. C. Thomas, 1975)
The Mouse in Biomedical Research, vol 1: History, Genetics and Wild Mice edited by H. L. Foster *et al.* (Academic Press, 1981). *Volume 2: Diseases* is in preparation at the time of writing)
The Nude Mouse in Experimental and Clinical Research edited by J. Foch and B. C. Giovanella (Academic Press, 1978)
Pathology of Tumours in Laboratory Animals, vol 2: Tumours of the Mouse edited by V. S. Turusov *et al.* (International Agency for Research on Cancer, 1979), again a comprehensive volume

Further information on other species include, for the hamster, *The Golden Hamster: its Biology and Use in Medical Research* by R. A. Hoffman, P. F. Robinson and H. Magalhaes (Iowa State University Press, 1968) and *The Pathology of the Syrian Hamster* edited by F. Homburger (Karger, 1972); for the guinea pig, the lavish *Anatomy of the Guinea Pig* by A. L. Schiller (Harvard University Press, 1975) and *The Biology of the Guinea Pig* edited by J. W. Wagner and P. J. Manning (Academic Press, 1976); for the rabbit, *The Biology of the Laboratory Rabbit* edited by S. H. Weisbroth *et al* (Academic Press, 1974); for the pig, *The Pig as a Laboratory Animal* by L. E. Mount and D. L. Ingram (Academic Press, 1971); and for the fowl, *Histology of the Fowl* by R. D. Hodges (Academic Press, 1974). Books relevant to the laboratory primate include:

An Atlas of Primate Gross Anatomy – Baboon, Chimpanzee and Man by D. R. Swindler and C. D. Wood (University of Washington Press, 1973)
Laboratory Primate Handbook by R. A. Whitney *et al.* (Academic Press, 1973)
Diseases of Laboratory Primates by T. C. Ruch (Saunders, 1959)

Comparative Pathology in Monkeys by B. A. Lapin and L. A. Yakovleva (C. C. Thomas, 1963)
Pathology of Simian Primates (in 2 parts) edited by R. N. Fiennes (Karger, 1972)

Special pathology

We now come to the consideration of special pathology. No exhaustive treatment can be attempted here: the intention is to give one or more recent sources for each subject, but to treat individual sections rather more liberally where this seems to be desirable.

Ageing

The morphological changes which accompany the ageing process in lower animals, sub-human mammals and man are described in *The Anatomy of Aging in Man and Animals* by A. Warren (Grune and Stratton, 1971). The effect of ageing on cells is dealt with in Aging and Cell Structure, vol 1 edited by J. E. Johnson, Jr, (Plenum, 1981) and *Time, Cells and Aging* by B. L. Strehler (2nd edn, Academic Press, 1977), and advances in research in *Frontiers in Aging Research* by various authors (Elsevier, 1979).

Blood

Articles on the morbid anatomy of the blood may be found in journals of haematology. These include *Acta Haematologica,* the American journal of haematology, *Blood* (New York), the *British Journal of Haematology* and *Folia Haematologica.* Three books on the erythrocyte are the comprehensive *The Red Cell: Production, Metabolism, Destruction, Normal and Abnormal* by J. W. Harris and R. Kellermeyer (Harvard University Press, 1970), *The Red Blood Cell* by D. MacN. Surgenor (2 vols, Academic Press, 1974–1975) and *The Pathology of Sickle Cell Disease* by J. Song (C. C. Thomas, 1971); the leucocyte is catered for by *The White Cell* by M. J. Cline (Harvard University Press, 1975), *Neutrophil Physiology and Pathology* edited by J. R. Humbert *et al.* (Grune and Stratton, 1975) and *Ultrastructure of Haemic Cells* by J. C. Cawley and F. G. Hayhoe (Saunders, 1973). Two recent books are *Blood and its Disorders* edited by R. M. Hardisty and D. Weatherall (2nd edn, Blackwell, 1982) and *Blood and its Diseases* by I. Chanarin *et al.* (2nd edn, Churchill Livingstone, 1980). The blood of children is catered for by *Paediatric Haematology* by M. L. N. Willoughby (Churchill Livingstone, 1977) and *Current Problems in*

ediatric Hematology edited by F. A. Oski *et al.* (Grune and Strat-
ɔn, 1975); that of the elderly by *Blood Disorders in the Elderly* by
. H. Thomas and D. E. B. Powell (Churchill Livingstone, 1971).
A recent book on the cytochemistry of the blood is *Haematological
ytochemistry* by F. G. J. Hayhoe and D. Quaglino (Churchill
ivingstone, 1980), and the leukaemia cell in *Leukemia: Cytology
nd Cytochemistry* by L. Kass (Lippincott, 1982), *The Leukemic
ell* edited by D. Catovsky (Churchill Livingstone, vol 1, 1976;
ol 2, 1981) and *Dynamic Morphology of Leukaemia Cells* by
I. Felix *et al.* (Springer-Verlag, 1978), which is a comparative
tudy by scanning electron microscopy and cinemicrography.

Atlases continue, deservedly, to be popular. Examples are:

tlas of Clinical Haematology by H. Begemann and J. W. Rastetter (3rd edn,
   Springer-Verlag, 1979)
tlas of Haematology by G. A. McDonald, T. C. Dodds and B. Cruickshank (4th
   edn, Churchill Livingstone, 1978)
tlas of the Blood and Bone Marrow by R. P. Custer (2nd edn, Saunders,
   1974)
Colour Atlas of Haematological Cytology by F. G. J. Hayhoe and R. J. Flemans
   (2nd edn, Wolfe Medical, 1982)
andoz Atlas of Haematology (2nd edn, 1973)

tlas of Blood Cells. Function and Pathology edited by D.
ucker-Franklin, M. F. Greaves, C. E. Grossi and A. M. Mar-
ront (2 vols, Lea and Febiger, 1981) is not so much an atlas as a
extbook, particularly well illustrated. A book on comparative
ilood cells is *Comparative Mammalian Haematology* by C. M.
Iawkey (Heinemann, 1975).

Blood vessels

he Pathology of Atherosclerosis by N. Woolf (Butterworths, 1981)

Bone and bone marrow

hondroid Bone, Secondary Cartilage and Metaplasia by W. A. Beresford (Urban
   and Schwarzenberg, 1980)
he Biology of Degenerative Joint Diseases by L. Sokoloff (University of Chicago
   Press, 1969)
Jltrastructure of Bone and Joint Diseases by K. Hirohata and K. Morimoto (Grune
   and Stratton, 1972)
*nternational Histological Classification of Tumours, No 6, Histological Typing of
   Bone Tumours* (World Health Organization, 1972)
omparative Pathology of Tumors of Bone by S. A. Jacobson (C. C. Thomas,
   1971)
Rone Tumours in Man and Animals by L. N. Owen (Butterworths, 1970)
Rone Marrow and Bone Tissue by R. Burkhardt (Springer-Verlag, 1971)
Iistopathology of the Bone Marrow by A. M. Rywlin (Little, Brown, 1976)

International Histological Classification of Tumours, No 14, Neoplastic Diseases of Haematopoietic and Lymphoid Tissues (World Health Organization, 1976)
An Atlas of Bone Marrow Pathology by M. C. G. Israels (4th edn, Heinemann, 1971)
Bone Marrow Biopsy by J. R. Krause (Churchill Livingstone, 1981)
Bone Marrow Interpretation by L. K. Kass (Lippincott, 1979)

Breast

Atlas of the Diseases of the Mammary Gland by I. Degrell (Karger, 1976); the text is duplicated in English and in German
Atlas of Breast Histopathology by R. M. Millis (MTP, 1982)
Colour Atlas of Breast Cytopathology by C. Grubb (HM+M, 1981)
Atlas of the Ultrastructure of Human Breast Diseases by A. Ahmed (Churchill Livingstone, 1978)
International Histological Classification of Tumours, No 2, Histological Typing of Breast Tumours (World Health Organization, 1968)

Cancer

This subject is well represented by specialist journals, and man countries have one or more journals devoted specifically to it. A example is the American *Cancer*, which contains, almost exclus ively, clinical papers. Examples of other American cancer journal are *Oncology* and the *Journal of Surgical Oncology*, which preser both clinical and experimental papers, and the *Journal of th National Cancer Institute* and *Cancer Research*, which are bot predominantly experimental. *Cancer Research* has considerabl antiquity, being first published in 1916 as the *Journal of Cance Research*, becoming the *American Journal of Cancer* in 1931, an adopting its present title in 1941.

Examples of European cancer journals are the *European Jour nal of Cancer and Clinical Oncology* (supported by a grant fror the Ministry of Education of Belgium) and which appended the la three words of its title in 1981, *Neoplasma* (Czechoslovakia), *Bu letin du Cancer* (France), the *Journal of Cancer Research and Cl nical Oncology* (Germany) which is the title adopted by *Zeitschri für Krebsforschung* (1903) in 1979, *Tumori* (Italy) and the *Britis Journal of Cancer* (United Kingdom). Perhaps here may be men tioned the *International Journal of Cancer*. This is the officia journal of the International Union Against Cancer, its editoria office being in Finland.

Asia also publishes specialist cancer journals. Examples are th *Indian Journal of Cancer*, and *Gann* and *Tumor Research*, bot from Japan.

Many of the general textbooks on cancer, such as *Cancer: Prir ciples and Practice of Oncology* edited by V. T. DeVita, Jr, *et a*

Lippincott, 1982), contain excellent sections on the pathology of tumours. Other texts include *Evan's Histological Appearances of Tumours* by B. J. B. Ashley (3rd edn, Churchill Livingstone, 1978) and the classic *Pathology of Tumours* by R. A. Willis (4th edn, Butterworths, 1977). More specialized are the *Histology of Borderline Cancer* by W. W. Park and J. W. Corkhill (Springer-Verlag, 1980), *Pathology of Soft-Tissue Tumours* by S. I. Hajdu (Lea and Febiger, 1979), *Diagnostic Electron Microscopy of Tumours* by F. N. Ghadially (Butterworths, 1980) and *Ultrastructural Appearances of Tumours* by D. W. Henderson and J. M. Papadimitriou (Churchill Livingstone, 1981). Atlases include the monumental *Atlas of Tumor Pathology* by various authors (Armed Forces Institute of Pathology, Washington, DC), the *International Histological Classification of Tumours* (World Health Organization), which is a large series of volumes with accompanying colour slides, the *UICC Illustrated Tumor Nomenclature* by H. Hamperl and L. V. Ackerman (2nd edn, Springer-Verlag, 1969) and *A Colour Atlas of Tumour Histopathology* by N. F. C. Gowing (Wolfe, 1980). The *TNM Classification of Malignant Tumours* (3rd edn, Geneva, UICC, 1978) has been usefully supplemented by the *TNM-Atlas: Illustrated Guide to the Classification of Malignant Tumours* edited by B. Spiessel and others (Berlin, Springer-Verlag, 1982).

Reference to books on the pathology of tumours of laboratory animals is to be found in the section on laboratory animals, but the attention of the reader is particularly drawn to the books published by the International Agency for Research on Cancer: *Pathology of Tumours of Laboratory Animals*, vol 1, parts 1 and 2; *Tumours of the Rat and Pathology of Tumours of Laboratory Animals*, vol 2; *Tumours of the Mouse* edited by V. S. Turusov *et al.* (International Agency for Research on Cancer 1972, 1976 and 1979, respectively).

Cytology

Two journals concerned with cytology are *Cell* and *Cell and Tissue Kinetics*. *The Cell* by D. W. Fawcett (2nd edn, Saunders, 1981) is a fine book, lavishly illustrated with excellent micrographs and, in the Current Histopathology Series, there is the *Atlas of General Cytology* by O. A. N. Husain (MTP, 1982). The following are concerned with diagnostic cytology: *Exfoliative Cytopathology* by Z. M. Naib (2nd edn, Little, Brown, 1976), the comprehensive *Diagnostic Cytology and its Histopathologic Bases* by L. G. Koss (2 vols, 3rd edn, Lippincott, 1979), *Handbook of Diagnostic Cytology* by

H. E. Hughes and T. C. Dodds (Churchill Livingstone, 1968), th
Dutch *Atlas of Clinical Cytology* by P. Lopes Cardozo (1975
emphasizing the use of Geimsa stain in diagnostic cytology, and th
concise *An Atlas of Diagnostic Cytology* by C. Gompel (Wile*
1978) which has good colour plates, but with the disadvantage tha
they are in a section in the middle of the book.

More specialized are *Cytological Atlas of Cerebrospinal Fluid* b
R. M. Schmidt (Johann Ambrosius Barth, 1978), the *Internation*
Histological Classification of Tumours, No 17, Cytology (
Non-Gynaecological Sites (World Health Organization, 1977) an
the encyclopaedic *The Chromosomes in Human Cancer and Leuk*
mia by A. A. Sandberg (Elsevier, 1980). Electron microscopy i
cytology is catered for by *Cell Structure: an Introduction to Biolog*
cal Electron Microscopy by P. G. Toner and K. E. Carr (Churchi
Livingstone, 1982), *Fine Structure of Cells and Tissues* by K. R. Po*
ter and M. A. Bonneville (Lea and Febiger, 1973), *Cell Fine Struc*
ture by T. L. Lentz (Saunders, 1971), which is an atlas of drawings c
whole-cell structure, *Microanatomy of Cell and Tissue Surfaces* b
P. Notta, P. M. Andrews and K. R. Porter (Lea and Febiger, 1977*
which is an atlas of cell structure using scanning methods. Ultra
structural pathology is served by *Ultrastructural Pathology of th*
Cell and Matrix by F. N. Ghadially (2nd edn, Butterworths, 1982*
Diagnostic Electron Microscopy by B. F. Trump and R. T. Jone
(vol 1, 1978; vol 2, 1979; vol 3, 1980, all Wiley) and *Atlas of Ultra*
structure, Ultrastructural Features in Pathology edited by C. H
Tseng (Appleton-Century-Crofts, 1980).

Ear

Pathology of the Ear by H. F. Schuknecht (Harvard University Press, 1974)
Pathology of the Ear by I. Friedmann (Blackwell, 1974)
Atlas of Histopathology of Ear Tumours by P. G. Gerlings (Lloyd-Luke, 1979)
An Atlas of Micropathology of the Temporal Bone by F. H. Linthicum and J. A
    Schwartzman (Saunders, 1974)

Eye

Ocular Pathology by C. H. Greer (3rd edn, Blackwell, 1979)
Ocular Pathology by M. Yanoff and B. S. Fine (2nd edn, Harper and Row, 1982)
Ocular Pathology Update edited by D. H. Nicholson (Masson, 1980)
Current Research in Ophthalmic Electron Microscopy (4 vols, Springer, 1981)
*International Histological Classification of Tumours, No 24, Tumours of the Eye and
    its Adnexa* (World Health Organization, 1980)

Forensic pathology

Two journals are the *American Journal of Forensic Medicine an(*

Pathology and *The Journal of Forensic Sciences*. General forensic texts include *Forensic Medicine* edited by C. O. Tedeschi (3 vols, Saunders, 1977), *Forensic Medicine* by K. Simpson (8th edn, Arnold, 1979), *Forensic Pathology: a Handbook for Pathologists* edited by R. S. Fisher and C. S. Petty (Castle House, 1978), and *Practical Forensic Medicine* edited by F. E. Camps and J. M. Cameron (2nd edn, Hutchinson, 1971). More specialized are:

Pathology of Injury – Current Knowledge and Future Development edited by A. C. Hunt (Harvey, Miller and Medcalf, 1972)
The Pathology of Trauma edited by S. Sevitt and H. B. Stoner (British Medical Association, 1970)
Fatal Civil Aircraft Accidents. Their Medical and Pathological Investigation by P. J. Stephens (Wright, 1970)
Pathology of Violent Injury by J. K. Mason (3rd edn, Year Book Medical Publishers, 1978)

Atlases include:

Color Atlas of Forensic Pathology by G. A. Gresham (Year Book Medical Publishers, 1978)
Colour Atlas of the Histopathology of Traumatic Injury by H. Fischer and C. J. Kirkpatrick (Harvey, Miller and Medcalf, 1982)
Atlas of Wounds by C. A. Gresham (MTP, 1982)

Finally, anyone with an interest in forensic matters, and who has not already done so, will want to read *Forty Years of Murder* by K. Simpson (Scribner, 1979).

Gastrointestinal Tract

The Gastrointestinal Tract edited by J. H. Yardley *et al.* (Williams and Wilkins, 1977) is a concise book written by 21 authors. Other general books are *Morphological Pathology of the Alimentary Canal. Gross, Radiographic and Microscopic* by A. M. Valdes-Dapena and G. N. Stein (Saunders, 1970), *Gastrointestinal Pathology* edited by B. C. Morson and I. M. P. Dawson (2nd edn, Blackwell, 1979) and *Pathology of the Gastro-intestinal Tract* edited by B. Morson (in *Current Topics in Pathology*; Springer-Verlag, 1976). More specialized are *Histopathologic Spectrum of Regional Enteritis and Ulcerative Colitis* by N. K. Mottoet (Saunders, 1971) and the *International Histological Classification of Tumours* (World Health Organization); *No 4, Histological Typing of Oesophageal Tumours* (1971); *No 18, Gastric and Oesophageal Tumours* (1977) and *No 15, Intestinal Tumours* (1976). Gastrointestinal cytology is covered by *Handbook and Atlas of Gastrointestinal Exfoliative Cytology* by J. C. Prolla and J. B. Kirsner (University of Chicago Press, 1972) and biopsy pathology by *Atlas of*

Gastrointestinal Biopsy Pathology by I. M. P. Dawson (MTP, 1982), *Biopsy Diagnosis of the Digestive Tract* by H. Rotterdom and S. C. Sommers (Raven Press, 1981), *Biopsy Diagnosis of the Digestive Tract* by J. D. Waye (Raven Press, 1981) and *Biopsy Pathology of the Small Intestine* by F. D. Lee and P. G. Toner (Chapman and Hall, 1980).

Gynaecology and obstetrics

A recent journal is *International Journal of Gynecological Pathology* (volume 1, 1982), General books include:

Gynaecological Pathology by M. Haines and C. Taylor (2nd edn, Churchill Livingstone, 1975)

Gynecologic and Obstetric Pathology: a Textbook edited by A. Blaustein (Springer-Verlag, 1977)

Pathology of the Female Genital Tract by A. Blaustein (2nd edn, Springer-Verlag, 1982)

Pathology in Gynecology and Obstetrics by C. Gompel and S. G. Silverberg (2nd edn, Lippincott, 1977)

Pathology for Gynaecologists by H. Fox and H. Buckley (Arnold, 1982)

Novak's Gynaecological and Obstetric Pathology by E. R. Novak and J. D. Woodruff (8th edn, Saunders, 1979)

Postgraduate Obstetrical and Gynaecological Pathology edited by H. Fox and F. A. Langley (Pergamon, 1972)

Books on surgical pathology include *Surgical Pathology of the Uterus* by S. G. Silverberg (Wiley, 1977), *Surgical Pathology of the Uterine Corpus* by M. R. Hendrickson and R. L. Kempson (Saunders, 1980) and *Surgical Pathology of the Endometrium* by H. Cove (Lippincott, 1981). Other books on the endometrium are *The Endometrium* by W. B. Robertson (Butterworths, 1981) and *Histopathology of the Endometrium* by G. Dallenbach-Hellwig (3rd edn, Springer-Verlag, 1981). Two other specialized text are *Corscaden's Gynecologic Cancer* by S. B. Gunsberg and H. C. Frick, II (5th edn, Williams and Wilkins, 1978) and *Pathology of the Placenta* by H. Fox (Saunders, 1978). Books involving diagnosis include:

International Histological Classification of Tumours (World Health Organization): *No 13, Histological Typing of Female Genital Tract Tumours* (1975); *No 9, Histological Typing of Ovarian Tumours* (1973) and *No 8, Cytology of the Female Genital Tract* (1973)

Atlas of Gynaecological Pathology by H. Fox (MTP, 1982)

Gynecological Cytopathology by M. J. Ayala and F. N. Ortiz (Year Book Medical Publishers, 1978)

Colour Atlas of Gynaecological Cytopathology by C. Grubb (HM & M, 1977)

Diagnostic Cytopathology of the Uterine Cervix by S. F. Patten (2nd edn, Karger, 1977)

Interpretation of Biopsy of Endometrium by A. Blaustein (Raven Press, 1980)

Head and neck

Pathology of the Head, Neck and Ear by L. Michaels *et al.* (Churchill Livingstone, 1980)

Heart

The Pathology of the Heart by A. Pomerance and M. J. Davies (Blackwell, 1975)
Cardiovascular Pathology edited by M. D. Silver (Churchill Livingstone, 1982)
Pathology of the Heart and Blood Vessels by S. E. Gould (3rd edn, C. C. Thomas, 1968)
Congenital Malformations of the Heart and Great Vessels by H. Bankl (Urban and Schwarzenberg, 1977)
Pathology of Congenital Heart Disease by A. E. Becker and R. H. Anderson (Butterworths, 1981)
Pathology of Cardiac Valves by M. J. Davies (Butterworths, 1980)
Histopathology of Cardiac Arrythmias by L. Rossi (2nd edn, Casa Edritice Ambrosiana, 1978)
A Colour Atlas of Cardiac Pathology by G. Farrer-Brown (Wolfe Medical, 1977)
Pathology of Ischaemic Heart Disease by Sir Theo Crawford (Butterworths, 1977)

Liver

General books include *Pathology of the Liver* edited by R. N. M. McSween *et al.* (Churchill Livingstone, 1977) and two atlases: *Clinical Histopathology of the Liver: an Atlas* by W. Wepler and E. Wildhirt (Grune and Stratton, 1972) and *Atlas of Liver Pathology* by D. G. D. Wight (MTP, 1982). More specialized are *International Histological Classification of Tumours, No 20, Tumours of the Liver, Biliary Tract and and Pancreas* (World Health Organization, 1978), *Ultrastructural Aspects of the Liver and its Disorders* by K. Tanikawa (Igaku Shoin, distributed by Springer-Verlag, 1968) and *Electron Microscopy in Human Disease, vol 8: The Liver, Gallbladder and Biliary Ducts* edited by J. V. Johannessen (McGraw-Hill, 1979). Three books on liver biopsies are *Atlas of Liver Biopsies* by H. Poulsen and P. Christoffersen (Munksgaard, 1979), *Biopsy Pathology of the Liver* by R. S. Patrick and J. O'D. McGee (Chapman and Hall, 1980) and *Liver Biopsy Interpretation* by P. Scheuer (3rd edn, Ballière Tindall, 1980).

Lung

Pathology of the Lung by H. Spencer (2 vols, 3rd edn, Pergamon, 1977)
Pulmonary Pathology by M. S. Dunnill (Churchill Livingstone, 1982)
The Pathology of Emphysema by L. Reid (Lloyd-Luke, 1967)
Surgical Pathology of Non-Neoplastic Lung Disease by A. L. A. Katzenstein and F. B. Askin (Holt Saunders, 1982)
Electron Microscopy in Human Medicine, vol 6: Nervous System, Sensory Organs and Respiratory Tract edited by J. V. Johannessen (McGraw-Hill, 1980)

Diagnostic Pulmonary Cytology by G. Saccomanno (American Society of Clinical Pathologists, 1978)
Atlas of Pulmonary Pathology by A. R. Gibbs and R. M. E. Seal (MTP, 1982)
International Histological Classification of Tumours, No 1: Histological Typing of Lung Tumours (World Health Organization, 1967)

Lymph nodes

The Histopathology of Lymphomas and Pseudolymphomas by J. R. Jackson (MTP, 1979)
Histopathology of Non-Hodgkin's Lymphomas by K. Lennert (1981)
An Atlas of Lymph Node Pathology by J. Arno (MTP, 1980)
A Colour Atlas of Thymus and Lymph Node Histopathology and Ultrastructure by K. Henry and G. Farrer-Brown (Wolfe Medical, 1981)
Electron Microscopy Atlas of Lymph Node Cytology and Pathology by Y. Mori and K. Lennert (Springer-Verlag, 1969)
Lymph Node Biopsy: a Diagnostic Atlas by A. H. T. Robb-Smith and C. R. Taylor (Miller Hayden, 1981)
Lymph Node Biopsy by H. L. Ioachim (Harper and Row, 1982)

Male reproduction

Atlas of Male Reproduction by I. D. Ansell (MTP, 1982)
Pathology of the Testis by R. C. B. Pugh (Blackwell, 1976)

Mouth

A relevant journal is the *Journal of Oral Pathology*. General textbooks include the comprehensive *Thoma's Oral Pathology* by R. J. Gorlin and H. M. Goldman (2 vols, 6th edn, Mosby, 1970), *A Textbook of Oral Pathology* by W. G. Shafer *et al.* (3rd edn, Saunders, 1974) and *Synopsis of Oral Pathology* by S. N. Bhaskar (6th edn, Year Book Medical Publishers, 1981). Atlases are well represented; examples are:

Atlas of Oral Pathology by R. B. Lucas (MTP, 1981)
Color Atlas of Oral Histopathology by E. A. Marsland and R. M. Browne (Year Book Medical Publishers, 1975)
Atlas of Oral Pathology by R. M. Smith *et al.* (Mosby, 1981)
Color Atlas of Oral Pathology by R. A. Colby *et al.* (3rd edn, Lippincott, 1974)

Books on oral tumours include:

Pathology of Tumours of the Oral Tissues by R. B. Lucas (4th edn, Churchill Livingstone, 1982)
International Histological Classification of Tumours (World Health Organization): *No 5, Histological Typing of Odontogenic Tumours, Jaw Cysts and Allied Lesions* (1971); *No 7, Histological Typing of Salivary Gland Tumours* (1972),
A Colour Atlas of Oral Cancers by A. Burkhardt and R. Maerker (Wolfe Medical, 1981)

Muscle

Two books are the American comprehensive textbook *Diseases of Muscle: a Study in Pathology* by R. D. Adams (3rd edn, Harper and Row, 1975) and *Skeletal Muscle Pathology* edited by F. L. Mastaglia (Churchill Livingstone, 1982).

Mycoses

A Colour Atlas and Textbook of the Histopathology of Mycotic Diseases by F. W. Chandler *et al.* (Wolfe Medical, 1980)

Neuropathology

Neuropathology has its specialist journals, including the *Journal of Neuropathology and Experimental Neurology* and *Neuropathology and Applied Neurobiology*. Some books are: *Greenfield's Neuropathology* by W. Blackwood and J. A. N. Corsellis (3rd edn, Arnold, 1976), *Histology and Histopathology of the Nervous System* edited by W. Haymaker and R. D. Adams (2 vols, C. C. Thomas, 1982), *A Guide to Neuropathology* by A. Hirano (1981), and the more specialized *Developmental Neuropathology* by R. L. Friede (Springer-Verlag, 1975), *Surgical Pathology of the Nervous System and its Coverings* by P. C. Burger and F. S. Vogel (2nd edn, Wiley, 1982) and *Electron Microscopy in Human Medicine, vol 6: Nervous System, Sensory Organs and Respiratory Tract* edited by J. V. Johannessen (McGraw-Hill, 1980). Atlases include *Atlas of Gross Neuropathology* by R. E. Shemmer (Green, 1980), *Atlas of Neuropathology* by N. Malamud and A. Hirano (2nd edn, University of California Press, 1974), which has a concise text with illustrative cases, *Colour Atlas of Neuropathology* by C. S. Treip (Wolfe, 1978) and *Atlas of Neuropathology* by M. V. Salmon (MTP, 1981).

Tumours are dealt with by the excellent *Pathology of Tumours of the Nervous System* by D. S. Russell and L. J. Rubinstein (4th edn, Arnold, 1977), *International Histological Classification of Tumours, No 21: Tumours of the Central Nervous* (World Health Organization, 1979) and *An Atlas of Tumours Involving the Central Nervous System* by R. O. Barnard *et al.* (Baillière Tindall, 1976). More specialized are *Atlas of the Histology of Brain Tumors* by K. J. Zulch (Springer-Verlag, 1971) and *Electron Microscopic Atlas of Brain Tumors* by Tung Pui Poon (Grune and Stratton, 1971). Other specialized books include:

Pathology of the Spinal Cord by J. Trevor Hughes (2nd edn, Lloyd-Luke, 1978)

Pathology of Peripheral Nerves by R. O. Weller and J. Cervos-Navarro (Butterworths, 1977)
Pathology of Peripheral Nerve by A. K. Asbury and P. C. Johnson (Saunders, 1978)
Ultrastructural Study of the Human Diseased Peripheral Nerve by C. Vital and J-M. Vallat (Masson, 1980)

Nose and sinuses

Pathology of Granulomas and Neoplasms of the Nose and Paranasal Sinuses by I. Friedmann and D. A. Osborn (Churchill Livingstone, 1982)
International Histological Classification of Tumours, No 19, Upper Respiratory Tract Tumours (World Health Organization, 1978)

Paediatrics

Paediatric Pathology edited by C. L. Berry (Springer, 1981)
Pathology of Infancy and Childhood by J. M. Kissane (2nd edn, Mosby, 1975)
Fetal and Neonatal Pathology: Perspectives for the General Pathologist edited by A. J. Barson (Praeger Scientific, 1982)
Pathology of the Fetus and the Infant by E. L. Potter (3rd edn, Year Book Medical Publishers, 1975)
Pediatric Surgical Pathology by L. P. Dehner (Year Book Medical Publishers, 1975)
The Pathology of the Perinatal Brain by L. B. Rorke (Raven Press, 1982)
Tumours of Infancy and Childhood edited by P. G. Jones and P. E. Campbell (Blackwell, 1976)

Palaeopathology

Paleopathology: An Introduction to the Study of Ancient Evidences of Disease by R. L. Moodie (AMS Press, 1923, reprinted 1975)
Paleopathology. Diseases and Injuries of Prehistoric Man by P. A. Janssens (John Baker, 1970)
Paleopathological Diagnosis and Interpretation: Bone Disease in Ancient Human Populations by R. T. Steinbock (C. C. Thomas, 1976)
Diseases in Antiquity: a Survey of the Diseases, Injuries and Surgery of Early Populations by D. R. Brothwell and A. T. Sandison (C. C. Thomas, 1967)

Prostate

The Prostate Cell: Structure and Function; part A, Morphologic, Secretory and Biochemical Aspects edited by G. P. Murphy *et al.* (Alan R. Liss, 1981)
Color Atlas of Cytodiagnosis of the Prostate by W. Staeler *et al.* (Year Book Medical Publishers, 1976)
International Histological Classification of Tumours, No 22, Prostate Tumours (World Health Organization, 1980)

Radiation

Radiation Histopathology by G. W. Casarett (2 vols, CRC Press, 1980)

Pathology of Irradiation by C. C. Berdjis (Williams and Wilkins, 1970)

Skin

Two journals are the *American Journal of Dermatopathology* and the *Journal of Cutaneous Pathology*. Books include *A Guide to Dermatohistopathology* by H. Pinkus and A. H. Mehregan (3rd edn, Appleton-Century-Crofts, 1981), *Histopathology of the Skin* by W. F. Lever and G. Schaumburg-Lever (5th edn, Lippincott, 1975), *An Introduction to the Diagnostic Histopathology of the Skin* by J. A. Milne (Arnold, 1972) and *Differential Diagnosis in Dermatopathology* by A. B. Ackerman *et al.* (Lea and Febiger, 1982). More specialized are the massive and sumptuous *Histological Diagnosis of Inflammatory Skin Diseases* by A. B. Ackerman (Lea and Febiger, 1978), *Malignant Melanoma: Clinical and Histological Diagnosis* by V. J. McGovern (Wiley, 1976), *International Histological Classification of Tumours, No 12, Histological Typing of Skin Tumours* (World Health Organization, 1974) and *Biopsy of Pigmented Lesions on the Skin* by V. J. McGovern (Raven Press, 1982). *Gross and Microscopic Pathology of the Skin* by M. R. Okun and L. M. Edelstein (2 vols, Dermatopathology Foundation Press, 1976) is a comprehensive reference atlas with concise text; other atlases include *Atlas of the Ultrastructure of the Human Skin* by A. S. Breathnach (Churchill Livingstone, 1971), *Atlas of Skin Pathology* by R. Marks *et al. (MTP, 1982)* and *Atlas of Tumors of the Skin* by A. W. Kopf *et al.* (Saunders, 1978).

Toxicology

Pathology of Drug-Induced and Toxic Diseases edited by R. H. Riddell (Churchill Livingstone, 1982)
Atlas of Toxic Reactions by R. Marks *et al.* (MTP, 1982)

Tropical medicine

Tropical Pathology by H. Spencer *et al.* (Springer-Verlag, 1973)
Pathology in the Tropics by G. M. Edington and H. M. Gillies (2nd edn, Arnold, 1976)
Pathology of Tropical and Extraordinary Diseases: an Atlas edited by C. H. Binford and D. H. Connor (2 vols, Castle House, 1979)

Urinary tract

General books include *Urologic Pathology* by M. Tannenbaum (Lea and Febiger, 1977), *Renal Pathology* edited by E. M. Darmady and A. MacIlver (Butterworths, 1980) and *Pathology of the*

Kidney by R. H. Heptinstall (3 vols, 3rd edn, Little, Brown, 1983). Ultrastructure is dealt with in *Electron Microscopy of the Kidney in Renal Disease and Hypertension* by A. K. Mandal (Plenum, 1979). Atlases include *Atlas of Renal Pathology* by R. A. Risdon and D. R. Turner (MTP, 1980), *Atlas of Glomerular Histopathology* by H. M. Schillings and J. H. Schuurmans Stekhoven (Karger, 1980), which is really a profusely illustrated textbook, and *Atlas of Glomerular Pathology* by P. M. Burkholder (Harper and Row, 1974). For cytology, *Atlas of Renal and Urinary Tract Cytology and its Histopathologic Bases* by G. B. Schumann and M. Weiss (Lippincott, 1980) and *Urinary Cytology* by H. J. de Voogt *et al.* (Springer-Verlag, 1977) are available. Tumours are dealt with in the *International Histological Classification of Tumours* (World Health Organization) *No 25, Kidney Tumours,* (1981) and *No 10, Histological Typing of Urinary Bladder Tumours* (1974), and renal biopsy by *Renal Pathology in Biopsy by H. U. Zollinger and M. J. Mihatsch (Springer-Verlag, 1978), Renal Biopsy Pathology with Diagnostic and Therapeutic Implications* by B. H. Spargo *et al.* (Wiley, 1980) and *Renal Biopsy* by D. B. Brewer (2nd edn, Arnold, 1973).

History of pathology

E. R. Long's *History of Pathology* (Williams and Wilkins, 1928; revised edn, Dover, 1965) is the first systematic history of the subject in English. Long also edited *Selected Readings in Pathology* (C. C. Thomas, 1929). E. Goldschmid's *Entwicklung und Bibliographie der pathologisch-anatomischen Abbildung* (Hiersemann, Leipzig, 1925) traces the development of pathological anatomical illustration and includes a chronological bibliography of all important publications containing illustrations of pathological conditions and an index of artists, printers and publishers. A short account is provided by E. D. Krumbhaar in his *Pathology,* published in the Clio Medica Series (Hoeber, 1937), and W. D. Foster has provided *A Short History of Clinical Pathology* (Livingstone, 1961).

The history of cancer is exhaustively covered in Jacob Wolff's classic *Die Lehre von der Krebskrankheit in den ältesten Zeiten bis zur Gegenwart* (4 vols, Fischer, 1907–1928), which is supplemented by C. D. Haagensen's *Exhibit of important books and memorabilia illustrating the evolution of the knowledge of cancer* published in the *American Journal of Cancer,* **18,** 42–126, 1933. P. M. Vaillancourt's *Bibliographic Control of the Literature of Oncology 1800–1960* (Scarecrow Press, 1969) includes a well-documented history.

In Chapter 1 libraries and their use are dealt with at length. There can be no doubt that the doctor, no matter in which part of the profession he practises, cannot keep himself properly informed without recourse to libraries, and the degree of efficiency he achieves in the use of a library will depend, primarily, upon his relationships with the library staff. The present author, not being a librarian, therefore intends to close this chapter with a few observations on librarians.

It is the librarian who controls and orders the information explosion, making possible the efficient exchange of information without which medical science cannot advance. He is an expert, primarily on documents: their identification, classification and cataloguing. He knows what is immediately available to him and how to obtain what is not. He can amass a body of relevant material for a particular purpose, but will not, normally, appraise its scientific value.

He is an expert, professional colleague and, if the reader, on first visiting the library, introduces himself and declares his interests, he will receive continuing support in his battle with the medical literature which this chapter cannot provide.

12

Medical microbiology

B. H. Whyte

Organizations

The scientific striving towards definition, consistency and comparability is nowhere greater than in the microbiological field. The organization which helps to promote these aims worldwide in this field is the International Association of Mircobiological Societies (IAMS), itself a division of the International Union of Biological Societies, working through its network of committees, commissions and federations. These are composed mainly of representatives of the various national member societies such as, in Britain, the Society for General Microbiology (SGM) and the Society for Applied Bacteriology (SAB), and, in the US, the American Society for Microbiology (ASM). Of special note within the IAMS are its International Association of Biological Standardization (IABS), concerned with criteria in the development of prophylactics, its International Commission on Microbiological Specifications for Foods (ICMSF), which seeks consensus on questions of food quality and testing methods, and its International Committees – on Systematic Bacteriology (ICSB) and on Taxonomy of Viruses (ICTV) – with their many subcommittees, which strive to preserve order in the taxonomic field. Also of interest in the IAMS are its World Federation of Culture Collections (WFCC) and its International Committee on Microbiological and Immunological Documentation (ICMID). International congresses have been run by the IAMS and its sections since 1930, and books, journals and symposia series are published by all the committees and member societies mentioned above, together forming a substantial part of the basic library of the microbiologist. The IAMS Directory is issued by ASM.

The Federation of European Microbiological Societies (FEMS) exists to encourage communication between national societies in Europe, and to facilitate rapid publication of journals.

The other area of international involvement for microbiologists, this time through national governments, is in the work of the World Health Organization (WHO), either at the individual level as members of expert committees and study groups, or at the laboratory level as designated collaborating centres. The overall purpose is the raising of health standards throughout the world, and infections, environmental problems and, again, biological standardization, are of particular concern. Reports of all kinds flow from these activities and journals include *Bulletin of the World Health Organization* with scientific content, and others that document health legislation and statistics.

The Department of Health and Social Security (DHSS) acts as a link in Britain with WHO activities and itself issues reports and memoranda on all matters of concern to the public health; certain series go back, in one form or another, for over a century. Collecting and publishing health statistics is the province of the Office of Population Censuses and Surveys (OPCS). The Commonwealth Agricultural Bureaux (CAB) publish a range of relevant abstract bulletins which are referred to.

The Medical Research Council (MRC) is involved in various specialized areas of virology and bacteriology. Many classic publications on microbiology are to be found in its earlier *Special Report Series*, its 9-volume *System of Bacteriology* (page 253) and elsewhere. Current work is outlined in its *Annual Report* and the functions of its various units in the *MRC Handbook*.

Microbiological work being done in the universities is documented in *Research in British Universities, Polytechnics and Colleges. II. Biological Sciences*, published by the British Library.

In England and Wales the Public Health Laboratory Service (PHLS) plays a central role in the control of infection, with its network of laboratories throughout the country and a full range of reference and special units, mainly held at its Central Public Health Laboratory (CPHL) at Colindale and at its Centre for Applied Microbiology and Research (CAMR) at Porton Down. Of special interest are the PHLS's Communicable Disease Surveillance Centre (CDSC), whose work is described by N. S. Galbraith and S. E. J. Young (*Commun. Med.*, **2**, 135, 1980), and its National

Collection of Type Cultures (NCTC), both at Colindale. The Service's history is described in *Half a Century of Medical Research* by A. Landsborough Thomson (**2**, 255, HMSO, 1975), and the extent of its diagnostic, reference, surveillance and research work is described in its annual reports, issued since 1962, where details of its *Monograph Series* can also be found. As with the MRC, most of its reports are now published in periodicals.

In America the Center for Disease Control (CDC) in Atlanta plays a somewhat similar role to that of the PHLS, and is a fruitful source of publications on specialist microbiological topics and infection surveillance. The Public Health Service (PHS) itself and its National Institutes of Health (NIH) at Bethesda have a long record of publication of outstanding journals and reports. The American Public Health Association (APHA) dates back to 1871 and is the source of a notable series of diagnostic handbooks.

Other sources of information are mentioned throughout the chapter.

Bacteriology

History

The earliest history of bacteriology is Friedrich Löffler's *Vorlesungen über die geschichtliche Entwickelung der Lehre von den Bacterien* published by Vogel of Leipzig in 1887, reissued in translation by Coronado Press (1983). D. H. Howard, its translator, describes it in *ASM News* (**48**, 297, 1982) as reasoning its way through the early 'spontaneous generation' and 'putrefaction' controversies and ending with a contemporary assessment of Koch's epoch-making work on wound infection.

W. Bulloch's *The History of Bacteriology* (Oxford University Press, 1938, reprinted 1960) is a scholarly account of the development of ideas, with an extensive bibliography and biographical notes. W. D. Foster's *A History of Medical Bacteriology and Immunology* (Heinemann, 1970) deals briefly with the early years and continues the subject from 1900, where Bulloch leaves off. P. Collard's *The Development of Microbiology* is a series of histories of such topics as media, sterilization, and genetics, each with its own chronological reference list. *Three Centuries of Microbiology* by H. A. Lechevalier and M. Solotorovsky (McGraw-Hill, 1965) links narrative with extensive quotations from original sources, and *Milestones in Microbiology* edited by T. D. Brock (Prentice-Hall, 1961, reprinted by ASM, 1975) is an anthology of classic papers, with descriptions of the Petri dish, the Gram stain and the so-called 'Koch's postulates' among them. An account of developments in the US is *Pioneer Microbiologists of America* by P. F. Clark (University of Wisconsin Press, 1961), and 'Early American publications relating to bacteriology' by L. S. McClung (*Bact. Rev.*, **8**, 119, 1944).

Dictionaries and encyclopaedic works

Dictionary of Microbiology by P. Singleton and D. Sainsbury (Wiley, 1978) includes some concise reviews and an appendix of microbial metabolic pathways. *A Dictionary of Microbial Taxonomy* by S. T. Cowan and edited by L. R. Hill (2nd edn, Cambridge University Press, 1978) is illuminating in its field.

Earlier encyclopaedias of historic reference value are *Kolle und Wassermann's Handbuch der pathogenen Mikroorganismen* edited by W. Kolle, R. Kraus und P. Uhlenhuth in 10 multipart volumes (3rd edn, Fischer, 1927–1931) and the MRC's *A System of Bacteriology in Relation to Medicine* edited by P. Fildes and J. C. G. Ledingham (9 vols, HMSO, 1929–1931).

CRC Handbook of Microbiology edited by A. I. Laskin and H. A. Lechevalier (2nd edn, 4 vols, CRC Press, 1977–1982) gives brief descriptions of the various classes of organisms with tabulated listings of associated infections in the first 2 vols, vols 3 and 4 being information sources on the chemistry of microbial composition. A similar type of compilation on diagnostic data is *CRC Handbook Series in Clinical Laboratory Science* edited by D. Seligson, Section E Clinical Microbiology (2 vols, CRC Press, 1977). *The Prokaryotes: a Handbook on Habitats, Isolation and Identification of Bacteria* edited by M. P. Starr, H. Stolph, H. G. Trüper, A. Balows and H. G. Schlegel (2 vols, Springer, 1981), after general introductory chapters, including a 50 page review of bacterial pathogenicity, treats each group of organisms under the specified headings, with identification keys and media details.

Systematics and culture collections

The international ordering of how bacteria should be named, identified and preserved is the work of the ICBS with its Judicial Commission. Its official organ is *International Journal of Systematic Bacteriology (IJSB)* and separate publications include *International Code of Nomenclature of Bacteria . . . 1976 Revision* edited by S. P. Lapage *et al.* (ASM, 1975) and *Approved Lists of Bacterial Names* edited by V. B. D. Skerman, V. McGowan and

P. H. A. Sneath (reprinted from *IJSB*, **30**, 225 by ASM, 1980). Names subsequently approved appear in *IJSB* in annual validation lists.

Parallel to this endeavour is the work sponsored by the Trust responsible for the production of *Bergey's Manual of Determinative Bacteriology*, a classification scheme which tends to receive universal acceptance because there is no other. The eighth edition is current, edited by R. E. Buchanan and N. E. Gibbons (Williams and Wilkins, 1974).A new 4-volume version of *Bergey's Manual of Systematic Bacteriology* is scheduled to start appearing in 1983 with vol 1, edited by N. R. Krieg (Williams and Wilkins). *Index Bergeyana*, edited by R. E. Buchanan *et al.* (Livingstone, 1966) and its *Supplement*, edited by N. E. Gibbons *et al.* (Williams and Wilkins, 1981) are compilations of thousands of names, including many inadequately authenticated.

Cowan's *Dictionary of Microbial Taxonomy* (*see* page 253) is a very readable guide to the fine tuning of the taxonomic field, with informative introductory chapters (one reviewing the history of bacterial classifications) and a bibliography of all the key work on systematics. V. B. D. Skerman's *A Guide to the Identification of the Genera of Bacteria, with Methods and Digests of Generic Characteristics* (2nd edn, Williams and Wilkins, 1967) seeks to integrate various individual approaches to the problem. An aspect necessary for computerization is dealt with in *Numerical Taxonomy* by P. H. A. Sneath and R. R. Sokal (Freeman, 1973).

Culture collections maintain and make available strains of bacteria representative of their taxa. S. P. Lapage describes their function and organization in *Biol. J. Linnean Soc., Lond.* **3**, 197, 1971, and preservation of microorganisms is dealt with by L. R. Hill in *Essays in Applied Microbiology* (*see* page 255). The UK collection, which includes bacteria of medical importance, is the National Collection of Type Cultures, housed at the Central Public Health Laboratory, Colindale.*Catalogue of the National Collection of Type Cultures* (6th edn, 1983) is issued by the PHLS. The equivalent US body is the American Type Culture Collection, Rockville, Maryland. The WFCC coordinates activities of culture collections and publishes *World Directory of Collections of Cultures of Microorganisms*, edited by V. F. McGowan and V. B. D. Skerman (2nd edn, World Data Center on Microorganisms, University of Queensland, Brisbane, 1982).

Standard textbooks

The definitive text and reference work is *Topley and Wilson's Principles of Bacteriology, Virology and Immunity* by Sir G. S. Wilson and Sir A. A. Miles, with additional authors (6th edn, 2 vols, Arnold, 1975). Scholarly and comprehensive, it covers the subject from a general standpoint in the first volume and its application to medicine and environmental hygiene in the second. A 7th edn, with expanded authorship, is at an advanced stage of preparation and scheduled to appear in four volumes about the end of 1983. *Microbiology* by B. D. Davis, R. Dulbecco, H. N. Eisen and H. S. Ginsberg (3rd edn, Harper and Row, 1980) is the best up-to-date teaching text, treating the subject within the context of modern biology and including large sections on molecular genetics and immunology. Of many other American texts, *Review of Medical Microbiology* by E. Jawetz, J. L. Melnick and E. A. Adelberg (14th edn, Lange, 1980) is the most popular. Updated every two years, it is comprehensive yet trimmed to the essentials for study or rapid reference. Undergraduate texts include the humbler *Medical Microbiology* by C. G. A. Thomas (4th edn, Baillière Tindall, 1979) and *A Short Textbook of Medical Microbiology* by D. C. Turk *et al.* (5th edn, Hodder and Stoughton, 1983). *Animal Microbiology* by A. Buxton and G. Fraser (2 vols, Blackwell, 1977) presents the subject to the veterinary reader. Texts are also available for other professional students such as dentists and nurses.

General microbiology

The fundamental study of bacteria is the breeding ground from which spring advances in the medical field, and so is of great relevance in the present context.

The Bacteria: a Treatise on Structure and Function originally a five-volume source on biological properties, from structure to heredity, is edited by I. C. Gunsalus and R. Y. Stanier (Academic Press, 1960–1964); additional volumes are being added under the editorship of Gunsalus, for example vol 6 on Bacterial Diversity (1978), and vol 7 on Mechanisms of Adaptation (1979). Two series of essays edited by J. R. Norris and M. H. Richmond and published by Wiley, *Essays in Microbiology* (1978) and *Essays in Applied Microbiology* (1981), have useful contributions on specialized, general and technological aspects. Similarly, *Companion to Microbiology: Selected Topics for Further Study* edited by A. T. Bull and P. M. Meadow (Longmans, 1978) treats topics with greater weight than in normal reviews to stimulate advanced study. A reliable text is *General Microbiology* by R. Y. Stanier, E. A. Adelberg and J. L. Ingraham (4th edn, Macmillan, 1977). Highly relevant ASM conference proceedings are annually assembled and edited by D. Schlessinger under the title *Microbiology – 1974, et seq.* Another regular meeting series is *Symposia Series of the Society for General Microbiology* (Cambridge University Press, 1949–). *Benchmark Papers in Microbiology* under the editorship of W. W. Umbreit was a series of collected classic reprints on such topics as growth and permeability, published by Dowden, Hutchinson and Ross in the early 1970s.

Special aspects are featured in the following:

Biochemistry of Bacterial Growth edited by J. Mandelstam, K. McQuillen and I. W. Dawes (3rd edn, Blackwell, 1982)
Diversity of Bacterial Respiratory Systems edited by C. J. Knowles (2 vols, CRC Press, 1980)
Microbial Physiology by A. G. Moat (Wiley, 1979)
Adsorption of Microorganisms to Surfaces edited by G. Bitton and K. C. Marshall (Wiley Interscience, 1980)
Microbial Cell Walls and Membranes by H. J. Rogers, H. R. Perkins and J. B. Ward (Chapman and Hall, 1980)
Microbial Toxins edited by S. J. Ajl, A. Ciegler, S. Kadis, T. C. Montie and G. Weinbaum (8 vols, Academic Press, 1970–1972)
Bacterial Toxins and Cell Membranes, edited by J. Jeljaszewicz and T. Wadström (Academic Press, 1978)

Microbial genetics is the experimental basis of the wider discipline of molecular biology which has brought immense impetus to its study. In the medical field such subjects as pathogenicity and drug resistance have been elucidated and manipulative techniques are revolutionizing the production of therapeutic substances. *Papers in Bacterial Genetics* edited by E. A. Adelberg (2nd edn, Little, Brown, 1966) is a collection of classic reprints. *Molecular Genetics: an Introductory Narrative* by G. S. Stent and R. Calendar (2nd edn, Freeman, 1978) presents the subject in the chronological sequence in which each discovery was made, and good background reading is *The Genetics of Bacteria and their Viruses* by W. Hayes (2nd edn, Blackwell, 1968). A simpler account is in *Bacterial and Bacteriophage Genetics: an Introduction* by E. A. Birge (Springer, 1981) and *Experiments in Molecular Genetics* by J. H. Miller (Cold Spring Harbor Laboratory, 1972) is a working handbook. Monographs include P. Broda's *Plasmids* (Freeman, 1979) and K. Hardy's *Bacterial Plasmids* (Nelson, 1981). Useful books on manipulative techniques are *Principles of Gene Manipulation: an Introduction to Genetic Engineering* by R. W. Old and S. B. Primrose (Blackwell, 1980) and *Genetic Engineering* edited by R. Williamson (4 vols, Academic Press, 1981–1983).

Bacteriophage, other than as a tool in genetics, has received little attention since M. H. Adams' classic *Bacteriophages* (Interscience, 1959), though the subject does receive scholarly treatment in *Topley and Wilson* (*see* page 254). Phage typing as an epidemiological tool is comprehensively covered in *Lysotypie und andere spezielle epidemiologische Laboratoriums-Methoden* edited by H. Rische (Fischer, 1973) and the later volumes of Norris and Ribbons' *Methods in Microbiology* (*see* below) cover special applications. A bibliography of the subject covering the years from its discovery to 1965 is *Bakteriophagie 1917 bis 1956* (2 vols, 1958) and *Bacteriophagy 1957–1965* (2 vols, 1967), compiled by H. Raettig and published by Fischer.

Technical methods

Methods in Microbiology edited originally by J. R. Norris and D. W. Ribbons, and latterly by T. Bergan and Norris (Academic Press, 1969–) is a multivolume compilation of specialized methods; some volumes are on a single theme and the last four (vols 10–13, 1978–1979) cover typing methods for various organisms. *Manual of Methods for General Bacteriology* edited by P. Gerhardt (ASM, 1981) assembles special methods for studying morphology, growth, genetics, etc. An earlier, valuable source in this area of work is *Theory and Practice in Experimental Bacteriology* by G. G. and E. Meynell (2nd edn, Cambridge University Press, 1970).

On the diagnostic side the successor to Mackie and McCartney's *Handbook of Practical Bacteriology* is now a comprehensive two-volume student text – *Mackie and McCartney Medical Microbiology, vol I Microbial Infections* edited by J. P. Duguid, B. P. Marmion and R. H. A. Swain (13th edn, 1978) and *vol. II The Practice of Medical Microbiology* edited by R. Cruickshank, J. P. Duguid, B. P. Marmion and R. H. A. Swain (12th edn, 1975), both published by Churchill Livingstone. Two outstandingly comprehensive American technical reference works are *Diagnostic Procedures for Bacterial, Mycotic and Parasitic Infections* edited by A. Balows and W. J. Hausler (6th edn, APHA, 1981) and *Manual of Clinical Microbiology* edited by E. H. Lennette, A. Balows, W. J. Hausler and J. P. Truant (3rd edn, ASM, 1980). The irregularly published *Cumitech* series keeps this latter volume updated between editions. Two other much respected diagnostic books are *Bailey and Scott's Diagnostic Microbiology* by S. M. Finegold and W. J. Martin (6th edn, Mosby, 1982) and *Clinical Bacteriology* by E. J. Stokes and G. L. Ridgway (5th edn, Arnold, 1980).

Visual identification is provided by atlases which include *A Colour Atlas of Microbiology* by R. J. Olds (Wolfe Medical, 1974) and *An Atlas of Medical Microbiology: Common Human Pathogens* by B. C. Stratford (Blackwell, 1977). *Colour Atlas and Textbook of*

Diagnostic Microbiology by E. W. Koneman, S. D. Allen, V. R. Dowell and H. M. Sommers (Lippincott, 1979) combines biochemical and metabolic pathway identification with visual identification. Other manuals of identification are:

Cowan and Steele's Manual for the Identification of Medical Bacteria by S. T. Cowan (2nd edn, Cambridge University Press, 1974), which details media, methods and diagnostic tables
Biochemical Tests for Identification of Medical Bacteria by J. F. MacFaddin (2nd edn, Williams and Wilkins, 1980)
Biotyping in the Clinical Microbiology Laboratory edited by A. Balows and H. D. Isenberg (C. C. Thomas, 1978), which gives typing by genetic composition
Microbial Classification and Identification edited by M. Goodfellow and R. G. Board (*SAB Symp. Ser. No 8*, Academic Press, 1980), which discusses newer methods

Special procedures and techniques are covered in the following:

Quality Assurance Practices for Health Laboratories edited by S. L. Inhorn (APHA, 1978)
Practical Methods in Electron Microsopy edited by A. M. Glauert (multivol, North-Holland, 1972–)
Cell and Tissue Culture by J. Paul (5th edn, Churchill Livingstone, 1975)
Fluorescent Protein Tracing by R. C. Nairn (4th edn, Churchill Livingstone, 1976)
Gel Electrophoresis of Proteins edited by B. D. Hames and D. Rickwood (IRL Press, 1981)
Gel Electrophoresis of Nucleic Acids edited by B. D. Hames and D. Rickwood (IRL Press, 1981)
Gas Chromatographic Applications in Microbiology and Medicine by B. M. Mitruka (Wiley, 1975)
Monoclonal Antibodies, Hybridomas: a New Dimension in Biological Analyses edited by R. H. Kennett, T. J. McKearn and K. B. Bechtol (Plenum, 1980).

Useful series on laboratory methods are *Broadsheets of the Association of Clinical Pathologists*, the *PHLS Monograph Series*, the *Society for Applied Bacteriology Technical Series*, and a variety of publications issued by WHO. *Rapid and Automated Methods in Microbiology and Immunology: a Bibliography 1976–1980* edited by W. J. Palmer was published by IRL in 1981.

Specific organisms

It is invidious to make a selection from the considerable literature on individual organisms and groups of organisms, their biology and the infections they cause. The following list is no more than an indication of the range:

Anaerobic Bacteria in Human Disease by S. M. Finegold (Academic Press, 1977)
Anaerobic Bacteriology: Clinical and Laboratory Practice by A. T. Willis (3rd edn, Butterworths, 1977)
The Biology of Mycobacteria edited by C. Ratledge and J. Stanford (vol 1–, Academic Press, 1982–)

The Biology of the Nocardiae edited by M. Goodfellow, G. H. Brownell and J. A. Serrano (Academic Press, 1976)
The Gonococcus edited by R. B. Roberts (Wiley, 1977)
New Developments on Pertussis edited by C. R. Manclark and J. C. Hill (Castle House Publishers, 1980)
Pseudomonas Aeruginosa: Clinical Manifestations of Infection and Current Therapy edited by R. G. Doggett (Academic Press, 1979)
The Genus Serratia edited by A. von Graevenitz and S. J. Rubin (CRC Press, 1980)
Yersinia Enterocolitica edited by E. J. Bottone (CRC Press, 1981)
Campylobacter: Epidemiology, Pathogenesis and Biochemistry edited by D. G. Newell (MTP, 1982)
Legionnaires' Disease by G. L. Lattimer and R. A. Ormsbee (Dekker, 1981)
The Biology of Parasitic Spirochaetes edited by R. C. Johnson (Academic Press, 1976)
The Mycoplasmas edited by M. F. Barile, S. Razin, J. G. Tully and R. F. Whitcomb (3 vols, Academic Press, 1979)
Rickettsiae and Rickettsial Diseases edited by W. Burgdorfer and R. L. Anacker (Academic Press, 1981)
Human Chlamydial Infections by J. Schachter and C. R. Dawson (PSG Publishing Co., 1978)

Conferences, reviews and bibliographies

International congresses for microbiology, held by IAMS since 1930, are now published only in abstract form. Another important conference volume regularly published is *Abstracts of the Annual Meeting of the American Society for Microbiology.*

Serials regularly publishing reviews include *Advances in Applied Microbiology, Advances in Microbial Physiology, Annual Review of Microbiology, Bulletin de l'Institut Pasteur, Critical Reviews in Microbiology, Current Topics in Microbiology and Immunology, Medical Microbiology* (vol 1–, Academic Press, 1982–), *Microbiological Reviews,* and the irregular series *Recent Advances in Medical Microbiology.*

Bibliographies on special topics include:

The Anaerobic Bacteria and their Activities in Nature and Disease: a Subject Bibliography, 1816–1938, compiled by E. McCoy and L. S. McClung (2 vols, University of California Press, 1939 with *Supplement 1938 and 1939* (1941); *1940–1969* (5 vols); *1970–1975* (2 vols) compiled by L. S. McClung (Dekker, 1982)
Haemophili in Medical Literature 1883–1978: an Indexed Bibliography of more than 1200 References compiled by D. C. Turk (Hodder and Stoughton, 1980)
Legionella Update edited by G. L. Jones and G. A. Hébert (CDC, 1980) covers 1978–1980; . . .*Update June – August 1980;* . . .*Update of Legionella Species* (1981)
Bibliograhy of Mycoplasma edited by E. S. Krudy and D. Shiers (IR, 1977), covers 1966–1975
Chronological References of Zoonoses: Leptospires and Leptospirosis by E. Ryu (2nd edn, Taipei, International Laboratory for Zoonoses), I 1812–1960 (1978); II 1961–1977 (1980)
Bibliography on Yaws 1905–62 (WHO, 1963)

Virology

The literature of virology reflects revolutionary advances in this field. The molecular study of the virus/cell interaction has revealed new principles of classification, shed new light on pathogenicity and spearheaded the development of specific chemotherapy. New techniques have speeded up diagnosis and opened up new possibilities for serological work, and genetic engineering has brought large-scale production of vaccines and antiviral substances within sight.

On the historical side *An Introduction to the History of Virology* by A. P. Waterson and L. Wilkinson (Cambridge University Press, 1978) has useful biographical notes and *The Virus: a History of the Concept* by S. S. Hughes (Heinemann, 1977) is a scholarly account of the development of the idea of the virus. J. R. Paul's *A History of Poliomyelitis* (Yale University Press, 1971) and W. I. B. Beveridge's *Influenza: the Last Great Plague* (Heinemann, 1977) are also interesting, and *Virus Hunters* by G. Williams (Hutchinson, 1960) is a popular account of the struggle to develop vaccines.

Reference works include *A Dictionary of Virology* by K. E. K. Rowson, T. A. L. Rees and B. W. J. Mahy (Blackwell, 1981), which includes references with the definitions, and the encyclopaedic series *Comprehensive Virology* edited by H. Fraenkel-Conrat and R. R. Wagner (Plenum, 1974–), which is nearing completion with vol 18. Each volume is on a different theme and includes lengthy reviews. Section H of the *CRC Handbook Series in Clinical Laboratory Science* edited by G.-D. Hsiung and R. H. Green (2 vols, CRC Press, 1978) is a reference compilation on virology and rickettsiology. The earlier encyclopaedia *Handbuch der Virusforschung* edited by R. Doerr and C. Hallauer (4 vols, Springer, 1938–1958) is continued in the series *Virology Monographs* (1968–). *Viruses of Vertebrates* by C. H. Andrewes, H. G. Pereira and P. Wildy (4th edn, Baillière Tindall, 1978) is a compilation of virus characteristics and a mine of references. The best atlas is *Ultrastructure of Animal Viruses and Bacteriophages* edited by A. J. Dalton and F. Hagenau (Academic Press, 1973).

Systematics is under constant review with the updated position published in *Intervirology* every few years; the fourth report of the ICTV appeared in *Intervirology,* **17,** 1–179, 1982. J. L. Melnick reviews the position annually in *Progress in Medical Virology.*

On fundamental research at the molecular level are *Introduction to Modern Virology* by S. B. Primrose and N. J. Dimmock (2nd edn, Blackwell, 1980), *The Biochemistry of Viruses* by S. J. Martin (Cambridge University Press, 1978), *The Molecular Biology of Animal Viruses* edited by D. P. Nayak (2 vols, Dekker, 1977, 1978) and the more specialized *Molecular Biology of Tumor Viruses* (2nd edn, 2 vols, Cold Spring Harbor Laboratory, 1980, 1982), with vol 1 edited by J. Tooze and vol 2 by R. Weiss, N. Teich, H. Varmus and J. Coffin.

On infections, the earlier, comprehensive *Viral and Rickettsial Infections of Man* edited by F. L. Horsfall and I. Tamm (4th edn, Pitman, 1965) still remains a useful background source on all but more recent knowledge and diseases; the best recent account is *Viral Infections of Humans: Epidemiology and Control* edited by A. S. Evans (2nd edn, Plenum, 1982). *Medical Virology* by F. Fenner and D. O. White (2nd edn, Academic Press, 1976) and D. M. McLean's *Virology in Health Care* (Williams and Wilkins, 1980) are good student texts, and *Human Diseases Caused by Viruses: Recent Developments* edited by H. Rothschild, F. Allison and C. Howe (Oxford University Press, 1978) is for clinicians. General microbiological and clinical texts also cover the subject extensively.

On prophylaxis and chemotherapy C. and H. Koprowski's *Viruses and Immunity* (Academic Press, 1975) and P. A. Bachmann's *Biological Products for Viral Diseases* (Taylor and Francis, 1981) cover vaccine prospects, and chemotherapy is dealt with at postgraduate level in D. J. Bauer's *The Specific Treatment of Virus Diseases* (University Park Press, 1977). Both theoretical and practical is *Chemotherapy of Viral Infections* edited by P. E. Came and L. A. Caliguiri (Springer, 1982), with full coverage of each antiviral, over 650 references to interferon, for example.

On diagnosis the comprehensive manual is *Diagnostic Procedures for Viral, Rickettsial and Chlamydial Infections,* edited by E. H. Lennette and N. J. Schmidt (5th edn, APHA, 1979) and a smaller practical bench book is *Diagnostic Methods in Clinical Virology* by N. R. Grist, E. J. Bell, E. A. C. Follett and G. E. D. Urquhart (3rd edn, Blackwell, 1979). The multivolume *Methods in Virology* edited by K. Maramorosch and H. Koprowski (Academic Press, 1967–) is added to as new methods develop. New and rapid techniques are dealt with in P. S. Gardner and J. McQuillin's *Rapid Virus Diagnosis: Application of Immunofluorescence* (2nd edn, Butterworths, 1980) and *New Developments in Practical Virology* edited by C. R. Howard (Liss, 1982).

On surveillance, *Viruses in Families* by J. P. Fox and C. E. Hall (PSG Publishing Co., 1980) reports on virus-watch programmes over many years. International surveillance, organized by WHO, is described in two chapters of E. and C. Kurstak's *Comparative Diagnosis of Viral Diseases* (Academic Press, vol 2, 1977, page 299; vol 3 1981, page 393). *WHO Yearly Virus Report* is issued in working document form.

On environmental aspects G. Bitton's *Introduction to Environmental Virology* (Wiley, 1980) includes coverage of food- and water-borne infection, and *Viruses and the Environment* edited by E. Kurstak and K. Maramorosch (Academic Press, 1978) deals with cancer hazards as well. Also of value are *Viruses in Water* edited by G. Berg, H. L. Bodily, E. H. Lennette, J. L. Melnick and T. G. Metcalf (APHA, 1976) and *Indicators of Viruses in Water and Food* edited by G. Berg (Ann Arbor Science Publishers, 1978).

On individual infections *Influenza: the Viruses and the Disease* by Sir C. H. Stuart-Harris and G. S. Schild (Arnold, 1976) is comprehensive and *Basic and Applied Influenza Research* edited by A. S. Beare (CRC Press, 1982) gives fuller coverage of vaccine developments. Hepatitis literature is extensive and includes *Hepatitis Viruses of Man* by A. J. Zuckerman and C. R. Howard (Academic Press, 1979), *Viral Hepatitis* by S. Krugman and D. J. Gocke (Saunders, 1978) and the symposia volumes *Viral Hepatitis: 1981 International Symposium* edited by W. Szmuness, H. J. Alter and J. E. Maynard (Franklin Institute Press, 1982) and *Hepatitis B Vaccine: INSERM Symposium* edited by P. Maupas and P. Guesry (Elsevier–North Holland, 1981). Herpes research is documented in *The Human Herpesviruses: an Interdisciplinary Perspective* edited by A. J. Nahmias, W. R. Dowdle and R. F. Schinazi (Elsevier, 1981), the clinical side in *Herpetic Infections of Man* by M. Juretić (University Press of New England, 1980), and tumour implications in *Oncogenic Herpesviruses* edited by F. Rapp (2 vols, CRC Press, 1980). Other works on special aspects are:

The Natural History of Rabies edited by G. M. Baer (2 vols, Academic Press, 1975)
Measles Virus and its Biology by K. B. Fraser and S. J. Martin (Academic Press, 1978)
Cytomegalovirus: Biology and Infection by M.Ho (Plenum, 1982)
Virus Infections of the Gastrointestinal Tract edited by D. A. J. Tyrrell and A. Z. Kapikian (Dekker, 1982)
Viral Diseases of the Skin, Mucous Membrane and Genitals by T. Nasemann (Saunders, 1977)
Viral Infections of the Nervous System edited by R. T. Johnson (Raven Press, 1982)
The Hazard from Dangerous Exotic Diseases by J. C. N. Westwood (Macmillan, 1980)

International congresses have been held under the auspices of IAMS since 1968, being previously included in the International Congresses for Microbiology.

Reviews and monographic series include *Advances in Virus Research, Progress in Medical Virology,* and the irregular *Modern Trends in Medical Virology* (Butterworths), *Monographs in Virology* (Karger), *Perspectives in Virology* (now Academic Press), *Recent Advances in Clinical Virology* (Churchill Livingstone) and *Virology Monographs* (Springer).

Bibliographies include:

A Bibliography of Infantile Paralysis 1789–1949 edited by M. Fishbein, E. M. Salmonsen and L. Hektoen (2nd edn, Lippincott, 1951), includes abstracts
Poliomyelitis Current Literature, monthly (1947–1958), later *Current Literature Poliomyelitis and Related Diseases,* (1959–1961) both financed by National Foundation for Infantile Paralysis
Poliomyelitis Immunity [1908–61] compiled by H. Raettig (2 vols, Fischer, 1963)
International Bibliography of Influenza 1930–1959 by C. G. Loosli, B. Portnoy and E. C. Myers (Univ. S. Calif. School of Medicine, 1978) to span the gap between the earlier bibliography 412 BC–1933 in *Annals of the Pickett–Thompson Laboratory* (vols 9–10, Baillière Tindal and Cox, 1933) and *Annotated Bibliography of Influenza,* quarterly (1960–1964; College of Physicians, Philadelphia)
Influenza Bibliography, monthly (1971–; WHO World Influenza Centre, National Institute for Medical Research, London)
A Decade of Viral Hepatitis: Abstracts 1969–1979 edited by A. J. Zuckerman (Elsevier–North Holland, 1980) arranged systematically with index
Bibliography of Creutzfeldt-Jakob Disease by C. J. Gibbs, C. L. Masters and D. C. Gajdusek (NIH, Bethesda, 1979)
Bibliography of Kuru by M. P. Alpers, D. C. Gajdusek and S. G. Ono (3rd rev., NIH, Bethesda, 1975)

Literature abstracts that specifically cover virology are *Excerpta Medica (Section 47) Virology,* 1971– (prior to which virology was included in *Section 4*) and *Virology Abstracts,* 1967–.

Mycology

Introduction to the History of Mycology by G. C. Ainsworth (Cambridge University Press, 1976) is a well-illustrated book for the professional reader which ends with a chapter on the history of books, journals, societies and culture collections. Also by Ainsworth is *Ainsworth and Bisby's Dictionary of Fungi* (6th edn, Commonwealth Mycological Institute, 1971).

Systematics are elucidated in *Mycologist's Handbook* by D. L. Hawksworth (CMI, 1971), which reprints the International Code of Botanical Nomenclature. *Bibliography of Systematic Mycology* and *Index of Fungi: a List of Names of New Genera . . .* are issued by CAB half-yearly. A British Society for Mycopathology Subcommittee produces *Nomenclature of Fungi Pathogenic to Man and Animals* (*MRC Memorandum No. 23*, 4th edn, HMSO, 1977).

Also of interest is *The Yeasts: a Taxonomic Study* edited by J. Lodder (2nd edn, North Holland, 1970). The National Collection of Pathogenic Fungi in Britain is held at the PHLS Mycological Reference Laboratory, housed at the London School of Hygiene and Tropical Medicine, and is a source of information on any specific question.

Mycology is included in all the larger works on microbiology. An excellent general text is *Smith's Introduction to Industrial Mycology* edited by A. H. S. Onions, D. Allsopp and H. O. W. Eggins (7th edn, Arnold, 1981), and student coverage is found in *Introduction to Modern Mycology* by J. W. Deacon (Blackwell, 1980). *The Yeasts* is a comprehensive three-volume work edited by A. H. Rose and J. S. Harrison (Academic Press, 1969–1971) and medical aspects are covered in *Medical Mycology* by C. W. Emmons, C. H. Binford, J. P. Utz and K. J. Kwon-Chung (3rd edn, Lea and Febiger, 1977) and *Medical Mycology: the Pathogenic Fungi and the Pathogenic Actinomycetes* by J. W. Rippon (2nd edn, Saunders, 1982).

Toxins are definitively treated in *Mycotoxic Fungi, Mycotoxins, Mycotoxicoses: an Encyclopaedic Handbook* edited by T. D. Wyllie and L. G. Morehouse (3 vols, Dekker, 1977–1978) and *Moulds, Toxins and Food* by C. Moreau (translated by M. Moss, Wiley, 1979), has a bibliography of over 3000 references. Useful brief coverage is given in *Mycotoxins* (*Environmental Health Criteria No 11*, WHO, 1979).

Diagnostic methods are dealt with in vol 4 of *Methods in Microbiology* edited by C. Booth (Academic Press, 1971), in *Laboratory Handbook of Medical Mycology* by M. R. McGinnis (Academic Press, 1980) and in *Medical Mycology Manual with Human Mycoses Monograph* by E. S. Beneke and A. L. Rogers (4th edn, Burgess, 1980). Serology is covered in *Serodiagnosis of Mycotic Diseases* by D. F. Palmer, L. Kaufman, W. Kaplan and J. J. Cavallaro (C. C. Thomas, 1977) and, of the many pictorial guides, Wolfe's complementary atlases *A Colour Atlas of Pathogenic Fungi* by D. Frey, R. J. Oldfield and R. C. Bridger (1979) and *A Colour Atlas and Textbook of the Histopathology of Mycotic Diseases* by F. W. Chandler, W. Kaplan and L. Ajello (1980) are outstanding.

Therapy is dealt with in *Antifungal Chemotherapy* edited by D. C. E. Speller (Wiley, 1980) and special topics are covered in *Fungal Infection in the Compromised Patient* edited by D. W. Warnock and M. D. Richardson (Wiley, 1982), *Candida and Candidosis* by F. C. Odds (Leicester University Press, 1979) and *Coccidioidomycosis* edited by D. A. Stevens (Plenum, 1980).

International IAMS Sectional Congresses combining Bacteriology and Mycology take place every four years and regular meetings are also held by the International Society for Human and Animal Mycology and the Pan American Health Organization.

Bibliography of Medical and Veterinary Mycological Manuals, Monographs and Symposia Issued in the Form of a Monograph up to the Year 1970 was compiled by H. Paldrok (Engellska Boktryckeriet, Stockholm, 1970).

Abstract bulletins dealing specifically with mycology are *Review of Medical and Veterinary Mycology* (CAB), *Biological Abstracts: Abstracts of Mycology* (BIOSIS) and *Microbiology Abstracts: Section C. Algology, Mycology and Protozoology* (IR).

Parasitology

Parasitology is normally linked with the study of tropical medicine, but even in temperate climates diseases caused by parasites, both imported and indigenous, cause problems and are given coverage in all comprehensive works on microbiology and infectious diseases. *A History of Parasitology* by W. D. Foster (Livingstone, 1965) is a good historical introduction to the subject. A comprehensive treatise is *Parasitic Protozoa* edited by J. P. Kreier (4 vols, Academic Press, 1977–1978), and teaching texts include *Parasitology: the Biology of Animal Parasites* by E. R. and G. A. Noble (Lea and Febiger, 1982) and *Medical Parasitology* by E. K. Markell and M. Voge (5th edn, Saunders, 1981). On the clinical side *Craig and Faust's Clinical Parasitology* by E. C. Faust, P. F. Russell and R. C. Jung (8th edn, Lea and Febiger, 1970) is still a mine of information and references. Useful information on the clinical side can also be found in *Manson's Tropical Diseases* by P. E. C. Manson-Bahr and F. I. C. Apted (18th edn, Baillière Tindall, 1982), and R. Knight's *Parasitic Disease in Man* (Churchill Livingstone, 1982) gives concise information on diagnosis, epidemiology and control of each infection. Diagnostic books include *Methods of Cultivating Parasites in vitro* by A. E. R. Taylor and J. R. Baker (2nd edn, Blackwell, 1978) and *Immunological Investigation of Tropical Parasitic Diseases* by V. Houba (Churchill Livingstone, 1980). Many atlases are of high quality – *Atlas of Medical Helminthology and Protozoology* by H. C. Jeffrey and R. M. Leach (2nd edn, Churchill Livingstone, 1975), *Atlas of Human Parasitology* by L. R. Ash and T. C. Orihel (American Society of Clinical Pathologists, 1980), and the complementary Wolfe productions, *A Colour Atlas of Tropical Medicine and Parasitology* by W. Peters and H. M. Gilles (2nd edn, 1981) and *A Colour Atlas of Clinical Parasitology* edited by T. Yamaguchi (1981). On immunology are *Immunology of Parasitic Infections* edited by S. Cohen and K. S. Warren (2nd edn, Blackwell, 1982) and *The Immunology of Parasitic Infections: a Handbook for Physicians, Veterinarians and Biologists* by O. O. Barriga (University Park Press, 1981). The British Society of Parasitology's Symposium No 18 is *Vaccines against Parasites* edited by A. E. R. Taylor and R. Muller (Blackwell, 1980), and 'Antiparasitic chemotherapy' is the subject of *Antibiotics and Chemotherapy*, vol 30, (Karger, 1981).

International congresses of Parasitology and of Protozoology take place every few years. As tropical parasitology is of great concern to WHO many studies and recommendations are published in its *Bulletin* and *Technical Report Series. Advances in Parasitology* publishes reviews on special aspects annually. Published bibliographies include:

Bibliography of Hookworm Disease (Ancylostomiasis) 1920–62 (WHO, 1965).
Schistosomiasis – a Bibliography of the World's Literature from 1852 to 1962 by K. S. Warren and V. A. Newill (Western Reserve University, 1967)
The African Trypanosomiases edited by H. W. Mulligan (Allen and Unwin, 1970)
Chagas's Disease (S. American Trypanosomiasis) compiled by M. A. Miles and J. E. Rouse (Bureau of Hygiene and Tropical Diseases, 1970)
Toxoplasmosis 1908–1967 by J. Jíra and V. Kozojed (2 vols, Fischer, 1970)

Abstract bulletins dealing specifically with parasitology are *Parasitological Abstracts* and *Helminthological Abstracts,* both produced by CAB, *Microbiology Abstracts: C Algology, Mycology and Protozoology* (IR) and *Tropical Diseases Bulletin (Bureau of Hygiene).*

Safety

Safe handling of pathogens has always been part of laboratory training, but new emphasis has been lent to the subject over the last ten years by the requirements of the Health and Safety at Work Act in the UK and by both real threats from treacherous viruses and conjectural ones connected with genetic engineering. Every aspect of work has been subject to scrutiny, with reports, regulations and codes seeking to preclude every hazard. A useful summary of the situation and of the range of research now being carried out is given in 'The containment of microorganisms' by J. Melling and K. Allner in *Essays in Applied Microbiology* (*see* page 255). 'The problems of virus containment' by A. E. Wright, G. J. Harper and D. I. H. Simpson can be found in *New Developments in Practical Virology*, page 305, edited by C. R. Howard (Liss, 1982). Both these papers come from the PHLS CAMR at Porton Down, where the Microbiological Safety Reference Laboratory is a source of specific information.

On pathogen hazards a key publication is *Code of Practice for the Prevention of Infection in Clinical Laboratories and Post- mortem Rooms* (the 'Howie Code') issued by the DHSS (HMSO, 1978). *A Guide to the Health and Safety (Dangerous Pathogens) Regulations 1981* (Booklet HS(R)12, HMSO, 1981) is one of the helpful guidance publications issued by the Health and Safety Executive, the body charged with implementing UK regulations. On genetic engineering the UK Genetic Manipulation Advisory Group (GMAG) disseminate information in their *GMAG Notes*. Their third report (Cmnd 8665, HMSO, 1982) prints the latest code of practice with a note on comparisons with that of US NIH. In 1981 the Royal Society produced *Safety in Research: a Study Group Report* which scrutinized the effects of legislative control on research. An appendix lists regulations affecting research in the UK. The need for rapid dissemination of information is stressed and the Royal Society of Chemistry is now producing *Laboratory Hazards Bulletin*.

Covering all general aspects of safety are *Handbook of Laboratory Safety* edited by N. V. Steere (2nd edn, CRC Press, 1971) and the more recent *Laboratory-acquired Infections: History, Incidence, Causes and Prevention*, by C. H. Collins (Butterworths, 1983), an excellent practical handbook for the laboratory with a comprehensive list of references. Laboratory infections are reviewed by R. M. Pike in *Hlth Lab. Sci.*, **13**, 105, 1976 and in *Annu. Rev. Microbiol.*, **33**, 41, 1979 and J. V. S. Pether gives a reasoned appraisal of the safety question in 'Prevention of laboratory-acquired infection' in *Recent Advances in Infection 2*, page 163, edited by D. S. Reeves and A. M. Geddes (Churchill Livingstone, 1982).

Environmental microbiology

The subject is featured in all major works on microbiology and, being of prime concern to WHO, many studies and recommendations can be found in its *Technical Report Series* and elsewhere. Good general coverage of the literature is given in *Abstracts on Hygiene and Communicable Diseases*.

Food

The Microbiology of Foods by F. W. Tanner (2nd edn, Garrard

Press, 1946) is an encyclopaedic source on earlier references; good modern texts are *Food Microbiology* by W. C. Frazier and D. C. Westhoff (3rd edn, McGraw-Hill, 1978) and *Microbiology of Foods* by J. C. Ayres, J. O. Mundt and W. E. Sandine (Freeman, 1980). The most useful current book on food poisoning is *Food-borne Infections and Intoxications* edited by H. Riemann and F. L. Bryan (2nd edn, Academic Press, 1979). Catering aspects are thoroughly covered in P. A. Alcock's *Food Hygiene Manual* (Lewis, 1980).

On laboratory methods the American approach can be found in *Compendium of Methods for the Microbiological Examination of Foods* edited by M. L. Speck (APHA, 1976), and the European standpoint is given coverage in *Isolation and Identification Methods for Food Poisoning Organisms* edited by J. E. L. Corry, D. Roberts and F. A. Skinner (*SAB Tech. Ser. No 17*, Academic Press, 1982). Working towards an international consensus is the series of books produced by the ICMSF, *Microorganisms in Foods* (vol 1, 2nd edn, University of Toronto Press, 1978; vol 2, University of Toronto Press, 1974; vol 3 Pts I and II, Academic Press, 1980). On special topics *Meat Microbiology* edited by M. H. Brown (1982), *Dairy Microbiology* edited by R. K. Robinson (2 vols, 1981), both from Applied Science Publishers, and *Standard Methods for the Examination of Dairy Products* edited by E. H. Marth (14th edn, APHA, 1978) are useful.

Surveillance reports on food poisoning in England and Wales have been published by the PHLS for 30 years, the latest location being *British Medical Journal. Food Poisoning* (*Memo 188/MED*, HMSO, 1982) on investigation and control of food infection in England and Wales is issued by DHSS, and gives regulations and notification procedures. Separate surveillance reports are issued annually by CDC and the Canadian Department of Health and Welfare.

Important regular meetings are the International Symposia on Food Microbiology held by the ICMFH, and the conferences of the World Association of Veterinary Food Hygienists. A review of the literature on food safety and food-borne illness is published each year in the annual report of the Food Research Institute of the University of Wisconsin. *Developments in Food Microbiology* (1982–) publishes reviews and literature coverage is found in *Food Science and Technology Abstracts* and *Dairy Science Abstracts* (CAB).

Water

The microbiological testing of water is dealt with in the American *andard Methods for the Examination of Water and Wastewater* lited by J. J. Connors, D. Jenkins and A. E. Greenberg (15th ln, APHA, 1981), and in Britain the standby remains the DHSS *ports on Public Health and Medical Subjects No 71,* the long vaited 5th edition of which, entitled *The Bacteriological Exami- ition of Drinking Water Supplies,* is due to be published in 1983. irveillance reports on water-borne infections are issued annually / the Canadian Department of Health and Welfare and by CDC. ι addition G. F. Craun reports on continuing surveillance each ar in *Journal of the American Water Works Association;* the ars 1971–1978 are covered in **73,** 360, 1981.

Sources of information and useful reports are, in Britain, the ational Water Council and, in America, the Environmental Pro- ction Agency, Cincinnati. The Water Research Centre at Mar- w produces *WRC Information,* a weekly abstract publication hich has taken the place of *Water Pollution Abstracts* since 1974. iruses in water are referred to on page 262.

isinfection and sterilization

ounteracting unwanted microorganisms in the environmental set- 1g is achieved by a variety of chemical and physical means, and e literature ranges from theoretical studies on destruction and hibition to practical advice on necessary sterility standards in idangered areas – the hospital environment, food and pharma- utical manufacture, the laboratory, the kitchen, swimming pools id spacecraft. Comprehensive texts include *Principles and Prac- e of Disinfection, Preservation and Sterilisation* edited by A. D. ussell, W. B. Hugo and G. A. J. Ayliffe (Blackwell, 1982) and isinfection, Sterilization and Preservation* edited by S. S. Block nd edn, Lea and Febiger, 1977). Still held in high regard is *A eview of Sterilisation and Disinfection as Applied to Medical, dustrial and Laboratory Practice* by S. D. Rubbo and J. F. Gard- :r (Lloyd-Luke, 1965), and it is understood that Gardner's 2nd lition may be published by Churchill Livingstone in 1983.

Bacteriological studies include *Inhibition and Destruction of the acterial Cell* edited by W. B. Hugo (Academic Press, 1971) and . D. Russell's *The Destruction of Bacterial Spores* (Academic :ess, 1982). On testing and application of disinfectants in a wide iriety of contexts is *Disinfectants: Their Use and Evaluation of ffectiveness* edited by C. H. Collins, M. C. Allwood, S. F. loomfield and A. Fox (*SAB Tech. Ser. No. 16,* Academic Press, ▸81).

Standards, guidelines and recommended practices for sterilizers

and disinfectants are issued by the British Standards Instituti(
and the US Association for the Advancement of Medical Instr
mentation, and reports on radiation sterilization are published I
the International Atomic Energy Agency. The DHSS reports a₁
makes recommendations from time to time on various medical a₁
pharmaceutical aspects, and the *British Pharmacopoeia* appe
dices deal with sterility standards.

Infectious diseases

History

Long before microbiology became a science people were recordi₁
outbreaks of infection and speculating as to their cause. Reference
R. H. Major's *Classic Descriptions of Disease* (3rd edn, Blackwe
1945) discloses observations on mumps and malaria by Hippocrate
A History of Epidemics in Britain by C. Creighton documen
recorded epidemics since 664 AD (2 vols, Cambridge Universi
Press, 1891, 1894, reprinted with additional bibliography, Fra₁
Cass, 1965). Tracing the gradual unravelling of ideas about infecti(
from the earliest times are *The Conquest of Epidemic Disease* I
C.-E. A. Winslow (Princeton University Press, 1944), *Pomp a₁*
Pestilence: Infectious Disease, its Origins and Conquest by R. Ha
(Gollancz, 1954) and A. Cockburn's *The Evolution and Eradicati(*
of Infectious Diseases (Johns Hopkins Press, 1963). Classics on ₁
study in the community are H. H. Scott's *Some Notable Epidem₁*
(Arnold, 1934), which re-examines the detective work in records
earlier outbreaks, M. Greenwood's *Epidemics and Crowd Diseas*
(Williams and Norgate, 1935), which bases the teaching of epiden₁
ology on historical study, *Papers of Wade Hampton Frost M. I*
edited by K. F. Maxcy (Commonwealth Fund/Oxford Universi
Press, 1941), which reflects varied experience in America during t₁
1910s to 1930s, and *Epidemiology in Country Practice* by W. ₁
Pickles (Wright, 1939), which records acute individual surveillan₁
in the small compass of Yorkshire village life over roughly the sam
period. On developments in treatment are P. E. Baldry's *The Bat₁*
against Bacteria – a Fresh Look (Cambridge University Press, 197€
H. F. Dowling's *Fighting Infection* (Harvard University Press, 197
and W. W. Spink's *Infectious Diseases: Prevention and Treatment*
the Nineteenth and Twentieth Centuries (Dawson, 1978). Specifica₁
on vaccination are H. J. Parish's *A History of Immunization* (196
and *Victory with Vaccines* (1968), both published by Livingstone.
Bibliography of Internal Medicine: Communicable Diseases by A. ₁

Bloomfield (University of Chicago Press, 1958) traces the history through key publications, giving translated abstracts of the more obscure papers.

Texts

Comprehensive textbooks on infectious diseases include *Principles and Practice of Infectious Diseases* by G. L. Mandell, R. G. Douglas and J. E. Bennett (2 vols, Wiley, 1979), *Infectious Diseases: a Modern Treatise of Infectious Processes* edited by P. D. Hoeprich (2nd edn, Harper and Row, 1977) and A. B. Christie's *Infectious Diseases: Epidemiology and Clinical Practice* (3rd edn, Churchill Livingstone, 1980) which gives good coverage of all the common diseases, is an excellent source of references and one of the few major texts still bearing the stamp of a single author. A classic text on the nature of infection and immunity is *Natural History of Infectious Disease* by F. M. Burnet and D. O. White (4th edn, Cambridge University Press, 1972). Among the many books for clinicians, *Microbial Disease: the Use of the Laboratory in Diagnosis, Therapy and Control* by D. A. J. Tyrrell, I. Phillips, C. S. Goodwin and R. Blowers (Arnold, 1979) directs the physician to the full range of laboratory services in the handling of each clinical syndrome. Of the many student texts, *The Biologic and Clinical Basis of Infectious Diseases* by G. P. Youmans, P. V. Paterson and H. M. Sommers (2nd edn, Saunders, 1980) is the most comprehensive.

Control of Communicable Disease in Man edited by A. S. Benenson (13th edn, APHA, 1981) is an outstanding ready reference handbook and, in the same field, *Infection* by R. T. D. Emond, J. M. Bradley and N. S. Galbraith (Grant McIntyre, 1982) is useful on UK control measures.

Atlases include *A Colour Atlas of Infectious Diseases* by R. T. D. Emond (Wolfe Medical, 1974) and *Infectious Diseases Illustrated: an Integrated Text and Colour Atlas* by H. P. Lambert and W. E. Farrer (Pergamon, 1982).

Special aspects

Animal and animal-borne infections are of recurring relevance, and comprehensive treatment is given in *CRC Handbook Series in Zoonoses* edited by J. H. Steele (7 vols, CRC Press, 1979–) and in *Diseases Transmitted from Animals to Man* edited by W. T. Hubbert, W. F. McCulloch and P. R. Schnurrenberger (6th edn, C. C. Thomas, 1975). Steele also contributes an excellent and well-referenced chapter in *The Theory and Practice of Public Health* edited by W. Hobson (5th edn, Oxford University Press, 1979) and special aspects are reported, at intervals, in *WHO Technical Report Series*. Access to veterinary and comparative literature is gained through *Index Veterinarius* and *Veterinary Bulletin*, both produced by CAB.

Hospital and surgical infections have received a great deal of attention in the last ten years and every aspect has come under scrutiny, from operating theatre procedures to infection control, nursing and hospital hygiene. The Second International Conference volume is *Nosocomial Infections* edited by R. E. Dixon (Yorke Medical Books, 1981), reprinted from *Amer. J. Med.*, **70**, 379, 631, 1981. Useful texts include *CRC Handbook of Hospital Acquired Infections* edited by R. P. Wenzel (CRC Press, 1981), *Hospital Infections* edited by J. V. Bennett and P. S. Brachman (Little, Brown, 1979) and *Occurrence Diagnosis and Sources of Hospital-associated Infections* edited by W. J. Fahlberg and D. Gröschel (Dekker, 1978), which contains a chapter on the history of hospital infection. Surgical aspects are treated in *Surgical Infectious Diseases* edited by R. L. Simmons and R. J. Howard (Appleton-Century-Crofts, 1982), *Hospital-acquired Infections in Surgery* edited by H. C. Polk and H. H. Stone (University Park Press, 1977) and *Surgical Sepsis* edited by C. J. L. Strachan and R. Wise (Academic Press, 1979).

Good sources on infection control are *Control of Hospital Infection: a Practical Handbook* edited by E. J. L. Lowbury, G. A. J. Ayliffe, A. M. Geddes and J. D. Williams (2nd edn, Chapman and Hall, 1981), its companion volume *Hospital-acquired Infection Principles and Prevention* by G. A. J. Ayliffe, B. J. Collins and L. J. Taylor (Wright, 1982), and *Infection: Prevention and Control* by E. C. Dubay and R. D. Grubb (2nd edn, Mosby, 1978). On basic questions of hygiene is I. M. Maurer's *Hospital Hygiene* (2nd edn, Arnold, 1978) and, on air hygiene, there is *Air Contamination Control in Hospitals* by J. R. Luciano (Plenum, 1977).

Infections in other specialist areas are dealt with in:

Oral Microbiology and Infectious Disease by G. W. Burnett, H. W. Scherp and G. S. Schuster (4th edn, Williams and Wilkins, 1976; student edn, 1978)

External Infections of the Eye: Bacterial, Viral and Mycotic by H. B. Fedukowicz (2nd edn, Appleton-Century-Crofts, 1978)

Infections of the Nervous System edited by P. J. Vincken and G. W. Bruyn (3 vols, North Holland, 1978)

Neurologic Infections in Children by W. E. Bell and W. F. McCormick (2nd edn, Saunders, 1981)

Infections in Obstetrics and Gynecology by D. Charles (Saunders, 1980)

Perinatal Infections edited by K. Elliot, M. O'Connor and J. Whelan (Excerpta Medica, 1980)

Microbial Skin Disease: its Epidemiology by W. C. Noble (Arnold, 1983)

Urinary Tract Infection by R. Maskell (Arnold, 1982)

The Challenge of Urinary Tract Infections by A. W. Asscher (Academic Press, 1980)
Sexually Transmitted Diseases by C. B. S. Schofield (3rd edn, Churchill Livingstone, 1979)
Recent Advances in Sexually Transmitted Diseases No 2 edited by J. R. W. Harris (Churchill Livingstone, 1981)
Venereal Diseases by A. King, C. Nicol and P. Rodin (4th edn, Baillière Tindall, 1980)

Epidemiology and surveillance

Texts on epidemiology include *Epidemiology: Principles and Methods* by B. MacMahon and T. F. Pugh (revised edn, Little, Brown, 1970), *Foundations of Epidemiology* by A. M. Lilienfeld (2nd edn, Oxford University Press, 1980), *An Introduction to Epidemiology* by M. Alderson (Macmillan, 1976), and the clinically orientated *Epidemiology of Diseases* edited by D. L. Miller and R. D. T. Farmer (Blackwell, 1982).

Central to the control of infection in the community is the surveillance and regular recording of its incidence, and many countries issue weekly bulletins giving statistical information and documenting current outbreaks. For England and Wales the PHLS Communicable Disease Surveillance Centre produces *Communicable Disease Report* (with restricted circulation), and the Scottish Home and Health Department issues *Communicable Diseases, Scotland.* Quarterly updatings from both these sources are published in *Community Medicine,* and the *Annual Report of the Chief Medical Officer of the DHSS* briefly reports on all important infections. Comparable information on animals can be found in *Animal Health,* the annual report of the Chief Veterinary Officer of the Ministry of Agriculture, Fisheries and Food. In the US *Morbidity and Mortality Weekly Report* is issued by CDC, as well as annual surveillance reports on many categories of infection. *Weekly Epidemiological Record* published by WHO highlights incidents reported from all countries, as well as international themes such as the spread of cholera and the eradication of smallpox. Annual statistics are published in the UK by the Office of Population Censuses and Surveys, and worldwide by WHO.

Immunity and immunization

The nature of infection and immunity is covered in most works on infectious diseases and in major microbiological texts. The subject is given comprehensive treatment, including immunodiagnosis and prevention, in the two-volume *Immunology of Human Infection* edited by A. J. Nahmias and R. J. O'Reilly (Plenum, 1981–1982). *Immunological Aspects of Infectious Diseases* edited by G. Dick (MTP 1979) also explores the subject and special aspects are covered in *The Pathogenesis of Infectious Diseases* by C. A. Mims (2nd edn, Academic Press, 1982), a useful student monograph, and in the conference volumes *Microbial Perturbation of Host Defences* edited by F. O'Grady and H. Smith (Academic Press, 1981) and *Immunomodulation by Bacteria and their Products* edited by H. Friedman, T. W. Klein and A. Szentivanyi (Plenum 1981).

Vaccination is dealt with in G. Dick's *Immunisation* (Update, 1978), in *Immunization in Clinical Practice* edited by V. A. Fulginiti (Lippincott, 1982) and in the DHSS guidelines *Immunisation against Infectious Diseases* (1982)

Therapy

The Molecular Basis of Antibiotic Action by E. F. Gale, E. Cundliffe, P. E. Reynolds, M. H. Richmond and M. J. Waring (2nd edn, Wiley, 1981) studies the mechanism of antibiotic action, and useful clinical manuals are *Antibiotic and Chemotherapy* by L. P. Garrod, H. P. Lambert and F. O'Grady (5th edn, Churchill Livingstone, 1981) and *The Use of Antibiotics: a Comprehensive Review with Clinical Emphasis* by A. Kucers and N. McK. Bennett (3rd edn, Heinemann, 1979). Methods of sensitivity testing and assay can be found in *Laboratory Methods in Antimicrobial Chemotherapy* edited by D. S. Reeves, I. Phillips, J. D. Williams and R. Wise (Churchill Livingstone, 1978) while *Antibiotics in Laboratory Medicine* edited by V. Lorian (Williams and Wilkins, 1980) combines methodology with documentation of sensitivity trends. The resistance problem is explored in L. E. Bryan's *Bacterial Resistance and Susceptibility to Chemotherapeutic Agents* (Cambridge University Press, 1982).

Reviews and secondary sources

Journals publishing regular reviews include *Epidemiological Reviews* and *Reviews of Infectious Diseases*, and the serial volumes of *Developments in Biological Standardization* publish proceedings of international meetings held by IUBS. Among many compilations of reviews are *Clinical Concepts of Infectious Diseases* edited by L. E. Cluff and J. E. Johnson (2nd edn, Williams and Wilkins, 1978), *Current Clinical Topics in Infectious Diseases* edited by R. S. Remington and M. N. Swartz (vol 1–, McGraw-Hill, 1980–),

Modern Topics in Infection edited by J. D. Williams (Heinemann, 1978) and *Recent Advances in Infection* edited by D. S. Reeves and A. M. Geddes (No 1–, Churchill Livingstone, 1979–).

Abstract bulletins that specifically cover infection and immunity are *Hospital Abstracts*, those abstracts contained in *American Review of Respiratory Disease* up to 1973, *Sexually Transmitted Diseases: Abstracts and Bibliography* and *Immunization: Abstracts and Bibliography*, both produced by CDC, *Immunology Abstracts*, and *Excerpta Medica (Section 26) Immunology, Serology and Transplantation*, in addition to those referred to at the end of the chapter.

Periodicals

Primary journals

It is 100 years since the first specialist journals in microbiology were founded. In 1883 Max von Pettenkofer decided to stop publishing his papers in the *Zeitschrift für Biologie* and to found a journal specific to the new science – *Archiv für Hygiene*. Three years later Robert Koch along with Carl Flügge started a rival publication – *Zeitschrift für Hygiene*. The following year, 1887, saw the foundation of a third German journal – *Centralblatt für Bakteriologie, Parasitenkunde, Infektionskrankheiten und Hygiene, Abteilung I*, and in Paris the Institut Pasteur launched the *Annales de l'Institut Pasteur*, 'publiées sous le patronage de M. Pasteur'. All these journals continue to flourish, the *Zeitschrift* as *Medical Microbiology and Immunology* and the *Archiv* as *Reihe B* of the *Zentralblatt* (spelling change, 1929) which retains its original volume numbering. Volume 175 contains a cumulative index which includes relevant papers from the earlier *Zeitschrift für Biologie*, covering the years 1865–1980. In 1902 the *Centralblatt*, which had previously included literature abstracts along with original papers, started publication of a separate *'Referate'* section, and in the following year, in France, a parallel abstract journal, *Bulletin de l'Institut Pasteur*, appeared – these too survive, though the *Bulletin* has since 1971, published reviews only. In Britain the Pathological Society launched *Journal of Pathology and Bacteriology* in 1893, but it was not till 1968 that the bacteriologists broke away to start their own journal, *Journal of Medical Microbiology*.

Twenty years ago the International Committee for Microbiological and Immunological Documentation of the IAMS undertook the task of compiling a world list of periodicals which 'regularly or sporadically publish material of microbiological or immunological interest'. It was published in 1969 as *Periodicals Relevant to Microbiology and Immunology* edited by G. Tunevall (Wiley Interscience). The information was gathered from national corresponding members and is somewhat uneven, but the resulting directory of 750 journals, with addresses and bibliographic details, and with separate national lists, is a useful compilation. A new edition is being prepared with the help of the National Library of Medicine in Washington, who will publish it.

A high proportion of microbiological journals are published by or on behalf of scientific societies, outstanding among which is the American Society for Microbiology which currently publishes seven major and four minor serials (in addition to the numerous textbooks and conference proceedings previously referred to), all of exceptional relevance and quality.

The list which follows is a selection of those specific to the field of medical microbiology and infectious diseases. No attempt has been made to include the general medical and specialty journals, the pages of which contain so many relevant papers, nor those concerned with general science, biochemistry or genetics, nor the purely immunological journals (many of which are also highly relevant), these subjects being properly covered in other chapters. A few veterinary journals are listed as they provide a source of comparative literature.

MICROBIOLOGY

Acta Microbiologica Academiae Scientiarum Hungaricae
Acta Pathologica et Microbiologica Scandinavica B. Microbiology
Annales de Microbiologie
Antonie van Leeuwenhoek Journal of Microbiology
Archives of Microbiology
Archives Roumaines de Pathologie Expérimentale et de Microbiologie
Canadian Journal of Microbiology
Clinical Microbiology Newsletter
Current Microbiology
European Journal of Clinical Microbiology
FEMS Microbiology Letters
Folia Microbiologica
Indian Journal of Medical Research
Indian Journal of Microbiology
Indian Journal of Pathology and Microbiology

International Journal of Systematic Bacteriology
Japanese Journal of Medical Science and Biology
Journal of Bacteriology
Journal of Clinical Microbiology
Journal of General Microbiology
Journal of Medical Microbiology
Journal of Microbiological Methods
Medical Microbiology and Immunology
Microbiologica
Microbiology and Immunology
Microbios
Microbios Letters
Revista de Microbiologia (S. Paulo)
Zentralblatt für Bakteriologie Mikrobiologie und Hygiene I Abt.
  A. Medizinische Mikrobiologie Infekiontskrankheiten und Parasitologie
  B. Umwelthygiene Krankenhaushygiene Arbeitshygiene Präventive Medizin

VIROLOGY

Acta Virologica
Annales de Virologie
Antiviral Research
Archives of Virology
Intervirology
Journal of General Virology
Journal of Medical Virology
Journal of Virological Methods
Journal of Virology
Soviet Progress in Virology
Virology

MYCOLOGY

Mycopathologia
Mykosen
Sabouraudia

PARASITOLOGY

American Journal of Tropical Medicine
  and Hygiene
Annals of Tropical Medicine and
  Parasitology
Journal of Helminthology
Journal of Parasitology
Journal of Protozoology
Parasitology
Transactions of the Royal Society of
  Tropical Medicine and Hygiene
Tropical and Geographical Medicine

INFECTIOUS DISEASES AND ANTIMICROBIAL THERAPY

American Journal of Infection Control
American Review of Respiratory
  Disease
Annales d'Immunologie
Antimicrobial Agents and
  Chemotherapy
Asian Journal of Infectious Diseases
British Journal of Venereal Diseases
Bulletin of the World Health
  Organization
Chemotherapy
Comparative Immunology Micro-
  biology and Infectious Diseases
Infection (Munich)
Infection Control
Infection and Immunity
International Journal of Epidemiology

International Journal of Zoonoses
Journal of Antimicrobial Chemotherapy
Journal of Epidemiology and
  Community Health
Journal of Hospital Infection
Journal of Infection
Journal of Infectious Diseases
Médecine et Maladies Infectieuses
Pediatric Infectious Diseases
Public Health
Revue d'Epidémiologie et de Santé
  Publique
Scandinavian Journal of Infectious
  Diseases
Sexually Transmitted Diseases
Tubercle

ENVIRONMENTAL MICROBIOLOGY

Applied and Environmental Micro-
  biology
Canadian Journal of Public Health
Dairy and Food Sanitation
Journal of Hygiene
Journal of Hygiene, Epidemiology,
  Microbiology and Immunology
Journal of Applied Bacteriology
Journal of Food Protection
Journal of Food Science
Water Research

LABORATORY TECHNOLOGY

American Journal of Clinical Pathology
American Journal of Medical
  Technology
Canadian Journal of Medical
  Technology
Journal of Biological Standardization
Journal of Clinical Pathology
Journal of Laboratory and Clinical
  Medicine
Laboratory Medicine
Laboratory Practice
Medical Laboratory Science
Public Health Laboratory

VETERINARY MEDICINE

American Journal of Veterinary Research
British Veterinary Journal
Canadian Journal of Comparative Medicine
Journal of the American Veterinary Medical Association
Journal of Comparative Pathology
Research in Veterinary Science
Veterinary Microbiology
Veterinary Record

Secondary sources

A full description of relevant abstract and index services, past as well as present, is given in 'Literature guide for microbiology' by E. C. Gergely on page 261 of the first volume of *Handbook of Microbiology (see* page 253). Another admirable source on earlier bibliographical information in the whole medical field is *A Handbook of Medical Library Practice* edited by J. Doe (American Library Association, 1943). (*See also Medical Reference Works*, edited by J. B. Blake and C. Roos, 1967, described on page 70.)

As in other fields of medicine, information on books and reports can be traced in the annual volumes of *NLM Current Catalog*, earlier material through the *Surgeon General's Catalog*, and currently available books in Bowker's *Medical Books in Print*. Theses can be found through *Dissertation Abstracts*, reviews through the review section of *Index Medicus*, and first descriptions through Garrison and Morton's *A Medical Bibliography*. Conferences can be located in the *BL Index to Conference Proceedings* and *Biological Abstracts/RRM* aims to index the contents of reports, reviews and meetings. Government publications can be traced through the *Annual Catalogue* (HMSO), and the indexed *Monthly Catalog of the US Government Publications*.

In the present chapter under each section dealing with a specialized subject area the appropriate secondary sources have been indicated, and only those covering the field generally are discussed here.

The prime tool for retrospective retrieval of titles in the medical field is *Index Medicus* (NLM), and for veterinary literature *Index Veterinarius* (CAB); the former goes back to 1879, the latter to 1933. *Current Contents, Life Sciences* and *Clinical Practice* sections, reprint a wide selection of contents pages, daunting for weekly scanning, but useful for tracking down references of the immediate past. To provide an updating service in the field of medical microbiology the Library of the Central Public Health Laboratory at Colindale has, for the last 30 years, issued a weekly

Library Bulletin of selected titles, with half-yearly indexes.

A range of abstract bulletins provide coverage of the literature of microbiology, from the weighty *Biological Abstracts* (1926–), covering the whole biological field, but with over a quarter of the sectional headings relevant to microbiological research, to the tailor-made *Microbiology Abstracts* (1965–), previously produced by Information Retrieval Ltd, now by Cambridge Scientific Abstracts, Bethesda. *Section A* covers *Industrial and Applied Microbiology*, and *Section B* covers *General Microbiology and Bacteriology*. At least 15 sections of *Excerpta Medica* (1947–) are said to have some relevant reference to the field, the most appropriate being *Section 4, Microbiology* and *Section 17, Public Health, Social Medicine and Hygiene*. *Abstracts on Hygiene and Communicable Diseases* (earlier *Bulletin of Hygiene*) (1926–) and *Tropical Diseases Bulletin* (1912–), both produced by the Bureau of Hygiene and Tropical Diseases, London, give good coverage of books and reports as well as journal articles in their respective fields and have a reputation for soundness. Many specialist bulletins produced by the Commonwealth Agricultural Bureaux have already been referred to, the last to be mentioned being *Veterinary Bulletin* (1931–), a valuable source of microbiological information.

In France, *Microbiologie, Virologie, Immunologie*, prepared by the CNRS and the Institut Pasteur forms Part 340 of the voluminous *Bulletin Signalétique,* published by Informascience. In Germany the *Referate* section of the *Zentralblatt für Bakteriologie, Mikrobiologie und Hygiene*, mentioned earlier, now has the majority of its abstracts in English. For retrospective searching this source along with the abstract sections in the earlier volumes of the *Zentralblatt* itself, dating back to 1887, and the *Bulletin de l'Institut Pasteur*, dating back to 1903, are an invaluable means of obtaining the gist of obscure early European papers. *Abstracts of Bacteriology 1917–25* (a precursor of *Biological Abstracts*) has poor coverage and inadequate entries. *British Abstracts AIII*, which included microbiology along with the rest of biology and medicine, ran from 1945 to 1953, and became first *British Abstracts of Medical Sciences*, and later *International Abstracts of Biological Sciences*.

Abstract bulletins are a vital necessity for scientists in isolated situations without sufficient primary publications to hand, and a long stop for all to catch up on papers they may have missed. Ideally, they should publish promptly, be reasonably complete in the field they purport to cover and provide the critical assessment of experts. The increasing tendency to cite by title only may indicate discriminating editorial policy, but has reached its *reductio ad absurdum* in *International Abstracts of Biological Sciences*, now little more than a list of titles. In one of a series of papers assessing the use of microbiological literature J. Carson and H. V. Wyatt (*ASM News*, **48**, 5, 1982) compare retrieval and rapidity of publication in *Index Medicus, Current Contents* and eight abstract bulletins. A significant fact to emerge from this small study is that, of the two bulletins from which one should expect full coverage, *Microbiology Abstracts B* retrieved 83 per cent, as against *Excerpta Medica* (Section 4) 29 per cent and (Section 17) 9 per cent. On promptness of publication *Abstracts on Hygiene and Communicable Diseases* equalled *Index Medicus* and *Biological Abstracts* with an average of 5 months time lapse. Quality is harder to assess, but most of the abstracts coming from the Bureau of Hygiene and CAB are still signed or initialled, as are most of those in the *Zentralblatt*.

Practically all the secondary sources mentioned throughout the chapter are, or will shortly be, accessible through DIALOG.

·Acknowledgement

The author wishes to thank kind friends in the Public Health Laboratory Service for helpful advice and to absolve them of any responsibility for mistakes or omissions.

13

Immunology and transplantation

D. N. H. Hamilton

Immunological research and the literature it brings forth still form a fairly compact division within the biomedical sciences and, fortunately, research workers can still comprehend the work and language of most other toilers in this vineyard. An international congress of immunologists is still a united meeting of wide interest to most participants, a happy situation long since departed in physiology or pathology. If any sub-divisions exist, however, it is between the clinical immunologists together with the transplant surgeons on the one hand, and on the other hand the laboratory immunologist. In the laboratory a further subtle separation of manpower and resources can be seen, into those interested in the problem of antibody formation (humoral immunity) and those working on cell-mediated immunological events (e.g. graft rejection, contact sensitivity, immuno-therapy, auto-immunity). These main streams of immunological endeavours are reflected in the published literature, and some journals often emphasize one aspect or the other.

Primary sources of information

The reader is well served by many journals for original articles and reviews. Experimental immunology has a well-defined series of journals, but tumour immunology and human transplantation studies are rather widely scattered in the literature:

Journal of Experimental Medicine. This journal, with its highly selective editorial policy, consistently publishes very important papers on immunological topics. According to a *Current Contents* survey this journal is the world's most quoted immunological journal, and comes third in the Life Sciences journals

Journal of Immunology. Papers contained here are grouped into the sub-divisions of immunology mentioned above. The origin of the papers is mostly in the US. According to *Current Contents*, this is the second most quoted journal in immunology

Immunology. This journal takes articles of wide immunological interest, mainly originating in Britain

Clinical and Experimental Immunology. The range of articles covered by this journal is, as the title suggests, with the clinical emphasis on auto-immune disease. Occasional short reviews on major topics are given

Transplantation. This journal restricts itself to articles on cell-mediated immunity and the mechanisms of graft rejection

Journal of the Reticulo-Endothelial Society. Articles covered are in general immunology and macrophage function

Transplantation Proceedings (*see* page 285)

Cellular Immunology. Papers in this journal are restricted to cell-mediated immunology

Infection and Immunity. Contributions largely on responses to microorganisms

European Journal of Immunology. This journal has a very attractive lay-out and attracts mostly studies of antibody formation

Tissue Antigens. A specialist journal serving tissue-typing and tumour antigen interests

Clinical Allergy. This journal is devoted to laboratory studies of human hypersensitivity

Journal of Immunological Methods. Started in 1972, the papers are devoted to immunological techniques

Medical Microbiology and Immunology. This German journal has contributors largely from Europe

Mouse News Letter. (formerly *Mouse News*). An informal collection of articles on new mouse strains, mutants and husbandry. Supplements are issued which describe inbred strains of mice

Immunological Communications. Started in 1972, this journal takes a wide range of immunological papers

IRCS Medical Science: Immunology and Allergy (IRCS)

Acta Pathologica et Microbiologica Scandinavica: Section C: Immunology

Clinical Immunology and Immunopathology

Cancer Immunology and Immunotherapy. A journal with emphasis on immunological manipulation of cancer

Molecular Immunology

Scandinavian Journal of Immunology

In the mid-1970s there was a remarkable production of new immunological journals, whose interest and specialist readership are hinted at in the titles.

Clinical Immunology Newsletter
Developmental and Comparative Immunology
Human Immunology
Immunobiology
Immunogenetics
Immunological Diseases

Immunology and Allergy Practice
Immunology of Reproduction
Immunopathology
International Journal of Immunopharmacology
Journal of Clinical Laboratory Immunology
Journal of Immunogenetics
Journal of Immunopharmacology
Journal of Neuroimmunology
Journal of Reproductive Immunology

Lastly, the informal *Immunology Today* monthly journal has reviews, book notices and letters.

The reader is well served by many excellent serial and other publications:

Advances in Immunology (Academic Press). Each volume contains a number of important reviews and a cumulative index

British Medical Bulletin. Occasional issues are devoted to immunological topics, e.g. *Immunological Tolerance* in 1976

Clinical Immunobiology. A series of invited review articles on human immunology and transplantation edited by F. H. Bach and R. A. Wood (4 vols, Academic Press, 1972–1980)

Clinical Immunology Reviews. vol 1, 1981 (Dekker)

Current Topics in Immunology (Arnold) is an important and continuing series of which sixteen titles have already appeared. The emphasis is clinical but many research workers also find these books of interest

Clinical Immunology Update: Reviews for Physicians is a new series of which the first volume, edited by E. C. Franklin (Churchill Livingstone, 1981), has recently appeared

Clinics in Immunology and Allergy. vol 1, 1981 (London, Saunders)

Comprehensive Immunology (Plenum) is an important series which commenced in 1977. Edited by R. A. Good and S. B. Day, several volumes on a variety of topics with various editors have so far appeared, the most recent being *Comprehensive Immunology: Vol 6. Cellular, Molecular, and Clinical Aspects of Allergic Diseases* edited by S. Gupta and R. A. Good (1979)

Contemporary Topics in Immunobiology (Plenum)

Contemporary Topics in Molecular Immunology (Plenum)

CRC Critical Reviews in Immunology (1981)

Current Perspectives in Allergy, subtitled *Contemporary Issues in Clinical Immunology and Allergy*, is a new Churchill Livingstone series of which vol 1, edited by E. J. Goetz and A. B. Kay, appeared in 1982

Current Topics in Microbiology and Immunology (Springer). Space is equally divided between classic microbiology, virology and experimental immunology

Monographs in Allergy (Karger). Each volume is devoted to a single topic

Progress in Allergy (Karger). Each of the volumes has a number of substantial review articles

Recent Advances in Clinical Immunology edited by R. A. Thompson, vol 1 (1977), vol 2 (1980) (Churchill Livingstone, irregular)

Research Monographs in Immunology is an irregular series published by Elsevier of which two titles have appeared: *Delayed Hypersensitivity* by J. L. Turk (3rd edn, 1980) and *Mitogenic Lymphocyte Transformation. A General Model for the Control of Mammalian Cell Proliferation* by D. A. Hume and M. J. Weidemann (1981)

The Antigens, a review of its subject, is edited by M. Sela (vols 1–5, 1973–1979; vol 6 in press, Academic Press)
Transplantation Reviews (Williams and Wilkins, Baltimore) Single topic volumes have been issued since 1969 and important volumes were vol 26 *(Suppressor T Cells),* vol 27 *(Antibody Suppression of Gene Products)* and vol 32 *(Complement).* The journal is now called *Immunology Reviews*

One rather distinctive feature of the immunological literature is the important role played by the published proceedings of international congresses, which may be devoted to single or multiple immunological topics. On single topics, some important volumes on antibody formation were published in the series *Advances in Experimental Medicine and Biology* (Plenum)

Other important series include the *Proceedings of the Leucocyte Culture Conferences,* the latest being the twelfth on *Cell Biology and Immunology of the Leukocyte Function* edited by M. R. Quastel (Academic Press, 1979), and the *Proceedings of the International Congresses of Immunology,* the most recent being entitled *Bacterial Endotoxins and Host Response: Proceedings of the 4th International Congress* edited by M. K. Agarwal (Elsevier – North Holland, 1980).

Many other conferences are published and details may be traced under title keywords in *Index of Conference Proceedings Received* published by BL, which appears monthly and cumulates annually. It is also available online from BLAISE.

The *Ciba Foundation Symposia (New Series),* published from 1972 to 1980 by Excerpta Medica and since 1981 by Pitman, contain invited authoritative contributions from established workers on a variety of subjects and include selected immunological topics, e.g. *Immunopotentiation* (1973), *Immunology of the Gut* (1977), *Microenvironments in Haemopoietic and Lymphoid Differentiation* (1981) and *Receptors, Antibodies and Human Disease* (1982).

The proceedings of the Brook Lodge meetings, where a small number of experts are brought together for discussion, have produced some volumes of interest to immunologists, which may be traced through the NLM *Current Catalog* under that heading.

Since these conferences tend to be highly selective of topics and speakers, the proceedings reflect well the growth points of immunology. Published proceedings give the reader a broad picture of the work going on throughout the world, and since there has been a recent tendency to print the delivered papers in an abbreviated form (perhaps only two pages in length), readers can find their way quickly through the whole proceedings. The most important works in this type of literature are the biannual meetings of what is now the Transplantation Society. These are published as special issues of *Transplanation Proceedings*. The first meeting was published as a book, *Advances in Transplantation* edited by J. Dausset (Munksgaard Copenhagen, 1967). Anyone interested in the historical development of current ideas in tissue transplantation and the many blind alleys explored will find endless interest in the earlier international congresses, which were all published as separate issues of the *Annals of the New York Academy of Sciences*. The last volume in this series (the Seventh International Transplantation Conference) was published in 1966, and earlier volumes appeared every two years previously. *Transplantation Proceedings* also undertakes to publish a number of volumes each year recording the proceedings of symposia and meetings devoted to transplantation. A similarly useful series of volumes containing the annual proceedings of the European Transplantation and Dialysis Association (ETDA) from 1964, was published by the Excerpta Medica Foundation and gives papers largely on clinical transplantation, renal dialysis and the equipment used for dialysis. Since 1973, they have been published as *Dialysis Transplantation and Nephrology* (Pitman Medical).

The Transactions of the corresponding American Society for Artificial Internal Organs (ASAIO) are also available.

Tumour immunology

Experimental laboratory studies on tumour immunology are to be found in many of the above-mentioned non-specialist journals. *Immunology* has a section in each issue for this topic, and the following specialist cancer journals may contain papers on immunology and, in particular, human immunology: *Journal of the National Cancer Institute, International Journal of Cancer, Cancer,* and *Cancer Research.*

Human transplantation

As mentioned above, *Transplantation* carries a number of human transplantation studies but the rest are to be found in general journals such as the *British Medical Journal, The Lancet, New England Journal of Medicine,* and also in the surgical journals – *Surgery, Gynecology and Obstetrics, Surgery, Annals of Surgery* and *Journal of Surgical Research.*

Brief communications

Short summaries of important work to be described in detail later appear regularly in *Nature* and *Transplantation*. *The Lancet* (which still holds the record for speed of publication) often publishes important clinical or basic immunological papers in its 'Preliminary Communication' or 'Hypothesis' sections, as does the rapid publication journal *Immunology Letters*.

Abstracting journals and indexes

Immunology is now well served for collections of current titles and abstracts. The most up to date is *Current Titles in Immunology, Transplantation and Allergy* (Pergamon), which runs only a month or so behind the original publication. *Excerpta Medica* has a section on *Immunology, Serology and Transplantation*. A new abstracting journal appeared in 1976 – *Immunology Abstracts* (Information Retrieval Ltd). The University of Sheffield Biomedical Information Service produces a regular list of *Titles in Renal Transplantation and Dialysis*. Abstracting is also given in the Immunology section of *Biological Abstracts* and the computerized multiple indexing system aids a search of the literature. Another set of immunological abstracts are given in the Immunology and Experimental Pathology section of *International Abstracts of Biological Sciences* (Pergamon).

As for clinical transplantation, the relevant papers are scattered thinly through a host of surgical journals, and the monthly *Surgery, Gynecology and Obstetrics* (the gynaecology and obstetrics papers were abandoned many years ago) provides a useful and well-written abstract section which includes a sub-section on transplantation. A useful abstracting service was formerly offered by *Transplantation* and covered broadly all articles relevant to transplantation, but this was discontinued in 1970.

As far as indexes go, the *Index Medicus* (described in Chapter 3) provides a comprehensive index to the immunological literature both in the English language and foreign languages. Many scientists prefer to read through the weekly journal *Current Contents Life Sciences* (and its weekly subject index), which simply reproduces the title pages of the current issues of all important scientific journals.

A similar service is given by the International Cancer Research Data Bank of the US National Cancer Institute, who publish a regular series of abstracts entitled *Clinical Cancer Immunology and Immunotherapy*.

Monographs and dictionaries

The language of immunology is generally agreed to present a considerable barrier to the beginner's understanding of the subject. Multiple alternative terminologies exist (e.g. syngeneic graft, isogeneic graft, autograft, all referring to grafts between genetically identical individuals), but fortunately there are two dictionaries to help the reader: *A Dictionary of Immunology* by W. J. Herbert and P. C. Wilkinson (2nd edn, Blackwell Scientific, 1977), and *Glossary of Immunological Terms* by W. J. Halliday (Butterworths, 1971).

The market for basic texts on immunology is a very competitive one and rapid publication of a new edition is an important sign of success.

The texts available include:

Basic and Clinical Immunology edited by H. H. Fudenberg *et al.* (3rd edn, Oxford University Press, 1980)
The Immune System: a Course on the Molecular and Cellular Basis of Immunity edited by I. McConnell *et al.* (2nd edn, Blackwell Scientific, 1981)
Basic Immunology by W. M. G. Amos (Butterworths, 1981)
Textbook of Immunology by B. Benecerraf and E. R. Unanue (2nd edn, Williams and Wilkins, 1982)
Immunologic Fundamentals by N. J. Bigley (2nd edn, Year Book Medical Publishers, 1981)
Essential Immunology by I. M. Roitt (4th edn, Blackwell Scientific, 1980)
Immunology for Undergraduates by D. M. Weir (4th edn, Livingstone, 1977)
Immunology, Immunopathology and Immunity by S. Sell (3rd edn, Harper and Row, 1980)

The following are monographs on immunological methods, the contents of which are indicated by their titles:

Standardization in Immunofluorescence: a Symposium edited by E. J. Holborow (Blackwell Scientific, 1970)
Fluorescent Protein Tracing by R. C. Nairn (4th edn, Livingstone, 1976)
Practical Immunology by L. Hudson and F. C. Hay (2nd edn, Blackwell, 1980)

For general texts on immunological methods, consult:

Handbook of Experimental Immunology by D. M. Weir (3rd edn, 3 vols, Blackwell Scientific, 1978)
Methods in Immunology and Immunochemistry edited by C. A. Williams and M. W. Chase (5 vols, Academic Press, 1967–1976)
In Vitro Methods in Cell Mediated Immunity edited by B. R. Bloom and P. R. Glade (Academic Press, 1971)
Laboratory Diagnosis of Immunologic Disorders by G. N. Vyas, D. P. Stites and G. Brecher (Grune and Stratton, 1975)
Methods in Immunodiagnosis by N. R. Rose and P. E. Bigazzi (2nd edn, Wiley, 1981)
Manual of Clinical Immunology by N. R. Rose and H. Friedman (2nd edn, American Society of Microbiology, 1980)

The *Practical Methods in Clinical Immunology* (Churchill Livingstone) is a useful series with several new volumes in preparation. Recently published are *Immunological Investigation of Renal Disease* by A. R. McGiven (1980) and *Investigation of Phagocytes in Disease* by S. D. Douglas and P. G. Quie (1981).

The following important monographs on immunology are available:

Clinical Aspects of Immunology edited by P. J. Lachman and D. K. Peters (4th edn, 2 vols, Blackwell Scientific, 1982). The emphasis of this book is on serology and antibody-mediated disease, rather than cell-mediated immunology

Immunology in Clinical Medicine by J. L. Turk (3rd edn, Heinemann, 1978). This slim book includes aspects of cell-mediated immunity

Immunological Diseases edited by Max Samter (3rd edn, 2 vols, Little, Brown, 1978). These two substantial volumes cover all aspects of immunology, including tumour immunology

Autoimmunity and Disease edited by L. I. Glynn and E. J. Holborow (2nd edn, Blackwell Scientific, 1973)

Cancer and the Immune Response by G. A. Currie (2nd edn, Arnold, 1980)

The Practice of Clinical Immunology by R. A. Thompson (2nd edn, Arnold, 1978)

T and B Lymphocytes: Origins, Properties and Roles in Immune Responses by M. F. Greaves, J. J. T. Owen and M. Raff (Excerpta Medica, 1973)

Clinical Immunology: A Clinician's Guide by A. Richter (2nd edn, Williams and Wilkins, 1982) is up to date and well organized, and there is also *Clinical Immunology in Medical Practice* edited by A. Basten (Blackwell, 1982)

Medical Immunology edited by W. J. Irvine (Teviot Scientific Publications, 1979)

The Mode of Action of Immuno-suppressive Agents by J. F. Bach (Excerpta Medica, 1975)

Immunologic Aspects of Anesthetic and Surgical Practice edited by A. Mathiev and B. D. Kahan (Grune and Stratton, 1975)

Viral Immunology and Immunopathology edited by A. L. Notkins (Academic Press, 1975)

Cancer and Transplantation edited by G. P. Murphy (Grune and Stratton, 1975)

Corynebacterium Parvum edited by B. Halpern (Plenum, 1975)

Immunology of the Gastro-intestinal Tract edited by P. Asquith (Churchill Livingstone, 1979)

Diagnosis and Treatment of Immunodeficiency Diseases by G. L. Asherson and A. D. B. Webster (Blackwell, 1980)

Obstetric and Perinatal Immunology by M. N. Cauchi (Arnold, 1981)

Immunology and Skin Diseases by R. H. Cormane and S. S. Asghar (Arnold, 1981)

The Interferon System by W. E. Stewart (2nd edn, Blackwell, 1981)

Lastly, useful texts on clinical transplantation are available:

Sociology and Legal Aspects of Transplantation (British Transplantation Society: *British Medical Journal* **1**, 251–255, 1975)

The Human Body and the Law by D. W. Meyers (Edinburgh University Press, 1970, Chapter 5).

Living and Dying: Adaptation to Haemodialysis by N. B. Levy (Thomas, Springfield, 1974)

The Courage to Fail: A Social View of Organ Transplants and Dialysis by R. C. Fox and J. P. Swazey (University of Chicago Press, 1974)

Immunology for Surgeons edited by J. E. Castro (MTP, 1976)

Clinical Transplantation edited by P. J. Morris (Churchill Livingstone, 1982)
Monoclonal Antibodies in Clinical Medicine by A. McMichael and J. Fabre (Academic Press, 1982)

History of immunology and transplantation

The history of immunology is now attracting attention and important reviews are given by B. H. Waksman in *J. Immunol.*, **107,** 617, 1971; J. Dausset in *Immunogenetics*, **10,** 1, 1980; W. F. Goebel in *Persp. Biol. Med.*, **18,** 419, 1975; and W. L. Ford in *Blood, Pure and Eloquent* edited by M. M. Wintrobe (McGraw-Hill, 1980).

For a review and bibliography of the history of clinical transplantation *see* D. N. H. Hamilton in *Clinical Transplantation* edited by P. J. Morris, (Churchill Livingstone, 1981, Chapter 1).

14

Clinical medicine

E. M. Read*; revised by
D. W. C. Stewart

A generation ago there appeared to be a clearly definable literature of clinical medicine which could be identified and described. There is, today, no frontier. Medicine, as an applied subject, is dependent on many disciplines and draws on the literature, not only of the biological and medical sciences such as biochemistry, genetics, immunology and immunochemistry, but also of the physical sciences and of the applied technologies.

The very great progress, in recent years, in the medical sciences and the advances of technology have profoundly affected medical practice and, because control of infections has made more apparent the importance of metabolic and genetic factors in disease, clinicians have been brought closer to their scientific colleagues, often as members of a research team, and make their own contribution in observation and description or (especially in such fields as endocrinology and immunology) as the investigators themselves. As a result, the literatures interlock and biochemical or experimental studies may be reported in clinical journals and case reports found in journals of clinical science. Similarly, within clinical medicine itself, specialties which are discussed separately herein are, in reality, interdependent. This chapter, therefore, does not stand alone but relies on most of the rest of the book to support it, and selection within it is, at times, arbitrary and must be taken as a pointer rather than as a comprehensive guide.

* Formerly Librarian, Royal Postgraduate Medical School, London

Periodicals

The intercommunication between the disciplines makes it difficult to discuss a periodical literature as extensive as that of medicine. An overview of it and of its subject distribution may be acquired from the *List of Journals Indexed in Index Medicus,* which is published annually in the January issue of the *Index Medicus* and is also issued in extended form as a separate publication with subject and geographical arrangement.

Among clinical research journals most are orientated to a specialty, but, in addition to the specialty journals, there is a group of general journals which cover the whole of internal medicine. Among the most important are *Acta Medica Scandinavica, American Journal of Medicine, Annals of Internal Medicine, Medicine, Archives of Internal Medicine* and *Quarterly Journal of Medicine.*

Of equal importance are the great English-language medical weeklies, *British Medical Journal, Journal of the American Medical Association, The Lancet* and *New England Journal of Medicine,* and the many comparable national journals of Europe and elsewhere, such as *Deutsche Medizinische Wochenschrift, Wiener Medizinische Wochenschrift, Medical Journal of Australia, Canadian Medical Association Journal* and *South African Medical Journal.* These are, to an extent, professional newspapers and have a wide currency. They publish papers, but also refresher-type material and professional news. Lastly, there is a small and decreasing group of hospital journals which, although publishing work which originates only from their own or an affiliated institution, have an international standing, such as *Journal of the Mount Sinai Hospital* and *Mayo Clinic Proceedings. Johns Hopkins Medical Journal* ceased publication in 1982 after many years and it is not likely that this type of publication can long survive in the present climate of publishing.

Between them these types of journal account for a very great portion of all that is important that is published outside the specialty journals. Most of them also publish case reports, for the case report holds a special place in medical reporting and is recognized as making an important contribution to medical progress, in that the careful description of a disease pattern is the first step towards its understanding.

However the periodical literature, along with much of the rest of clinical publication, has a markedly two-tiered structure which reflects a dual function. A majority of workers in medicine are practitioners and not researchers. They are interested in the utilization of existing knowledge and in the practical application of advances, not in the advancement itself. They need rapid access to information in order to keep themselves up to date and abreast of current practice. The literature reporting original work is, therefore supported by a substructure of secondary publications which digests and disseminates, often with remarkable speed. There is a range of periodicals devoted entirely to this form of publication and, beyond them, reviews, seminars, clinics and symposia. To some extent the professional weeklies have a foot in both camps. There are many state-of-the-art journals often directed to particular professional groups – for instance, *The Practitioner* and *Update* for the general practitioner, and *British Journal of Hospital Medicine* and *Hospital Update* for the hospital doctor. *Medicine International* is a journal which started life as a part work whose issues were intended to build up into a multi-volume handbook, and it is still published with each issue covering a specific topic. Special editions are published for Australia, the Middle East and other places containing items of more local interest. Some of these journals are distributed free to selected groups of medical practitioners, but all are available on subscription to those who wish to have them.

There is a multiplicity of news-sheets and reporting services (often from drug houses), drug house journals (some of which publish reviews of good quality), and industry-supported alerting and abstracting services.

Indexing and abstracting services

The general indexing and abstracting services are dealt with fully in Chapter 3. Most of them are relevant to clinical medicine, but the two which are most important in current clinical situations are *Index Medicus* and *Excerpta Medica*.

Index Medicus provides good coverage for the clinician and is, almost invariably, the first tool of resort. Its separate listing of review articles (*Bibliography of Medical Reviews*) can offer a quick way in to the literature and appears as part of each monthly issue. The accompanying thesaurus, *Medical Subject Headings (MeSH)* is a relatively easy key to the headings used, though care must be exercised in its use in some areas, especially in the difficult one of eponyms, and it can be advisable to use a dictionary of eponyms to define search terms before using the *Index Medicus*. *Index Medicus* covers some 2700 journal titles worldwide, but there is a bias towards American material and it is a little weak in coverage of journals on health services and related topics. There is also an

Abridged Index Medicus which covers 118 titles more closely related to clinical practice. Both versions index only and do not include abstracts.

Excerpta Medica both indexes and provides an English-language abstract of papers covered. Few libraries are able to stock the complete service, but because it is published in about 50 sub-sections, any one of which may be purchased separately, it is very useful in hospitals or institutes with particular areas of interest. Specific sections are mentioned later in this chapter and elsewhere in the book.

Most of the indexing and abstracting services are available as computer-based online systems and these are also discussed elswhere in the book.

Current awareness

No comprehensive, general alerting service is possible over so wide a field. *Current Contents, Clinical Practice (CCCP)* and *Current Contents, Life Sciences (CCLS)* offer partial and overlapping coverage. *CCCP* lists the contents of some 700 clinical journals while *CCLS* covers some of them, but includes, in addition, experimental, medical science and laboratory medicine material which the clinical researcher also needs. Now that the traditional line between clinician and medical scientist has gone, increasing value is placed on the many special lists and bibliographies devoted to specific subject fields. The University of Sheffield Biomedical Information Service is a good example of the type of publication which is produced to meet specific needs. Its range of current awareness bulletins covers some 121 topics and is based both on the scanning of the primary literature and on secondary sources.

A selective service designed with the practitioner in mind rather than the researcher is provided by the series *Current Medical Literature* published by CML Ltd and the Royal Society of Medicine. Each journal issue lists by title of relevant papers, in some cases providing an abstract or an evaluative editorial note which can sometimes be critical of the paper reviewed. Subjects represented by journals in the series are Cardiovascular Medicine, Gastroenterology, Rheumatology and Dermatology.

Another service designed to help the specialist is the *Core Journals in . . .* series published by Excerpta Medica. Subjects covered are *Cardiology* (11) 1980–, *Clinical Endocrinology* (12) 1982–, *Clinical Pharmacology* (10) 1983–, *Gastroenterology* (12) 1980–,

Clinical Neurology (10) 1978–, *Obstetrics/Gynecology* (14) 1977–, *Ophthalmology* (10) 1978– and *Pediatrics* (14) 1977–. Figures in brackets indicate the number of specialist journals covered. Each monthly issue contains a 'coreview' column – relevant abstracts from six of the foremost general medical journals (*British Medical Journal, The Lancet* (UK), *New England Journal of Medicine, Journal of the American Medical Association* (US), *Deutsche Medizinische Wochenschrift* (Germany), *Nouvelle Presse Médicale* (France)) followed by abstracts of all articles in the leading journals in the appropriate specialty.

Reviews

Reviews are always valuable in a rapidly developing subject and are especially so in an applied subject such as clinical medicine, which not only takes account of its own advances, but is also affected by advances throughout the basic sciences. The term review here covers a wide range of publications, reflecting once again the differing needs of researcher and practitioner. It embraces the full, scholarly review of the literature of a specific topic, the survey of recent progress, and the subject digest by an authoritative writer for the practising clinician.

Most of the regular review series are specialty-based. They may often be recognized by their distinctive titles, which contain such words as *Advances in. . ., Recent Progress in. . ., Seminars in. . ., Clinics in. . ., Topics in. . . or Modern Problems in. . .* Outside these review serials there are, of course, many individual reviews published in other journals or as special supplements which may be traced (as, indeed, may they all) by means of the *Bibliography of Medical Reviews*, a by-product of *Index Medicus*. They form a valuable starting point, especially if the topic is too narrow to be helped much from textbook or monograph sources.

General review serials are *Advances in Internal Medicine* and *Annual Review of Medicine*. Both of these assume a considerable subject knowledge and are reviews for the specialist. The company Annual Reviews Inc. publishes a number of uniform review volumes in various specialties, all of which are of high quality and reasonable price. Regular overviews of the year's work are the *Year Book* series, published by Year Book Medical Publishers. There are over 20 titles, including *Year Book of Medicine* and *Year Book of Family Medicine*, and they are arranged by topics and reproduce, in the form of abstracts with editorial comment, the significant periodical publications of the year. As each divides its subject into a number of broad chapters, they offer a quick way in to the recent literature of a subject (*see* page 72).

Progress in Clinical Medicine edited by A. Horler and J. B. Foster (7th edn, Churchill Livingstone, 1978) is published every six years or so and reviews current developments for the general physician. A similar review is *Recent Advances in Medicine – 18* edited by A. M. Dawson, (Churchill Livingstone, 1981). In addition to medicine the *Recent Advances* series covers some 37 other more specialized topics, including *Recent Advances in Community Medicine* edited by A. Smith (No 2, 1982).

Related to orthodox reviews are symposia, which are produced in ever greater numbers and form a very mixed group of publications of variable quality. Many are published in answer to the need to provide the physician with up-to-date, high-quality information in an easily assimilable form. In this category are the volumes in the *Clinics* series published by Saunders, each issue of which is a separate symposium. They are similar in style and intent to *Medical Clinics of North America* from the same publisher, which was one of the prototypes for this kind of journal. Quality is uniformly good as is physical presentation. *British Medical Bulletin* (published for the British Council by Churchill Livingstone, four issues a year) produces high-quality overviews of important topics of current interest. Recent issues, for example, have been on *Alcohol and Disease* and *Regulatory Peptides of Gut and Brain*. The publications described above are generally not true symposia in the sense that they are not the result of a meeting of the contributors, but that in no sense diminishes their value as publications.

The proceedings of actual meetings and symposia come in many forms and are not always easy to trace and identify. The annual *Advanced Medicine* symposia published by Pitman are the proceedings of meetings held at the Royal College of Physicians and are published in a straightforward way. Some of the volumes in Excerpta Medica's *International Congress Series* can also be of importance to clinicians. Other conferences may be published as parts of issues of journals, as supplements, as series, or as one-off publications. The *Index to Conference Proceedings received by the British Library Lending Division* is a keyword index to proceedings held in that Library either as single volumes or as parts of journals. It covers all subject fields, but with emphasis on the sciences and applied sciences, and is published in serial form monthly with periodic cumulations now available on microfiche. It is, however, not an index to individual papers within a symposium but to the symposium as a whole. Individual papers are indexed in *Index Medicus* if the symposium has published in a journal covered by the *Index*. For several years up to 1980 the *Index Medicus* also indexed each month a number of one-off conference and symposia volumes. A comprehensive index of conference proceedings is the Institute for Scientific Information's *Index to Scientific and Technical Proceedings,* which covers over 3000 proceedings from books and journals as well as the contents of selected books other than conference proceedings. All items are indexed at chapter level and the file is also available online. *World Meetings: Medicine* is primarily a list of forthcoming meetings, but it also lists, when known, where the proceedings or the programme will be published and can thus provide pre-publication information.

General reference works

For reference works dealing with data books, nomenclature, synonyms, eponyms, and classic descriptions, *see* Chapter 4.

General textbooks and monographs

With new knowledge being applied and new techniques employed so fast that for something to be in print it must almost be out of date, multi-volume treatises belong to the basic sciences rather than to clinical medicine. Large, general systems of medicine have given place to the one-volume reference text though in some case the work may be available in a choice of a one- or two-volume format, making it perhaps a better buy for the bookshelf of a group practice. There are three of equal standing: *Cecil's Textbook of Medicine* edited by J. B. Wyngaarden and L. H. Smith (15th edn, Saunders, 1982), the *Oxford Textbook of Medicine* edited by D. J. Weatherall (2 vols, Oxford University Press, 1982) and *Harrison's Principles of Internal Medicine* edited by R. G. Petersdorf *et al.* (10th edn, McGraw-Hill, 1983). The *Harrison* textbook is being supported by a series of *Update* volumes, the third of which was published in 1982.

Diagnosis and methods

Physical examination is the first step towards clinical care. *Differential Diagnosis: the Interpretation of Clinical Evidence* by A. M. Harvey and J. Bordley (3rd edn, Saunders 1979), is a clear exposition with illustrative cases and tables of the process involved in the interpretation of symptoms. *Hutchison's Clinical Methods* by S.

Mason and M. Swash (17th edn, Baillière Tindall, 1980), provides details of many investigative procedures; and *Clinical Physiology* edited by E. J. M. Campbell, C. J. Dickinson and J. D. H. Slater (4th edn, Blackwell, 1975), gives a means of evaluating what is normal function. Good colour illustrations of many clinical conditions are assembled in the *Ciba Collection of Medical Illustrations* prepared by Frank. H. Netter (1954).

The assessment of treatment assumes a need to quantify: *Statistical Methods in Medical Research* by P. Armitage (2nd edn, Blackwell, 1982), is a thorough introduction to the needed expertise. *Medical Surveys and Clinical Trials* by L. J. Witts (2nd edn, Oxford University Press, 1964) remains a classic work which deals with the manner and method of acquiring clinical data; the 1964 edition has an excellent bibliography on observer variability.

Clinical skill

Clinical skill is dependent on a more than simple knowledge. Relevant here are *Clinical Judgement* by A. R. Feinstein (Williams and Wilkins, 1967), a personal and discursive exposition of the application of scientific principles to clinical activity; *Controversy in Internal Medicine* edited by F. J. Ingelfinger *et al.* (Saunders, I: 1966; II: 1974); and *Richard Asher Talking Sense. A Collection of Papers. . .* edited by Sir Francis Avery Jones (Pitman, 1972).

Metabolic and genetic disorders

Now that the major infectious diseases have been brought for the most part under control, the importance of metabolic and genetic factors in many disease situations has become clearer. Together with immunology, they are relevant to most of clinical medicine, and so the following are standard reference works for every clinician: *Metabolic Control and Disease* (formerly *Duncan's Diseases of Metabolism*) edited by P. K. Bondy (8th edn, 2 vols, Saunders, 1980); *The Metabolic Basis of Inherited Disease* by J. B. Stanbury *et al.* (5th edn, McGraw-Hill, 1982), which reviews 14 000 references; *Mendelian Inheritance in Man: Catalogs of Autosomal Dominant, Autosomal Recessive, and X-linked Phenotypes* by V. A. McKusick (5th edn, Johns Hopkins Press, 1978); and *Human Cytogenetics* by J. L. Hamerton (2 vols, Academic Press, 1971).

Specialties

Cardiology

Advances in techniques and in electrophysiological research, as well as in drug therapy, have been responsible for recent rapid progress in cardiology and for increased publication. There are three groups of journals which are, between them, the source of original work:

(1) The journals of general medicine.
(2) Those devoted to clinical cardiology – *American Heart Journal, American Journal of Cardiology, Angiology, Archives des Maladies du Coeur et des Vaissaux, Atherosclerosis, British Heart Journal, Cardiology, Circulation, Coeur et Médecine Interne, European Heart Journal, Current Concepts in Cardiology, Journal of Cardiovascular Medicine,* and *International Journal of Cardiology.*
(3) A group concerned with basic cardiovascular research – *Cardiovascular Research, Circulation Research, Journal of Cellular and Molecular Cardiology, Journal of Cerebral Blood Flow and Metabolism,* and *Microvascular Research.*

All the journals published by the American Heart Association are of high quality and all contain material of interest to the clinician.

There are a number of special literature sources. Abstracting journals are *Excerpta Medica Section 18: Cardiovascular Diseases and Cardiovascular Surgery* and *Section 6: Internal Medicine.* The year's work is reviewed by the *Year Book of Cardiology* and the *Year Book of Medicine* between them. A regular list of review articles, retrieved in co-operation with NLM from the *Bibliography of Medical Reviews,* appears among the back pages of *American Journal of Cardiology. Progress in Cardiovascular Diseases* provides bi-monthly topical reviews for the postgraduate. *Progress in Cardiology* edited by P. M. Yu and J. F. Goodwin (Lea and Febiger, 1972–) is an annual volume for the cardiologist and *Modern Concepts in Cardiovascular Disease,* a topic-a-month style leaflet or brief essay, assumes for the most part a similar specialist interest. Reviews of recent progress which are published every few years are *Recent Advances in Cardiology–8* edited by J. Hamer (Churchill Livingstone, 1981) and in the *Cardiology* volumes published in *Butterworths International Medical Reviews* series.

HISTORY

Multi-volume systems in clinical medicine are soon invalidated but, because of its full bibliographies and detailed descriptions, *Cardiology: an Encyclopedia of the Cardiovascular System* edited by A. Luisada (5 vols, McGraw-Hill, 1959–1961) is still an interesting source of background and historical information. Knowledge of the heart and circulation is rather recent in terms of medical history, but perhaps for that reason it is well documented and many landmarks in cardiology are available in reprint (e.g. Harvey, Withering, Starling). Two of the many books which summarize its progress and the people involved are *A History of the Heart and Circulation* by F. A. Willius and T. J. Dry (Saunders, 1948) and *Cardiac Classics* edited by F. A. Willius and T. E. Keys (Mosby, 1941), reprinted as *Classics of Cardiology* (Dover, 1961), which reproduces papers in English from Harvey to Herrick. Three classic reference works which have now attained an historical importance are *An Atlas of Acquired Diseases of the Heart and Great Vessels* by J. E. Edwards (3 vols, Saunders, 1961); Helen Taussig's *Congenital Malformations of the Heart* (2nd edn, 2 vols, Harvard University Press for Commonwealth Fund, 1960–1961), probably the most respected work in its field, and Maude Abbott's *Atlas of Congenital Cardiac Disease* (American Heart Association, 1936; reprinted 1954).

DATA AND NOMENCLATURE

As a source of basic physiological data, the FASEB biological handbook *Respiration and Circulation* (Bethesda, Maryland 1971) is valuable for the clinician as well as for the scientist. Each table and chart is supported by source references for the data quoted. There are data on the vascular system and blood distribution, and on the heart and pumping action. A guide to nomenclature is the New York Heart Association's *Diseases of the Heart and Great Vessels; Nomenclature and Criteria for Diagnosis* (7th edn, Little, Brown, 1973), which gives full definitions of terminology and frequently lists signs. An atlas of heart conditions is provided by vol 5 of the *Ciba Collection of Medical Illustrations* and by *A Colour Atlas of Cardiac Pathology* by G. Farrer-Browne (Wolfe Medical, 1977). *Scientific Foundations of Cardiology* edited by P. Sleight (Heinemann, 1982) provides a comprehensive overview of the scientific background to the diagnosis and management of heart disease and maintains the high standards of the earlier works on other topics in this series.

TEXTBOOKS

There are several excellent textbooks. Notable among them is *The Heart, Arteries and Veins* by J. W. Hurst *et al.* (5th edn, McGraw-

Hill, 1981), the earlier edition of which was supported by occasional update volumes on special topics to maintain currency. Others of importance are *Diseases of the Heart* by C. K. Friedberg (4th edn, Saunders, 1982), *Heart Disease* by E. Braunwald (Saunders, 1980), *Medical and Surgical Cardiology* by W. Cleland, J. Goodwin, L. McDonald and D. Ross (Blackwell, 1969), and *Heart Disease* by E. N. Silber and L. M. Katz (Macmillan, 1975). *Cardiac and Vascular Diseases* edited by H. L. Conn and O. Horwitz (Lea and Febiger, 1971), admirably synthesizes basic science and clinical information, and still part of the British scene is Paul Wood's near-classic *Diseases of the Heart and Circulation*. First published in 1931 and now revised and enlarged by his friends and colleagues (3rd edn, Eyre and Spottiswoode, 1968), it has lost its highly personal flavour but is still strong on symptoms and physical signs and has a synthesis of work on ischaemic heart disease. For the general physician *Clinical Heart Disease* by S. Oram (2nd edn, Heinemann, 1981), is a very practical book with a strong bedside bias. It is written in a clear, firm, sometimes dogmatic style, and each chapter has a select guide to further reading which often includes early classic work – for instance Sir Thomas Lewis's *Mechanism and Graphic Registration of the Heart Beat* (3rd edn, Shaw, 1925) and Mackenzie's *The Study of the Pulse* (Pentland, 1902). For heart disease in children there are *Heart Disease in Paediatrics* by S. C. Jordan and Olive Scott (2nd edn, Butterworths, 1981); *Heart Disease in Infancy* by J. H. Moller and W. A. Neal (Appleton-Century-Crofts, 1981); *Pediatric Cardiology* by A. S. Nadas and D. C. Fyler (3rd edn, Saunders, 1972) and the older, but still valuable, *Paediatric Cardiology* by H. Watson (Lloyd-Luke, 1968). A. E. Becker and R. H. Anderson's *Pathology of Congenital Heart Disease* (Butterworths, 1981) is a comprehensive work which complements the series *Paediatric Cardiology* also edited by Becker (vol 3, 1981). *Modern Management of Congestive Heart Failure* by J. Hamer (Lloyd-Luke, 1982) provides good treatment of its subject.

MONOGRAPHS IN SERIES

The American Heart Association publishes a series of monographs which include reviews, symposia and conference proceedings, and covers many special topics. They are mostly published as supplements to *Circulation* and *Circulation Research*. *Cardiovascular Clinics* edited by A. N. Brest (Davis, 1969–) is a further monograph series, but is concerned with current concepts in treatment and management, e.g. *Complex Methods in Electrocardiology* edited by C. Fisch (1974), *Cardiac Diagnosis and Treatment* edited by N. O. Fowler (1975) and *Pericardial Disease* by D. Spodick (1976).

SPECIAL AREAS

Many special areas have their own literature. For cardiovascular physiology *Cardiovascular Dynamics* by R. F. Rushmer (4th edn, Saunders, 1976) is valuable and may be supported, for more detailed information, by the *Handbook of the American Physiological Society,* now in the process of publishing its second edition.

There is much published on methods of diagnosis, investigation and measurement:

Angiography by H. L. Abrams (2nd edn, 2 vols, Churchill Livingstone, 1971)
An Atlas of Cardiology, Electrocardiograms and Chest X-rays by N. Conway (Wolfe Medical, 1977)
Echocardiography by H. Feigenbaum (3rd edn, Lea and Febiger, 1981)
Clinical Cardiac Radiology by K. Jefferson and S. Rees (2nd edn, Butterworths, 1980)
Two-Dimensional Echocardiography edited by J. A. Kisslo (Churchill Livingstone, 1980)
Auscultation of the Heart and Phonocardiography by A. Leatham (Williams and Wilkins, 1976)
Cardiac Catherization and Angiography by D. Verel and R. G. Grainger (3rd edn, Churchill Livingstone, 1978)
Non-invasive Cardiology edited by A. M. Weissler (Grune and Stratton, 1974)

For the sub-specialty of electrocardiography the principal journal, additional to the major cardiology journals, is *Journal of Electrocardiography.* A specialist review is *Advances in Electrocardiology* edited by R. C. Schlant and J. W. Hurst (Grune and Stratton, 1972). There are several good general introductions, among them *Principles of Clinical Electrocardiography* by M. J. Goldman (10th edn, Lange, 1979). The electrophysiological background can be provided by *Electrical Phenomena in the Heart* edited by W. C. DeMello (Academic Press, 1972) and by *The Conduction of the Cardiac Impulse* by P. F. Cranefield (Futura, 1975). For work on dysrhythmias *see Clinical Disorders of the Heart Beat* by S. Bellet (3rd edn, Lea and Febiger, 1971), *Disorders of Cardiac Rhythm* by L. Schamroth (2nd edn, Blackwell, 1980), *Extrasystoles and Allied Arrhythmias* by D. Scherff and A. Schott (2nd edn, Heinemann, 1973) and *Cardiac Arrhythmias: the Modern Electrophysiological Approach* by D. M. Krikler and J. F. Goodwin (Saunders, 1975). For work on conduction impulses there is *His Bundle Electrocardiography* by O. S. Narula (Davis, 1975).

Works for other special areas are *Intensive Coronary Care* edited by M. F. Oliver and D. G. Julian (WHO, Copenhagen, 1976), *The Myocardium: Failure and Infarction* by E. Braunwald

(Hospital Practice Publishing, 1974), *Peripheral Vascular Disease* edited by J. F. Fairbairn *et al;* (5th edn, Saunders, 1980), and *Venous Thrombosis and Pulmonary Embolism* by M. Hume and D. P. Sevitt (Oxford University Press, 1970).

For work on hypertension, Pickering's text, *High Blood Pressure* (2nd edn, Churchill, 1968), is now classic and has extensive bibliographies. Early literature is consolidated by *Bibliography of the World Literature on Blood Pressure, 1920–1950* edited by E. K. Koller and J. Katz (3 vols, Commonwealth, 1952) and current publication is indexed by the bi-monthly MEDLARS-based *Recurring Bibliography of Hypertension* from the American Heart Association.

Clinical haematology

Much of the publication on disorders of the blood is concerned with it as a laboratory subject, but the roles of clinician and laboratory worker are not always well defined and a considerable body of publication is of importance to them both.

The major journals for the clinician are *Blood, British Journal of Haematology* and *Scandinavian Journal of Haematology;* and the journals of internal medicine and of cancer.

For current awareness *Current Literature of Blood* is issued weekly from the Blood Information Service, Buffalo. Monthly abstracting services are *Excerpta Medica, Section 25: Hematology* and *Leukemia Abstracts* from the John Crerar Library in Chicago.

There are several review serials. Of interest to both the pathologist and the clinician are the quarterly *Seminars in Hematology,* the annual *Progress in Hematology* and *Recent Advances in Haematology-3* edited by A. V. Hoffbrand (Churchill Livingstone, 1982); *Topical Reviews in Haematology* edited by S. Roath (No 2, Wright, 1982) gives similar coverage. *Clinics in Haematology* is produced largely for the clinician.

Basic data on blood and its constituents, both normal and abnormal may be derived from:

The FASEB biological handbook: *Blood and other body fluids* (1961) *Sandoz Atlas of Haematology* (2nd edn, Sandoz Ltd, 1973)
Living Blood Cells and Their Ultrastructure by M. Bessis (Springer, 1973)
The Red Cell by J. W. Harris and R. W. Kellermeyer (revised edn, Harvard University Press for Commonwealth Fund, 1970)
Man's Haemoglobins by H. Lehmann and R. G. Huntsman (North Holland, 1974)

Comprehensive textbooks for the clinician are:

Postgraduate Haematology by A. V. Hoffbrand (2nd edn, Heinemann, 1981)
Blood and its Disorders, by R. M. Hardisty and D. J. Weatherall (2nd edn, Blackwell, 1982)

Clinical Hematology by M. M. Wintrobe *et al.* (8th edn, Lea and Febiger, 1981)
Hematology by W. J. Williams *et al.* (2nd edn, McGraw-Hill, 1977)

Books on special topics are:

Genetic Markers of Human Blood by E. R. Giblett (Blackwell, 1969)
Leukemia edited by F. Gunz and A. G. Baikie (3rd edn, Grune and Stratton, 1974)
The Megaloblastic Anaemias by L. Chanarin (2nd edn, Blackwell, 1979)
The Thalassaemia Syndromes by D. J. Weatherall and J. B. Clegg (3rd edn, Blackwell, 1981)
Drug-induced Blood Disorders by G. C. de Gruchy (Blackwell, 1975)
Human Blood Coagulation, Haemostasis and Thrombosis by R. Biggs (2nd edn, Blackwell, 1976)
Blood Transfusion in Clinical Medicine by P. L. Mollison (7th edn, Blackwell, 1982)
The Bleeding Disorders by G. I. C. Ingram (2nd edn, Blackwell, 1982)

Two useful histories of the subject are *Einführung in die Geschichte der Hämatologie* edited by K. G. von Boroviczeny (G. Thieme, 1974) and *Blood, Pure and Eloquent* a detailed account edited by M. M. Wintrobe (McGraw-Hill, 1980).

Respiratory disease

So many developments have occurred in respiratory medicine in recent years that it has changed its face completely. There has been a revolution in the treatment of tuberculosis and more has become known about viral infections and about bronchogenic cancer. The result has been a concentration of work on the understanding of respiratory physiology and the clinical significance of the facts of lung function. Journals have broadened their scope or changed their titles. The primary journals are *American Review of Respiratory Disease, British Journal of Diseases of the Chest, Chest, European Journal of Applied Physiology, Journal of Applied Physiology, Respiration, Scandinavian Journal of Respiratory Disease, Thorax, Tubercle,* along with such journals as *Clinical Allergy* and *Journal of Allergy and Clinical Immunology,* as well as the general journals. Work on respiratory viral infections is also included in the wide coverage of the *Journal of Infectious Diseases,* which publishes clinical as well as experimental material.

Current abstracting services are *Excerpta Medica, Section 15: Chest, Diseases, Thoracic Surgery and Tuberculosis* and *Section 6: Internal Medicine,* and (for cardiopulmonary disease) *18: Cardiovascular Diseases and Cardiovascular Surgery,* and also sections of the *Smoking and Health Bulletin.* For earlier literature *Chest Disease Index and Abstracts, including Tuberculosis 1946–45* (initially called *Tuberculosis Index*) had a wider periodicals coverage than *Index Medicus* and also included monographs and reports.

Reviews are to be found in such general review serials as *Advances in Internal Medicine* and *Year Book of Medicine,* and as supplements to the specialty journals; *BTTA Review* has been published as an irregular supplement to *Tubercle* and a new series has begun, *Recent Advances in Respiratory Medicine* (Churchill Livingstone, 1976–).

There are two fine textbooks which are current and comprehensive: *Respiratory Disease* by J. Crofton and A. Douglas (3rd edn, Blackwell, 1981) and *Textbook of Pulmonary Diseases* edited by G. L. Baum (2nd edn, Little, Brown, 1974). *Scientific Foundations of Respiratory Medicine* edited by J. G. Scadding and G. Cumming (Heinemann, 1981) presents the scientific background to clinical practice and discusses current hypotheses now being tested. It is rich in clinical and epidemiological data. *Thoracic Medicine* edited by P. Emerson (Butterworths, 1981) groups descriptions of disease by gross radiological features.

Respiratory Function in Disease by D. V. Bates, P. T. Macklem, and R. V. Christie (2nd edn, Saunders, 1971) considers function in disease states with discussion of clinical, pathological and radiological findings, and has about 4000 literature references. *Respiratory Physiology* by J. B. West (2nd edn, Blackwell, 1979), is a good beginner's introduction to the background physiology, and has suggestions for further reading. It may be supplemented by *Handbook of Physiology, Section 3: Respiration* by the American Physiological Society (Williams and Wilkins, 1964–1965), *Ventilation/Blood Flow and Gas Exchange* by J. B. West (3rd edn, Blackwell, 1971) and *The Respiratory Muscles* by E. J. M. Campbell et al. (2nd edn, Lloyd-Luke, 1970). *Respiratory Physiology* by N. B. Slomin (4th edn, Year Book Medical Publishers, 1981) complements these works.

Applied Respiratory Physiology by J. F. Nunn (2nd edn, Butterworths, 1977) is a work designed to bridge the gap between pure respiratory physiology and the treatment of patients. Basic data is found in the FASEB biological handbook *Circulation and Respiration* (1971). For lung function tests themselves, *The Lung: Clinical Physiology and Pulmonary Function Tests* by J. H. Comroe et al. (Year Book Medical Publishers, 1962), is a clinician's working text which provides detail of tests and discusses specific respiratory disabilities. *Lung Function: Assessment and Application in Medicine* by J. E. Cotes (4th edn, Blackwell, 1979) combines theoretical text with practical manual and evaluates function in health as well as disease.

X-ray findings play a significant part in diagnosis and all textbooks give them prominence, for example *A Colour Atlas of*

Respiratory Diseases by D. G. James and P. R. Studdy (Wolfe Medical, 1981). Good guide-books are *Portfolio of Chest Radiographs* and *Second Portfolio of Chest Radiographs* by B. T. Le-Roux and T. C. Dodds (Livingstone, 1964, 1968). These atlas volumes provide between them hundreds of X-ray photographs and overcome the main disadvantage of an atlas by giving clinical data with each picture. As a complement to them, *Chest Roentgenology* by B. Felson (Saunders, 1973) and *Principles of Chest X.-Ray Diagnosis* by G. Simon (4th edn, Butterworths, 1978) are good diagnostic texts.

Bronchoscopy is essential to the study of thoracic disease for it can provide information obtainable in no other way from the living patient. A well-illustrated guide to use is *Diagnostic Bronchoscopy* by P. Stradling (4th edn, Churchill Livingstone, 1981).

Occupational disease of the lung is a large and growing problem. The bibliographical sources for occupational health are treated in depth in Chapter 8. A well-referenced text for the physician is *Occupational Lung Disorders* by W. R. Parkes (2nd edn, Butterworths, 1982).

Paediatric aspects are well covered in *Pediatric Respiratory Disease* by J. Gerbeaux (2nd edn, Wiley, 1982) and in *Respiratory Illness in Children* by P. D. Phelan, L. I. Landau and A. Olinsky (2nd edn, Blackwell, 1982).

Work on respiratory failure is found in the literature of anaesthesia as well as of respiratory medicine. A practical manual on management, which also has a well-selected reference list to further reading, is *Respiratory Failure* by M. K. Sykes, M. W. McNicol and E. J. M. Campbell (2nd edn, Blackwell, 1976).

Infections are still responsible for much respiratory disease. Although tuberculosis no longer holds the stage as once it did, there is still a tuberculosis problem, especially in the developing countries, and the traditional picture still needs to be described. This is done well in about 100 pages in *Respiratory Diseases* by J. Crofton and A. Douglas (3rd edn, Blackwell, 1981). *Modern Drug Treatment in Tuberculosis* by J. D. Ross and N. W. Home (5th edn, Chest, Heart and Stroke Association, 1976) is a useful pamphlet.

A series of special issues of the *Bulletin of WHO* spread over the years 1959 to 1970 deal with special aspects; and there is still one international, English-language journal, *Tubercle*.

Gastroenterology

Gastroenterology has a very wide literature. It involves that of biochemistry, genetics and immunology, as well as of digestive disease and nutrition. The gastroenterologist is essentially a general physician and important work is to be found in the general journals, such as *British Medical Journal, The Lancet, American Journal of Medicine, New England Journal of Medicine,* and *Annals of Internal Medicine;* in the specialty journals, such as *American Journal of Digestive Diseases, American Journal of Gastroenterology, Digestion, Gastroenterology, Gut,* and *Scandinavian Journal of Gastroenterology;* in the journals of clinical nutrition, such as *American Journal of Clinical Nutrition* and *Journal of Human Nutrition;* in the basic nutrition journals, such as *British Journal of Nutrition* and *Journal of Nutrition;* and in journals of clinical immunology and biochemistry. Gastroenterology is a specialty which employs an increasing range of diagnostic and therapeutic techniques and much of importance is also published in such journals as *Journal of Clinical Investigation, Journal of Laboratory and Clinical Medicine* and *Laboratory Investigation.*

Review serials are, therefore, especially important. Annual volumes in general medicine series such as *Advances in Internal Medicine, Annual Review of Medicine* and *Year Book of Medicine* are relevant, as well as the occasional reviews: *Modern Trends in Gastroenterology* edited by A. E. Read (vol 5, Butterworths, 1975), *Progress in Gastroenterology* edited by G. B. J. Glass (Grune and Stratton, 1968, 1970), *Recent Advances in Gastroenterology – 4* by J. Badenoch and B. Brooke (Churchill Livingstone 1980) and *Topics in Gastroenterology No 9* edited by D. P. Jewell and E. Lee (Blackwell, 1981). A series of symposia is *Clinics in Gastroenterology* (Saunders, 1972–).

Journal literature is indexed by *Gastroenterology Abstracts and Citations,* a MEDLARS-based monthly, which lists approximately 1000 citations a month of which about one-third have accompanying abstracts, and by *Excerpta Medica, Section 48: Gastroenterology* and *Section 6: Internal Medicine.* Neighbouring overlapping fields are covered by *Nutrition Abstracts and Reviews* and the *Feeding and Weight Abstracts,* and by *Intestinal Absorption,* a monthly abstracting service from the University of Sheffield Biomedical Information Service.

The leading reference textbook is now *Gastrointestinal Disease, Pathophysiology – Diagnosis – Management* edited by M. H. Sleisenger and J. Fordtran (2nd edn, Saunders, 1978). It has the edge over the fuller *Gastroenterology* edited by H. L. Bockus (3rd edn, 4 vols, Saunders, 1974–1976). Good, shorter texts include *Gastroenterology* by I. A. D. Bouchier (3rd edn, Baillière Tindall, 1982) and H. J. Dworkin's *Gastroenterology* (Butterworths,

1982). Among the older books still of interest is a good, very personal text, *Clinical Gastroenterology* by H. M. Spiro (2nd edn, Macmillan, 1976) and, notable among the smaller introductions, are *Diseases of the Digestive System* by S. C. Truelove and P. C. Reynell (3rd edn, Blackwell, 1983) and *Clinical Gastroenterology* by F. A. Jones, P. Gummer and J. E. Lennard-Jones (2nd edn, Blackwell, 1968). A detailed colour atlas is provided in the *Ciba Collection of Medical Illustrations Vol 3: Digestive Systems* (3 parts, 1959–1962).

For normal function *Physiology of the Digestive Tract* by H. W. Davenport (5th edn, Year Book Medical Publishers, 1982) provides a straightforward background review; the *Handbook of Physiology, Section 6: The Alimentary Canal* of the American Physiological Society (5 vols, Williams and Wilkins, 1967–1968), together with *Intestinal Absorption in Man* by I. McColl and G. E. Sladen (Academic Press, 1975) give greater depth. Comprehensive coverage is provided by the two volumes of L. R. Johnson's *Physiology of the Gastrointestinal Tract* (Raven Press, 1981) while *Scientific Foundations of Gastroenterology* edited by W. Sircus and A. N. Smith (Heinemann, 1980) covers both normal and pathological conditions.

For diagnosis *Clinical Tests of Oesophageal Function* by R. Earlam (Crosby Lockwood Staples, 1976) and *Fibre-optic Endoscopy* by P. R. Salmon (Pitman, 1975) support *Techniques of Clinical Gastroenterology* by H. W. Boyce and E. D. Palmer (C. C. Thomas, 1975) and *Clinical Investigation of Gastrointestinal Function,* by M. Bateson and I. A. D. Bouchier (2nd edn, Blackwell, 1982).

Books on special topics are

Gastrointestinal Pathology by B. C. Morson and I. M. P. Dawson (2nd edn, Blackwell, 1979)
Paediatric Gastroenterology by C. M. Anderson and V. Burk (Blackwell, 1975)
The Neurology of Gastrointestinal Disease by C. A. Pallis and P. D. Lewis (Saunders, 1974)
Coeliac Disease edited by W. T. J. M. Hekkens and A. S. Pena (MTP, 1975)
Inflammatory Bowel Disease by J. B. Kirsner and R. G. Shorter (2nd edn, Lea and Febiger, 1980)
The Metabolic Basis of Inherited Disease by J. B. Stanbury, J. B. Wyngaarden and D. S. Fredrickson (5th edn, McGraw-Hill, 1982)
Human Nutrition and Dietetics by Sir Stanley Davidson *et al.* (7th edn, Churchill Livingstone, 1979).

J. H. Baron and F. G. Moody's *Foregut* (Butterworths, 1981) is the first of a planned series of special topic reviews in gastroenterology.

The standard works on the liver are Sheila Sherlock's *Disorders of the Liver and Biliary System* (6th edn, Blackwell, 1981) and

Diseases of the Liver by L. Schiff (5th edn, Harper and Row, 1982). A review of recent advances is provided every few years by *Progress in Liver Diseases No 7* edited by H. P. Popper and F. Shaffner (Grune and Stratton, 1982). *Atlas of Liver Pathology* by D. G. D. Wight (MTP, 1982) is a well-illustrated reference work as is *A Colour Atlas of Liver Disease* by Sheila Sherlock and J. A. Summerfield (Wolfe Medical, 1979).

Work on hepatitis commands attention and is fast-moving enough to have its own MEDLARS-based annual literature index, *Hepatitis Bibliography*.

Renal disease

That complicated structure, the kidney, has an involvement with most systems of the body, and papers tend to be dispersed throughout the literature of general medicine, laboratory medicine and immunology, as well as published in the specialty journals. The more important of these are *Clinical Nephrology, Kidney International, Nephron, Scandinavian Journal of Urology and Nephrology, Transactions: American Society for Artificial Internal Organs* and *Transplantation*.

There is one abstracting service specific to renal medicine which covers the whole field, *Excerpta Medica, Section 28: Urology and Nephrology*. There are several which are more limited. *Abstracts: Renal Insufficiency* is a quarterly from Extracorporeal Medical Specialities, which abstracts periodical literature and conference reports, and also summarizes meetings. Two of the series from the University of Sheffield Biomedical Information Project are relevant, *Renal Physiology* and *Renal Transplantation and Dialysis*. There is also a quarterly MEDLARS-based index, *Artificial Kidney Bibliography*.

Although there is no range of special review serials, it is a rapidly advancing subject and there is wide review coverage from the general and special journals, from the general review serials, from the symposia in series (such as *Medical Clinics of North America, British Medical Bulletin*) and from conference reports. An annual volume appears under the editorship of J. Hamburger, *Advances in Nephrology from the Necker Hospital (Paris)* (Year Book Medical Publishers, 1971–). What might yet be a British occasional series, *Recent Advances in Renal Disease* edited by N. F. Jones (Churchill Livingstone, 1975), has produced only one volume so far.

There are two comprehensive English-language textbooks: *Diseases of the Kidney* edited by M. B. Strauss and L. G. Welt (3rd edn, 2 vols, Little, Brown, 1979) and *Renal Disease* edited by Sir Douglas Black (4th edn, Blackwell, 1979). The loose-leaf *Nephrologie* by J. Hamburger *et al.* (2 vols, Editions Médicales Flammarion, 1966–) is updated every year, but appeared in a one-off English-language version as *Nephrology* (Wiley, 1979).

Standards for nomenclature and diagnostic criteria are now, for the first time, available in *A Handbook of Kidney Nomenclature and Nosology: Criteria for Diagnosis. . .* prepared by the International Committee for Nomenclature and Nosology of Renal Disease (Little, Brown, 1975). It marks a beginning for world-wide communication.

For atlases there are the *Ciba Collection of Medical Illustration, Vol. 6: Kidneys, Ureters and Urinary Bladder* prepared by F. H. Netter and *A Colour Atlas of Renal Diseases* by G. Williams (Wolfe Medical, 1973; 3rd impression 1979).

For work on physiology and fluid balance *Physiology of the Kidney and Body Fluids* by R. F. Pitts (3rd edn, Year Book Medical Publishers, 1974) is a good introduction, which may be supported by J. R. Robinson's *Fundamentals of Acid-Base Regulation* (5th edn, Blackwell, 1975) and *Clinical Disorders of Fluid and Electrolyte Metabolism* by M. H. Maxwell and C. Kleeman (3rd edn, McGraw-Hill, 1980). Wider coverage of both normal and pathological conditions is provided by *Scientific Foundations of Urology* edited by G. D. Chisholm (2nd edn, Heinemann, 1982).

Books on special topics are:

The Challenge of Urinary Tract Infections by A. W. Asscher (Grune and Stratton, 1980)
The Kidney by H. E. de Wardener (5th edn, Churchill Livingstone, in press)
Pathology of the Kidney by R. H. Heptinstall *et al* (3rd edn, 3 vols, Little, Brown, 1983)
Urinary Tract Infection: Symposium Proceedings edited by W. Brumfitt and A. W. Asscher (Oxford University Press, 1973)
The Renal Unit by A. J. Wing and M. Magowan (Macmillan, 2nd edn in preparation)

L. T. J. Murphy has written an excellent *History of Urology* (C. C. Thomas, 1971).

Endocrinology and metabolism

Clinical endocrinologists are themselves usually engaged in basic investigation, with endocrine disorders regarded as problems in pathologic physiology. There tends, therefore, to be no clear dividing line between the literature of basic and of clinical endocrinology, and several journals publish in both fields. Among basic sources are *Endocrinology, Journal of Endocrinology, Steroids,*

Annales d'Endocrinologie (Paris) and *Acta Endocrinologica;* and the review serials *Recent Progress in Hormone Research* and *Memoirs of the Society for Endocrinology*.

Work on the clinical aspects of endocrine disorders is found in *Calcified Tissue International, Clinical Endocrinology, Hormone Research, Journal of Clinical Endocrinology, Metabolism: Clinical and Experimental, Neuroendocrinology,* and *Diabetes,* but also throughout journals of general medicine, and, especially, in paediatric journals.

The volume of publication and the spread of the journals involved makes *Endocrinology Index* especially valuable. It is a MEDLARS-based monthly with 4000–5000 entries per issue arranged by subject and by author. It groups subject entries in broad categories, but excludes endocrine pancreas because this is itself the subject of a separate bibliography, *Diabetes Literature Index*. The annual collection of abstracts *Endocrine Society Programme of the . . . Annual Meeting* serves as an additional source, as does *Calcified Tissue Abstracts,* for work on bone metabolism.

In addition to the *Year Book of Endocrinology,* reviews may be found in *Advances in Internal Medicine* and *Advances in Metabolic Disorders. Clinics in Endocrinology* (Saunders, 1972–) produces symposia on current methods of management. Occasional reviews are *Recent Advances in Endocrinology and Metabolism – 2* edited by J. L. H. O'Riordan (Churchill Livingstone, 1982) and the new *Butterworths' International Medical Review* series, the first clinical endocrinology volume of which is *The Pituitary* edited by C. Beardwell and G. L. Robertson (Butterworths, 1981). This new series takes the place of the older *Modern Trends in Endocrinology, Vol 4,* edited by F. T. G. Prunty and H. Gardiner-Hill (Butterworths, 1972). *Clinical Endocrinology* edited by E. B. Astwood and C. E. Cassidy (Grune and Stratton; 1960; II, 1968), though somewhat old, still merits a place on the library shelves.

A one-volume, well-referenced clinical textbook which also gives fair coverage to general principles is *Textbook of Endocrinology* edited by R. H. Williams (6th edn, Saunders, 1981). *Fundamentals of Clinical Endocrinology* by R. Hall, G. A. Smart and M. Besser (3rd edn, Pitman Medical, 1980) is a useful introduction, good on thyroid, hormonal control of metabolism and diabetes. A more comprehensive work is *Endocrinology* edited by L. J. de Groot (3 vols, Grune and Stratton, 1979). A very valuable source is *Genetic Disorders of the Endocrine Glands* by D. L. Rimoin and R. N. Schimke (Kimpton, 1971). Combined aspects are covered by *Medical and Surgical Endocrinology* by D. A. D. Montgomery and R. B. Welbourne (Arnold, 1975).

Until recently the only history of endocrinology was the section in Sir Humphry Rolleston's *The Endocrine Organs in Health and Disease* (London, Oxford University Press, 1936), but the field is now extremely well served by V. C. Medvei's *History of Endocrinology* (MTP, 1982). It is arranged chronologically and ends with three chapters that discuss present trends and the outlook for the future, arranged by topics. These three chapters in themselves run to 150 pages and cite over 600 references to form a useful survey of current problems. The book is illustrated and also contains a section of biographies of endocrinologists.

As an atlas the *Ciba Collection of Medical Illustrations Vol. 4: Endocrine System and Selected Metabolic Diseases* prepared by F. H. Netter (1965) is still useful, but the clinical features of endocrine disorders are well illustrated in *A Colour Atlas of Endocrinology* by R. Hall, D. Evered and R. Greene (Wolfe Medical, 1979). The Wolfe series of colour atlases, which now covers most clinical fields, is generally to be recommended and the publishers are now producing more specialized atlases in the series, such as *A Colour Atlas of Thymus and Lymph Node Histopathology with Ultrastructure* by K. Henry and G. Farrer-Brown (Wolfe Medical, 1981). Here too, should be mentioned *Methods in Investigative and Diagnostic Endocrinology* edited by S. A. Berson and R. S. Yalow (3 vols, North Holland, 1972–1975).

Three works on metabolic disorders are indispensable to the endocrinologist: *Metabolic Control and Disease* edited by P. K. Bondy and L. E. Rosenberg (8th edn, Saunders, 1980), formerly *Duncan's Diseases of Metabolism, The Metabolic Basis of Inherited Disease* by J. B. Stanbury *et al.* (5th edn, McGraw-Hill, 1982), and *Clinical Disorders of Fluid and Electrolyte Metabolism* edited by M. H. Maxwell and C. R. Kleeman (3rd edn, McGraw-Hill, 1980).

Among monographs on disorders of specific systems are:

The Pituitary Gland by G. W. Harris and B. T. Donovan (3 vols, Butterworths, 1966)

The Hypothalamus and Pituitary in Health and Disease by W. C. Locke and A. V. Shally (C. C. Thomas, 1968)

The Thyroid: a Fundamental and Clinical Text by S. C. Werner and S. H. Ingbar (4th edn, Harper and Row, 1978)

The Thyroid and its Diseases by L. J. Groot and J. B. Stanbury (4th edn, Wiley, 1975)

Adrenal Steroids and Disease by C. L. Cope (2nd edn, Pitman, 1972), a comprehensive review with over 3000 references

The Adrenal Cortex edited by A. B. Eisenstein (Little, Brown, 1967)

Aldosterone and Aldosteronism by E. J. Ross (Lloyd-Luke, 1975)

Intersexuality edited by C. Overzier (Academic Press, 1963)

Hermaphroditism, Genital Anomalies and Related Endocrine Disorders by H. W.

Jones and W. W. Scott (2nd edn, Williams and Wilkins, 1971), which was written
  for physician and surgeon and succeeds H. H. Young's classic monograph *Genital
  Abnormalities, Hermaphroditism and Related Adrenal Diseases* (Williams and
  Wilkins, 1937)
Calcium Disorders by D. A. Heath (Butterworths, 1982)
Calcium Metabolism and the Bone by L. P. R. Fourman and P. Boyer (2nd edn,
  Blackwell, 1968)
Metabolic Bone and Stone Diseases by B. E. Nordin (Williams and Wilkins, 1973)

The complications of diabetes mellitus are so widespread that they
concern every physician no matter what his or her specialty. Now
that clinical management is so successful and diabetic pregnancies
are no longer a rarity, it is also a disease which is on the increase.
Although there are specialist journals – *Diabète et Metabolisme,
Diabetes, Diabetologia* – papers on all aspects of fundamental
research are widely scattered throughout the biochemistry and
endocrinology journals, and clinical papers are found throughout
the journals of general medicine and paediatrics. *Diabetes Care* is
a bi-monthly journal of the American Diabetes Association aimed
specifically at clinicians.

Index Medicus is the general means of approach, but a more
comprehensive coverage is obtained from *Diabetes Literature
Index* (1966–), especially where diabetes is present as a complicating factor and is not the principle topic of the paper. The listing is
based on MEDLARS and has an hierarchical, keyword and an
author index. It succeeds *Diabetes Related Literature Index*
(1960–1964), which was produced as a supplement to *Diabetes*. As
a current alerting service, abstracts (30–50) of papers in
non-diabetic journals are published in *Diabetes* each month.

Much of the recent literature has been in the form of conference
proceedings on research topics, but *Clinical Diabetes Mellitus*
edited by G. P. Kozak (Saunders, 1982) is a good, modern text
which may become standard. The long-standing reference work,
with an emphasis on treatment, is *Joslin's Diabetes Mellitus*, edited
by A. Marble *et al.* (11th edn, Lea and Febiger, 1971). Also of value
are *Diabetes and its Management* by W. G. Oakley, D. A. Pyke and
K. W. Taylor (3rd edn, Blackwell, 1978), *Clinical Diabetes Mellitus*
by J. M. Malins (Eyre and Spottiswoode, 1968) and *Complications
of Diabetes* by H. Keen and J. Jarrett (2nd edn, Arnold, 1982).

Clinical immunology

Immunology has implications for ever wider areas of medicine and
surgery. As both a laboratory and a clinical subject, it is dealt
with in depth in Chapter 13. Some general sources for the working
clinician are listed below.

JOURNALS

Clinical Allergy
Journal of Allergy and Clinical Immunology
Clinical and Experimental Immunology
Clinical Immunology and Immunopathology

REVIEWS

Current Topics in Immunology (Arnold) produces short reviews on topics of special interest to clinicians. Earlier volumes include:

The Practice of Clinical Immunology by R. A. Thompson (vol 1, 1974)
Cancer and the Immune Response by G. A. Currie (vol 2, 2nd edn, 1980)
Allergic Drug Reactions by H. E. Amos (vol 3, 1976)

and most recently published are:

Immunology and Skin Diseases by R. H. Cormane and S. S. Asghar (vol 15, 1981)
Obstetric and Perinatal Immunology by M. N. Cauchi (vol 16 1981)

BOOKS

Essential Immunology by I. M. Roitt (4th edn, Blackwell, 1980)
Clinical Aspects of Immunology by P. J. Lachmann and D. K. Peters, (2 vols, 4th edn, Blackwell, 1982)
Immunological Diseases edited by M. Samter (3rd edn, 2 vols, Little, Brown, 1978)
Autoimmunity and Disease edited by L. E. Glynn and E. J. Holborow (2nd edn, Blackwell, 1973)

Dermatology

The primary journals in dermatology are *Acta Dermato-Venereologica, Archives of Dermatology, British Journal of Dermatology, Journal of the American Academy of Dermatology, Clinical and Experimental Dermatology* and *Journal of Investigative Dermatology. Cutis* is a lesser, but useful, clinical journal. Since skin disorders are not infrequently a manifestation of systemic disease or connected with the immune response, work is also found in the general journals and the journals of immunology.

In spite of this scatter of publication, or perhaps because of it, the literature of dermatology is well organized. *Index of Dermatology* is a MEDLARS-based monthly which lists everything that has implications for dermatology, irrespective of its main emphasis. It is, thus, more comprehensive than the information printed under the skin headings in *Index Medicus*. A regular, monthly abstracting service is provided by *Excerpta Medica, Section 13: Dermatology and Venereology.*

Among reviews, *Year Book of Dermatology* not only highlights important work in the periodical literature, but also contains at the end of each section a list of recommended review articles. Other reviews are *Current Problems in Dermatology* (Basle), which publishes detailed and critical reviews by international authors at intervals of a little over a year; and *Progress in Diseases of the Skin vol 1* edited by R. Fleischmeier (Grune and Stratton, 1981) and *Recent Advances in Dermatology – 5* edited by A. Rook (Churchill Livingstone, 1980).

A comprehensive reference textbook which is also a guide to the literature, both periodical and monographic, is *Textbook of Dermatology* edited by A. Rook, D. S. Wilkinson and F. J. G. Ebling (3rd edn, 2 vols, Blackwell, 1979). It integrates for the physician the growing knowledge of biology of the skin and pathological processes with practical clinical considerations and descriptions. *Andrew's Diseases of the Skin* edited by A. N. Domonkos (7th edn, Saunders, 1982) is a clinically orientated working text designed for desk-top rather than library use with a very good coverage in its 1100 pages, though references are only given in a selective way. Another good, standard American textbook is *Dermatology in General Medicine* by T. B. Fitzpatrick (2nd edn, McGraw-Hill, 1979) augmented by update volumes.

A series of monographs, *Major Problems in Dermatology* (Saunders and Lloyd-Luke), provides for many special subjects, e.g. *Dermatitis Herpetiformis* by J. O'D Alexander (1975), *Microbiology of Human Skin* by W. C. Noble (2nd edn, 1981), *Urticaria* by R. P. Warin and R. H. Champion (1974), *Gonorrhoea* by R. S. Morton (1977), and *Vasculitis* by K. Wolff and R. K. Winkelmann (1980).

Other books on special topics are:

Neuro-Cutaneous Disease by J. A. Aita (C. C. Thomas, 1966)
Skin signs of systemic disease by I. M. Braverman (2nd edn, Saunders, 1981)
Clinical Tropical Dermatology by O. Canizares (Blackwell, 1975)
Contact Dermatitis by E. Cronin (Churchill Livingstone, 1981)
Lupus Erythematosus by E. L. Dubois (2nd edn, University of Southern California Press, 1974)
Medical Mycology by C. W. Emmons *et al.* (3rd edn, Lea and Febiger, 1977)
Histopathology of the Skin by W. F. Lever (5th edn, Pitman, 1975)
Dermatological Photobiology by I. A. Magnus (Blackwell, 1976)
The Nails in Disease by P. D. Samman (3rd edn, Heinemann, 1978)

For older literature, *Handbuch der Haut- und Geschlechtskrankheiten* edited by J. Jadassohn (23 vols, Springer, 1927–1934: Erganzungswerk, 1959–), is a very detailed source. Some classic descriptions have been grouped into an anthology of selected and translated excerpts, with critical notes, as *Classics in Clinical Dermatology, with Biographical Sketches* by W. B. Shelley and J. T. Crissey (C. C. Thomas, 1953) and there is an earlier *History of*

Dermatology by W. A. Pusey (C. C. Thomas, 1933; reprinted, 1976).

Illustration is important in dermatology. A short, but definitive, work is *Dermatology: an Illustrated Guide* by L. Fry (2nd edn, Update, 1978). An extensive and very beautiful atlas is *Atlas de Dermatologie* by P. Graciansky and S. Boulle (10 vols, Maloine, 1952–1968); later adapted by M. B. Sulzberger into an American edition (4 vols, Year Book Medical Publishers, 1955–1960). In the Wolfe colour atlas series is *A Colour Atlas of Dermatology* by G. M. Levene and C. D. Calnan (1974). Without colour, but with discussion and literature reviews, is *Consultations in Dermatology I* and *II* with Walter B. Shelley (Saunders, 1973–1974).

The practice of dermatology rests on knowledge of the biology of normal skin. Useful series are *Advances in Biology of the Skin,* a series of monographs edited by W. Montagna (Pergamon) and *The Physiology and Pathophysiology of the Skin* edited by A. Jarrett (6 vols, Academic Press, 1973–1980).

Rheumatology

Rheumatology is very much an interdisciplinary subject and uses the literature of general medicine, immunology and orthopaedics besides its own specialty journals, *Annals of the Rheumatic Diseases, Arthritis and Rheumatism, Journal of Rheumatology (Toronto), Revue du Rhumatisme et des Maladies Ostéo-Articulaires* and *Scandinavian Journal of Rheumatology.*

For current literature searching rheumatologists rely on *Index Medicus* and other general sources, but for retrospective searching there is the annual *Index of Rheumatology,* based on MEDLARS and issued by the American Rheumatism Association. Abstracts are provided by *Excerpta Medica, Section 31: Arthritis and Rheumatism.*

Because of the interdisciplinary nature of the subject, there are several review series. *Rheumatology, An Annual Review* publishes an annual symposium on a specific theme. *Seminars in Arthritis and Rheumatism* is a quarterly which covers both medical and surgical aspects. A title in the *Clinics* series, *Clinics in Rheumatic Diseases,* produces three issues a year and *Reports on Rheumatic Diseases,* issued by the Arthritis and Rheumatism Council, is a series of brief summaries (about four a year) on specific topics. Earlier *Reports* back to 1959, are periodically revised and issued with an index in booklet form. These last are state of the art publications, however, and have no references to the literature. Reviews, symposia and conference reports are issued as occasional supplements to *Annals of the Rheumatic Diseases,* and there is a more frequent series of supplements to the *Scandinavial Journal of Rheumatology.* There are three occasional review series: *Recent Advances in Rheumatology – 2* edited by W. W. Buchanan and W. C. Dick (Churchill Livingstone, 1981), *Progress in Rheumatology* edited by I. Machtey (Wright, 1982) and *Topical Reviews in Rheumatic Diseases* edited by V. Wright (vol 1, Wright, 1982).

There are three major textbooks: *Textbook of Rheumatology* by W. N. Kelley *et al.* (Saunders, 1981); *Copeman's Textbook of the Rheumatic Diseases* by J. T. Scott (5th edn, Churchill Livingstone, 1978), and *Arthritis and Allied Conditions: a Textbook of Rheumatology* edited by D. J. McCarthy *et al.* (9th edn, Lea and Febiger, 1979). Kelley's textbook is a very substantial one-volume work which fills the need for a comprehensive text in this rapidly developing area of research and practice. The bulk of the book deals with clinical problems, but there is a substantial section on the scientific basis of rheumatology. This latter aspect is dealt with in *The Scientific Basis of Rheumatology* by G. S. Panayi (Churchill Livingstone, 1982). *Textbook of Pediatric Rheumatology* by J. T. Cassidy (Wiley, 1982) covers an aspect of the subject not dealt with elsewhere in a single volume.

Helpful supporting sources are:

Kidney and Rheumatic Disease by P. Bacon (Butterworths, 1982)
Applied Drug Therapy of the Rheumatic Diseases by H. A. Bird and V. Wright (Wright, 1982)
Legg-Calvé-Perthes Disease by A. Catterall (Churchill, 1982)
Laboratory Diagnostic Procedures in the Rheumatic Diseases edited by A. S. Cohen (2nd edn, Lea and Febiger, 1972)
Atlas of Rheumatology and Rheumatic Disease by J. Dequeher (Wolfe Medical, 1982)
Lupus Erythematosus by E. L. Dubois (2nd edn, University of Southern California Press, 1974)
Pathology of Rheumatic Diseases by H. G. Fassbender (translated by G. Loewi, Springer, 1975)
Connective Tissue Diseases by G. R. V. Hughes (2nd edn, Blackwell, 1979)
Metabolic Degenerative and Inflammatory Diseases of Bone and Joints by H. L. Jaffe (Lea and Febiger, 1972)
Heritable Disorders of Connective Tissue by V. A. McKusick (4th edn, Mosby, 1972)

Neurology

Neurology is a great stronghold of clinical medicine, observing and interpreting the symptoms of disturbed function in terms of normal anatomy and physiology; the immense fascination of its complexity has given rise to a vast and often elegant literature. The clinician is now, however, more affected than heretofore by the work of the neuroscientist and the literatures are becoming very much interconnected. Neuroscientific literature is well covered in Chapter 6 and this section attempts to deal only with the clinical.

Formerly one periodical literature catered for both neurology and psychiatry, and several periodical titles still reflect the past. In the last 25 years, however, the disciplines have moved to separate publication (and psychiatry is the subject of Chapter 17). Important journals for the neurologist include:

Acta Neurologica Scandinavica
Annals of Neurology
Archives of Neurology
Brain
Diseases of the Nervous System
Epilepsia
Headache
Journal of Nervous and Mental Disease
Journal of Neurology (Berlin)
Journal of Neurology, Neurosurgery and Psychiatry
Neurology
Paraplegia
Revue Neurologique

INDEXING AND ABSTRACTING SERVICE

Neurology, as a whole, relies on the general indexing and abstracting services, *Index Medicus* and *Excerpta Medica: Section 8: Neurology and Neurosurgery* and, for current awareness, on *Concise Clinical Neurology Review,* a bi-weekly abstracting service based on 816 journals and produced as part of the National Institute of Neurological Diseases information network. But the literature of certain specialized fields is very well defined and lends itself to separate organization: for instance, *Muscular Dystrophy Abstracts* and *Epilepsy Abstracts* are both published by Excerpta Medica. *Parkinson's Disease and Related Disorders, Citations from the Literature and Cerebrovascular Bibliography* are based on MEDLARS.

Electroencephalography is fully covered. Current literature is indexed by *Electroencephalology and Clinical Neurophysiology: Index to Current Literature* (a quarterly supplement to the journal, which may be purchased separately). Retrospective coverage is provided by a series of volumes: *Bibliography of Encephalography 1875–1948* by M. A. B. Brazier (*Electroencephalography and Clinical Neurophysiology, Suppl No 1,* 1959), *KWIC Index of EEG Literature 1949–64* by R. G. Bickford *et al.* (Elsevier, 1965) and *KWIC Index to EEG and Allied Literature 1964–66; 1966–69* from the Brain Information Service at UCLA.

Research on headache and facial pain is being channelled by the journal *Headache* which has an abstracting section, and the review serial *Research and Clinical Studies in Headache.*

The Spastics Society is responsible for the thorough indexing of literature on spasticity and neurological and development disorders of childhood generally. Its journal *Developmental Medicine and Child Neurology* carries a regular literature section and publishes, as a supplement, an annual *Bibliography of Developmental Medicine and Child Neurology.* The Society also publishes *Clinics in Developmental Medicine,* a series of monographs.

REVIEWS

Among reviews, the year's work is summarized in *Year Book of Neurology and Neurosurgery,* while *Progress in Neurology and Psychiatry* (Grune and Stratton) also gave annual coverage until 1973. Occasional volumes were published in *Modern Trends in Neurology vol 6* edited by D. Williams (Butterworths, 1975) and *Recent Advances in Clinical Neurology – 3* edited by W. B. Matthews (Churchill Livingstone, 1982); this last is the successor to *Recent Advances in Neurology and Neuropsychiatry.* Pitman publishes a *Progress in Neurology* series, each volume of which deals with a specific topic, such as *Metabolic Disorders of the Nervous System* edited by F. C. Rose (1981). Conference proceedings, reviews and monographs appear in several named series. One such is *Research Publications of the Association for Research in Nervous and Mental Disease (ARNMD).* These are the proceedings of its annual conference and cover a wide range of topics, including the scientific and the psychiatric as well as the clinical neurological. A most important series of this kind is *Advances in Neurology* (Plenum), which has produced over 30 volumes in ten years including, for example, *Huntington's Chorea, 1872–1972, vol 1,* edited by D. B. Calne (1973) and, more recently, *Brain Edema (vol 28)* by J. Cervos-Navarro (1980) and *Headache* edited by Macdonald Critchley (vol 33, 1982). The *Contemporary Neurology Series* (F. A. Davis) is also a useful review publication.

OTHER SECONDARY SOURCES

Among other secondary sources, the starting point for many years to come will be *Handbook of Clinical Neurology* edited by P. J. Vinken and G. W. Bruyn (North Holland, 1968–, over 43 vols to date). Begun in 1968 it is still in progress and aims at complete coverage. Inevitably, knowledge, and with it, practice, are already moving ahead of the contents, but it will remain a source book and some volumes (e.g. *Basal Ganglia, vol 6*) will not be supplanted for some time. The progress of neurology, more than of some other disciplines, is signposted by great names and their story can provide the key to its bibliography. An entry point is *Founders of Neurology: One Hundred and Forty-six Biographical Sketches . . .* edited by W. Haymaker and F. Schiller (2nd edn, C. C. Thomas, 1970), supported by *Neurological Classics,* compiled by R. H. Wilkins and I. A. Brody (Johnson Repr. Corp., 1973), which gathers together some classic descriptions in translation, previously published in *Archives of Neurology.*

The Doctrine of the Nerves by J. D. Spillane (Oxford University Press, 1981) is a history of neurology whose intention is to show the newcomer to neurology the lie of the land. It can be recommended as a good modern history of the subject.

TEXTBOOKS

There are several good textbooks. The acknowledged standard in the UK has long been *Brain's Diseases of the Nervous System* edited by J. N. Walton (8th edn, Oxford University Press, 1977); but complementary publications are *Brain's Clinical Neurology* edited by R. Bannister (5th edn, Oxford University Press, 1978), and *Essentials of Neurology* by J. N. Walton (4th edn, Pitman Medical, 1975). Two books at undergraduate level for reading rather than reference provide a good background. They are *Diseases of the Nervous System* by W. B. Matthews and H. Miller (3rd edn, Blackwell, 1979), and *Practical Neurology* by W. B. Matthews (3rd edn, Blackwell, 1975).

Books on diagnosis and examination are:

Neurological Examination in Clinical Practice by E. R. Bickerstaff (4th edn, Blackwell, 1980)
Electrodiagnosis and Electromyography by S. Licht (3rd edn, Licht, 1971)
An Atlas of Clinical Neurology by J. D. Spillane (3rd edn, Oxford University Press, 1982)
Diagnostic Neuroradiology by J. M. Taveras and E. H. Wood (2nd edn, 2 vols, Williams and Wilkins, 1976)

The following are important sources of reference:

Genetics of Neurologic Disorders by M. Baraitser (Oxford University Press, 1967)
Greenfield's Neuropathology edited by W. Blackwood and J. A. N. Corsellis (3rd edn, Arnold, 1976)
A Centennial Bibliography of Huntington's Chorea, 1872–1972 G. W. Bruyn and N. C. Myrianthopoulos (Nijhoff, 1974)
Scientific Foundations of Neurology edited by M. Critchley, J. O'Leary and B. Jennett (Heinemann, 1972)
Tropical Neurology edited by J. D. Spillane (Oxford University Press, 1973)

Clinical Neuro-Ophthalmology by F. B. Walsh and W. F. Hoyt (4th edn, Williams and Wilkins, 1982)

Disorders of Voluntary Muscle edited by J. N. Walton (4th edn, Churchill Livingstone, 1981).

15

General practice

M. Hammond

General practice must be one of the most difficult areas of medical literature to discuss. The needs and special interests of family doctors, their involvement as clinical assistants in hospital, their work as medical officers to commercial firms or sporting organizations, their involvement in emergency care, their work on committees, and their newer role as teachers in vocational training and audit must cover every facet of medical literature.

Since the formation of the College of General Practitioners in 1952 there has been a considerable growth in the literature designed specially for general practice, and it is this material that is discussed in this chapter. Books mentioned here are arranged in chronological order to show the development of the literature because there are a number of items which, although not readily available, nevertheless merit attention.

Indexes

The *Index Medicus* has a heading *Family Practice,* but this covers the subject only superficially. Since 1980 the World Organization of National Colleges, Academies and Academic Associations of General Practitioners/Family Physicians (WONCA) has been producing, in co-operation with the National Library of Medicine, FAMLI (*Family Medicine Literature Index*). This appears quarterly and is cumulated at the end of the year. It includes the information stored in the Medical Literature Analysis and Retrieval System (MEDLARS) of the National Library of Medicine as well as a supplement containing references to family medicine journals not included in this system. The 1981 cumulated edition also contains a keywords thesaurus in family medicine and a list of family medicine books published during 1979–1981.

New Reading for General Practice, published by the Royal College of General Practitioners Library, is a current-awareness publication covering material seen in the library, arranged under subject headings – cumulated to the end of each year after three quarterly issues, with an annual author index. Journal articles, reports, and books are included in this publication. Many entries have a brief description of content which is concentrated on British material but includes references to major works from overseas.

Current Literature on General Medical Practice and *Current Literature on Health Services,* both produced monthly by the Department of Health and Social Security Library, list material under subject headings seen in that library. Chapters 2 (Primary sources of information) and 3 (Indexes, etc.) expand this section.

Reviews and yearbook

The only major review of general practice is *Primary Health Care* by D. Hicks, which was commissioned in June 1973 by the Operational Research Service of the Department of Health and Social Security and published in 1976 by HMSO. Four hundred and thirty references are cited.

Health surveys and related studies (Pergamon, 1979) by M. Alderson and R. Dowie of the Royal Statistical Society and the Social Science Research Council is vol. 9 in the series *Reviews of United Kingdom Statistical Sources,* and includes much non-clinical, general-practice material. On a smaller scale, *Trends in General Practice 1979* by the Royal College of General Practitioners (*British Medical Journal,* 1979), a collection of essays on general practice, is the most recent publication in the *Present State and Future Needs* series. Also available is *The General Practitioner's Yearbook* (Winthrop Laboratories).

Journals

Material of interest to general practitioners appears in a vast range of periodicals, while material written especially for them has snowballed almost beyond control in recent years. The throw-away journal, a type of material which many consider lightweight, is, according to readership surveys (J. Cowhig, The medical newspaper, *Brit. med. J.*, **285**, 109–111, 1982), the most widely read type of all weekly publications by British general practitioners. The free circulation newspapers *Pulse* and *General Practitioner* head this list. *Doctor, Medical News* and *World Medicine* are similar in content in that they give a very up-to-date résumé of what is going on in general practice, as well as reporting superficially on topical clinical subjects. *Practitioner, Medical Digest, Medicine International* (which is in a three-yearly, monthly add-on format) *Modern Medicine, Update, Modern Geriatrics, British Journal of Sexual Medicine,* and *Journal of Maternal and Child Health* have more clinical content, but are again distributed free of charge. *Medeconomics* deals with the business side of practice organization. *Trainee* has been aimed at vocational training schemes. Drugs are covered by *MIMS, Drug and Therapeutics Bulletin, Prescribers' Journal* and the *British National Formulary. Health Trends*, published by the Department of Health and Social Security and the Welsh Office, is distributed free to doctors in the National Health Service as a semi-official publication – the Scottish equivalent, *Health Bulletin,* is issued by the Scottish Home and Health Department.

Pharmaceutical companies issue additional material and there are numerous supplements and additions to many of the newspapers and journals mentioned above. Another category of journal is the periodical obtained as part of a subscription paid to a society. This traditional type of journal includes the *British Medical Journal*, with a Practice Observed section which was started in 1981, the *Journal of the Royal College of General Practitioners* and the *Journal of the Royal Society of Medicine. The Lancet* and *New England Journal of Medicine* are also taken by some general practitioners.

Foreign periodicals of general practice are not taken by many general practitioners, but where the system of family practice has similarities with Britain a number of these periodicals contain useful and applicable information for British general practitioners; the *Journal of Family Practice*, the *Canadian Family Physician* and the *New Zealand Family Physician* are the best examples in this category. Organizations of general practice in other countries usually produce a journal and these are listed below.

British journals of particular interest to general practitioners

BMA News (Review) (BMA, 1966–)
British Journal of Sexual Medicine (Medical News Tribune Ltd, 1973–)

British National Formulary (BMA and Pharmaceutical Society of Great Britain, 1981–)
British Medical Journal: Practice Observed (BMA, 1981–)
Doctor (Sutton-Siebert Publications, 1971–)
Drug and Therapeutics Bulletin (DHSS,1963–)
General Practitioner (Medical Publications, 1963–)
Geriatric Medicine (Maclean-Hunter, 1979–), formerly *Modern Geriatrics* (1970–1979)
Health Bulletin (Scottish Home and Health Department, 1941–)
Health Trends (DHSS and Welsh Office, 1969–)
Journal of Maternal and Child Health (Barker Publications Ltd, 1975–)
Journal of the Royal College of General Practitioners (RCGP, 1967–), formerly *Journal of the College of General Practitioners* (1952–1967)
Journal of the Royal Society of Medicine (RSM 1978–), formerly *Proceedings of the Royal Society of Medicine* (1907–1977)
The Lancet (1823–)
Medeconomics (Medical Publications, 1980–)
Medical Digest (MacLean Hunter, 1956–)
Medicine International (Medical Education International Ltd, 1981–) formerly *Medicine* (1971–1980)
MIMS (Medical Publications, 1959–)
Mims Magazine (Medical Publications, 1974–)
Modern Medicine (Modern Medicine Publications, 1956–)
Practitioner (Morgan Grampion, 1868–)
Prescribers' Journal (DHSS, 1961–), formerly *Prescribers' Notes* (1952–1960)
Pulse (Morgan Grampion, 1959–)
Trainee (Update Publications Ltd, 1981–)
Update (Update Publications Ltd, 1968–)
World Medicine (IPC Business Press Ltd, 1965–)

Foreign journals of particular relevance to British general practitioners

Canadian Family Physician (College of Family Physicians of Canada, 1967–) formerly *Journal of the College of Family Physicians of Canada* (1954–1967)
Journal of Family Practice (Appleton-Century-Crofts, 1974–)
New England Journal of Medicine (Massachusetts Medical Society, 1812–)
New Zealand Family Physician (Royal New Zealand College of General Practitioners, 1974–)

Some journals of other colleges of general practice

Allgemeinmedizin International General Practice (International General Practice, 1971–)
American Family Physician (American Academy of Family Physicians, 1970–), formerly *G. P.* (1950–1969)
Australian Family Physician (Royal Australian College of General Practitioners, 1972–), formerly *Annals of General Practice* (1956–1971)
Family Physician (Israel) (Kupat-Holim Health Insurance Institution of the General Federation of Labour in Israel, 1970–)
Family Practitioner (College of General Practitioners, Malaysia, 1974–)
Filipino Family Physician (Philippine Academy of Family Physicians 1963–)

GP (Singapore) (College of General Practitioners, Singapore, 1973–)
Hong Kong Practitioner (Hong Kong College of General Practitioners, 1978–)
Huisarts en Wetenschap (Nederlands Huisartsen Genootschap, 1958–)
Singapore Family Physician (College of General Practitioners, Singapore, 1975–)
Sri Lankan Family Physician (College of General Practitioners, Sri Lanka, 1979–)

Monographs and textbooks

An Introduction to General Practice by D. Craddock (3rd edn, Lewis, 1970), first published in 1953, is an invaluable compendium of practical experience backed by references to the literature. *General Practice for Students of Medicine* by R. Harvard Davis (Academic Press, 1975) describes the objectives and features of a system of primary and continuing care. *General Practice Medicine* edited by J. H. Barber and F. A. Boddy (Churchill Livingstone, 1975) is an excellent, shortish practical handbook on the diagnosis and management of common conditions, including comments on broader topics such as terminal illness. *A Handbook of Treatment* edited by H. W. Proctor and P. S. Byrne (MTP, 1976) is a reference source on therapeutics with a distinguished authorship and comprehensive coverage. *A Textbook of Medical Practice* edited by J. Fry, P. S. Byrne and S. Johnson (MTP, 1976) is a large work which discusses common clinical problems in family medicine. *A New Approach to Medicine: Principles and Priorities in Health Care* by J. Fry (MTP, 1978) raises serious and important questions concerning the cost-effectiveness of existing health programmes. *Scientific Foundations of Family Medicine* edited by J. Fry, E. Gambrill and R. Smith (Heinemann, 1978) is weighty, but authoritative, with 73 chapters and over 100 contributors. *Towards Earlier Diagnosis* by K. Hodgkin (4th edn, Churchill Livingstone, 1978) emphasizes the different incidence of problems occurring in general practice vis-à-vis hospital practice, and gives management advice. *A Guide to General Practice* by the Oxford GP Trainee Group (Blackwell, 1979) provides a collection of data for everyday use, not easily found elsewhere and essential for the new GP. *Clinical Thinking and Practice, Diagnosis and Decision in Patient Care* by H. J. Wright and D. B. MacAdam (Churchill Livingstone, 1979) is a short introduction to the concept of clinical method. *Common Diseases, Their Nature, Incidence and Care* by J. Fry (2nd edn, MTP, 1979) is an important book which contains information not easily found elsewhere. *Introduction to General Practice* by M. Drury and R. Hull (Baillière Tindall, 1979) is a small volume in the *Concise Medical Textbook Series*, primarily designed for students. *A Primer of Primary Care* by S. G. Marshall and A. P. R. Eckersley (Lloyd-Luke, 1980) is written specifically for the doctor new to general practice. *Lecture Notes on Medicine in General Practice* by C. M. Harris (Blackwell, 1980) is a short, down-to-earth account covering morbidity, psychosocial aspects, resources, specific skills and the clinical roles of the GP. *Primary Care* edited by J. Fry (Heinemann, 1980) is a comprehensive book with contributions from 29 international experts, particularly useful for course organizers and trainees. *An Introduction to Family Medicine* by I. R. McWhinney (Oxford University Press, 1981) is a small volume that provides a core of knowledge and emphasizes principles and methods required by the family physician. *An Introduction to Primary Medical Care* by D. C. Morrell (2nd edn, Churchill Livingstone, 1981) uses case histories to demonstrate how the new GP can evaluate the needs of patients. *Manual of Primary Health Care* by P. Pritchard (2nd edn, Oxford University Press, 1981) is a unique, practical book of the 'who, why, what, where, when and how' variety. *General Practice* by E. Gambrill (Heinemann, 1982) provides an overview of general practice for the trainee and trainer. *Practice* by J. Cormack, M. Marinker and D. Morrell (Kluwer, 1976–1982) is an attractive and useful add-on series written by GPs for GPs.

General practice as a way of life is criticized or revealed in *The GP: What's Wrong?* by D. Cargill (Gollancz, 1967) and *The Longest Art* by K. Lane (Allen and Unwin, 1969). *A Fortunate Man* by J. Berger and J. Mohr (Allen Lane, 1967) is an account of a country doctor's relationship with his patients and practice, with beautiful photographs. *Limits to Medicine. Medical Nemesis: The Expropriation of Health* by I. Illich (Marion Boyars, 1976), opens with the words 'The medical establishment has become a major threat to health' and sets forth a radical, thought-provoking thesis. In *Medicine: The Forgotten Art?* (Pitman, 1978) C. Elliott-Binns turns to Hippocrates' writings, distilling from them lessons applicable to modern medicine, while in *The Doctor, Father Figure or Plumber?* (Croom Helm, 1979) J. McCormick expresses his feelings about his work.

General practice has a rapidly-expanding literature which cannot all be considered here; a further useful selection of recent important titles is found in the regularly revised *Medical Textbook Review* edited by V. Daniels (5th edn, Cambridge Medical Books, 1982).

Prevention and screening

Screening in General Practice edited by C. R. Hart (Churchill Livingstone, 1975) evaluates the present status of medical screening in general practice in the UK and is a state of the art report. In *Self-Care in Health* by J. D. Williamson and K. Danaher (Croom Helm, 1978) the many aspects of self-care are examined and analyzed in a wide-ranging manner. *The Family Good Health Guide. Common Sense on Common Health Problems* by J. Fry, A. Moulds, G. Strube and E. Gambrill (MTP, 1982) distils the expertise of a group of general practitioners. *Health and Prevention in Primary Care* by the Royal College of General Practitioners' Council Working Party (RCGP, 1981) is an RCGP policy statement.

Clinical

Night Calls. A Study in General Practice by M. B. Clyne (Tavistock, 1961), *Family Ill Health. An Investigation in General Practice* by R. Kellner (Tavistock, 1963), and *Asthma: Attitude and Milieu* by A. Lask (Tavistock, 1966) are all based on work by general practitioners. *Bronchial Asthma: A Genetic, Population and Psychiatric Study* by D. Leigh and E. Marley (Pergamon, 1967) is based on data taken from two London general practices. An early work is *Geriatrics and the General Practitioner Team* by M. K. Thompson (Baillière Tindall and Cassell, 1969). *Medicine Takers, Prescribers and Hoarders* by K. Dunnell and A. Cartwright (Routledge and Kegan Paul, 1972) is a study in 14 parliamentary constituencies in Britain, made with the co-operation of 326 general practitioners. *Psychopharmacology in Family Practice* by D. Wheatley (Heinemann, 1973) is a descriptive account of the programme of the General Practitioner Research Group. *Oral Contraception and Health. An Interim Report from the Oral Contraception Study of the Royal College of General Practitioners* (Pitman, 1974) records data contributed by 1400 general practitioners on some 46 000 women for this interim report; later reports have appeared in various medical journals.

The Hidden Alcoholic in General Practice. A Method of Detection Using a Questionnaire by R. H. Wilkins (Elek, 1974) elaborates on work with selected patients attending a health centre in Manchester, where an Alcoholic Risk Register was developed. *Contraception, Abortion and Sterilization in General Practice* is by K. L. Oldershaw (Kimpton, 1975). *Coronary Care in the Community* edited by A. Colling (Croom Helm, 1977) is the proceedings of a national workshop held for general practitioners in March 1976. *Laboratory, a Manual for the Medical Practitioner* edited by H. W. K. Acheson (Kluwer, 1978; updated, 1982) is a nicely prepared reference source. *Obesity and its Management* by D. Craddock (3rd edn, Churchill Livingstone, 1978) is written from the author's own experience in treating patients over a period of ten years. *The Care of the Elderly in the Community* by I. Williams (Croom Helm, 1979) is a practical work concentrating on care in the home. *Hypertension* by J. Tudor Hart (1980), *Rheumatology in General Practice* by M. Rogers and N. Williams (1981), *Renal Medicine and Urology* by D. Brooks and N. Mallick (1982) are all volumes in the useful Library of General Practice Series published by Churchill Livingstone. *Treatment. A Handbook of Drug Therapy* edited by V. W. M. Drury, O. L. Wade, L. Beeley and P. Alesbury (Kluwer, 1978; updated, 1982) is regularly updated and well produced. *Geriatric Problems in General Practice* by G. K. Wilcock, J. A. M. Gray and P. M. M. Pritchard (Oxford University Press, 1982) and *Paediatric Problems in General Practice* by M. Modell and R. Boyd (Oxford University Press, 1982) cover day-to-day problems in general practice.

Children

The Catarrhal Child by J. Fry (Butterworths, 1961), *Presenting Symptoms in Childhood* by J. Fry (Butterworths, 1962) and *Absent. School Refusal as an Expression of Disturbed Family Relationships* by M. B. Clyne (Tavistock, 1966) are older but interesting studies. *Today's Three-Year-Olds in London* by M. Pollak (Heinemann, 1972) is an important study and *Paediatric Care. Child Health in Family Practice* by S. Carne (MTP, 1976) is a general text on the management of child health. *Nine Years Old* by M. Pollak (MTP, 1979), written from personal experience, is an account of the development of children in a London practice containing many immigrant families. *The First Year of Life* by G. C. Jenkins and R. C. F. Newton (Churchill Livingstone, 1981) deals specifically with health and development during the first twelve months. *Child Care in General Practice* edited by C. Hart (2nd edn, Churchill Livingstone, 1982) covers all common complaints, *Healthier Children – Thinking Prevention* is a report by a Royal College of General Practitioners Council Working Party (RCGP, 1982).

Psychiatry in general practice

Depressive Disorders in the Community by C. A. H. Watts (Wright, 1966) is a study of 16 years' work, while *Neurosis in the Ordinary Family*, by A. Ryle (Tavistock, 1967) is a psychiatric survey documenting research into 112 working-class families. The work grew out of a casework experiment involving a psychiatrist, a psychiatric social worker and a general practitioner. *Common Neuroses in General Practice, A Behavioural Approach* by J. C. M. Wilkinson and K. Latif (Wright, 1974) is a concise handbook for those wishing to employ behaviour therapy. *Psychosocial Disorders in General Practice* edited by P. Williams and A. Clare (Academic Press, 1979) is a collection of 23 papers illustrating the development of psychiatric research in general practice. *Psychiatric Illness in General Practice* by M. Shepherd, B. Cooper, A. C. Brown and G. Kalton (2nd edn, Oxford University Press, 1981) is an account of the work and findings of the General Practice Research Unit at the Institute of Psychiatry, London.

Doctor–patient relationship

The Doctor, His Patient and the Illness by M. Balint (2nd Edn, Pitman, 1964), now a classic, remains a most influential work. *One Man's practice. Effects of Developing Insight on Doctor–Patient Transactions* by R. S. Greco and R. A. Pittinger (Tavistock Publications, 1966) is an account of how training in communication skills based on the teaching of Michael Balint altered a general practitioner's approach to his patient. *Doctors and Patients. A relationship examined* by M. Hodson (Hodder and Stoughton, 1967) is a work based on twenty-two years' experience. *Patient-Centred Medicine* edited by P. Hopkins (Regional Doctor Publications, 1972) reported on the First International Conference of the Balint Society in Great Britain. *Complaints Against Doctors. A Study in Professional Accountability* by R. Klein (Charles Knight, 1973) discusses the system for dealing with patients' complaints. A sociological analysis is provided by *Going to See the Doctor. The Consultation Process in General Practice* by G. Stimson and B. Webb (Routledge and Kegan Paul, 1975). *Doctors Talking to Patients. A Study of the Verbal Behaviour of General Practitioners Consulting in their Surgeries* by P. S. Byrne and B. E. L. Long (HMSO, 1976) is a study based on tapes containing consultations with nearly 2500 patients. *Language and Communication in General Practice* edited by B. Tanner (Hodder and Stoughton, 1976) deals with these skills and is derived from a symposium organized by the Royal College of General Practitioners. A useful introductory text is *Patients, Practitioners and Medical Care: Aspects of Medical Sociology* by D. Robinson (2nd edn, Heinemann, 1978). *Doctor/Patient Relationship. A Study in General Practice* by F. Fitton and H. W. K. Acheson (HMSO, 1979) is the result of a two-year research project investigating the visits of 320 patients to two general practitioners. All consultations in this study period were recorded on audiotape and interactions between receptionists and patients, nurses and patients' expectations and quality of relationships with doctors were studied. *The Human Face of Medicine* edited by P. Hopkins (Pitman, 1979) is based on the Fourth International Conference (1978) of the Balint Society in Great Britain on the Aims, Achievement and Assessment of Balint training.

Patient participation

The rationing of resources within the National Health Service has increased the interest in preventive medicine and patient participation in primary care. Early works are *General Practice: a Consumer Commentary* prepared by E. Hutchinson (Research Institute for Consumer Affairs, 1963) and *Patients and their Doctors. A Study of General Practice* by A. Cartwright (Routledge and Kegan Paul, 1967). A survey of the views of nearly 1400 patients on their doctors is reported in *The Process of Becoming Ill* by D. Robinson (Routledge and Kegan Paul, 1971) and is based on a study of families in a South Wales general practice. *The Move to Henfield Health Centre. A Study of Patients' Views* by K. S. Dawes, R. Dowie and J. M. Bevan (*Health Services Research Unit Report No. 16,* University of Kent at Canterbury, 1975) is one of a series of publications on the same subject area. *Access to Primary Care* by R. Simpson (*Royal Commission on the National Health Service Research Paper Number 6,* HMSO, 1979) is a report on a survey into services for children and old people in Stoke Newington and West Cumbria, while *Changes in the Structure of General Practice: the Patient's Viewpoint,* by S. Arber and L. Sawyer (2 vols, DHSS, 1979) is a report from interviews of 1084 patients selected in their own homes. Views on appointment systems, the role of receptionists and doctors are documented. *Access to Primary Health Care* by J. Ritchie, A. Jacoby and M. Bone (HMSO, 1981) is an enquiry carried out on behalf of the United Kingdom Health Departments on patients' experience of and views about the accessibility of primary health care services. *General Practice Revised. A Second Study of Patients and their Doctors* by A. Cartwright and R. Anderson (Tavistock, 1981) is a follow-up survey to Cartwright's original work, mentioned above. *Patient Participation in General Practice* edited by P. Pritchard (*Occasional Paper No. 17,* Royal College of General Practitioners, 1981) and *Patients's Rights. A Guide to the Rights and Responsibilities of Patients and Doctors in the NHS* by National Consumer Council (NCC, 1982) represent views from both ends of the spectrum.

Education for general practice

The development of vocational training for general practice was first suggested in *General Practice and the Training of the General Practitioner,* Report of a Committee of the British Medical Association (BMA, 1950), accepted by the *Royal Commission on Medical Education 1965–68. Report* (Chairman Lord Todd; HMSO, 1968), and an account of its implementation and working appears in *Training for General Practice* by The Joint Committee on Postgraduate Training for General Practice (JCPT, 1982). The following educational texts have been produced:

A Study of Doctors, Mutual Selection and the Evaluation of Results in a Training Programme for Family Doctors by M. Balint, E. Balint, R. Gosling and P. Hildebrand (Tavistock, 1966) describes in detail a 14-year postgraduate training scheme for general practitioners in the field of psychological medicine which was developed by Michael Balint at the Tavistock Clinic

The Future General Practitioner: Learning and Teaching by the Royal College of General Practitioners (BMJ, 1972) reported the results of a working party who studied the content of training for general practitioners

Learning to Care, Person to Person by P. S. Byrne and B. E. L. Long (Churchill Livingstone, 1975)

The Assessment of Postgraduate Training in General Practice by J. Freeman and P. S. Byrne (2nd edn, Society for Research into Higher Education Ltd, 1976)

An Opportunity to Learn. An International Study of Learning and Teaching in General Practice by E. V. Kuenssberg (*Occasional Paper 2;* Royal College of General Practitioners, 1976) is an account of the author's visits to Europe and North America as the Wolfson Visiting Professor, 1974

Focus on Learning in Family Practice by W. E. Fabb, M. W. Heffernan, W. A. Phillips and P. Stone (Royal Australian College of General Practitioners, Family Medicine Programme, 1976)

Medical Education and Primary Health Care edited by H. Noack (Croom Helm, 1976) is based on a conference in 1976 planned by the Institute for Research in Education and Evaluation at the Medical Faculty of the University of Bern

General Practice and University edited by J. C. van Es (Scheltema and Holkema, 1979)

General Practitioners and Postgraduate Education in the Northern Region by B. L. E. C. Reedy, B. A. Gregson and M. Williams (*Occasional Paper 9,* Royal College of General Practitioners, 1979)

Education for Co-operation in Health and Social Work. Papers from the Symposium on Interprofessional Learning, University of Nottingham, July 1979 edited by H. England (*Occasional Paper 14,* Royal College of General Practitioners, 1980)

Section 63 Activities by J. Wood and P. S. Byrne (*Occasional Paper 11,* Royal College of General Practitioners, 1980) is a history of the development of opportunities offered to general practitioners in the UK to pursue their education, with a detailed analysis of the North-Western Region and recommendations for future action

Fourth National Trainee Conference, Report, Recommendations and Questionnaire, Exeter, 1980 edited by C. Ronalds, A. Douglas, D. P. Gray and P. Selley (*Occasional Paper 18,* Royal College of General Practitioners, 1981)

Teaching General Practice edited by J. Cormack, M. Marinker and D. Morrell (Kluwer, 1981)
In-Service Training by P. Freeling and S. Barry (NFER – Nelson, 1982) is an account and evaluation of the RCGP Nuffield courses started in 1974
Training for General Practice by D. J. P Gray (MacDonald and Evans, 1982) is an account of the organization and running of a vocational training scheme.

The RCGP examination has inspired the following texts:

Problem-centred Learning, The Modified Essay Question in Medical Education by K. Hodgkin and J. D. E. Knox (Churchill Livingstone, 1975)
The MRCGP Examination. A Comprehensive Guide to Preparation and Passing by A. J. Moulds, T. A. Bouchier Hayes and K. H. M. Young (MTP, 1978)
MCQ Tutor for the MRCGP Exam by A. J. Moulds and T. A. I. Bouchier Hayes (Heinemann, 1981)
The MRCGP Study Book by T. A. I. Bouchier Hayes, J. Fry, E. Gambrill, A. Moulds and K. Young (Update, 1981).

General practitioners' use of literature has been surveyed in *The Use of Medical Literature: a Preliminary Survey* by G. Ford, V. Maguire and P. Walker (British Library Research and Development Reports, 1980), and *Information and the Practice of Medicine: Report of the Medical Information Review Panel* by P. A. Cockerill (British Library Research and Development Reports, 1981), which again includes specific research on general practitioners.

Government and official statements

While any policy document on the health service is likely to have implications for general practice, the documents listed here are a selection of the major reports since the early 1950s. References within the report obviously lead to wider coverage. Reports on a specific area come under that section:

Report of the Committee on General Practice within the National Health Service by Central Health Services Council (Chairman Henry Cohen, HMSO, 1954)
Royal Commission on Doctors' and Dentists' Remuneration 1957–1960. Report (Chairman Harry Pilkington, HMSO, 1960)
A Review of the Medical Services in Great Britain; the report of a Committee sponsored by Royal College of Physicians of London (Social Assay, 1962)
The Field of Work of the Family Doctor. Report of the Sub-Committee by Central Health Services Council (Chairman Annis Gillie, HMSO, 1963)
Commentaries of the Working Party on General Practice by Department of Health and Social Security (HMSO, 1964)
General Practice. Report of a WHO Expert Committee (*Technical Report Series 267*, WHO, 1964)
A Charter for the Family Doctor Service by British Medical Association (BMA, 1965)
Domiciliary Midwifery and Maternity Bed Needs. Report of the Sub-Committee by

Department of Health and Social Security and Welsh Office (Chairman Sir John Peel, HMSO, 1970)

Primary medical care by British Medical Association, Planning Unit (*Report No. 4*, BMA, 1970)

The Report of the Joint Working Party on the General Medical Services 1973 by Department of Health and Social Security (Chairman George Godber, HMSO, 1974)

Report of the Committee of Inquiry into the Regulation of the Medical Profession (Chairman A. W. Merrison, HMSO, 1975)

Competence to Practise. Report of a Committee of Enquiry set up for the Medical Profession in the United Kingdom by Committee of Enquiry into Competence to Practise (Chairman E. A. J. Alment, HMSO, 1976)

Primary Health Care. A Joint Report by the Director-General of the World Health Organization and the Executive Director of the United Nations Children's Fund (Alma-Ata conference, WHO, 1978)

Royal Commission on the National Health Service. Report (Chairman Sir Alec Merrison, HMSO, 1979)

Patients First. Consultative Paper on the Structure and Management of the National Health Service in England and Wales by the Department of Health and Social Security and the Welsh Office (HMSO, 1979)

Inequalities in Health. Report of a Research Working Group (Chairman Douglas Black, DHSS, 1980)

Statistics and research

Details of general practice content and workload appear in the following publications. The development of the collection of morbidity statistics by general practitioners from their own practices is as follows:

General Practitioners' Records. An Analysis of the Clinical Records of Eight Practices during the Period April 1951 to March 1952 by W. P. D. Logan, (*General Register Office Studies on Medical and Population Subjects No. 7*, HMSO, 1953) which followed on from the series *Supplement on General Morbidity, Cancer and Mental Health* from the Registrar General's Statistical Review of England and Wales

General Practitioners' Records. An Analysis of the Clinical Records of Some General Practices during the Period April 1952 to March 1954 (*General Register Office Studies on Medical and Population Subjects No. 9*, HMSO, 1955)

Morbidity Statistics from General Practice. Volume 1 (General) by W. P. D. Logan and A. A. Cushion (*General Register Office Studies on Medical and Population Subjects No. 14*, HMSO, 1958)

Morbidity Statistics from General Practice. Volume 11 (Occupation) by W. P. D. Logan (*General Register Office Studies on Medical and Population Subjects No. 14*, HMSO, 1960)

Morbidity Statistics from General Practice. Volume III (Disease in General Practice) by Research Committee of the Council of the College of General Practitioners (*General Register Office Studies on Medical and Population Subjects No 14*, HMSO, 1962)

Morbidity Statistics from General Practice. Second National Study 1970–1971 by Royal College of General Practitioners, Office of Population Censuses and

Surveys and Department of Health and Social Security (*Studies on Medical and Population Subjects No 26,* HMSO, 1974)

Trends in National Morbidity. A Comparison of Two Successive National Morbidity Surveys from the Birmingham Research Unit of the Royal College of General Practitioners (*Occasional Paper 3,* RCGP, 1976)

Morbidity Statistics from General Practice. 1971–1972. Second National Study by Royal College of General Practitioners, Office of Population Censuses and Surveys and Department of Health and Social Security (*Studies on Medical and Population Subjects No 36* (HMSO, 1979)

Morbidity Statistics from General Practice 1970–71. Socio-economic Analyses by Royal College of General Practitioners, Office of Population Censuses and Surveys and Department of Health and Social Security (HMSO, 1982)

Individual practice accounts appear in the following:

Epidemiology in Country Practice by W. N. Pickles (Wright, 1939)

An Analytical Study of North Carolina General Practice 1953–1954 by O. L. Peterson, L. P. Andrews, R. S. Spain and B. G. Greenberg (*Journal of Medical Education,* **31,** No 12 Part 2, 1956), included because this is one of the first overall surveys of general practice

Illness and General Practice. A survey of Medical Care in an Inland Population in South-East Norway by B. G. Bentsen (Universitets Forlaget, Oslo 1970)

Family Medicine. The Medical Life History of Families by F. J. A. Huygen (Dekker and Van de Vegt, 1978)

The Symptom Iceberg. A Study of Community Health by D. Rainsford Hannay (Routledge and Kegan Paul, 1979), a study based on 1344 home interviews with patients

Information from patients concerning their sickness is contained in:

The Survey of Sickness 1943 to 1952 by W. P. D. Logan and E. M. Brooke (*General Register Office Studies on Medical and Population Subjects No 12,* HMSO, 1957)

Health and Sickness: the Choice of Treatment. Perceptions of Illness and Use of Services in an Urban Community by M. E. J. Wadsworth, W. J. H. Butterfield and R. Blaney (Tavistock, 1971)

The General Household Survey. Introductory Report by Office of Population Censuses and Surveys (HMSO, 1973)

The General Household Survey, 1974, 1975, 1976, 1977, 1978, 1979, 1980 by Office of Population Censuses and Surveys (HMSO, 1977, 1978, 1979, 1980, 1981, 1982, 1983)

Information about general practice can be found in:

Health and Personal Social Services Statistics for England (with summary tables for Great Britain 1978) by Department of Health and Social Security. (HMSO, 1980)

Compendium of Health Statistics by Office of Health Economics (4th edn, OHE, 1981)

Methods of carrying out this research are covered in:

A Handbook for Research in General Practice edited by T. S. Eimerl and A. J. Laidlaw (Livingstone, 1969)

Evaluating Primary Care. Some Experiments in Quality Measurement in an Academic Unit of Primary Medical Care by E. M. Clark and J. A. Forbes (Croom Helm, 1979) is an account of auditing general practice work

Research in General Practice by J. G. R. Howie (Croom Helm, 1979) updates the
   Eimerl and Laidlaw book
The Measurement of the Quality of General Practitioner Care by C. J. Watkins
   (*Occasional Paper 15,* Royal College of General Practitioners, 1981) lays down
   guidelines for individual audit

   Classification is covered by:

*ICHPPC-2 International Classification of Health Problems in Primary Care (1979
Revision)* by Classification Committee of World Organization of National Colleges,
Academics and Academic Association of General Practitioners/Family Physicians
(Oxford University Press, 1979)

Practice organization

In 1951 the Nuffield Provincial Hospitals Trust invited Dr Stephen
Taylor to conduct a non-statistical survey of 94 general practitioner practices. His report, *Good General Practice, A Report of a
Survey* (Oxford University Press, 1954) has become a classic and
started a growing literature in this area. Later books include:

The Payment of the General Practitioner. Some European Comparisons by J.
   Hogarth (Pergamon, 1963)
Appointment Systems in General Practice by J. M. Bevan and G. J. Draper (Oxford
   University Press, 1967)
*Medical Records, Medical Education and Patient Care. The Problem-Oriented
   Record as a Basic Tool* by L. L. Weed (Press of Case Western Reserve Univer-
   sity, 1969)
The New General Practice and The New General Practice 2, collections of articles
   published in the British Medical Journal (BMA, 1968 and 1970)
Group Practice by J. S. Clark (E. & S. Livingstone, 1971)
*The Organization of Group Practice. A Report of a Sub-Committee of the Standing
   Medical Advisory Committee* (The Harvard Davis Report, HMSO, 1971)
Family Doctors and Public Policy. A Study of Manpower Distribution by J. R. But-
   ler (Routledge and Kegan Paul, 1973)
Administration in General Practice by H. Owen (Arnold, 1975)
*Innovations in Medical Records in the United Kingdom. Report to King Edward's
   Hospital Fund on a survey in the U.K.* by D. H. H. Metcalfe, A. L. Rector, A. D.
   Clayden and L. Hallam (1977)
Medical Records in General Practice by L. I. Zander, S. A. A. Beresford and P.
   Thomas (*Occasional Paper 5,* Royal College of General Practitioners, 1978)
Running a Practice. A Manual of Practice Management by R. V. H. Jones, K. J.
   Bolden, D. J. Pereira Gray and M. S. Hall (2nd edn, Croom Helm, 1978)
Sick Health Centres – and How to Make them Better by G. Beales (Pitman, 1978)
An Analysis of Primary Medical Care. An International Study by W. J. Stephen
   (Cambridge University Press, 1979)
*Providing Primary Care from Health Centres and Similar Premises: Aspects of the
   Experience and Opinions of Patients and General Practitioners* by J. Bevan and
   G. Baker (*Health Service Research Unit Report No. 40,* University of Kent at
   Canterbury, 1979) is one of a series of reports on the same subject
Doctors on the Move by J. Bevan, D. Cunningham and C. Floyd (*Occasional Paper*

7, Royal College of General Practitioners, 1979) is an account of the organization of a doctor–nurse team

The Quality of Life. The Peckham Approach to Human Ethology by I. H. Pearse (Scottish Academic Press, 1979) is a health centre experiment of the 1940s, reviewed

Computing in General Practice. A Report for the General Medical Services Committee of the British Medical Association by P. Palmer and C. Rees (Scicon, 1980)

Computers and the General Practitioner edited by A. Malcolm and J. Poyser (Pergamon, 1982)

Health Centres in Devon. A Report to Devon Area Health Authority by J. Lyons (DAHA, 1982)

Premises

The Doctor's Surgery. A Practical Guide to the Planning of General Practice edited by W. A. R. Thomson (*Practitioner*, 1964) is a collection of articles from that journal

Design Guide for Medical Group Practice Centres by National Building Agency and College of General Practitioners (NBA, 1966)

Health Centres. A Design Guide by Department of Health and Social Security and Welsh Office (HMSO, 1970)

Design Guide: Health Centres in Scotland by Scottish Home and Health Department (HMSO, 1973)

Primary Health Care Buildings. Briefing and Design Guide for Architects and their Clients by R. Cammock (Architectural Press, 1981)

Staffing

Social Casework in a General Medical Practice by J. Collins (Pitman 1965)

Feeling the Pulse. A Survey of District Nursing in Six Areas by L. Hockey (Queen's Institute of District Nursing, 1966)

Social Casework in General Practice by J. A. S. Forman and E. M. Fairbairn (Oxford University Press, 1968)

Co-operation in Patient Care. Studies of District Nurses Attached to Hospital and General Medical Practices by L. Hockey and A. Buttimore (Queen's Institute of District Nursing, 1970)

The Evaluation of a Direct Nursing Attachment in a North Edinburgh Practice by S. W. MacGregor, M. A. Heasman and E. V. Kuenssberg (Scottish Health Service Studies, 1971)

Social Work in General Practice by E. M. Goldberg and J. E. Neill (Allen and Unwin, 1972)

Use or Abuse? A Study of the State-enrolled Nurse in the Local Authority Nursing Services by L. Hockey (Queen's Institute of District Nursing, 1972)

A Family Visitor. A Descriptive Analysis of Health Visiting in Berkshire by J. Clark (Royal College of Nursing and National Council of Nurses of the United Kingdom, 1973)

Dietitians in the Community. Report of an Exploratory Study by K. S. Dawes (Health Services Research Unit, University of Kent at Canterbury, 1974)

The Work of the Nursing Team in General Practice by M. Gilmore, N. Bruce and M. Hunt (Council for the Education and Training of Health Visitors, 1974)

The GP and the Primary Health Care Team by N. D. Mackichan (Pitman, 1976)

The Health Visitor in Primary Health Care. A General Study of Health Visitors in Two Health Centres and a Detailed Survey of the Contrasting Work Patterns in One Centre by E. Dautrey (Polytechnic of North London, 1976)

Team Care in General Practice by G. Marsh and P. Kaim-Caudle (Croom Helm, 1976)

Treatment Room Nursing. A Handbook for Nursing Sisters Working in General Practice, Schools and Industry by S. M. Jacka and D. G. Griffiths (Blackwell, 1976)

Physiotherapy in the Community. A Descriptive Study of Fourteen Schemes by C. J. Partridge and M. D. Warren (Health Services Research Unit, University of Kent at Canterbury, 1977)

Teamwork for Preventive Care by N. Bruce (Wiley, 1980)

Towards Team Care edited by J. H. Barber and C. R. Kratz (Churchill Livingstone, 1980)

Delegation in General Practice. A Study of Doctors and Nurses by A. Bowling (Tavistock, 1981)

The Medical Secretary's and Receptionist's Handbook by M. Drury (4th edn, Baillière Tindall, 1981)

The Primary Health Care Team. Report of a Joint Working Group of the Standing Medical Advisory Committee and the Standing Nursing and Midwifery Advisory Committee (DHSS, 1981)

Receptionists' Handbook by Department of Health and Social Security (DHSS, 1981)

Social Work and General Medical Practice, Collaboration or Conflict? by J. Huntington (Allen and Unwin, 1981)

An Evaluation of Health Visiting by J. Robinson (Council for the Education and Training of Health Visitors, 1982).

History

History in general is dealt with in Chapter 22, but the following may be useful additions:

The Growth of the General Practitioner of Medicine in England by N. G. Horner (Bridge and Co., 1922)

'The evolution of the general practitioner in England' by W. J. Bishop, in *Science, Medicine and History* edited by E. A. Underwood (vol 2, page 351, Oxford University Press, 1953)

Medical Practice in Modern England: The Impact of Specialization and State Medicine by R. Stevens (Yale University Press, 1966)

The Changing Scene in General Practice by I. Dopson (Johnson, 1971)

'Evolution of medical practice' by J. Brotherston, in *Medical History and Medical Care, A Symposium of Perspectives* edited by G. McLachlan and T. McKeown (Oxford University Press 1971)

The Division in British Medicine. A History of the Separation of General Practice from Hospital Care 1911–1968 by F. Honigsbaum (Kogan Page, 1979)

A Doctor for the People: 2000 Years of General Practice in Britain by J. Cule (Update, 1980)

The Family Doctor, His Life and History by R. Gibson (Allen and Unwin, 1981).

A History of the Royal College of Practitioners: the First 25 Years, edited by J. Fry *et al.* (MTP Press, 1983)

Two particularly interesting general-practice autobiographies or biographies are *Country Doctor* by G. Barber (Boydell Press, 1973) and *Will Pickles of Wensleydale. The Life of a Country Doctor* by J. Pemberton (Bles, 1970).

16

Information for patients and public

R. B. Tabor and R. E. Gann

Traditionally, medical libraries have been concerned with medical literature for professional use, with patients and public being excluded. Shapiro (Health education horizons and patient satisfaction, *Am. J. Public Health*, **62**, 229, 1972) described a new shape for health which included comprehensive health care, a focus on preventive medicine and patient satisfaction. An official view in the report *Prevention and Health, Everybody's Business: a Reassessment of Public and Personal Health* (HMSO, 1976) echoes and develops the theme that individuals must be responsible for their own health. Certainly, patients are rarely merely passive recipients of medical treatment and are expected to carry out therapeutic measures, including their own medication as advised by their doctor. These are some indications that patients and the public require to be better informed about health and medical matters. As an endorsement for this view there has been an increasing number of publications on medicine and health written with the public in mind.

Concurrent with this increase in commercial publication has developed a considerable body of 'literature' intended for patients and issued by hospitals, institutions and pharmaceutical companies. Most of this may be regarded as ephemera; generally it is part of a local hospital's patient education programme and changes with medical practice. M. Philbrook's *Medical Books for the Lay person: an Annotated Bibliography* (Boston Public Library, 1976) is an early attempt to list the range of books available. The staff of the library of the Health Sciences at the University of Illinois Medical Center have prepared a useful guide, *Sources of Health Information for Public Libraries* (University of Illinois Medical Center, 1976) as a result of a workshop conducted by Irwin Pizer for the Chicago Public Library system. This interest and concern that the public should have access to medical literature was expressed by the American Academy of Family Physicians; in 1975 the Academy issued a screened list of useful and free or inexpensive items, *Compendium of Patient Education Materials* (Kansas City, AAFP Reprint b-3500, 1975)

The use of popular medical literature in patient education programmes has been the subject of numerous articles by doctors and nurses. A. M. Rees edited a collection of accounts of such programmes, *Developing Consumer Health Information Services* (Bowker, 1982) in which are described several aspects of the 'new medical consumerism', together with reports of seven programmes where libraries were involved (both public and medical libraries). In this book Rees goes on to consider aspects of developing library services for patient/health education, including a section on networks and networking. A similar work by M. E. Madnick, *Consumer Health Education: a Guide to Hospital Based Programs* (Nursing Resources, 1980) concentrates on patient education activities and information sources. It is noteworthy that most of this literature is American and the programmes and sources described are not always readily transferable to British or European practice. A useful compilation of American practice in patient education was issued as vol 6, December 1971, of the *Nursing Clinics of North America: Symposium on Teaching Patients.* In *Self-care in Health* J. D. Williamson and K. Danaher (Croom Helm, 1978) explore the many aspects of self-care in an attempt to open up the subject for wider discussion. In particular they demonstrate the importance of the field of self-care in national, economic and personal health terms.

Patient compliance

The underlying purpose of this stream of patient education programmes is that of 'compliance' – getting the patient to carry out the instructions of the doctor. There is an authoritarian ring to much of this literature and some doctors prefer to use the term 'adherence' rather than compliance. The wide variation in terms used is an indicator of the differences of opinion about providing information for patients and the public. A particularly useful study of compliance is *Compliance with Therapeutic Regimens* by D. L. Sackett and R. B. Haynes (Johns Hopkins University Press, 1976). This book developed out of a workshop/symposium with the same title held at McMaster University Medical Center in May 1974. It contains several interesting chapters on individual behaviour relating to illness and complying with medical advice.

Underlying the theme of compliance lies the concept of informed consent and it has been regarded as a basic right for the patient to be informed about medical care. In the UK the Patients' Association has made some suggestions regarding such rights, but no formal declaration within the National Health Service has been declared. On the other hand, in America the Joint Commission on Accreditation of Hospitals has issued a statement of basic rights for patients, *Accreditation Manual for Hospitals* Joint Commission on Accreditation of Hospitals, 1980). This topic has received continuing attention in the periodical literature and forms a basis for the 1980 Reith Lectures,: *Unmasking of Medicine* by I. Kennedy (Allen and Unwin, 1981)

Primary sources

Directories and reference works

There is a considerable number of directories of voluntary organizations, patient associations and self-help groups, of varying quality. The most useful general directory of voluntary organizations is *Voluntary Organisations: an NCVO Directory* (National Council for Voluntary Organisations, 1982) which lists over 500 national organizations in alphabetical order, with a subject index. The directory covers all fields of voluntary activity, but there is a good health content. Of the directories dealing with health topics, *Directory for the Disabled* (3rd edn, Woodhead–Faulkner, 1981) is an indispensable guide to organizations, services and information materials for disabled people and those who work with them. Useful brief guides to health organizations include *Help! I Need Somebody* compiled by S. Knight (3rd edn, Kimpton, 1980) and *Self Help and the Patient: a Directory of National Organisations Concerned with Various Diseases and Handicaps* (8th edn, Patients' Association, 1982). Addresses of voluntary health care organizations change so frequently that directories can be out-of-date a year after publication. *The King's Fund Directory of Organisations for Patients and Disabled People* (King's Fund, 1979) was enormously useful on publication, but is no longer an essential work.

Social Services Year Book (Longman, annual) is worth the expense as a guide to addresses of statutory agencies (health, social services, social security, education) as well as voluntary bodies. *Charities Digest* (Family Welfare Association, annual) remains useful, if only for the many benevolent associations, while *Directory of Grant-making Trusts* (8th edn, Charities Aid Foundation, 1983) provides guidance through the maze of 2200 grant-making bodies.

For more specific groups of patients, the *Mental Health Year Book* (MIND, 1981) is a unique directory of government departments, health and local authorities, and voluntary organizations in the mental health field. Services for the blind are listed in *Directory of Agencies for the Blind in the British Isles and Overseas* (Royal National Institute for the Blind, 1980). Detailed information on financial help for disabled people is provided in *Disability Rights Handbook* (Disability Alliance, annual), complete with updating supplements. Aids are comprehensively described and illustrated in *Equipment for the Disabled* (Oxford Regional Health Authority, frequently updated).

Books

Popular medical publishing is a boom area and it is not possible here to list titles comprehensively. Instead, some general works are cited together with indications of other important series.

Written particularly for the patient is *The Penguin Medical Encyclopaedia* by P. Wingate (3rd edn, Penguin, 1983). Two useful works for anyone about to undergo surgery are *A Dictionary of Operations; A Handbook for Patients* by A. Stanway (Granada, 1981) and *A Patient's Guide to Operations* by D. Delvin (Penguin, 1981). A major work remains *Instructions for Patients* by H. Winter-Griffith (2nd edn, Saunders, 1975). This is a loose-leaf compilation of 350 instruction sheets of general information, treatment and warning signs on a wide variety of conditions for use in patient education. The sheets may be removed for photocopying and a copy given to the patient. The same author has produced a similar work on drug information designed for use by doctors and clinics, entitled *Drug Information for Patients* (Saunders, 1978), which is again in loose-leaf format. The intention is to take out the relevant page and photocopy it for the patient when medication is prescribed. The information given includes precautions, side-effects, storage, effects on daily living, and overdosage. A comparable British publication is *Medicines, A Guide for Everybody* by P. Parish (4th edn, Penguin, 1982).

An interesting alternative approach is provided by D. M. Vickery and J. F. Fries's *Take Care of Yourself: a Practical Do It Yourself Guide to Medical Care* (British edition adapted by J. A. M. Gray and S. A. Smail, Unwin, 1979). This uses algorithms to take the patient through key questions on common health problems and advises when to contact the doctor.

An encyclopaedic approach is taken in *Symptoms: the Complete Home Medical Encyclopedia* edited by S. Miller (Thomas Y. Crowell Co, 1979). This is in two parts, a listing of symptoms (using common names for them) and a well-illustrated list of diseases.

For specific health topics, several publishers have impressive lists of titles. The Oxford University Press *The Facts* series is written by leading consultants and gives authoritative descriptions of major conditions for the lay person. Titles include *Alcoholism, Arthritis and Rheumatism, Asthma, Back Pain, Breast Cancer, Cancer, Childhood Diabetes, Coronary Heart Disease, Depression, Epilepsy, Kidney Disease, Migraine, Multiple Sclerosis, Parkinson's Disease, Rabies, Sexually Transmitted Diseases* and *Stroke.*

Churchill Livingstone's *Patient Handbooks*, including *The Diabetic Child, You after Childbirth, Epilepsy Explained, Help for Bedwetting, High Blood Pressure*, and *All About Heart Attacks*, and the *Pocket Health Guides* published by Hamlyn, with *Allergies, Arthritis and Rheumatism, Back Pain, Children's Illnesses, Depression and Anxiety, Diabetes, Heart Trouble, The Menopause, Premenstrual Tension*, and *Skin Troubles*, all offer expert advice to the patient.

Other important publishers of books on health for patients and the public are the Consumer's Association, the Souvenir Press *Human Horizons* series and Penguin Books who, with titles like *Our Bodies Ourselves* and *Make it Happy* can provide a more stimulating antidote to a sometimes conservative field. Typical of the latter is the BMA *Family Doctor* series of 40 booklets for a lay readership, available through chemists' shops.

The Health Education Council and Scottish Health Education Group are responsible for a wide range of booklets, leaflets and posters on topics related to the promotion of good health (alcohol, smoking, diet, keeping fit, family planning and sex education). Most specialist patient organizations produce booklets on coping with specific handicaps and illnesses: the British Diabetic Association, the Chest, Heart and Stroke Association, the Association for Spina Bifida and Hydrocephalus, the Spastics Society, MENCAP and MIND all do so.

Access to the wealth of American literature on health topics, in the form of booklets and leaflets from government bodies, voluntary organizations, insurance companies and pharmaceutical firms, can now be had through a micropublishing venture *Consumer Health Information Service* (Microfilming Corporation of America).

Journals

Popular health topics abound in the press. Magazines devoted entirely to health for the lay person include *Doctor's Answers* (Marshall Cavendish) and *Advice* (Whinfrey Strachan). Both are intended to be collected in weekly parts to form a 'home medical encyclopaedia'. The *Home Medical Guide* (Hamlyn) is another part work, this time in a more useful card index form. *Mind and Body* (Marshall Cavendish) was issued during 1971–1973 as a popular background study, in serial form, to describe human anatomy and physiology for the layman. News of health education campaigns, new leaflets, posters and other information materials are given in the free and attractive *Health Education News* (Health Education Council). Also from the Health Education Council, *Health Education Journal* contains original articles describing and evaluating projects. Most useful in the professional literature is *Community Care* (IPC Business Press), a journal for social workers with original articles, news and reviews, usually with a reasonable health content. The monthly supplement to *Nursing Times*, *Community Outlook*, is particularly valuable for details of new lay health literature, with the emphasis on preventive health education rather than management of illness. Lively perspectives on voluntary activity in general are provided by *Voluntary Action* (National Council for Voluntary Organisations) and *Involve* (Volunteer Centre).

A new international journal (in English) appeared in 1979, *Patient Counselling and Health Education*, which is published quarterly by Excerpta Medica (Princeton, US). This periodical is intended for a professional audience and contains articles on patient education programmes.

Handicapped Living (A. E. Morgan Publications) adopts the popular magazine format for a wide range of features, reviews and information on all aspects of living with disability. *New Age* (Age Concern) is a similarly lively and glossy publication on issues affecting the elderly. Care of the child in hospital and the role of the parent are sympathetically covered in *NAWCH News* (National Association for the Welfare of Children in Hospital), while the rights and representation of the adult patient are aired in *Patient Voice* (Patients Association). Aimed at Community Health Councils,

CHC News (Association of Community Health Councils) is also valuable for patients' rights in hospital and community.

Most voluntary organizations and self-help groups publish journals or, at least, newsletters. These form a vital part of patient information, giving details of new advances in treatment and research, practical advice on self-care and notification of new publications and new addresses. In many cases a journal or newsletter is supplied as one of the benefits of membership of the organization. Particularly notable are *Spinal Injuries Association Newsletter,* a bulletin of practical information on self-care and social aspects of disability; *Parents Voice* (MENCAP), a readable journal for parents and professionals involved in mental handicap and *Balance* (British Diabetic Association), a newspaper for diabetics with features on research, diet, recreation and personal care. *Exchange* (National Eczema Society) and *Beyond the Ointment* (Psoriasis Association) are two well-produced and informative magazines for sufferers from skin disorders. For the past nine years *Mind Out* (MIND) has provided stimulating reading for all involved in mental health. Unfortunately this has now ceased publication but may be revived in another form.

Other periodicals of note include:

Arthritis News (Arthritis Care)
Communication and *Newsletter* (National Society for Autistic Children)
Talk Back (Back Pain Association)
Spastics News (Spastics Society)
Action (National Fund for Research into Crippling Diseases)
Cystic Fibrosis News (Cystic Fibrosis Research Trust)
Hearing (Royal National Institute for the Deaf)
Newsletter of the Down's Children's Association
Epilepsy News (British Epilepsy Association)
Fax (Friedreich's Ataxia Group)
Contact (RADAR)
Possability (Possum Users Association)
Progress (Disablement Income Group)
Responaut
Newsletter of the Association to Combat Huntington's Chorea
MS News (Multiple Sclerosis Society)
Muscular Dystrophy Group Journal
The Parkinson Newsletter (Parkinson's Disease Society)
News and Views (National Society for Phenylketonuria and Allied Disorders)
Newsletter of the National Association for Deaf, Blind and Rubella Handicapped
Newsletter of the Schizophrenia Association
AFASIC Newsletter (Association for Speech-Impaired Children)
Link (Association for Spina Bifida and Hydrocephalus),
Hope (Chest, Heart and Stroke Association)

Three more periodicals are worthy of special mention because of their interesting format. *Communications* (MENCAP) is a package containing briefing sheets on aspects of mental handicap together with copies of leaflets from a wide range of organizations. Summaries of features from the BBC Radio 4 programme for the blind, *In Touch,* are available in bulletin form or on tape cassette. Finally, as an example of a gold mine of information in a cheap duplicated format, there is the newsletter for parents of handicapped children, also called *In Touch* (edited by Mrs Ann Worthington from her home in Cheshire). It contains information not readily found elsewhere, including shared advice on coping with practical child care problems and personal contacts for a large number of very uncommon syndromes.

Broadcasting media

For many professionals, and certainly for patients and the public, television and radio are prime sources of health information and education.

Television programmes such as *Medical Express* (BBC 1) and *Where there's life . . .* (Yorkshire) present topical medical themes, but may be low on factual information. *Grapevine* (BBC 2) reports on self-help and the programmes are backed up with very informative fact sheets. Channel 4's *Wellbeing* concentrates on positive health and is also supported by information sheets.

On radio *Medicine Now* (Radio 4) is a magazine programme on new treatments and research. *Does he take sugar?* (Radio 4) provides practical advice and information, coupled with challenging features on disablement. *In Touch* (Radio 4) provides similar news and facts for blind people.

Viewdata systems have considerable potential for the provision of health and social information, particularly to disabled and housebound people. However, we are still waiting for the potential to be realized. *Prestel* carries a limited amount of health information from information providers, including the Health Education Council, British Medical Association and individual voluntary organizations. *Ceefax* (BBC) and *Oracle* (IBA) are chiefly useful for providing subtitles for the hard of hearing.

The Volunteer Centre's Media Project has looked at the role of broadcasting in the broad field of social action. A periodical, *Media Project News,* and the *Directory of Social Action Programmes* describe national and local television and radio programmes on health topics.

Secondary sources

Indexes and abstracts

Popular Medical Index (Clover Publications) is a unique index to health literature at a lay level in the form of books, selected professional journals *(BMJ, Lancet, Nursing Times, Nursing Mirror, Scientific American)* and popular magazines, including women's magazines. Positive health, illness and disability, medical treatment and alternative medicine are all covered. It is published quarterly with an annual cumulation.

The literature of voluntary activity, including health and social welfare, is covered by *Voluntary Forum Abstracts* (NCVO Volunteer Centre); included are books, reports and descriptions of projects in the journal literature.

Current awareness

Abstracts of published reports of health education and patient information activities and descriptions of ongoing projects appear in *Current Awareness in Health Education Abstracts* (US Department of Health and Human Services: Center for Health Promotion and Education). The emphasis is on American projects, but there is also coverage of British and European practice.

The Health Education Council lists, *Recent Additions to the Library* and *Recent Additions to the Resource Centre,* provide current awareness of print and audio-visual material, respectively, which might be used in patient education. Material for primary prevention and the management of illness is included. Also from the Health Education Council is *Journal Articles of Interest to Health Educators* which lists reports of educational and information activities in the professional literature.

In the specific field of mental handicap, *BIMH Current Awareness Service* (British Institute of Mental Handicap) lists current book and journal literature for patients, parents and professionals.

The monthly guide to medical literature, *British Medicine* (Pergamon), includes a 'miscellaneous' section listing books for the lay person.

There are several indispensable information bulletins providing up-to-date details of publications, organizations and events. *Information Service for the Disabled* (Disabled Living Foundation) is essential. It consists of a current-awareness newsletter and a set of constantly updated information sheets on all aspects of disabled living, in particular aids and equipment. *RADAR Bulletin* (Royal

Association for Disability and Rehabilitation) and *MSS Bulletin* (Multiple Sclerosis Society) provide valuable current information on physical disability, while *MIND Information Bulletin* covers the field of mental health.

Information Service for Voluntary Organisations (National Council for Voluntary Organisations) is an updating service on all spheres of voluntary activity, and lists new organizations and publications. Abstracts of research and summaries of reports in the field of childhood and adolescence may be found in *Highlights* (National Children's Bureau).

Bibliographies and source lists

Among the American source guides to health information is a specific group of publications on self-help. These include information on self-diagnosis and self-treatment. Mostly these are intended to be complementary to advice from doctors, but the self-help approach is strongly emphasized.

Medical Self-care: Access to Health Tools edited by T. Ferguson (Summit Books, 1980) is a popular guide to self-help resources. This is a compilation of the first eight issues of *Medical Self-care*, which is a continuing popular health magazine, specially interesting for its *Whole Earth Catalog* format and its crisp presentation – at least for the American audience.

A most important and complementary guide to self-help is *Health: a Multimedia Source Guide* by J. Ash and M. Stevenson (R. R. Bowker, 1976). This is a guide to groups, companies, government agencies, libraries and research institutes which can provide information on specialist aspects of health or medicine. If the answer to a health enquiry is not found in the literature, this guide indicates where else the information may be found.

A useful compendium of information designed for libraries to assist them in selecting relevant information materials is *Serving Physically Disabled People: an Information Handbook for all Libraries* by R. A. Velleman (R. R. Bowker, 1979). A valuable first section introduces the problems of disability and this is followed by separate sections on the public library, the special rehabilitation library and school and university libraries. The book is more than a guide to resources, containing as it does much background information which puts the resources mentioned into context.

Health information

American material on health information for patients and the public has been surveyed in some detail by A. M. Rees and B. A. Young in *The Consumer Health Information Sourcebook* (Bowker, 1981). This authoritative guide reviews the needs of 'consumers' for health information and goes on to provide an annotated guide to reference works, bibliographies and primary sources for patient education. English language and Spanish materials are included.

The National Institutes of Health of the US Department of Health and Human Services are major publishers of lay health literature. *Health Information Resources in the Department of Health and Human Services* (National Health Information Clearinghouse, 1980, DHHS (PHS) Publication No 80–50146) is a directory of Federal and Federally-sponsored health information resources and their publications. Also available is *NIH Publications List* (National Institutes of Health, 1979, NIH Publication No 80–6), a list of booklets for health professionals and the public arranged by the issuing body.

In Britain there are no overall sources guides to health information for the public. *Health Education Council Publications List*, coupled with *Scottish Health Education Group Material Catalogue*, provides access to a wide range of largely free health education publications. The Health Education Council also publishes a series of excellent source lists on individual topics. Other publication lists worth mentioning are those issued by Disabled Living Foundation, RADAR (an essential directory of access guides) and MIND.

The Wessex Regional Library and Information Service series, *Communication*, is a unique set of guides to information suitable for patients on individual medical conditions. A brief general outline of the condition is followed by details of helpful organizations, publications, audio-visual materials and background reading. Also from Wessex, *Getting Started: Collecting and Organising Patient Information* by R. E. Gann (WRLIS, 1982) is an information pack containing a core bibliography of patient information literature together with advice on collecting, organizing and keeping up-to-date with literature and organizations.

While concentrating on civil rights and social welfare, *Know How to Find Out Your Rights* by G. Morby (2nd edn, Pluto Press, 1982) has a useful health section of particular relevance to mental health. Health information in the languages of ethnic minorities can be hard to trace. *Community Information (Asian Languages) Directory* (National Association of Citizens Advice Bureau and Commission for Racial Equality, 1980) and *Directory of Information Materials in non-Asian Languages* (London Voluntary Service Council, 1981) are therefore invaluable. A guide to the literature of alternative medicine is available in *Alternative Medicine: Readers' Guide* compiled by I. Thompson (Library Association Public Libraries Group, 1981)

Biography and fiction can provide an insight into the experience of illness and disability for professional and patient alike. *Reflections: a Subject Guide to works of Fiction, Biography and Autobiography on Medical and Related Topics* edited by R. B. Tabor (2nd edn, Wessex Regional Library Information Service, 1983) is an extensive guide to English-language material. More specifically for children's literature is *Notes from a Different Drummer: a Guide to Juvenile Fiction Portraying the Handicapped* by B. H. Baskin and K. H. Harris (Bowker, 1977). Meanwhile, *Dying, Grief and Death: a Critically Annotated Bibliography* by M. A. Simpson (Plenum, 1979) includes many fictional and biographical works.

17

Psychiatry

H. Marshall*; revised by H. E. Taylor

Psychiatry is a medical discipline and its literature is part of the literature of medicine. It therefore draws heavily upon the usual medical and biological sciences, but at the same time it extends further than most of its fellow medical disciplines into the behavioural and social sciences, as well as into the arts and humanities. In what follows the basic literature of medicine and biology is taken for granted: it is assumed that readers interested in psychiatric literature have recourse to the journals, abstracts, indexes, reviews textbooks and reference works that form the staple medical bibliographical tools. *Index Medicus* and *Science Citation Index,* for example, are just as useful in psychiatry as in the rest of medicine and the special sources dealt with in this chapter supplement, but do not supplant, the general medical sources covered elsewhere in the book. The information explosion, too, has been taken for granted and it is not considered necessary to stress that psychiatry is affected by it in the same way as the rest of the medical field.

Figure 17.1 shows the main areas and topics covered by psychiatry and its related disciplines. The material quoted in the present chapter is for the most part confined to the 'inner circle' of *Figure 17.1,* with fewer side glances towards medicine and biology which are covered by other sections of the book, than towards the behavioural and social sciences, with which the user of medical literature may be less familiar. A search for information in psychiatry can lead readers along strange paths. They may find

* Formerly Librarian, Institute of Psychiatry, University of London

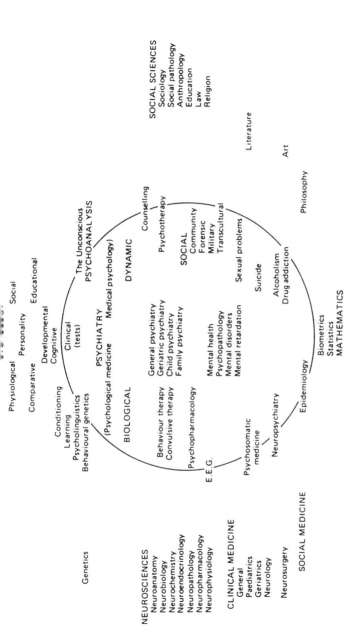

Figure 17.1 Psychiatry and its related disciplines (adapted from Elliot, 1971)

themselves involved in molecular pharmacology or in hallucinogenic art; in the intricacies of repertory grid techniques or in the latest in existentialist thought; in a study of biogenic amines in sleep or in Freudian analysis of the content of dreams. This chapter, while trying to help readers on their way, pays less attention to biochemical maturation of the brain, say, than to disorders of childhood behaviour.

Psychiatry has been fortunate in its documentalists, who have included psychiatrists, psychologists and librarians. Hack Tuke, a nineteenth-century psychiatrist and member of a famous family of psychiatrists, compiled a very useful *Dictionary of Psychological Medicine* (1892), which included signed articles by contributors from many countries, synonyms in four languages, notes on bibliographical aids and on societies interested in psychiatry, lists of periodicals and a chronological bibliography of important publications from 1584 to 1892. C. M. Louttit, a psychologist and one-time editor of *Psychological Abstracts,* published a comprehensive *Handbook of Psychological Literature* (1932) which contained much that is still of psychiatric relevance. In more modern times C. K. Elliott, a psychologist, prepared a *Guide to the Documentation of Psychology* (Bingley, 1971); B. Ennis, a psychiatrist, published a *Guide to the Literature in Psychiatry* (1971); and E. Cosyns-Verhaegen, a Belgian librarian, has compiled a union catalogue of psychiatric works in Belgian libraries which provides a useful bibliography of psychiatry and general psychopathology, geriatric psychiatry, drug dependence and criminology (1972–1974).

This chapter begins with the main sources of information in general psychiatry, goes on to deal with special divisions of psychiatry and related fields, and ends with a brief guide to biographical and historical literature. Most of the items mentioned are well documented by Elliott or Ennis, as well as by Blake and Roos in their *Medical Reference Works, 1679–1966* (Medical Library Association, 1967) and supplements (*see* page 70).

General psychiatry

Periodicals

The general psychiatric journals reflect the history and nature of the subject. Traditionally, they began as the journals of professional bodies concerned with the care of the mentally ill, and most of the leading national journals of psychiatry are still the organs of the corresponding national association. Their changes in title, like those of their parent societies, indicate changing concepts of and attitudes towards mental illness. The *British Journal of Psychiatry* is a typical example; beginning life in 1853 as the *Asylum Journal of Mental Science,* it changed its title in 1859 to *Journal of Mental Science* and again in 1963 to the *British Journal of Psychiatry.* Its sponsoring body, which was originally the Association of Medical Officers of Asylums and Hospitals for the Insane, later became the Medico-Psychological Association, then the Royal College of Psychiatrists. The American Psychiatric Association and its journal, the *American Journal of Psychiatry,* have been undergoing similar changes since 1844, always in the general direction of acceptability and respectability.

Traditionally, too, psychiatric periodicals used to cover both psychiatry and neurology, but in the last two decades many such journals have split into two separate publications. The *Archives of Neurology and Psychiatry,* for example, divided in 1959 into the *Archives of Neurology* and the *Archives of General Psychiatry,* while *Acta Psychiatrica et Neurologica Scandinavica* similarly changed, in 1961, to *Acta Psychiatrica Scandinavica* and *Acta Neurologica Scandinavica.* This divorce of general psychiatry from general neurology has been accompanied by an increase in interdisciplinary journals of a more specialized kind, many in what have come to be called the neurosciences. *Psychopharmacology* (1959–) (formerly *Psychopharmacologia), Neuropsychologia* (1963–), *Psychophysiology* (1964–), *Physiology and Behavior* (1966–), *Pharmacology, Biochemistry and Behavior* (1973–) and *Journal of Clinical Neuropsychology* (1979–) are examples of such periodicals reporting material from new, hybrid disciplines. They are usually not confined to one country or continent and sometimes publish papers in more than one language: many are commercially published journals with editorial boards that include distinguished workers from several countries, from more than one discipline, and from many centres of research. They come into being when their area of interest reaches a stage at which, as the introductory editorial of *Psychophysiology* put it, a worker has 'to search through more than eighty different journals to find all the articles being written by his colleagues'; and they help scientists in neighbouring disciplines to find out what is going on in their field.

In addition to this overlap with the neurosciences, psychiatry has, of course, always had its subdivision, as well as an intimate and intricate relationship with psychology and later with psychoanalysis. Some of its branches are esoteric, semantically confusing and often subtle, as journal titles sometimes show. Thus one might expect a journal of 'medical psychology' to be slanted towards 'dynamic' psychiatry and psychoanalysis, and a journal of 'psychological medicine' to be more concerned with biological psychiatry. Within the dynamic, psychoanalytical area, 'psychoanalysis' in a title implies a Freudian approach, 'individual psychology' the school of Adler, and 'analytical psychology' the school of Jung. 'Psychosomatic' may imply psychological or dynamic interpretations of physical disorders, or it may cover the more general concept of psychophysical relations. The second half of this century has seen the emergence of more obvious and increasingly autonomous disciplines within psychiatry, each with its own body of literature: there are thus journals which specialize in child psychiatry, geriatric psychiatry and social psychiatry, and in particular methods of treatment, such as group analysis or behaviour therapy.

With the advent of so many special journals, the general journals of psychiatry inevitably now contain less original material from the borderlands and special divisions of the subject. Some of them have become, perhaps, more 'clinical' in their choice of original papers and, particularly if they are the journals of national associations, they have come to act also as alerting or secondary sources of information by publishing review articles, supplements and special publications devoted to particular areas of interest. The following are the main general psychiatric journals, with indications, where appropriate, of their sponsoring bodies.

ENGLISH LANGUAGE

Acta Psychiatrica Scandinavica (and *Supplements*)
American Journal of Orthopsychiatry (American Orthopsychiatric Association; originally specialized in child psychiatry, but is now more general)
American Journal of Psychiatry (American Psychiatric Association)
Archives of General Psychiatry (American Medical Association)
Australian and New Zealand Journal of Psychiatry (Royal Australian and New Zealand College of Psychiatrists)
Biological Psychiatry (Society of Biological Psychiatry)
British Journal of Medical Psychology (British Psychological Society)
British Journal of Psychiatry (Royal College of Psychiatrists)
Canadian Journal of Psychiatry (formerly *Canadian Psychiatric Association Journal;* publishes in French and English)
Comprehensive Psychiatry (American Psychopathological Association)
International Journal of Mental Health
Journal of Clinical Psychiatry (formerly *Diseases of the Nervous System*)
Journal of Nervous and Mental Disease
Journal of Neurology, Neurosurgery and Psychiatry (British Medical Association)
Journal of Psychiatric Research
Psychiatric Quarterly (New York School of Psychiatry)
Psychiatry (William Alanson White Psychiatric Foundation: mainly socioanalytic)
Psychological Medicine (and *Supplements*)

OTHER LANGUAGES

Annales Médico-Psychologiques (Société Médico-Psychologique)
Evolution Psychiatrique
Fortschritte der Neurologie, Psychiatrie und ihrer Grenzgebiete
Nervenarzt (Deutsche Gesellschaft für Psychiatrie und Nervenheilkunde)
Perspectives Psychiatriques
Psychiatria Clinica (accepts papers in English, French and German)
Psychiatrie, Neurologie und Medizinische Psychologie (Gesellschaft für Psychiatrie und Neurologie)
Schweizer Archiv für Neurologie, Neurochirurgie und Psychiatrie (Schweizerische Neurologische Gesellschaft und Schweizerische Gesellschaft für Psychiatrie; publishes in French and German, and occasionally in Italian and English)
Zhurnal Nevropatologii Psikhiatrii imeni S. S. Korsakova

It is a measure of the acceptance of English as an international language that some of the above foreign-language journals accept papers in English and that in some countries psychiatric journals in English appear regularly (*Indian Journal of Psychiatry, Israel Journal of Psychiatry and Related Sciences* and *Psychiatria Fennica* – a Finnish yearbook of psychiatry).

More complete lists of journals are to be found in Elliott (1971) and Ennis (1971), and in the annual *List of Journals Indexed in Index Medicus.*

Abstracts, indexes, bibliographies

The global abstracting services most relevant to psychiatry are *Psychological Abstracts* and *Excerpta Medica (Section 32: Psychiatry)* and, to a lesser extent, *Biological Abstracts, Chemical Abstracts (Biochemistry Section)* and *Sociological Abstracts.* The most important general indexes are *Index Medicus, Science Citation Index* and *Current Contents* (especially *Current Contents, Life Sciences* and *Current Contents, Social and Behavioral Sciences*).

Few journals of general psychiatry now publish abstracts of current literature: they tend more to issue abstracts of papers scheduled to appear in forthcoming numbers of their own journal. Of the services which are still provided, the most comprehensive is that given by the *Annales Médico-Psychologiques.* The privately published *Digest of Neurology and Psychiatry* (Institute of Living, 200 Retreat Avenue, Hartford, Conn. 06107 US) appears 10 times per annum and is supplied free of charge to physicians throughout the world: with about 450 descriptive abstracts a year, it is naturally highly selective, but it is useful and includes book reviews. The *Zentralblatt für die gesamte Neurologie und Psychiatrie – Neurology-Psychiatry* issues critical abstracts in psychiatry and neurology: its coverage is international and includes chapters from books, but there is a fairly long time-lag before abstracts appear.

The Hall-Brooke Foundation (Professional Library, 47 Long Lots Rd, Westport. Conn. 06881, US) issues a monthly *Selected List of Tables of Contents of Psychiatric Periodicals,* for which a small charge is now made, and Cleveland State Hospital provides a similar monthly listing of neuropsychiatric literature. Both these publications are supported in part by the pharmaceutical industry.

Several regular current-awareness services are helpful. For example, the British Department of Health and Social Security (DHSS) issues *Current Literature on Health Services* monthly, which has sections on both Psychiatric Services and the Mentally Handicapped, while the Humberside Health Authority's Information and Reference Service publishes *Care of the Mentally Disordered,* a free, monthly annotated list covering mental handicap, mental illness and psychogeriatrics. Current psychiatric bibliographies can most usefully be obtained from periodical articles, reviews and monographs, and the Royal College of Psychiatrists, London, issues a *Reading List,* now appearing in a new series (1979) of general and specialist lists covering a wide area of the psychiatric field. Three American psychiatrists (J. B. Woods *et al, Bull. Med. Libr. Ass.,* **56,** 404, 1968) have published a list of basic psychiatric literature (articles and article sources) obtained from the recommended reading lists in 140 training programmes. The writers found that, out of the 4000 articles recommended, about 300 received a third of the total recommendations, and these they list in their article. They also found that many of the articles came from books such as the *American Handbook of Psychiatry* or the *Standard Edition* of Freud, and by concentrating on 26 such publications they claimed that the 'purchase of relatively few works will enable a small library to obtain a significant amount of the basic material in psychiatry'. The selection has a distinct American and psychoanalytic bias and, while admittedly compiled along very different lines, shows surprisingly little overlap with the Royal College of Psychiatrists list.

Older bibliographies may be found in Blake and Roos (1967) and some special bibliographies are included under the appropriate divisions covered below.

Reviews

There are not many review journals in psychiatry. *Seminars in Psychiatry* (1969–1972) devoted each of its issues to a specific topic, providing good current surveys of the areas covered. Since the journal ceased publication, the series has been continued in book form as *Seminars in Psychiatry*, a monograph series issued irregularly by Grune and Stratton. *Psychiatric Clinics of North America* (1978–), appearing three times a year, covers a single subject in each issue: August 1982, for example, deals with Pediatric Liaison Psychiatry. *Fortschritte der Neurologie und Psychiatrie* provides, in addition to original papers, planned coverage of special subjects; for example, a review of the literature on obsessions (1947–1970) took over from a similar review published in the same journal in 1949 covering the years 1918 to 1947. The Group for the Advancement of Psychiatry, a division of the American Psychiatric Association, publishes its *Reports and Symposia* in journal form, each issue reviewing a topical theme. Many of the general psychiatric journals run regular or occasional reviews or 'current status' articles, and the British Journal of Psychiatry issues *Special Publications* which have, to date, surveyed areas such as psychogeriatrics, schizophrenia and the affective disorders. The *Acta Psychiatrica Scandinavica Supplements*, while publishing original material, often supply good incidental reviews.

The main annual publications are *Progress in Neurology and Psychiatry* (Grune and Stratton, 1946–), in which specialists review different fields, including the basic sciences, each being covered at least biennially, and the *Year Book of Psychiatry and Applied Mental Health*, which separated in 1970 from the *Year Book of Neurology, Psychiatry and Neurosurgery* (Year Book Publications).

Conferences, monographs, books

Conferences on psychiatric themes are numerous and their proceedings, like so many conference proceedings, are often tantalizingly difficult to run to earth. Sometimes the journals published by relevant associations provide the only clue and perhaps the only published reports that appear. The World Psychiatric Association organizes a World Congress every five years, of which six have now been held and the proceedings of which are published, latterly by Excerpta Medica. Many other organizations publish annual proceedings, one of the most important being the Association for Research in Nervous and Mental Disease, whose proceedings have appeared regularly since 1920. Each year a specific topic is covered: for example, *Social Psychiatry* (No 47), *Addictive States* (No 46) or *Brain Dysfunction in Metabolic Disorders* (No 53). Most of its publications go out of print very quickly, but some have been reprinted by Hafner. They are quoted variously under their individual editors and titles, or as *ARNMD Transactions*, or just as *ARNMD*, but recent volumes give their official abbreviation as *Res. Publ. Assoc. Res. nerv. ment. Dis.* and this is how they are indexed in *Index Medicus*. *Recent Advances in Biological Psychiatry* used to appear as the annual conference report of the Society of Biological Psychiatry, but changed in 1969 to the bi-monthly journal, *Biological Psychiatry*. Another regular series is issued by the American Psychopathological Association, whose annual meetings are again devoted to a single theme: they are often quoted by editors and title, the editors for many years being P. H. Hoch and J. Zubin.

Monograph series in psychiatry include the *Nervous and Mental Disease Monographs*, which began in 1907 and of which Ennis (1971) lists 85 up to the end of 1954. They provided translations of many of the early German works in psychoanalysis. The *Maudsley Monographs*, published by Oxford University Press for the Institute of Psychiatry, began in 1955 and have now reached No 26.

The number of books published on psychiatric topics is increasing enormously. Psychiatry is clearly popular with the lay as well as with the professional reader, and paperbacks now abound. Guides to new books are to be found principally in the review section of journals and in their lists of books received. *Contemporary Psychology*, which is the book review journal published by the American Psychological Association, is a good source of psychiatric book reviews. Another useful publication was the *Mental Health Book Review Index* (1956–1973), which annually listed books that had had three or more reviews in some 225 journals scanned for the purpose by an editorial committee and their librarian collaborators. It ceased publication in 1973, but has had a welcome resurrection as the *Chicorel Index to Mental Health Book Reviews* (1976–). For the years already covered, it provided valuable information, and those interested in the documentation of psychiatry will also find in it unusual editorials with titles such as 'The developmental sciences: a bibliographical analysis of a trend', or 'Lectureships in the behavioural sciences: an introduction to socio-bibliography'. Book catalogues issued by booksellers are also of interest: the psychiatry section of H. K. Lewis's *Medical Book List* and H. Karnac's *Psychoanalysis and Psychotherapy*, and H. K. Lewis's catalogue on *Psychology, Psychoanalysis and Allied Subjects* deserve special mention.

A more comprehensive list of books is given in K. Menninger's *Guide to Psychiatric Books in English* (3rd edn, Grune and Stratton, 1972) which lists books under 17 main headings and 26 sub-headings. Ennis (1971) also gives a book list, under 53 headings. Cosyns-Verhaegen's union catalogue of psychiatric books in Belgian libraries has already been mentioned. J. B. Woods *et al.*, whose list of basic articles was cited under Bibliographies above, also compiled a list of the most frequently recommended books. From 87 reading lists (nearly 2500 books and neary 10 000 recommendations) which were considered by their sponsors to cover the basic literature that a psychiatric resident should read in the course of three years' training, they arrived at 104 books which received one-third of the total recommendations. They list these books under ten broad headings, the most popular subjects being psychoanalytic theories of personality, schizophrenia, psychotherapy and child psychiatry (*Bull. Med. Libr. Ass.*, **56**, 295, 1968). The Royal College of Psychiatrists, London, has issued a *List of Books Suitable for a Psychiatric Library (Brit. J. Psychiat. Spec. Publ. No. 12*, 1977), which ranges widely over topics considered by a committee of the College to be of interest and relevance to psychiatrists; it is, however, now somewhat out of date.

The author catalogue of the Tavistock Joint Library, London, was published in 1975 by G. K. Hall. It lists approximately 10 000 books and 5500 pamphlets, the main areas covered being psychology, psychiatry, psychoanalysis, sociology and the study of organizations. The library now has a very full subject index and a subject catalogue will shortly be published by G. K. Hall.

It is difficult to select individual books for mention here, and the short list given below is therefore limited to textbooks which can range from the clinical notes issued by university psychiatric departments for the use of their undergraduate medical students to comprehensive multi-volume and highly expensive publications. The following are some of the standard current titles:

American Handbook of Psychiatry (2nd edn, 6 vols, Basic Books, 1972–1975)
Companion to Psychiatric Studies by A. Forrest (2nd edn, Churchill Livingstone, 1978)
Comprehensive Textbook of Psychiatry edited by H. I. Kaplan *et al.* (3rd edn, 3 vols, Williams and Wilkins, 1980)
Henderson and Gillespie's Textbook of Psychiatry revised by I. Batchelor (10th edn, Oxford University Press, 1969)
Guide to Psychiatry by M. Sim (4th edn, Churchill Livingstone, 1981)
Clinical Psychiatry by Mayer-Gross *et al.* (3rd edn by E. Slater and M. Roth, Baillière Tindall, 1969).

Chapters on psychiatry in general textbooks of medicine should not be overlooked. Mention might also be made of the 'up-dating' publications entitled *Recent Advances in Clinical Psychiatry* (1 by K. Granville-Grossman, 2, 3 and 4 edited by K. Granville-Grossman, Churchill Livingstone, 1971, 1976, 1979, 1982).

As books in libraries are usually classified, it is perhaps appropriate to mention that the bibliographical classification of psychiatry often presents difficulties. Special libraries devoted to psychiatry and its related disciplines are sometimes tempted to abandon the general or medical classification schemes discussed in an earlier chapter and to evolve schemes of their own. One such scheme is used in psychiatric libraries in Belgium (*Classification Psychiatrique Belge*, Cosyns-Verhaegen *et al.*, Brussels, Fondation Julie Renson, 1967). Another has been devised by the Royal College of Psychiatrists, London, and is used in its book list mentioned above. The Belgian scheme is a simple one, with seven main categories and not many subdivisions, except in psychiatry. The Royal College of Psychiatrists scheme has 25 main categories and more elaborate subdivisions in psychiatry and in its related fields.

Reference works

Encyclopaedias and dictionaries of psychiatry are well covered by Ennis (1971), Elliott (1971) and Menninger (1972). The definitions provided in them are apt to vary according to the point of view of the authors or editors and it is as well for the uninitiated to consult more than one. English-language dictionaries of psychiatry and psychology include H. B. and A. C. English's *Comprehensive Dictionary of Psychological and Psychoanalytical Terms* (Longmans, 1958); M. Calman's *Dictionary of Psychoanalysis* (W. H. Allen, 1979); L. E. Hinsie and R. J. Campbell's *Psychiatric Dictionary* (5th edn, Oxford University Press, 1981); *A Concise Encyclopaedia of Psychiatry* edited by D. Leigh *et al.* (MTP, 1977); the *Encyclopaedia of Psychology* edited by H. J. Eysenck *et al.* (3 vols, Search Press, 1972), which has appeared in German as *Lexikon der Psychologie* as well as in French, Italian, Portuguese and Spanish; and B. B. Wolman's *International Encyclopaedia of Psychiatry, Psychology, Psychoanalysis and Neurology* in 12 vols (Van Nostrand Reinhold, 1977).

An important American publication on diagnostic classification is the *Diagnostic and Statistical Manual of Mental Disorders DSM-III* (American Psychiatric Association, 1980). English glossaries have been published by the General Register Office (revised by the Office of Population Censuses and Surveys) – *Glossary of Mental Disorders* (1968; amended 1973); by the American Psychiatric Association – *A Psychiatric Glossary* (5th edn, 1980); and by the World Health Organization – *Mental Disorders: a Glossary and Guide to their Classification in accordance with the Ninth Revision of the International Classification of Diseases* (1978). The WHO glossary is available in all the main languages and is the basis of most of the official national glossaries and classifications. The World Psychiatric Association has issued *Common Psychiatric Terms* in four languages – English, French, German, Spanish (Sandoz, for the WPA, 1971), a similar publication being L. Moor's *English–French–German Glossary for Psychiatry, Child Psychiatry and Abnormal Psychology* (Expansion Scientifique Française, 1965). An interesting French publication is the psychiatric section of the *Encyclopédie Médico-Chirurgicale*, which is loose-leaf and decimally paginated, so that it can be kept up to date by supplementary pages and replacement of entire articles. A standard German dictionary is Ch. Müller's *Lexicon der Psychiatrie* (Springer, 1973).

The *Directory of World Psychiatry*, issued by the World Psychiatric Association in 1971 with a supplement in 1977, lists hospitals and institutions dealing with the mentally ill in 89 countries and Van Nostrand Reinhold publish a *Mental Health Year Book Directory* edited by J. Norback (1979–1980). A new venture by MIND (National Association for Mental Health, London) is the *Mental Health Year Book* (1981/82) which brings together a wide range of information on British mental health services and voluntary organizations, together with background articles, a glossary of psychiatric terms and a selected reading list and list of relevant journals.

Another recent useful publication is Bette Greenberg's *How to Find Out in Psychiatry: a Guide to Sources of Mental Health Information* (Pergamon, 1978).

Special divisions of psychiatry

The sources of information already mentioned are, of course, relevant also for special divisions of psychiatry, as are sources in general medicine. Thus, the *Annual Review of Pharmacology* should not be overlooked in a search for recent information in psychopharmacology, while *Progress in Neurology and Psychiatry* may well contain a good review of child psychiatry, and *The Lancet* and the *British Medical Journal* publish articles and reviews in special areas of psychiatry as well as in more general medical and psychiatric fields.

Alcoholism and drug addiction

There has always been a steady flow of literature on this subject, but the recent increase of interest in addictive and hallucinogenic drugs has caused this area to have a small information explosion of its own. The main periodicals are the *American Journal of Drug and Alcohol Abuse*, the *British Journal of Addiction*, the *International Journal of the Addictions*, the *Journal* (formerly *Quarterly Journal) of Studies on Alcohol*, which also publishes a supplement at irregular intervals (now at No 8) and the United Nations' *Bulletin on Narcotics*.

So far as alcoholism is concerned, the *Journal of Studies on Alcohol* provides the chief secondary source of information, alternate issues being devoted entirely to documentation of current literature. The Center of Alcohol Studies of Rutgers University, which sponsors this journal, have also published the *International Bibliography of Studies on Alcohol* edited by M. Keller (3 vols, 1966) which covers the periods 1901–1950 and 1951–1960 with Index, and until 1976 they issued abstracts on punched cards under the title *Classified Abstract Archive of the Alcohol Literature (CAAAL)*. The *Alcoholism Digest Annual* provides yearly reviews. Early bibliographies are to be found in what are still standard texts on the subject: E. M. Jellinek's *Alcoholic Addiction and Chronic Alcoholism* (Yale University Press, 1942) and the same author's *Disease Concept of Alcoholism* (Hillhouse Press, 1960).

Abstracts on drug abuse and addiction are provided in *Drug Dependence* (Excerpta Medica, Section 40, 1972–), in *Criminology and Penology Abstracts*, in *Criminal Justice Abstracts (*formerly *Crime and Delinquency Literature)* and in the usual psychiatric abstracting journals. There are many special bibliographies within the general area of drug abuse and addiction, including *Drugs of Addiction and Non-addiction, their Use and Abuse. A Comprehensive Bibliography, 1960–1969* (Whitston, 1970) and a supplement, *Drug Abuse Bibliography, 1970* (1971), L. A. Moore's *Marijuana (Cannabis) Bibliography, 1960–1968* (Bruin Humanist Forum, 1969), the US National Clearinghouse for Mental Health Information's *Bibliography on Drug Dependence and Abuse, 1928–1966* (1969) and Unesco's *Cannabis Bibliography* (1965). The official reports of the Advisory Committee on Drug Dependence (*Cannabis*, HMSO, 1968, and *Amphetamines and Lysergic Acid Diethylamide*, HMSO, 1970) are also worth mentioning.

Child psychiatry, child psychology and allied disciplines

Child psychiatry and child psychology are so interwoven and so closely allied to other disciplines that most of their periodicals cover a fairly wide range of subjects. The main journals are the *Journal of the American Academy of Child Psychiatry*, the *Journal of Child Psychology and Psychiatry and Allied Disciplines*, the *Journal of Abnormal Child Psychology* and *Acta Paedopsychiat-*

rica. The *American Journal of Orthopsychiatry,* which began as a journal of child psychiatry, still publishes many articles in this field. In related disciplines the most relevant periodicals are *Child Development, Developmental Psychology, Developmental Medicine and Child Neurology, Early Child Development and Care, Exceptional Children,* the *Journal of Experimental Child Psychology* and the *Merrill-Palmer Quarterly – Journal of Developmental Psychology.* Journals of education and of paediatrics are also of interest, as are journals of sociology such as *Family Process* and *Journal of Marriage and the Family.*

Abstracts appear in *Acta Paedopsychiatrica,* in *Child Development Abstracts and Bibliography* (which includes book reviews and lists of books received) and in *Developmental Medicine and Child Neurology.* Annual reviews are found in *Psychoanalytic Study of the Child* (Yale University Press, now at vol 36), which has a useful *Abstracts and Index* volume covering the first 25 years; in *Annual Progress in Child Psychiatry and Development* (Brunner-Mazel, 1968–), which is an annual collection of reprints; in *Advances in Child Development and Behavior* (Academic Press, 1963–); in the *Minnesota Symposia on Child Psychology* (University of Minnesota Press, 1967–); and in *Review of Child Development Research* (University of Chicago Press, now at vol 5). The *Monographs of the Society for Research in Child Development* have been appearing since 1935. *A Multi-Axial Classification of Child Psychiatric Disorders* by M. Rutter *et al.* was published by the World Health Organization in 1975.

Forensic psychiatry

The care of the mentally ill has legal implications and criminal law has likewise a close relationship with psychiatry. Most textbooks of psychiatry include a chapter on the laws relating to mental illness, sometimes combined with general administrative psychiatry, and usually also a section on criminal responsibility and the psychiatric connotations of crime. The periodicals which cover this inter-disciplinary area are legal, medical and psychiatric, those of special relevance including the *British Journal of Criminology, Delinquency and Deviant Social Behaviour,* the *Bulletin of the American Academy of Psychiatry and the Law,* the *Howard Journal of Penology and Crime Prevention,* the *International Journal of Offender Therapy and Comparative Criminology,* the *International Journal of the Sociology of Law* (formerly the *International Journal of Criminology and Penology)* and the *Journal of Research in Crime and Delinquency.* Abstracts are found in *Criminology and Penology Abstracts,* which includes also expert review articles, and in *Criminal Justice Abstracts*. For further information the reader is referred to *Use of Criminology Literature* edited by M. Wright (Butterworths, 1974).

Mental retardation

Like child psychiatry, to which it is closely linked, this is an area in which psychology, psychiatry and the developmental sciences are closely allied and in which the neurosciences and social sciences also play an important part. The main periodicals are the *American Journal of Mental Deficiency*, the *British Journal of Mental Subnormality*, the *Journal of Mental Deficiency Research* and *Mental Retardation*. Abstracts appear in *Developmental Disabilities Abstracts* (formerly *Mental Retardation Abstracts*). Review publications include *Advances in Mental Handicap Research* (John Wiley, 1979–), the *International Review of Research in Mental Retardation* (Academic Press, 1966–) and *Mental Retardation and Developmental Disabilities, an Annual Review* (Brunner-Mazel, 1970–). A comprehensive *Bibliography of World Literature on Mental Retardation, 1940–1963* was published in 1963 by the US Department of Health, Education and Welfare, and a supplement to this appeared in 1965 covering March 1963 to December 1964. American government publications include many useful items; those put out by the President's Committee on Mental Retardation deserve particular mention.

The British Institute of Mental Handicap produces a monthly *Current Awareness Service on Mental Handicap*, indexed under some 30 headings, and it has over 70 reading lists available on all aspects of care and treatment. It also publishes reports of conferences. The British Library Automated Information Service (BLAISE) has a monthly offline bibliographic citation list under the heading *Mental Retardation*, but this is not indexed.

Neuropsychiatry

As has been mentioned, neurology and psychiatry were traditionally regarded as a single area of study. While this is now less frequently the case. many of the sources listed under general psychiatry cover the neurological borderlands too. Neuropsychiatric topics of particular interest include epilepsy, head injury, disorders of the brain and nervous system, and psychosurgery. Most textbooks of psychiatry contain relevant sections. Special mention may be made of *Epilepsia, Electroencephalography and Clinical Neurophysiology* (the *EEG Journal*), *Epilepsy Abstracts*, the *KWIC Indexes of Electroencephalographic Literature*, the *Hand-*

book of Electroencephalography and Clinical Neurophysiology
edited by A. Rémond (Elsevier, 1971–), and certain volumes of
the *Handbook of Clinical Neurology* edited by P. J. Vinken and G.
W. Bruyn (North Holland, 1969–).

Psychoanalysis and related schools

Ennis (1971) introduces her section on 'The journals in theoretical
systems' by saying that 'psychoanalytic journals are not generally
recommended for persons with easy-reading proclivities . . . They
are written in a highly specialised professional language which
requires of the reader trained clinical observation, background
knowledge, and experience.' Nevertheless psychoanalysis is a
popular subject, as the proliferation of books and paperbacks tes-
tifies. It has its own history, its own schools and its own bibliographical aids; some of its literature, especially the writings of
Freud, is dealt with almost on biblical concordance lines. Even its
spelling is open to confusion: the hyphenated version is, strictly
speaking, correct in works of British origin, the unhypenated spelling is American; and although James Strachey, Freud's principal
translator, said towards the end of his enormous labours that if he
were to start again he would probably suppress the tiresome
hyphen, it is still retained in the title of the *International Journal of
Psycho-Analysis* and in the name of its parent body, the International Psycho-Analytical Association.

Ennis gives a clear account of the various journals in psychoanalysis and related schools and of their splits and diver-
gencies. The chief periodicals in Freudian psychoanalysis are the
International Journal of Psycho-Analysis, the *International Review
of Psycho-Analysis*, the *Journal of the American Psychoanalytic
Association*, *Psychoanalytic Quarterly* and *Psychoanalytic Review*.
The organ of the Jungian school is the *Journal of Analytical Psychology* and that of the Adlerian school the *Journal of Individual
Psychology*. Of the general psychiatric journals, the *British Journal of Medical Psychology* and *Psychiatry* are particularly relevant.

The *Annual Survey of Psychoanalysis* (International Universities Press, 1950–) aims to give definitive reviews of each year's
work, but it is relatively unconcerned with the passage of time and
the volume which appeared in 1971 covers the literature of 1959. A
comprehensive index of psychoanalytic writings was begun in
Index Psychoanalyticus, 1893–1926 edited by J. Rickman (Hogarth
Press, 1928). This has been revised and brought up to date by A.
Grinstein in his *Index of Psychoanalytic Writings* (14 vols,
International Universities Press, 1956–1975). The *Chicago*

Psychoanalytic   Literature   Index   1920–1970,   1971–1974,   and quarterly, cumulating annually thereafter, reproduces the author and subject card index of the Chicago Institute for Psychoanalysis, and covers books, symposia and reviews, as well as abstracts and articles in professional journals.

The writings of Freud and Jung occupy a special place and many English translations have appeared. The *Standard Edition of the Complete Psychological Works of Sigmund Freud* translated by J. Strachey and published by the Hogarth Press, runs to 24 vols, the last being devoted entirely to indexes and bibliography. Jung's *Collected Works*, translated by R. F. C. Hull, are published in English by Routledge and Kegan Paul and run to 20 vols, of which vol 19 has a general bibliography and vol 20 the Index.

The *International Psycho-Analytical Library* (Hogarth Press) has issued nearly 100 vols on psychoanalysis, including many translations and reprints of papers previously published elsewhere. Other series include the *Psychoanalytic Study of Society* (International Universities Press, 1960–), which 'acts as a meeting ground for psychoanalysts and social scientists', and *Science and Psychoanalysis* (Grune and Stratton, 1958–), which publishes the transactions of the American Academy of Psychoanalysis, whose aim is to 'broaden research in human understanding and effective modes of therapy'.

Dictionaries include J. Laplanche and J.-B. Pontalis's *Language of Psycho-Analysis* (translated from the French, Hogarth Press, 1973), C. Rycroft's *Critical Dictionary of Psycho-Analysis* (Nelson, 1958) and A. Strachey's *New German-English Psycho-Analytical Vocabulary* (Baillière, Tindall and Cox, 1943).

Psychosomatic medicine

The first journal in this area was *Psychosomatic Medicine*, organ of the American Psychosomatic Society, which began in 1938. *Psychotherapy and Psychosomatics*, published by the International Federation for Medical Psychotherapy, came next in 1953; followed by *Psychosomatics* (Academy of Psychosomatic Medicine) in 1960; *Psychiatry in Medicine*, now the *International Journal of Psychiatry in Medicine*, (1965–); and the *Journal of Psychosomatic Research* (Society for Psychosomatic Research, 1956–).

Psychosomatic medicine is closely related to general medicine and also, from some points of view, to psychoanalysis and psychotherapy. Its secondary sources are those of medicine, general psychiatry, psychology and psychoanalysis.

Social psychiatry

To quote the first issue of the journal of the same name, social psychiatry is 'concerned with the effects of social conditions upon behaviour and the relationship between psychiatric disorder and the social environment'. Its special journals are *Hospital and Community Psychiatry* (1950–), *Community Mental Health Journal* (1965–), the *International Journal of Social Psychiatry* (1955–), *Social Psychiatry* (1966–) and *Transcultural Psychiatric Research Review*, which has been appearing, under slightly varying titles, since 1956. *Community Mental Health Review* (1976–) gives summaries, reviews and an index to world literature in the subject. For other secondary sources the reader should turn to the general medical, psychiatric, psychological and sociological tools.

Treatment: General

Treatment is, of course, covered throughout the literature, but some of its divisions may usefully be dealt with separately, and here the general annual review *Current Psychiatric Therapies* (Grune and Stratton, 1961–) deserves mention. Previously called *Progress in Psychotherapy* (1955–1960), it now covers the whole range of treatment, its aim being 'to re-evaluate traditional modes of psychiatric therapy and to explore promising new techniques'. In 1975, in addition to reviews of longer established methods such as psychopharmacology, it included chapters on the clinical use of meditation, poetry therapy in groups and pet-facilitated psychotherapy (PFP): the editor hoped that these 'new modalities . . . will not be adopted as disparate cults, but will instead be combined with the best of the old into a biologically, psychodynamically, socially comprehensive and resourceful organon of psychiatric treatment'.

Treatment: psychopharmacology

There has been a striking increase in the literature of psychopharmacology during the last decade, but it is still rather widely scattered. The general medical and psychiatric journals report, on the whole, clinical material, while more specialized literature appears in the pharmacological journals and in such periodicals as *Neuropharmacology*, *Psychopharmacology* and *Pharmacology, Biochemistry and Behavior*. The US National Clearinghouse for Mental Health Information issues the quarterly *Psychopharmacology Abstracts*, and the same organization also publishes the

Psychopharmacology Bulletin, designed to 'facilitate the dissemination and exchange of information, with an emphasis on rapid, informal reporting', rather than to provide a substitute for publication in journals. It includes much useful information, good bibliographies and a regular index of the current literature.

The Collegium Internationale Neuropsychopharmacologicum holds annual conferences, the proceedings of which are published in book form. The earlier volumes appeared under different titles and with different editors, although they are often quoted as *Neuropsychopharmacology*, with year and volume number, so that citations look deceptively like journal references. More recent proceedings have been published by Excerpta Medica. *Modern Problems of Pharmacopsychiatry* is a monograph series issued by Karger under the general editorship of F. Freyhan. *Advances in Biochemical Psychopharmacology* is another series, published by Raven Press since 1969. The literature up to 1967 is summarized in *Psychopharmacology: A Review of Progress* edited by Dr Efron *et al.* and published as *US Public Health Service Publication No 1836*.

Treatment: psychotherapy and behaviour therapy

Although these two methods of treatment have, on the whole, their own literature, it is convenient to deal with them together. Their close relationship is illustrated by the title of the (British) Association for Behavioural Psychotherapy.

Psychotherapy was first on the scene with the *American Journal of Psychotherapy* (Association for the Advancement of Psychotherapy, 1947–), *Psychotherapy, Theory, Research and Practice* (Psychotherapy Division of the American Psychological Association, 1963–), the *International Journal of Group Psychotherapy* (American Group Psychotherapy Association, 1951–) and *Group Analysis* (Group-Analytic Society, 1967–). The *International Journal of Psychoanalytic Psychotherapy*, after absorbing the *International Journal of Psychiatry*, put out its fifth volume in 1976 as a hardbacked annual, although it retains its journal title. The journals of psychoanalysis are of great relevance here and the general literature of psychiatry and psychology provides most of the secondary sources of information.

Behaviour therapy now has several periodicals – *Behaviour Research and Therapy* (1963–), *Behavior Therapy* (Association for the Advancement of Behavior Therapy, 1970–), the *Journal of Behavior Therapy and Experimental Psychiatry* (Behavior Therapy Research Society, 1970–) and *Behavioural Analysis and Modification* (Urban and Schwarzenberg, 1975–). *Advances in Beha-*

vior Therapy (Academic Press, 1969–) reports the conference proceedings of the Association for the Advancement of Behavior Therapy, and *Progress in Behaviour Therapy* (Springer, 1975–) has so far reported the proceedings of a meeting organized jointly by the European Association for Behaviour Therapy and the Behavioural Engineering Association. There is also *Annual Review of Behavior Therapy, Theory and Practice* (Brunner-Mazel, 1973–), while the Aldine Press publishes a yearly collection of reprints which is now called *Behavior Change,* earlier volumes of which have borne the title *Psychotherapy,* or *Psychotherapy and Behavior Change.* W. R. Morrow prepared an annotated *Behavior Therapy Bibliography, 1950–1969,* which was published by the University of Missouri Press in 1971, and M. R. Britt has published privately a *Bibliography of Behavior Modification, 1924–1973,* listing nearly 7000 entries. B. B. Wolman's *Dictionary of Behavioral Science* was published in 1973 by Van Nostrand Reinhold.

Before leaving these disciplines within psychiatry, it may be appropriate to mention a few more special topics and publications. There is a *Journal of Geriatric Psychiatry* (1968–) and bibliographies of geriatric psychiatry are included in the recurring bibliographies on ageing which appear in the *Journal of Gerontology.* C. Müller has edited *Bibliographia Gerontopsychiatrica: Bibliography of Geriatric Psychiatry* (H. Habner Verlag, 1973). At least two serial publications are devoted to schizophrenia – the *Schizophrenia Bulletin* (1969–), issued by the National Institute of Mental Health, and the *Annual Review of the Schizophrenic Syndrome* (Brunner-Mazel, 1971–), which is an anthology of what are considered to be the important papers published during the year. L. Bellak has been responsible for reviews of the schizophrenia literature covering three decades: *Dementia Praecox (1936–1946), Schizophrenia* (1946–1956) and *The Schizophrenic Syndrome* (edited by L. Bellak and L. Loeb), covering 1956–1966. They were published by Grune and Stratton (1948), Logos Press (1958) and Grune and Stratton (1969), respectively. A much newer concept in psychiatry is biofeedback, on which the Aldine Publishing Company issues a yearly anthology entitled *Biofeedback and Self-control* (1971–).

Another fairly recent development is the emergence of a vigorous school of 'anti-psychiatry' – a term which has not yet found its way into the indexing languages but which is certainly appearing in the literature. Its best-known exponents are D. Cooper, R. D. Laing and T. S. Szasz, and it is dealt with in some of the newer textbooks.

Related fields

Art and psychiatry

Confinia Psychiatrica, the organ of the International Society of Art and Psychotherapy, publishes papers in this and other borderland areas. It has, for example, published the proceedings of the *6th International Congress of Psychopathology of Expression,* other volumes of which have been published by Excerpta Medica. A similar series of colloquia is issued by Karger under the title *Psychiatry and Art.* The proceedings of the *World Congress of Psychiatry* usually include a symposium on the same or a similar theme. The classic monograph is H. Prinzhorn's *Bildnerei der Geisteskranken* (1922), an English translation of which was published by Springer in 1972 under the title *Artistry of the Mentally Ill.*

N. Keill's bibliography of *Psychiatry and Psychology in the Visual Arts and Aesthetics* was published by the University of Wisconsin Press in 1965, and a useful indication of current writings can be obtained from the *Liste des Acquisitions* issued twice yearly by the Centre International de Documentation Concernant les Expressions Plastiques, Paris (CIDEP), which details the books and periodical articles added to that library.

Art therapy, a different area, is documented in the *American Journal of Art Therapy* and in *Art Psychotherapy,* or in the annual *Current Psychiatric Therapies,* now at vol 20.

The neurosciences

The *Journal of the Neurological Sciences* defines its subject matter as 'all those sciences which underlie modern concepts of nervous structure and functioning'. They are basic to many medical disciplines and are not dealt with in detail here. Relevant journals include *Brain, Brain Research,* the *Canadian Journal of Neurological Sciences,* the *Journal of the Neurological Sciences, Neuroscience, Neurosciences Research* and the *Neurosciences Research Program Bulletin* (anthologies from which are published in the *Neurosciences Research Symposia Summaries*). The Massachusetts Institute of Technology, which is responsible for the *Neurosciences Research Program Bulletin,* also publishes a series entitled *Neurosciences: A Study Program,* of which three volumes have now appeared (Rockefeller University Press and M.I.T. Press, 1967–). The *Annual Review of Neuroscience* appeared first in 1978, while *Developments in Neuroscience* and the multidisciplinary review

Trends in Neurosciences both appeared in 1977. Some of the inter-disciplinary journals that are closely related to psychiatry have already been mentioned.

Psychology

The relationship between psychology and psychiatry is particularly close, and no one interested in the one subject can afford to ignore the literature of the other. The following journals are especially relevant: The *British Journal of Social and Clinical Psychology*, now split into *British Journal of Clinical Psychology* and *British Journal of Social Psychology*, the *Journal of Abnormal Psychology*, the *Journal of Clinical Psychology*, the *Journal of Consulting and Clinical Psychology*, and the *Journal of Counseling Psychology*. *Biological Psychology*, the *Journal of Experimental Social Psychology*, the *Journal of Personality*, the *Journal of Personality and Social Psychology*, the *Journal of Personality Assessment*, the *Journal of Research in Personality and Social Behavior*, and *Personality* are important too, as are *Psychological Bulletin*, *Educational and Psychological Measurement*, *Language and Speech* and the *Journal of Verbal Learning and Verbal Behavior*.

Review media include the *Annual Review of Psychology* and *Progress in Clinical Psychology*. The *Handbook of Abnormal Psychology* edited by H. J. Eysenck *et al.* is now in its second edition (Pitman Medical, 1972), and, like G. Lindzey and E. Aronson's *Handbook of Social Psychology* (2nd edn, 5 vols, Addison-Wesley, 1968), is a useful source of information.

Psychological Abstracts (1927–) is as relevant to psychiatry as *Index Medicus*. It has cumulated author and subject indexes and, with its predecessor *Psychological Review Index*, covers the literature from 1894 to the present day. For recent years it, too, is available online. The *Psychological Reader's Guide* (Elsevier Sequoia, Lausanne) provides a monthly list of the contents of more than 200 journals in psychology.

Psychological and psychiatric tests, rating scales and questionnaires present peculiar and usually difficult problems, although O. K. Buros has accomplished wonders by editing a most helpful series of aids: *Mental Measurement Yearbook*, of which eight editions have appeared since 1938, mostly published by the Gryphon Press, which, with the earlier *Educational, Psychological and Personality Tests, gives coverage back to 1933; Tests in Print* (2nd edn, 1974); *Reading Tests and Reviews* (1968); and *Personality Tests and Reviews* (1970). Buros describes tests in full bibliographical detail, provides expert reviews and gives bibliographies on the use of each test. The eighth edition of the *Yearbook* covers 1184 tests, with 898 original reviews. Even so, not all tests can be included, and priority is not unnaturally given to those which are commercially available in the US. *Psychological Abstracts* also gives information about tests, and catalogues are issued by Swets and Zeitlinger, Western Psychological Services (Los Angeles), the Consulting Psychologists Press (Palo Alto), the Psychological Corporation (New York), Psychological Assessment Resources (Odessa, Florida) and in the UK by the University of London Press, the English Universities Press and the National Foundation for Educational Research. But a relatively new or not-much-quoted test, scale or questionnaire can still be a very small needle in a large number of haystacks.

Sociology

As the emergence of a discipline of social psychiatry shows, sociology has become of increasing interest to psychiatrists. Periodicals of relevance are the *British Journal of Social Work, Family Process*, the *Journal of Health and Social Behavior*, the *Journal of Marriage and the Family*, the *Journal of Social Issues*, the *Milbank Memorial Fund Quarterly – Health and Society, Social Forces, Social Problems* and *Social Work Today*.

   Sociological Abstracts is useful, especially in such areas as drug addiction. *Current Sociology* (Mouton, 1953–1975, now Sage Pubns) is an irregular series, each issue of which is devoted to the sociology of a special topic: in 1973, for example, one number was devoted to a trend report and bibliography of alienation as a concept in the social sciences. The *International Bibliography of the Social Sciences – Sociology* (Tavistock, 1951–) provides an annual listing of important scientific publications in sociology and is indexed by subject in French and English; it is international in coverage, selection being made by national correspondents as well as by the editorial staff.

Biography and history of psychiatry

Biography

Current directories of psychiatrists include the *Biographical Directory of Fellows and Members of the American Psychiatric Association* and the annual lists of members put out by most of the national organizations and by such bodies as the International

Psycho-Analytic Association. The *Proceedings of the World Congress of Psychiatry* generally include a useful list, with addresses, of all participants. Ennis (1971) gives details of selected obituary notices that appeared in the main American journals between 1922 and 1966, and the cumulated indexes of the *Journal of Mental Science* also guide one to this kind of information; unfortunately they do not extend beyond 1939.

Kurt Kolle's *Grosse Nervenärzte* (a three-volume publication now partly in its second edition, Thieme, 1956–1963) gives fairly full biographies and portraits of 65 great men in neurology and psychiatry, including not only clinicians and therapists, but also research workers 'who may never have seen a patient'. The selection is international, including the usual famous names such as Jean-Martin Charcot, Jean-Etienne Esquirol, Henry Head, John Hughlings Jackson, Emil Kraepelin, Adolf Meyer, Henry Maudsley and Philippe Pinel. Early French psychiatrists are also well covered in R. Semelaigne's *Les Pionniers de la Psychiatrie Française avant et après Pinel* (2 vols, Baillière, 1930).

L. Zusne's *Names in the History of Psychology* (Hemisphere, 1975) contains short biographies and, where possible, photographs of and biographical references to 526 individuals arranged chronologically from Heraclitus, born *ca* 540 BC, to Carl Hovland, born 1912. The names were selected from over 1000 submitted to a panel of judges who rated them according to their own knowledge of the men in question on a three-point scale of 'lasting fame'. Psychiatry is well represented, most of the classic names being there, as well as more recent figures such as Melanie Klein. There are entries, too, for distinguished men and women in related areas – for example, Emil Durkheim, Alfred Kinsey, and Margaret Mead. The *History of Psychology in Autobiography*, which is now in its sixth volume (Prentice-Hall, 1974), also features a few psychiatrists. Other anthologies of interest are R. McKown's *Pioneers in Mental Health* (Dodd, Mead, 1961) and H. Mannheim's *Pioneers in Criminology* (Steven, 1960).

Kolle and Zusne naturally both include biographies of Freud, about whom more has been written than anyone else in the field: his definitive biography is Ernest Jones's *Life and Work of Sigmund Freud* (3 vols, Hogarth Press, 1953–1959).

History

The reader wishing an introduction to the history of psychiatry might well begin with the historical chapters in some of the main textbooks of psychiatry and with the highly relevant periodical, the

Journal of the History of Behavioral Sciences. H. Ellenberger's chapter in the *American Handbook of Psychiatry* (2nd edn, Basic Books, 1972–1975) and G. Mora's in the *Comprehensive Textbook of Psychiatry* by H. I. Kaplan *et al.* (3rd edn, Williams and Wilkins, 1980) are scholarly contributions that set the scene well, while those interested in historiography could have their appetite whetted by Mora's paper in the first issue of the journal ('The historiography of psychiatry and its development, a re-evaluation', *J. Hist. Behav. Sci.,* **1**, 43, 1965). Similar contributions are H. Schipperges's chapter in vol 3 of *Psychiatrie der Gegenwart* (2nd edn, Springer, 1975), Henri Ey's chapter in his *Manuel de Psychiatrie* (4th edn, Masson, 1974) or the historical introduction, again by Henry Ey, to the psychiatric section of the *Encyclopédie Médico-Chirurgicale.*

As might be expected, there are as many approaches and divisions in the history of psychiatry as there are in the subject itself. Most psychiatric historians recognize, if they do not all attempt to deal with, the many contrasting strands – theoretical, philosophical, biological, neurological, clinical, psychological, psychoanalytical and social – that make up the complex weave, as well as the chronological and geographical variants that give it added colour and interest. The references they give naturally vary, but on some books there is a clear consensus – even though Dr Schipperges sadly includes one German source chiefly because of the esteem in which it is held in Anglo-American countries. The following lists of books in English are not, of course, comprehensive, nor are the broad categories mutually exclusive: histories in other languages are well documented in, for example, Mora's chapter in the *Comprehensive Textbook of Psychiatry.*

GENERAL ACCOUNTS

A Short History of Psychiatry by E. G. Ackerknecht (translated from the German, 2nd edn, Hafner, 1968)
Roots of Modern Psychiatry: Essays in the History of Psychiatry by M. D. Altschule (2nd edn, Grune and Stratton, 1965)
One Hundred Years of Psychiatry by E. Kraepelin (translated from the German (1916), Owen, 1962)

DYNAMICALLY ORIENTATED

The History of Psychiatry: An Evaluation of Psychiatric Thought and Practice from Prehistoric Times to the Present by F. G. Alexander and S. T. Selesnick (Harper and Row, 1966)
Man above Humanity: A History of Psychotherapy by W. Bromberg (Lippincott, 1954)
The Discovery of the Unconscious: The History and Evolution of Dynamic Psychiatry by H. Ellenberger (Basic Books, 1970)
The Unconscious before Freud by L. L. Whyte (Basic Books, 1966)

Depth Psychology by D. Wyss (translated from the German (1916), Allen and
  Unwin, 1966)
A History of Medical Psychology by G. Zilboorg and G. W. Henry (Norton, 1941)

GEOGRAPHICALLY ORIENTATED

US:

One Hundred Years of American Psychiatry by American Psychiatric Association
  (Columbia University Press, 1944)
Psychiatry and the Community in Nineteenth Century America by R. B. Caplan
  (Basic Books, 1969)
*The Mentally Ill in America: A History of their Care and Treatment from Colonial
  Times* by A. Deutsch (2nd edn, Columbia Press, 1949)

Great Britain:

*Lunacy, Law and Conscience, 1744–1845. The Social History of the Care of the
  Insane* by K. Jones (Routledge, 1954)
Mental Health and Social Policy, 1845–1959 by K. Jones (Routledge, 1960)
A History of the Mental Health Services by K. Jones (Routledge, 1972)
The Historical Development of British Psychiatry: 18th and 19th Centuries by D.
  Leigh (Pergamon, 1961)
*Madhouses, Mad-doctors and Madmen: the Social History of Psychiatry in the
  Victorian Era* by A. Scull (Athlone, 1981)
Chapters in the History of the Insane in the British Isles by D. H. Tuke (Paul,
  Trench, 1882)

World:

World History of Psychiatry edited by J. G. Howells (Baillière, Tindall and Cassell, 1975); contains chapters on the history of psychiatry in 29 countries

HISTORY OF HOSPITALS

*The State and the Mentally Ill: A History of the Worcester State Hospital in
  Massachusetts, 1830–1920* by G. N. Grob (University of North Carolina Press,
  1966)
The Story of Bethlehem Hospital from its Foundation in 1247 by E. G. O'Donoghue
  (Unwin, 1914)
*The Trade in Lunacy: A Study of Private Madhouses in England in the 18th and 19th
  Centuries* by W. L. Parry-Jones (Routledge, 1972)

SPECIAL TOPICS

A History of the Care and Study of the Mentally Retarded by L. Kanner (C. C. Tho-
  mas, 1964)
The History and Philosophy of Knowledge of the Brain and its Functions edited by
  F. N. L. Poynter (Blackwell, 1958)
The Falling Sickness: A History of Epilepsy by O. Temkin (2nd edn, Johns Hopkins,
  1971)
Hysteria: the History of a Disease by I. Veith (Chicago University Press, 1965)

SOURCE BOOKS AND EARLY MATERIAL

Documentary History of Psychiatry: a Source Book on Historical Principles by C.
  E. Goshen (Vision Press, 1967)

Three Hundred Years of Psychiatry, 1535–1860: a History Presented in Selected English Texts by R. A. Hunter and I. MacAlpine (Oxford University Press, 1963)

Historical Notes on Psychiatry (Early Times to End of 16th Century) J. R. Whitwell (Lewis, 1935)

Useful anthologies of classic papers have been published by M. Rosen *et al.* *(The History of Mental Retardation: Collected Papers.* 2 vols, University Park Press, 1976) and by V. Skultans *(Madness and Morals: Ideas on Insanity in the 19th Century,* Routledge, 1975), while S. R. Hirsch and M. Shepherd have edited a selection of European texts, translated mostly from French and German *(Themes and Variations in European Psychiatry,* Wright, 1974). Early bibliographies can be found in Tuke (1892), in H. Laehr's *Literatur der Psychiatrie, Neurologie und Psychologie* (3 vols, Reimer, 1900), in O. Bumke's *Handbuch der Geisteskrankheiten* (11 vols, Springer, 1928–1930) and, of course, in the indispensable *Index-Catalogue of the Library of the Surgeon General's Office.*

Since much of this early work is in French and German, translations are of considerable importance. Ennis (1971) comments on some of the problems involved and gives a partial list of translated works.

Conclusion

Ellenberger closes his chapter in the *American Handbook of Psychiatry* with a note on the 'psychiatric explosion' that, since 1920, has given rise to so many almost autonomous disciplines within the subject. He recalls Henry Ey's warning that such boundless expansion would inevitably lead to a reaction in the form of the dissolution of psychiatry and suggests that this is what we are witnessing today. 'Pan-psychiatry' has led to 'anti-psychiatry' and the outcome of 25 centuries of effort is that the basic principles of the subject need careful revision. No doubt the literature of psychiatry will reflect this and its bibliographical control will need revision too.

Acknowledgements

My thanks to those members of staff at the Library of the Institute of Psychiatry and the Tavistock Joint Library who have helped me in the revision of this chapter.

References

Blake, J. B. and Roos, C. (eds) (1967), *Medical Reference Works 1679–1966*, Medical Library Association

Borchardt, D. H. (1968), *How to Find Out in Philosophy and Psychology*, Pergamon

Cosyns-Verhaegen, E. (1972–1974), *Psychiatrie et Santé Mentale: Catalogue Collectif des Ouvrages. Bibliographica Belgica 125*, 4 vols, Fondation Julie Renson

Elliott, C. K. (1971), *A Guide to the Documentation of Psychology*, Clive Bingley

Ennis, B. (1971), *Guide to the Literature in Psychiatry*, Partridge Press

Greenberg, B. (1978), *How to Find Out in Psychiatry: a Guide to Sources of Mental Health Information*, Pergamon

Louttit, C. M. (1932), *Handbook of Psychological Literature*, Principia Press

Menninger, K. (1972), *A Guide to Psychiatric Books in English*, 3rd edn, Grune and Stratton

Tuke, D. Hack. (1892), *A Dictionary of Psychological Medicine*, Churchill

18

Surgery and anaesthesia

A. M. Rodger

The literature of surgery

In common with other branches of medicine, scientific and technical progress has created new areas of surgical specialties which
have undergone rapid development in recent years. The basic
principles of the craft of surgery remain the same, but advances in
recent times have made many of the old textbook divisions irrelevant. Over the past decades the most obvious changes have
involved the shift in emphasis away from infectious complications
and on to the new techniques in cardiac and transplant surgery.
This, however, is a change in emphasis only because advances in
treatment nearly always provide new problems, as in antibiotic
therapy where the causative organisms of infection develop strains
resistant to existing medication. Both the rapid progress in current
research and the wide range of specialties limit the utility of textbooks of general surgery. Most of the primary information is
found in the periodical literature and the stocks of many medical
libraries now consist predominantly of journals, which are the
main source of new surgical information, and of review articles,
which survey recent developments in specialized subjects. The
journal reader is aided by abstracting services, which provide a
summary of the most outstanding current contributions to the periodical literature. Information on progress in surgical specialties
may also be obtained from monographs, i.e. books dealing with
one selected topic, and from publications in book form which aim

to present advances in particular aspects of surgery. The journal remains the principal source of new information.

Journals

In addition to the many journals catering for the specialist, there are a number which carry articles on all aspects of surgery. These are usually nationally or geographically orientated, e.g. *Acta Chirurgica Scandinavica, American Journal of Surgery, American Surgeon, Australian and New Zealand Journal of Surgery, British Journal of Surgery, European Surgical Research, World Journal of Surgery* and *Surgical Clinics of North America,* which concentrates on a single topic per issue.

Other journals of a similar type are produced which are without a national emphasis in the title but whose content may reflect the country of origin. Sometimes such commercially produced journals are the official organ of a society or group. Examples here are *Annals of Surgery* (official publication of the American Surgical Association), *Archives of Surgery* (official publication of the International Cardiovascular Society and Western Surgical Association), *Journal of Surgical Research* (official organ of the Association for Academic Surgery), *Surgery* (journal of the Society of University Surgeons) and *Surgical Forum.* This last is hardly a periodical in the accepted sense. It is an annual publication and takes the form of the proceedings of the American College of Surgeons Forum on fundamental surgical problems.

There are the weekly medical publications which not only disseminate news and current research, but also carry articles of surgical import. Such journals include the *British Medical Journal, The Lancet, Journal of the American Medical Association* and the *New England Journal of Medicine.* Yet another group of journals are published under the aegis of a single institution, often with an international reputation. Among such journals are *Annals of the Royal College of Surgeons of England, Lahey Clinic Bulletin, Journal of the Mount Sinai Hospital, Journal of the Royal College of Surgeons of Edinburgh* and *Mayo Clinic Proceedings.*

As with most other areas in medicine, the journals together constitute the most important source of surgical information, covering as they do communications regarding new discoveries, reviews of the literature or state-of-the-art appraisals, case reports, advances in technique, etc.

Indexes and abstracts

To peruse regularly even a selection of journals is too time consuming for the individual. For bibliographical search purposes, *Index Medicus* is the standard and most widely used aid. In addition, the separate listing of the *Bibliography of Medical Reviews* is useful for selecting major review articles on a given topic. MEDLARS computer tapes can be tapped through the data base MEDLINE when a manual search of *Index Medicus* is considered insufficient or inappropriate to the search requirements.

In surgery the most comprehensive abstracting service is provided by *Excerpta Medica* (*see* page 63). Of its 42 sections, those relevant to surgery are:

Surgery (Section 9)
Neurology and Neursurgery (Section 8)
Plastic Surgery (Section 34)
Orthopaedic Surgery (section 33)
Cardiovascular Diseases and Cardiovascular Surgery (Section 18)
Cancer (Section 16)
Gastroenterology (Section 48)
Chest Diseases: Thoracic Surgery and Tuberculosis (Section 15)
Urology and Nephrology (Section 28)
Oto-rhino-laryngology (Section 11)
Ophthalmology (Section 12)

International Abstracts of Surgery is published as part of the monthly journal *Surgery, Gynecology and Obstetrics*. About 4000 abstracts appear each year, arranged anatomically and indexed bi-annually. The *Zentralorgan für die gesamte Chirurgie und ihre Grenzgebiete* is a comprehensive journal publishing 5400 abstracts a year. It has a subject arrangement and several volumes are published annually with subject and author indexes.

Abstracts and reviews of relevant literature are published in certain specialty journals, e.g. *Diseases of the Colon and Rectum, British Journal of Urology* and *Journal of Pediatric Surgery*.

The *Audio Journal Review* is published in two sections *(General Surgery* and *Ophthalmology)* by Grune and Stratton and was first produced in 1972, giving abstracts of general surgery in tape form. It is compiled from surveys of major surgical and medical journals. Twelve cassettes, each lasting sixty minutes, are issued annually and current material can become available in this form before its appearance in printed reviews and abstracting journals.

The plethora of journals and the increasing number of new periodicals launched each year make a speedy alerting service difficult to maintain. A reasonable international cover is provided by *Current Contents: Life Sciences* and *Current Contents: Clinical Practice*, which between them provide the reader with the tables of contents of virtually all the major surgical journals.

British Medicine was formerly published under the aegis of the British Council, but since the May 1980 issue has been published by Pergamon. This journal provides a monthly guide to current medical literature published in Britain. As well as listing journal contents this publication covers monographs, textbooks and government reports. In addition it gives lists of forthcoming conferences.

Reviews

The review publication is a useful way of keeping track of recent advances or trends in certain areas of medicine and surgery. Review publications are invaluable guides, not only to workers whose specialty may be the subject reviewed, but also to specialists in ancillary fields, keeping them up to date with major developments. Many such publications tend to concentrate on specific topics and examples of these are mentioned in the relevant sections. One such publication of general surgical interest is *Recent Advances in Surgery – 10* edited by S. Taylor (Churchill Livingstone, 1980), which contains articles on such diverse topics as vascular surgery, breast carcinoma, peptic ulcer and a review of the current treatment of fractures. *Surgical Reviews – 2* edited by J. S. P. Lumley and J. L. Craven (Heinemann, 1981) is one of a review series aimed at the postgraduate reader. *International Medical Reviews* is a new series, of which vol 1 is *Trauma* edited by D. Carter and H. C. Polk (Butterworths, 1981). A notable example of this type of publication is the *Current Surgical Practice, vol 3* edited by J. Hadfield and M. Hobsley (Arnold, 1981). This series comprises a selection of lectures given at the Royal College of Surgeons of England and emphasizes areas of surgery in which there have been important advances in recent years. The most recent volume contains lectures on various aspects of gastrointestinal surgery, renal transplantation, surgery of the rheumatic hand and breast cancer, as well as a variety of other topics. Previous volumes in this series were published in 1976 and 1978. The American firm, Year Book Medical Publishers, produce annual reviews in a number of subjects, e.g. *Year Book of Surgery* currently edited by S. I. Schwartz. The same publishers also produce *Advances in Surgery,* an annual volume of which the latest is *Advances in Surgery – 15* edited by G. L. Jordan (Year Book Medical Publishers, 1982). In the same category is *Surgery Annual 1982* edited by L. M. Nyhus (Prentice Hall International)

Textbooks: general surgery

The single-volume textbook covering all aspects of surgery suffers from the faults expected of a textbook that deals with evolving and diversifying subject matter; principally obsolescence, often before publication, and uneven weighting when attempting to discuss all specialties. Nevertheless, such works are essential as basic training texts. There are a number of textbooks of high reputation, gained through the popularity of successive editions with generations of students. One of the best known is *Bailey and Love's Short Practice of Surgery* revised by A. J. H. Rains and H. D. Ritchie (18th edn, Lewis, 1981). *Current Surgical Diagnosis and Treatment* edited by J. E. Dunphy and L. W. Way (5th edn, Lange Medical Publishers, 1981) is a popular American textbook with an international reputation. It is comprehensive and deals with specialized subjects as well as filling the requirements of a basic text. One of the notable features of this book is the currency of the references, many being cited in the same year as the book is published and the majority less than three years old. *Surgical Treatment* by C. Illingworth (Pitman, 1980) is for senior students and registrars. It is a short book assuming some surgical knowledge by the reader. As usual with this author the style is clear and concise. Useful for general revision are *Lecture Notes on General Surgery* by H. Ellis and R. Y. Calne (5th edn, Blackwell, 1977) and *A Synopsis of Surgical Anatomy* by D. J. Du Plessis (11th edn, Wright, 1975). A useful book for background reading for Surgical Fellowship candidates is *Scientific Foundations of Surgery* edited by J. Kyle and J. D. Hardy (3rd edn, Heinemann, 1981).

Textbooks: operative surgery

A standard work for many years has been *Hamilton Bailey's Emergency Surgery* edited by H. A. F. Dudley (10th edn, Wright, 1977). This book advises when to operate and when not to, and how to operate in emergencies. It is especially valuable to the surgeon working in isolation. *Farquharson's Textbook of Operative Surgery* edited by R. F. Rintoul (6th edn, Churchill Livingstone, 1977) is a standard work for those working for higher surgical qualifications.

General Surgical Operations edited by R. M. Kirk (Churchill Livingstone, 1978) is a practical manual for the general surgeon. The essential reference work for the library shelves is the series *Operative Surgery* under the general editorship of C. Rob and R. Smith (3rd edn, Butterworths, 1976–1982). This comprises a seventeen-volume series with each volume being compiled by a specialist editor. The cost is prohibitive for the individual but it is essential material for the library reference shelves. Of use to postgraduates is *Tutorials in Surgery – 3: Operative Surgery* by F. G. Smiddy (Pitman 1982). Previous volumes in this series appeared in 1977 and 1979.

Orthopaedics

The correction of diseases and injuries to the locomotor system forms a large branch of surgery, and here dramatic changes have taken place in the organization and techniques employed in accident surgery, and, in particular, the management of trauma. There has been an increasing realization of the importance of cross connections with other disciplines, particularly in the area of rheumatology and the use of artificial prostheses to replace diseased joints.

JOURNALS

In addition to the general surgical journals listed at the beginning of the chapter a number of journals cater specifically for the orthopaedic surgeon. The most important are *Acta Orthopaedica Scandinavica, Hand, Injury: British Journal of Accident Surgery, Journal of Trauma, Reconstructive Surgery and Traumatology, Journal of Bone and Joint Surgery* and *Spine. Injury* and the *Journal of Trauma* carry a short selection of abstracts relating to orthopaedics.

REVIEWS

There are several survey publications in orthopaedics including *Recent Advances in Orthopaedics – 3* edited by B. McKibbin (Churchill Livingstone, 1979), which contains articles on a number of subjects including spinal tuberculosis, osteosarcoma and hip surgery. There is also the *Year Book of Orthopedics and Traumatic Surgery* edited by M. B. Coventry (Year Book Medical Publisher, 1981) and the *Postgraduate Orthopaedic Series,* of which two recent issues have been *Biochemical Disorders of the Skeleton* by R. Smith, (Butterworths, 1979) and *Hip Disorders in Children* by G. C. Lloyd-Roberts and A. H. C. Ratcliff (Butterworths, 1978). The American Academy of Orthopedic Surgeons produces an occasional selective bibliography of some 3000 article titles of interest to orthopaedic surgeons, *Selective Bibliography of Orthopedic Surgery* (3rd edn, Kimpton, 1975). A relatively new series is *Current Problems in Orthopaedics,* of which the last is *Current Problems in Orthopaedics: Bone Repair and Fracture Healing in Man* by S. Sevitt (Churchill Livingstone, 1981).

TEXTBOOKS AND MONOGRAPHS

The most comprehensive work is *Campbell's Operative Orthopaedics* edited by A. S. Edmondson and A. H. Crenshaw (6th edn,

Year Book Medical Publishers, 1980). This is a two-volume work priced at over £100, but it is the definitive work for reference shelves. Other general works which may be considered essential reading are *A System of Orthopaedics and Fractures* by A. G. Apley (6th edn, Butterworths, 1982) and *Mercer's Orthopaedic Surgery* edited by R. B. Duthie and G. Bentley (8th edn, Arnold, 1983). Another comprehensive text is *Watson-Jones Fractures and Joint Injuries,* edited by J. N. Wilson (6th edn, 2 vols, Churchill Livingstone, 1982).

Some recommended texts on regional orthopaedic surgery are *Surgery of the Foot* by H. Du Vries and edited by V. I. Inman (4th edn, Kimpton, 1978), *Injuries of the Knee Joint* by I. S. Smillie (5th edn, Churchill Livingstone, 1978), *Manual of Spinal Surgery* by D. H. R. Jenkins, R. D. Weeks, A. C. Yau and R. R. Du (Butterworths, 1982) and the latest work in a rapidly developing specialty is *Operative Hand Surgery* edited by D. P. Green (Churchill Livingstone, 1982). A useful work for revision study is *Lecture Notes on Orthopaedics and Fractures* by T. Duckworth (Blackwell, 1980)

Paediatric surgery

The information sources contained in the chapter on Paediatrics (page 430) are appropriate also to paediatric surgery. Abstracts are published in *Excerpta Medica, Section 10: Pediatrics and Pediatric Surgery.* Review publications dealing with medical paediatrics also contain information for the surgeon, e.g. the series *Modern Problems in Paediatrics* edited by F. Falkner, N. Kretchmer and E. Rossi (Karger); vol 18 in this series is the latest and it deals with paediatric neurosurgery. Other publications of this type are *Advances in Pediatrics vol 27* edited by L. A. Barness (Year Book Medical Publishers, 1981) and the *Postgraduate Paediatric Series* edited by J. Apley and published by Butterworths. *Surgical Conditions in Paediatrics* by H. H. Nixon (Butterworths, 1978) is one of this series.

Monographs and textbooks on paediatric surgery include *Surgery in Infancy and Childhood* edited by W. M. Dennison (3rd edn, Churchill Livingstone, 1974), a general textbook for students and junior hospital staff, *Handbook of Pediatric Surgical Emergencies* by D. B. Groff (Kimpton, 1981), and *Paediatric Surgery* edited by H. H. Nixon (Butterworths, 1978). This book is one of Butterworths *Operative Surgery* series (3rd edn). Other recent publications include *Pediatric Surgery* by T. M. Holder and K. W. Ashcroft (Saunders, 1980), which deals with general paediatric surgery. More condensed is *A Handbook of Pediatric Surgery* by J. L. Ternberg, M. J. Bell and R. J. Bower (Williams and Wilkins, 1980) which is more a pocketbook than a handbook. A popular comprehensive text is the encyclopaedic *Pediatric Surgery* by M. M. Ravitch *et al.* (3rd edn, Year Book Medical Publishers, 1979).

Thoracic and cardiovascular surgery

The primary specialist journals in this section are the *Journal of Cardiovascular Surgery, Journal of Thoracic and Cardiovascular Surgery, Scandinavian Journal of Thoracic and Cardiovascular Surgery, Thorax* and *Annals of Thoracic Surgery*.

The American Journal of Cardiology publishes abstracts of the conference proceedings of the American College of Cardiology, usually in advance of presentation. Also the American Heart Association publishes monographs under the series title, *Cardiovascular Surgery*. A recent review publication is *The Present State of Cardiothoracic Surgery* edited by J. A. Dyde and R. E. Smith (Pitman, 1981). This volume comprises the proceedings of the 5th Coventry Conference on this subject and is a good update on the topic.

Among books currently available are *D'Abreu's Practice of Cardiothoracic Surgery* edited by J. L. Collis, D. B. Clarke and R. A. Smith (4th edn, Arnold, 1976). Two books of note in the *Operative Surgery* series are *Cardiothoracic Surgery* edited by J. W. Jackson (Butterworths, 1978) and *Vascular Surgery* edited by C. Rob (Butterworths, 1976). The former volume is particularly strong on adult heart disease. Although nearly 10 years old *Arterial Surgery* by H. H. Eastcott (2nd edn, Pitman, 1973) is a summation of a lifetime's work in the field.

Recent works on vascular surgery include *Surgical Management of Vascular Disease* by C. Jamieson (Heinemann, 1982), *Operative Arterial Surgery* by P. R. F. Bell and W. Barrie (Wright, 1981), which is of value to postgraduate trainees, while *A Practice of Vascular Surgery* by R. C. Kester and S. H. Leveson (Pitman, 1981) covers most aspects of peripheral arterial surgery and is aimed at the same market. *Operative Techniques in Vascular Surgery* edited by J. J. Bergan and J. T. Yao (Grune and Stratton, 1980) is the published proceedings of a symposium held in the US and, consequently, represents a variety of individual viewpoints. Also recommended is *Tissue Heart Valves* by M. I. Ionescu (Butterworths, 1979).

Neurosurgery

The neurosurgeon tends to work in a distinct field with the emphasis on head injuries and lesions of the intervertebral disc, which require close co-operation with the orthopaedic surgeon. There are a number of journals concerned with this specialty, particularly the *Journal of Neurology, Neurosurgery and Psychiatry* and the *Journal of Neurosurgery*. Relevant information is also to be found in:

Acta Neurologica Scandinavica
Archives of Neurology
Brain
Diseases of the Nervous System
Electroencephalography and Clinical Neurophysiology
European Neurology
Journal of Neurological Sciences
Neurology

Review publications include the *Neurosurgical Review* which is published approximately every four years by Walter de Gruyter. Two other series published by Springer are *Advances and Technical Standards in Neurosurgery*, of which the latest is vol 8 (Springer, 1981), and *Advances in Neurosurgery*, of which the latest is vol 10 edited by W. Driesen, M. Brock and M. Klinger (Springer, 1982). The American Congress of Neurosurgeons publishes its annual proceedings under the title *Clinical Neurosurgery* edited by P. W. Carmel (vol 27, Williams and Wilkins, 1981).

Standard textbooks and monographs in neurosurgery include *An Introduction to Neurosurgery* by B. Jennett (3rd edn, Churchill Livingstone, 1977), *Neurosurgery* edited by L. Symon (3rd edn, Butterworths, 1979), and *Current Surgical Management of Neurological Disease* edited by C. B. Wilson and J. T. Hoff (Churchill Livingstone, 1980), which includes sections on congenital disorders, neoplastic diseases, vascular disorders and trauma. *Essentials of Neurosurgery* by R. R. Smith (Harper and Row, 1980) is a concise but clear general text on the subject. Also to be recommended are *Management of Acute Head Injuries* by R. Hayward (Blackwell, 1980) and *Spinal Cord Injuries, Comprehensive Management and Research* by L. Guttmann (2nd edn, Blackwell, 1976).

Plastic surgery

This is a very distinct and, arguably, one of the oldest branches of surgery. Burn injuries remain one of the main reasons for surgical repair as do hand injuries and the repair of cleft lip and palate. Immunological research is of paramount importance to the plastic surgeon, especially in the areas of skin homografts and cartilage grafts.

JOURNALS

The specialist journals in this subject include *Acta Chirurgiae Plasticae, British Journal of Plastic Surgery, Burns, Journal of Maxillo-Facial Surgery, Hand, Plastic and Reconstructive Surgery,* which carries a selection of International Abstracts, and the *Scandinavian Journal of Plastic and Reconstructive Surgery.*

REVIEWS

One of the current review publications is *Recent Advance in Plastic Surgery – 2* edited by I. T. Jackson (Churchill Livingstone, 1981). This edition covers a number of topics, including hand surgery, reconstruction of the ear and a concise resumé of present techniques of breast reconstruction. Year Book Medical Publishers produce the *Year Book of Plastic and Reconstructive Surgery,* at present edited annually by F. J. McCoy *et al.* The American Society of Plastic and Reconstructive Surgeons produces a series of educational symposia of which the latest is vol 21, *Symposium on Pediatric Plastic Surgery* edited by D. Kernahan and H. D. Thomson (Mosby, 1981)

TEXTBOOKS

General textbooks in plastic surgery include *Fundamental Techniques of Plastic Surgery and their Surgical Application* by I. A. McGregor (7th edn, Churchill Livingstone, 1981). This book has proved itself as essential reading for surgical training through successive editions and it has maintained a high standard of clear text and illustration since it first appeared nearly twenty years ago. *Operative Plastic and Reconstructive Surgery* edited by J. N. Barron and M. N. Saad (Churchill Livingstone, 1980–1981) is a three-volume work, the first two dealing with general plastic and reconstructive techniques while the third is devoted to surgery of the hand. In the *Operative Surgery* series there is *Plastic Surgery* edited by J. Watson and R. M. McCormack (3rd edn, Butterworths, 1978). Another comprehensive work is *Plastic Surgery: a Concise Guide to Clinical Practice* edited by W. C. Grabb and J. W. Smith (3rd edn, Little, Brown, 1980) which is designed for senior students and surgeons in training. More specialized current monographs include *Plastic Surgery in Infancy and Childhood* edited by J. C. Mustardé (2nd edn, Churchill Livingstone, 1978) and *Advances in the Management of Cleft Palate* edited by M. Edwards and A. C. H. Watson (Churchill Livingstone, 1980). One of the most rapidly developing fields is that of hand surgery and there is a journal devoted to developments in this area. Neverthe-less, there are a number of books which deal comprehensively with the subject. They include *Hand Surgery* edited by J. E. Flynn (3rd edn, Williams and Wilkins, 1982), *The Practice of Hand Surgery* edited by D. W. Lamb and K. Kuczynski (Blackwell, 1981) and, although it is now dated, *The Hand: Diagnosis and Indications* by G. Lister (Churchill Livingstone, 1977) is useful for its outline of the principles of treatment and clinical examination rather than operation techniques. *Burns, A Team Approach* edited by C. P. Artz *et al.* (Saunders, 1979) can be recommended as the summa-tion of work by 43 recognized authorities on the subject.

Urological surgery

Some of the principal journals of interest to the urological surgeon are the *British Journal of Urology, Journal of Urology, Urologic Clinics of North America, Nephron, Scandinavian Journal of Urology* and *Nephrology*. The *British Journal of Urology* also carries a select list of appropriate articles appearing in a range of periodi-cals. This is *Current Urological Literature: Select Bibliography* and it is arranged anatomically.

An up-to-date review publication is *Recent Advances in Urology – 3* edited by W. F. Hendry (Churchill Livingstone, 1981) with chapters on prostatectomy in the 1980s, treatment of urologic can-cer and repair of hypospadias.

Current Trends in Urology is a new series, vol 1 being edited by M. I. Resnick (Williams and Wilkins, 1981) which covers a range of some 10 subjects, including vaso-vasotomy.

There are several comprehensive textbooks of surgical urology. Some of the best known are *Campbell's Urology* edited by J. H. Harrison *et al* (4th edn, Saunders, 1979) and *Current Operative Urology* edited by E. D. Whitehead and E. Leiter (2nd edn, Har-per and Row, in preparation). Less recent, but still in current use, are *Operative Urology* by J. Blandy (Blackwell, 1978), *Urologic Surgery* edited by J. F. Glenn and W. H. Boyce (Harper and Row, 1975) and *Urology* edited by D. Innes Williams (Butterworths, 1977). This last is in the *Operative Surgery* series. Background reading for Surgical Fellowship candidates is provided by *Scientific Foundations of Urology* edited by G. D. Chisholm and D. Innes Williams (Heinemann, 1982). More specialized texts include *Renal Transplantation. Theory and Practice* edited by J. Hamburger *et al.* (2nd edn, Williams and Wilkins, 1981), a compact useful reference book, and *Endoscopic Operative Urology* by J. P. Mitchell (Wright, 1981). 'Genitourinary problems' in *Pediatrics* by A. B.

Belman and G. W. Kaplan (Holt-Saunders, 1981) is a suitable review of current practice in a rapidly developing specialty.

Abdominal surgery

The preserve of the general surgeon includes abdominal surgery, and relevant articles are to be found in the standard surgical journals, as well as in the specialist journals such as *Digestive Diseases and Sciences, American Journal of Gastroenterology, Diseases of the Colon and Rectum, Gastroenterology* and *Gut.*

A comprehensive index to the journal literature in gastroenterology is provided by *Gastroenterology Abstracts and Citations,* which is MEDLARS-based and appears monthly. A number of the more important citations carry abstracts. Selective abstracts are provided by *Excerpta Medica, Section 48: Gastroenterology.*

Some of the books currently available in this area of surgery are the following: *Abdominal Operations* edited by R. Maingot (7th edn, Prentice Hall International, 1980), a good practical guide but expensive for the individual pocket. *Manual of Lower Gastrointestinal Surgery* by C. E. Welch, L. W. Ottinger and J. P. Welch (Springer, 1980) is one of a series from this publisher under the general title of *Comprehensive Manuals of Surgical Specialties.* Two other works which can be recommended for postgraduate study are *Surgery of the Alimentary Tract* by R. T. Shackleford and G. D. Zuidema (2nd edn, Saunders, 1981–1982) and *Gastrointestinal Surgery* by J. S. Najarian and J. P. Delaney (Year Book Medical Publishers, 1979). This last has multiple-choice question tests at the end of each chapter, which makes it beneficial to Fellowship candidates. Three shorter and more concise works may be recommended: *Cope's Early Diagnosis of the Acute Abdomen* edited by W. Silen (15th edn, Oxford University Press, 1979), the *Acute Abdomen for the Man on the Spot* by J. C. Angell (3rd edn, Pitman, 1978), both of which are ideal for the house surgeon or junior registrar, and a recent American work, *Introduction to Abdominal Surgery: Fifty Clinical Studies* by C. J. Schein (Harper and Row, 1981). More specific textbooks include:

Surgery of the Anus, Rectum and Colon by J. C. Goligher (4th edn, Ballière, Tindall and Cassell, 1980)
Intestinal Obstruction by H. Ellis (Prentice Hall, 1982)
Surgery of the Gall Bladder and Bile Ducts by Lord Smith of Marlow and S. Sherlock (2nd edn, Butterworths, 1981)
Hepatic, Biliary and Pancreatic Surgery edited by J. S. Najarian and J. P. Delaney (Year Book Medical Publishers, 1980)

History of surgery

Probably the best known source book of historical information is *Garrison and Morton's Medical Bibliography* by L. T. Morton (4th edn, Gower, 1983). The National Library of Medicine in the US produces a *Bibliography of the History of Medicine*, which is currently available in two five-year cumulations, one covering 1970–1974 and the other covering 1975–1979. There are several good texts on the history of surgery. Two recent publications are the *Rise of Surgery* by O. W. Wangensteen and S. D. Wangensteen (Dawson, 1978) and *The Healers, a History of Medicine in Scotland* by D. Hamilton (Canongate, 1981). Older standard texts include *The History and Literature of Surgery* by J. S. Billings (Argosy Antiquarian, 1970), a reprint of a classic text initially published in 1895 as part of *A System of Surgery* by F. S. Dennis; *An Introduction to the History of Surgery* by R. H. Meade (Saunders, 1970) is useful as a basis for further study and contains an excellent bibliography; *Great Ideas in the History of Surgery* by L. M. Zimmerman and J. Veith (Baillière, Tindall and Cox, 1962) contains extracts from antiquarian texts and verbatim reports as they originally appeared; *Milestones in Modern Surgery* by A. Hurwitz and G. A. Degenshein (Cassell, 1958) is, perforce, dependent upon the American authors' concept of a milestone, but the criteria used for selection ensure a reasonable survey; *The Development of Modern Surgery* by F. E. Cartwright (Arthur Baker, 1967) covers the last 150 years and is designed for the lay reader as well as the student of medical history. A classic which has been reprinted and is again available since its appearance 50 years ago is *A Short History of Surgery* by D'Arcy Power (New York, A. M. S. Press, 1981). Information on the history of surgery is also to be found in the histories of some great institutions, e.g. *The Royal College of Surgeons of England – A History* by Z. Cope (Blond, 1959) and in the biographies of famous surgeons.

   In addition to the volumes already mentioned, there are a number of books dealing with the historical aspect of surgical specialties. Examples of this type are *History of Urology* by L. S. Murphy (C. C. Thomas, 1972), an exhaustive treatise on the subject. *A History of the Acute Abdomen* by Z. Cope (Oxford University Press, 1965) is a compact work crammed with well organized information and *A History of Thoracic Surgery* by R. Meade (Blackwell, 1961) runs to 1000 pages and carries an extensive bibliography. Plastic surgery is served by *The Source Book of Plastic Surgery* by F. McDowell (Williams and Wilkins, 1977). However, no resumé of the history of this specialty would be complete without mention of *McDowell Indexes of Plastic Surgery* edited by F. McDowell (Williams and Wilkins, 1977–1981). This monumental five-volume work covers citations in journal or book form from 900 BC to 1976 and must rank as an astonishing piece of historical research.

The literature of anaesthesia

Within the last few decades the scope of anaesthetics has enlarged from the concept of the ether bottle, and now includes not only a more sophisticated range of anaesthetic agents, but also changes in the method of induction, including intravenous anaesthetic drugs and relaxants. Improved methods as well as advances in physiology and pharmacology have enabled the surgeon to gain access to deeper structures and to explore more extensively and with greater safety than before. The modern anaesthetist must have a considerable knowledge, anatomical and functional, of the respiratory, cardiovascular and nervous system. Metabolism, excretion and endocrine function also have aspects related to the efficient practice of anaesthetics. Techniques have become specialized for anaesthetists in oto-rhino-laryngology, dental surgery, pulmonary operations, neurosurgery, ophthalmology and electroconvulsive therapy. Special care units – respiratory and coronary – and intensive care therapy units now involve a large contribution from the anaesthetist.

The principal English language journals of anaesthesia are:

Acta Anaesthesiologica Scandinavica
Anaesthesia
Anesthesia and Analgesia
Anesthesiology
Anaesthesia and Intensive Care
British Journal of Anaesthesia

Anaesthesia contains *Anaesthetic Literature* which is a classified list of recent articles pertaining to anaesthetics. This journal also carries reviews of appropriate audio-visual material available.

Abstracting and indexing services

Excerpta Medica Section 24: Anesthesiology
Anesthesia Abstracts
Anesthesiology Bibliography, is quarterly service provided by the National Library of Medicine in the US through the Wood Library–Museum of Anesthesiology, and is useful as a quick-reference tool

Textbooks and monographs

Comprehensive textbooks have the disadvantage of being out of date, often by the time of publication, but they do have the merit of gathering together current concepts and practice in one or two volumes. A reasonably up-to-date and comprehensive textbook is *Anaesthesia* edited by R. D. Miller, (2 vols, Churchill Livingstone, 1981). *General Anaesthesia* edited by T. C. Gray, J. F. Nunn and J. E. Utting, (2 vols, 4th edn, Churchill Livingstone, 1979) is another two volume work; vol 1 covers the basic sciences while vol 2 deals with clinical practice. Another standard reference work, *A Practice of Anaesthesia* edited by H. C. Churchill Davidson (4th edn, Lloyd-Luke, 1978) is popular, although its examples and citations tend to ignore the European literature. The preceding three texts are all suitable for postgraduate specialist study in this field and, in addition, *The Scientific Foundations of Anaesthesia* edited by C. Scurr and S. Feldman (3rd edn, Heinemann, 1982) may be recommended to those taking higher examinations in anaesthesia. There are a number of good monographs dealing with anaesthesia under a variety of conditions and occasions and, while there are many such monographs, among the more recent and well received are:

Anaesthesia for Cardiac Surgery and Allied Procedures by M. A. Branthwaite (2nd edn, Blackwell, 1980)
Paediatric Anasthesia by H. T. Davenport (3rd edn, Heinemann, 1980)
Neurosurgical Anaesthesia and Intensive Care by T. V. Campkin and J. M. Turner (Butterworths, 1980)
Obstetric Anaesthesia and Analgesia by D. D. Moir (2nd edn, Ballière Tindall, 1980)

History of anaesthesia

The last few decades have seen some considerable developments in anaesthesia and this comparatively recent history is covered by *Anesthesiology Progress since 1940* by E. M. Papper, S. H. Ngai and L. C. Mark (University of Miami Press, 1973). An earlier period is dealt with in *Essays on the First Hundred Years of Anaesthesia* by W. S. Sykes (Churchill Livingstone, 1961). This two-volume work has been re-issued under the Krieger imprint in 1972, meanwhile a new, third volume of the *Essays* edited by R. Ellis was published by Churchill Livingstone in 1982. *Foundations of Anesthesiology* by A. Faulconer and T. E. Keys (C. C. Thomas, 1965) is a compilation of some 150 reprints of famous papers on anaesthesia and related topics. Another compilation of first-hand accounts is *Milestones in Anesthesia* by F. Cole (University of Nebraska Press, 1965) which covers the period 1665–1940. *The Evolution of Anaesthesia* by M. H. Armstrong Davidson (John Sherratt, 1965) is a history in which the author sets out to dispel some of the 'romantic myths' of the 'conquest of pain'. B. M. Duncum's *The Development of Inhalation Anaesthesia* (Oxford University Press, 1947) deals with the period 1846–1900. An earlier work which has been updated by additional material is *History of Surgical Anesthesia* by T. E. Keys (Krieger, 1978). In conclusion the history of the extensive range of anaesthetic equipment is explored in *The Development of Anaesthetic Apparatus* by K. B. Thomas (Blackwell, 1975). This is a history based on the Charles King collection of the Association of Anaesthetists of Great Britain and Ireland.

19

Obstetrics and gynaecology

P. C. Want

It is inadvisable even to attempt to isolate the literature of any
medical specialty, since each embraces an indefinable 'grey' area
of closely related subjects which must be included in any worthwhile survey. Obstetrics and gynaecology is no exception and,
under the umbrella of this general heading, such topics as embryology, endocrinology, infertility, female urology and family planning are included, in addition to texts dealing with the main topics
of pregnancy and diseases of women. Texts on medical sexology
and andrology, subjects hitherto somewhat neglected, are of
increasing interest to gynaecologists. The published work of
experts in other fields, for example anaesthetics, is important when
written with the special needs of the pregnant patient in mind.

Indexes and abstracts

The prime bibliographic tool is *Index Medicus* and its annual
cumulations, described in Chapter 3. There are also a number of
indexes and abstracts which are more specialized and can be consulted in conjunction with, or instead of, *Index Medicus.*

A new bi-monthly current-awareness publication in the *Ad
Referendum* series is now available. This is *Ad Referendum:
Obstetrics and Gynaecology* (Infomed, 1982–) which comprises the
collected contents lists of selected core journals and bibliographical details of relevant articles from certain other publications. It is

available free to interested medical practitioners on application. *Core Journals in Obstetrics/Gynecology* (Excerpta Medica, 1977–) contains abstracts from some 14 leading specialist periodicals and six or so general medical journals, with the intention of providing, within one month of publication, notification of important clinical papers. A companion series entitled *Core Journals in Clinical Endocrinology* was first published in 1982.

The *Bibliography of Reproduction: a Classified Monthly List of References Compiled from the Research Literature; Vertebrates including Man* (Reproduction Information Service, 1963–) cites selected books and theses as well as certain journals not included in *Index Medicus*, and is, as the title suggests, aimed particularly at research workers. It is an official publication of the Society for the Study of Fertility (UK), the Society for the Study of Reproduction (US), the Australian Society for Reproductive Biology and the Blair Bell Research Society. Published monthly, in two volumes per annum, each issue carries author and animal indexes and each volume a subject index referring to individual citation numbers. It is more up-to-date than *Index Medicus* and is designed for current rather than retrospective searching. Several thousand journals are covered and 50 per cent of the papers indexed are in foreign languages, translations of the titles being provided. Entries are grouped under broad subject headings, each paper being cited in only one place and allotted a serial number which may be quoted as a cross-reference elsewhere. Within each subject section books and monographs are listed first, followed by papers in a hierarchy running from humans through to fishes. Addresses of authors are included wherever possible. The absence of any cumulation of the monthly indexes hampers retrospective searching when checking for example, details of an item which has not appeared in *Index Medicus*, but which has appeared elsewhere. Special subject bibliographies are included in certain issues and are also available separately. Every few months a useful list of future meetings pertaining to reproductive biology is issued. The Reproduction Research Information Service, commencing with the literature of 1963, operates a literature search service based on an information store with over 260 000 references (December 1982) which is growing at a rate of 1400–1800 per month.

Abstracting publications tend to be more selective in their coverage and often concentrate on the more important papers appearing in the major medical journals of the world. The most comprehensive abstracting publication is *Excerpta Medica; Section 10: Obstetrics and Gynecology* (1948–). This now appears in two volumes per annum, each consisting of ten issues in which author and keyword subject indexes are provided both cumulating in the final issue. Abstracts are generally short and often comprise the summary already published at source. Nonetheless, this is a useful source of information, often eliminating the need to pursue the original paper. The *Human Genetics* (1963–) and *Endocrinology* (1947–) *Sections,* numbered 22 and 3 respectively, are also useful. The *Year Book of Obstetrics and Gynecology* (Year Book Medical Publishers, 1902–) often contains a review paper and many of the summaries are substantial, with occasional accompanying editorial comment. An effort is made at rough subject grouping which is helpful in reviewing recent work on a particular topic. *Obstetrical and Gynecological Survey* (Williams and Wilkins, 1946–) provides a survey of recently published literature. Each monthly issue contains a good review article in addition to substantial summaries of important papers. Editorial comment accompanies each summary, often at length. Each December issue comprises a five-year cumulated author and subject index to both reviews and abstracts, providing a useful quick reference guide to recent literature.

The International Abstracts of Surgery section of *Surgery, Gynecology and Obstetrics* (American College of Surgeons) appeared in the latter publication from 1913, vol 16 onwards. It contains signed abstracts on the 'Surgery of the female reproductive system' which is subdivided into: uterus and adnexa; ovaries; external genitalia; pregnancy and complications; and placenta, fetus and newborn. Emphasis throughout is, however, on general surgery and the periodical itself cannot be regarded as a primary journal in the subject field of obstetrics and gynaecology. The abstracts are, therefore, of limited value since non-subscribers are unlikely to take the trouble to check them.

A new publication of a more specialized nature is *Obstetric Anesthesia Digest* (Elsevier Biomedical, 1981–). It appears quarterly and is particularly useful to the specialist library which may not be able to justify subscriptions to journals in the field of anaesthetics, since good summaries of important papers are provided together with critical commentaries. The obstetric anaesthetist may find it of sufficient interest for his or her personal library, especially since it is published ready-punched for a ring binder and takes up very little space.

Similar publications originate overseas. These include:

Berichte über die gesamte Gynäkologie und Geburtshilfe sowie deren Grenzgebeite (Berlin, 1923–)
Meditsinskii Referativnyi Zhurnal (Moscow, 1957–)
Gynäkologische Rundschau (Basle, 1964–)
Rassegna Bibliografica della Stampa Ostetrico–Ginecologica (Rome, 1949–)

Sekai Sanfujinka Soran [Survey of World Obstetrics and Gynaecology] (Tokyo, 1958–)

Dictionaries

Although it cannot be considered a dictionary in the usual sense of the term, *Obstetric-Gynecologic Terminology* edited by E. C. Hughes (Davis, 1972) is a most useful reference tool. It has a subject arrangement, with an index providing the key to the whole. A brief definition is given, together with any known synonyms for each term and, generally, more detail is included than in conventional medical dictionaries. A polyglot dictionary is available, prepared by N. C. Louros and entitled *Obstétrique et Gynécologie: glossaire des termes obstétricaux et gynécologiques en français, latin, anglais, russe, allemand, espagnol, italien, grec* (Elsevier, 1964). A selection of dictionaries intended for midwives has been published, the most recent being *Baillière's Midwives Dictionary* by V. Da Cruz and M. Adams (6th edn, Baillière Tindall, 1976).

Directories

Publications of this nature have a limited 'life', even when updated at regular intervals. Among the more useful directories are the *Royal College of Obstetricians and Gynaecologists, Register of Fellows and Members (RCOG, 1966–)*, published bi-annually. Arrangement is alphabetical, with separate sections for Fellows and Members, and each section contains a geographical breakdown. The counterpart for the US is the American College of Obstetricians and Gynecologists' *Directory of Fellows, with By-Laws, Councils, Commissions, Committees and Task Forces,* the most recent edition (1983–4) being issued from the new home of the College in Washington, DC. Continental publications include *Gynäkologen deutscher Sprache. Biographie und Bibliographie* (Stuttgart), published under various titles since 1928.

Periodicals

Numerous important papers are, of course, to be found in leading general medical journals, such as the *New England Journal of Medicine, British Medical Journal* and *The Lancet.* Periodicals devoted specifically to obstetrics, gynaecology and closely related subjects, such as infertility and endocrinology, not only exist in abundance but are also increasing with the addition of some two or three new titles each year that require serious consideration. Listed below, and grouped roughly by subject, are a selection of the most important titles, with emphasis on British and American publications. Representative journals from other countries are noted, as are details of a number of newer titles which at present may not easily be traced in checklists elsewhere.

Obstetrics and gynaecology

Acta Obstetrica et Gynecologica Scandinavica (Umea, 1926–)
American Journal of Obstetrics and Gynecology (St. Louis, 1920–)
Archives of Gynecology (Munich, 1978–)
Asia-Oceania Journal of Obstetrics and Gynaecology (Tokyo, 1980–)
Australian and New Zealand Journal of Obstetrics and Gynaecology (Melbourne, 1961–)
Biology of Reproduction (Champaign, 1969–)
British Journal of Obstetrics and Gynaecology (Oxford, 1975–)
Clinical Obstetrics and Gynecology (Philadelphia, 1958–)
Clinics in Obstetrics and Gynaecology (Eastbourne, 1974–)
Contemporary Ob/Gyn (Oradell, 1975–)
Diagnostic Gynecology and Obstetrics (New York, 1979–)
Early Human Development (Amsterdam, 1977–)
European Journal of Obstetrics, Gynaecology and Reproductive Biology (Amsterdam, 1973–)
Geburtshilfe und Frauenheilkunde (Stuttgart, 1939–)
Gynecologic Investigation (Basle, 1970–)
Gynecologic Oncology (New York, 1972–)
International Journal of Biological Research in Pregnancy (Munich, 1980–)
International Journal of Gynecological Pathology (New York, 1982–)
International Journal of Gynaecology and Obstetrics (Limerick, 1969–)
Journal de Gynécologie, Obstétrique et Biologie de la Reproduction (Paris, 1972–)
Journal of Obstetrics and Gynaecology (Bristol, 1980–)
Journal of Perinatal Medicine (Berlin and New York, 1973–)
Journal of Reproductive Immunology (Amsterdam, 1980–)
Journal of Reproductive Medicine (Chicago, 1968–)
Maturitas (Amsterdam, 1979–)
Minerva Ginecologica (Torino, 1950–)
Obstetrics and Gynecology (New York, 1953–)
Placenta (Eastbourne, 1980–)
Prenatal Diagnosis (New York, 1981–)
Seminars in Perinatology (New York, 1977–)
Surgery, Gynecology and Obstetrics (Chicago, 1905–)
Toko-ginecologica Practica (Madrid, 1936–)
Zeitschrift für Geburtshilfe und Perinatologie (Stuttgart, 1972–)
Zentralblatt für Gynäkologie (Leipzig, 1877–1944; 1947–)

Fertility, sterility and contraception

Acta Europaea Fertilitatis (Padua, 1969–)
British Journal of Family Planning (London, 1977–)
Clinical Reproduction and Fertility (Oxford, 1982–)
Contraception (Los Altos, 1970–)
Fertility and Sterility (Birmingham, 1950–)
Infertility (New York, 1978–)
International Journal of Fertility (Lawrence, 1955–)
Journal of Reproduction and Fertility (Cambridge, 1960–)

Endocrinology

Acta Endocrinologica (Valby, 1948–)
Clinical Endocrinology (Oxford, 1972–)
Endocrinology (Baltimore, 1917–)
Journal of Clinical Endocrinology and Metabolism (Baltimore, 1941–)
Journal of Endocrinology (Colchester, 1939–)

Human genetics

American Journal of Human Genetics (Baltimore, 1949)
Annals of Human Genetics (Cambridge, 1954–)
Journal of Medical Genetics (London, 1964–)

Serials and series in book form

A number of serials, generally hardback publications, are particularly useful for reviews or special topic studies within the subject field. Extensive bibliographies may be included. A recent example is *Progress in Obstetrics and Gynaecology* edited by J. W. W. Studd (vol 3, Churchill Livingstone, 1983). Content is divided equally between the two subject fields and chapters are contributed by specialists on topics of current interest. *Recent Advances in Obstetrics and Gynaecology* edited by John Bonnar (vol 14, Churchill Livingstone, 1982) has appeared under various editors since 1947, but individual chapters are not necessarily revised in new editions. A similar publication from America that is devoted to gynaecology is M. L. Taymor and T. H. Green's *Progress in Gynecology* (the latest being vol 6, Grune and Stratton, 1975). *Obstetrics and Gynecology Annual* (vol 12, Appleton-Century-Crofts, 1983) contains review articles on various topics and has an American bias. Long bibliographies at the end of most papers are a significant and useful feature. The two titles *Clinics in Obstetrics and Gynaecology,* published by Saunders, and *Clinical Obstetrics and Gynecology,* published by Harper and Row, are a perpetual cause of reference confusion, especially when quoted in abbreviated form, since the distinction between British and American spelling is often overlooked. The difference in volume numbers is the most useful guide as only one volume is produced annually in each case. *Clinical Obstetrics* was first published in 1958 and appears quarterly, whilst the volumes in the *Clinics* series appear in three parts per annum, commencing in 1974. The latter has proved popular with postgraduate students preparing for primary examinations in the specialty, since most of the contributors are known specialists in their subject field. Each part generally consists of two main sections containing a selection of papers on a major topic. The American series has a similar arrangement of a selection of papers on two or three topics.

Among the small number of more specialized publications are *Reviews in Perinatal Medicine* edited by E. M. Scarpelli and E. V. Cosmi (vol 4, Raven Press, 1981); *Clinics in Perinatology* (vol 1, Saunders, 1974, in progress), which is similar in format to *Clinics in Obstetrics and Gynaecology;* and *Advances in Reproductive Physiology* (vol 5, Academic Press, 1971).

Some hardback publications that appear as series are separately advertised as monographs and cited under author and volume title. An example is *Clinics in Obstetrics and Gynaecology* and others are:

Contributions to Gynecology and Obstetrics (Karger, 1961–)
Major Problems in Obstetrics and Gynecology (Saunders, 1970–)
Developments in Obstetrics and Gynecology (Nijhoff, 1980–)
Butterworths International Medical Reviews: Obstetrics and Gynaecology (1981–)

Textbooks and monographs

In the sections below an attempt has been made at a logical progression from general to specific, but books on more than one subject are allotted the earliest appropriate placing without subsequent repetition.

Obstetrics with gynaecology

Standard reference works include C. J. Dewhurst's *Integrated Obstetrics and Gynaecology for Postgraduates* (3rd edn, Blackwell, 1981); *Combined Textbook of Obstetrics and Gynaecology* edited by J. Walker, I. MacGillivray and M. C. MacNaughton (9th edn, Churchill Livingstone, 1976); J. C. M. Browne's *Postgraduate Obstetrics and Gynaecology* (4th edn, Butterworths, 1973); *Obstet-*

rics and Gynecology by J. R. Willson and E. R. Carrington (6th edn, Mosby, 1979) and D. N. Danforth's *Obstetrics and Gynecology* (4th edn, Harper and Row, 1982). Among the smaller paperbacks available are J. Willocks' *Essential Obstetrics and Gynaecology for Postgraduates* (2nd edn, Churchill Livingstone, 1982) and M. M. Anderson's *A Handbook of Obstetrics and Gynaecology for the House Officer* (Faber, 1981). Two useful texts for foundation studies for primary examinations are *Scientific Foundations of Obstetrics and Gynaecology* edited by E. E. Philipp, J. Barnes and M. Newton (2nd edn, Heinemann, 1977) and *Scientific Basis of Obstetrics and Gynaecology* edited by R. R. Macdonald (2nd edn, Churchill Livingstone, 1978). For undergraduates the available texts include D. Llewellyn-Jones' *Fundamentals of Obstetrics and Gynaecology; vol 1, Obstetrics; vol 2, Gynaecology* (3rd edn, Faber, 1982); R. W. Taylor and M. G. Brush's *Obstetrics and Gynaecology* (Baillière Tindall, 1978); B. G. Wren's *Handbook of Obstetrics and Gynaecology* (Baillière Tindall, 1979); G. V. P. Chamberlain and C. J. Dewhurst's *Practice of Obstetrics and Gynaecology* (Pitman, 1977) and *Undergraduate Obstetrics and Gynaecology* edited by H. G. Dixon (Wright, 1980). These are, on the whole, also quite adequate for revision purposes at Diploma level, if supplemented by the larger texts as necessary.

Tropical medicine is covered by the textbook *Obstetrics and Gynaecology in the Tropics and Developing Countries* by J. B. Lawson and D. B. Stewart (Arnold, 1967) and a number of publications are available on the subject of obstetrical and gynaecological emergencies as follows:

Handbook of Obstetric Emergencies: a Guide for Emergencies in Obstetrics and Gynecology by R. H. Schwarz (2nd edn, Kimpton, 1977)
Emergencies in Gynecology and Obstetrics (Year Book Medical Publishers, 1981) translated by H. E. Kaiser from the second German edition (Thieme, 1974)
Manual of Gynecologic and Obstetric Emergencies by B.-Z. Taber (Saunders, 1979)
Emergencies in Obstetrics and Gynecology by A. W. Cohen (Churchill Livingstone, 1981)

The two branches of the specialty are often treated separately for greater emphasis on one or the other. They are divided below for easier reference as this may be helpful to those called upon to make the distinction. One or two titles from each section probably complement the general texts sufficiently for most purposes.

OBSTETRICS

The more comprehensive textbooks are *Williams' Obstetrics* by J. A. Pritchard and P. C. MacDonald (16th edn, Appleton-Century-

Crofts, 1980); J. P. Greenhill and E. R. Friedman's *Biological Principles and Modern Practice of Obstetrics* (Saunders, 1974), which is the successor to *Greenhill's Obstetrics* (13th edn, 1965); *Beck's Obstetrical Practice and Fetal Medicine* by E. S. Taylor (10th edn, Williams and Wilkins, 1976) and a new two-volume work *Principles and Practice of Obstetrics and Perinatology* edited by L. Iffy and H. Kaminetzky (Wiley, 1981). On the whole the equivalent British publications are less substantial in their content, but are favoured for reference by those familiar with British obstetric practice. Such titles are *Holland and Brews' Manual of Obstetrics* by.R. Percival (14th edn, Churchill Livingstone, 1980) and *Obstetrics by Ten Teachers* edited by S. G. Clayton, T. L. T. Lewis and G. Pinker (13th edn, Arnold, 1980). *Obstetrics and the Newborn* by N. A. Beischer and E. V. Mackay (Saunders, 1978) originally appeared in Australia in 1976 and makes easy reading, as does *Obstetrics Illustrated* by M. M. Garrey, A. D. T. Govan, C. Hodge and R. Callander (3rd edn, Churchill Livingstone, 1980). Handbooks and quick-reference works are readily available, among which may be noted G. V. P. Chamberlain's *Lecture Notes on Obstetrics* (4th edn, Blackwell, 1980); G. J. Amiel's *Essential Obstetric Practice* (MTP, 1981); S. Bender and V. R. Tindall's *Practical Student Obstetrics* (Heinemann, 1980); *Obstetrics* by G. M. Stirrat (Grant McIntyre, 1981); and *Pocket Obstetrics* by Sir Stanley Clayton and J. R. Newton (Churchill Livingstone, 1979). Two reference texts suitable for midwives are M. F. Myles' *Textbook for Midwives* (9th edn, Churchill Livingstone, 1981) and J. Towler and R. Butler-Manuel's *Modern Obstetrics for Student Midwives* (Lloyd-Luke, 1973). Obstetric complications are dealt with in Professor Ian Donald's *Practical Obstetric Problems* (5th edn, Lloyd-Luke, 1979) and *Obstetric Emergencies* by D. Cavanagh, R. E. Woods and T. C. O'Connor (3rd edn, Harper and Row, 1982). Other titles of interest in this general section include *Textbook for Midwives in the Tropics* by O. A. Ojo and E. B. Briggs (2nd edn, Arnold, 1982) and, for those interested in the application of computers to the specialty, O. J. S. Van Hemel's *An Obstetric Data Base: Human Factors, Design and Reliability* (Thesis, Free University of Amsterdam, 1977), copies of which are available from the Department of Medical Informatics.

GYNAECOLOGY

Those interested in the diseases of women may consult Sir Norman Jeffcoate's *Principles of Gynaecology* (4th edn, Butterworths, 1975) as a standard reference work. Alternatively, two American publications worth noting are *Novak's Textbook of Gynecology* by H. W. Jones and G. S. Jones (10th edn, Williams and Wilkins, 1981) and L. Parsons and S. C. Sommers' *Gynecology* (2nd edn, Saunders, 1978). Also useful is *Gynaecology by Ten Teachers* under the direction of S. G. Clayton and edited by S. G. Clayton, D. Fraser and T. L. T. Lewis (13th edn, Arnold, 1980), which has appeared regularly since 1919 when it bore the title *Diseases of Women*. Few other comparable publications have appeared in new editions in recent years as new titles have succeeded them in importance. Two texts that are profusely illustrated in colour recently appeared on the market almost simultaneously; namely, N. A. Beischer and E. V. Mackay's *Colour Atlas of Gynaecology* (Saunders, 1981) and V. R. Tindall's *Colour Atlas of Clinical Gynaecology* (Wolfe, 1981). A popular volume with examination candidates at various levels is *Gynaecology Illustrated* by M. M. Garrey, A. D. T. Govan, C. H. Hodge and R. Callander (2nd edn, Churchill Livingstone, 1978) and 'pocket' reference works include *Lecture Notes on Gynaecology* by Dame Josephine Barnes (5th edn, Blackwell, 1983); *Pocket Gynaecology* by Sir Stanley Clayton and J. R. Newton (9th edn, Churchill Livingstone, 1979) and *Guidelines to Gynaecology* by M. D. Read and S. Mellor (Blackwell, 1982). *Everywoman: a Gynaecological Guide for Life* by J. D. Llewellyn-Jones (3rd edn, Faber, 1982) is intended for the laywoman.

Obstetrics and gynaecology related to childhood, adolescence and the ageing woman

Of the various publications available the following are particularly useful: *The Gynecology of Childhood and Adolescence* by J. W. Huffman, Sir C. John Dewhurst and V. J. Capraro (2nd edn, Saunders, 1981); *Practical Pediatric and Adolescent Gynecology* by Sir John Dewhurst with a contribution by G. V. P. Chamberlain (Dekker, 1980), and *The Ageing Reproductive System* edited by E. L. Schneider (Raven Press, 1978). Unless the reader is particularly interested in the sociological aspects of adolescent pregnancy most of the books on the pregnant teenager may be ignored since they contain little of interest to the clinician. An exception is *Adolescent Obstetrics and Gynecology* edited by A. K. K. Kreutner and D. R. Hollingsworth (Year Book Medical Publishers, 1978) which has a large section on the subject. Texts on particular aspects of the above subjects are also mentioned under appropriate headings later in the chapter.

Anatomy and physiology, diagnosis, pathology, surgery and therapy related to obstetrics and gynaecology

Only the more general works are dealt with in this section; those on specific topics are included in the relevant categories.

ANATOMY AND PHYSIOLOGY

A basic reference book is *Gynaecological and Obstetrical Anatomy* by C. F. V. Smout, F. Jacoby and E. W. Lillie (4th edn, Lewis, 1969) and a simpler text, more suitable for undergraduates and midwives, is C. W. F. Burnett's *Anatomy and Physiology of Obstetrics* revised by M. M. Anderson (6th edn, Faber, 1979). Another standard text is *Clinical Physiology in Obstetrics* edited by F. E. Hytten and G. V. P. Chamberlain (Blackwell, 1980), previously published as *The Physiology of Human Pregnancy*. The proceedings of a workshop have been published as *Development and Function of the Reproductive Organs* edited by A. G. Byskov and H. Peters (Excerpta Medica, 1981). The most recent publication on pelvic anatomy is *Moloy's Evaluation of the Pelvis in Obstetrics* by C. M. Steer (3rd edn, Plenum, 1975) and the lymphatic system of this region is dealt with in *Lymphatic System of the Female Genitalia* by A. A. Plentl and E. A. Friedman (Saunders, 1971), which is the second volume in the series entitled *Major Problems in Obstetrics and Gynecology*.

DIAGNOSIS

Developments in ultrasound and peritoneoscopy have resulted in a surge of publications on these subjects, only a selection of which are given here; it should be borne in mind that many others are available. Useful books are M. J. Bennett and S. J. Campbell's *Real Time Ultrasound in Obstetrics* (Blackwell, 1980); R. G. Law's *Ultrasound in Clinical Obstetrics* (Wright, 1980); M. Kobayashi's *Illustrated Manual of Ultrasonography in Obstetrics and Gynecology* (2nd edn, Igaku Shoin, 1980) and P. A. Athey and E. P. Hadlock's *Ultrasound in Obstetrics and Gynecology* (Mosby, 1981). The proceedings of a scientific meeting of the Royal College of Obstetricians and Gynaecologists, 2nd December, 1977, were published as *The Current Status of Fetal Heart Rate Monitoring and Ultrasound in Obstetrics* edited by R. W. Beard and S. Campbell (RCOG, 1978). *Progress in Medical Ultrasound: Reviews and Comments* by A. Kurjak (vol 1, Excerpta Medica, 1980, in progress) has now reached vol 3 and has useful chapters devoted to obstetrics and gynaecology which contain numerous references for further reading. *Fetal Ultrasonography: the Secret Prenatal Life* by F. Borruto, M. Hansmann and J. W. Wladimiroff (Wiley, 1982), the proceedings of a meeting, is now available and contains chapters on topics such as fetal biometry, prenatal diagnosis of malformations, and prenatal behaviour, as well as more specialized material.

Of the books available on endoscopy and peritoneoscopy the following should be noted: P. C. Steptoe's *Laparoscopy in Gynecology* (Livingstone, 1967), which still awaits a long-promised new edition; S. Dexeus, J. M. Carrera and F. Coupez' *Colposcopy* (Saunders, 1977), translated from the Spanish edition of 1973 and vol 10 in the series *Major Problems in Obstetrics and Gynecology;* H. Bauer's *Color Atlas of Colposcopy* (Igaku Shoin, 1979), translated by A. Schaetzing and containing approximately 100 colour illustrations; and M. Coppleson, E. Pixley and B. Reid's *Colposcopy: a Scientific and Practical Approach to the Cervix and Vagina in Health and Disease* (2nd edn, C. C. Thomas, 1978). Two popular atlases are P. Kolstad's *Atlas of Colposcopy* (3rd edn, Universitetsforlaget; University Park Press; 1982) and the beautifully produced volume by R. Cartier entitled *Practical Colposcopy* (Karger, 1977).

Radiology is covered by J. G. B. Russell's *Radiology in Obstetrics and Antenatal Paediatrics* (Butterworths, 1973) and *Radiography in Obstetrics* by A. S. Fisher and J. G. B. Russell (Butterworths, 1975).

Books on cytodiagnosis are no longer as widely available as in past years, so a few older but still useful titles are mentioned here. A forerunner was the classic *Atlas of Exfoliative Cytology* by G. N. Papanicolaou (Harvard University Press, 1954), to which supplements were issued in 1956 and 1960. Later publications were E. G. Wachtel's *Exfoliative Cytology in Gynaecological Practice* (2nd edn, Butterworths, 1969) and *Cytology of the Female Genital Tract* by G. Riotton and W. M. Christopherson in collaboration with R. Lunt (WHO, 1973), published as No 8 in the series *International Histological Classification of Tumours.* More recently, the following have appeared: C. Grubb's *Colour Atlas of Gynaecological Cytopathology* (HM & M, 1977); *Gynecological Cytopathology* edited by M. J. Ayala and F. N. Ortiz, translated from the Spanish by M. D. R. Canner (Mosby, 1978), which contains numerous coloured plates; and *Gynaecological Cytopathology* by M. E. Boon and M. L. Tabbers-Bourmeester (Macmillan, 1980).

PATHOLOGY

The best known publications are *Novak's Gynecologic and Obstetric*

Pathology by E. R. Novak and J. Donald Woodruff (8th edn, Saunders, 1979); H. Fox and F. A. Langley's *Postgraduate Obstetrical and Gynaecological Pathology* (Pergamon, 1973); and *Gynaecological Pathology* by M. Haines and C. W. Taylor (2nd edn, Churchill, 1975). In addition there is a most useful large reference work, *Pathology of the Female Genital Tract* edited by A. Blaustein (2nd edn, Springer, 1982), which contains over 1200 illustrations, some in colour, and numerous references to the literature.

Among the books dealing generally with benign diseases that affect the female are:

Infections in Obstetrics and Gynaecology by D. Charles (Saunders, 1980) (Major Problems in Obstetrics and Gynecology; vol 12)
Infectious Diseases in Obstetrics and Gynecology by G. R. G. Monif *et al.* (Harper and Row, 1974);
Gynecologic Disorders: Differential Diagnosis and Therapy edited by C. J. Pauerstein (Grune and Stratton, 1982)
Chronic Pelvic Pain in Women edited by M. Renaer (Springer, 1981)
Genital Infection by Chlamydia Trachomatis by J. D. Oriel and G. L. Ridgway (Arnold, 1982)

Tumours, benign and malignant, are the subject of numerous monographs. Those relating to specific organs are dealt with under the appropriate headings and among the many books published on general gynaecological oncology may be mentioned:

Gynecologic Oncology: Fundamental Principles and Clinical Practice by M. Coppleson (2 vols, Churchill Livingstone, 1981)
Corscaden's Gynecologic Cancer by S. B. Gusberg and H. C. Frick, II (5th edn, Williams and Wilkins, 1978)
Gynaecological Malignancy edited by M. G. Brush and R. W. Taylor (Baillière Tindall, 1975), which concentrates on the endometrium, cervix and ovary
Clinical Gynecologic Oncology by P. J. Disaia and W. T. Creasman (Mosby, 1981)
Malignancies of the Ovary, Uterus and Cervix by R. S. Bush (Arnold, 1979)
Gynecologic Oncology by L. McGowan (Appleton-Century-Croft, 1978)
Gynecological Cancer edited by N. Thatcher (Pergamon, 1979), which concentrates primarily on cancer of the uterus, breast and ovary
Management of Complications in Gynecologic Oncology edited by G. Delgado and J. P. Smith (Wiley, 1982)
Gynecologic Oncology; Controversies in Cancer Treatment by S. Ballon (Hall, 1981)
Modern Concepts of Gynecologic Oncology by J. R. Van Nagel (Wright, 1982)
Controversies in Gynaecological Oncology, the proceedings of a scientific meeting of the Royal College of Obstetricians and Gynaecologists held in February, 1980, and edited by J. A. Jordan and A. Singer (RCOG, 1980)

SURGERY

Among the established textbooks are *R. W. Te Linde's Operative Gynecology* by R. F. Mattingly (5th edn, Lippincott, 1977);

Shaw's Textbook of Operative Gynaecology (4th edn, revised by J. Howkins and C. N. Hudson, 1977) and *Bonney's Gynaecological Surgery* by J. Howkins and Sir John Stallworthy (8th edn, Bailière Tindall, 1974). Several atlases are available, but perhaps the most lavish are the series of six volumes by D. H. Lees and A. Singer entitled *A Colour Atlas of Gynaecological Surgery* (Wolfe, 1978–1982) comprising vol 1, *Vaginal Operations;* vol 2, *Abdominal Operations for Benign Conditions;* vol 3, *Operations for Malignant Disease;* vol 4, *Surgery of Vulva and Lower Genital Tract;* vol 5, *Infertility Surgery;* and vol 6, *Surgery of Conditions Complicating Pregnancy.* Each volume contains a series of colour photographs illustrating, step-by-step, innumerable operative techniques. Other less elaborate but useful reference atlases are J. H. Nelson's *Atlas of Radical Pelvic Surgery* (2nd edn, Appleton-Century-Crofts, 1977); *Gynaecology and Obstetrics* edited by D. W. T. Roberts (3rd edn, Butterworths, 1977), which is part of the series edited by C. Rob and Sir Rodney Smith entitled *Operative Surgery: Fundamental International Techniques;* and L. Parsons and U. Ulfelder's sizeable *Atlas of Pelvic Operations* (2nd edn, Saunders, 1968). More specific are J. H. Bellina's recent book *Gynecologic Laser Surgery* (Plenum, 1981) and P. L. Martin's *Ambulatory Gynecologic Surgery* (PSG, 1979). Two texts are especially devoted to obstetrics, the best known being *Munro Kerr's Operative Obstetrics* edited by P. R. Myerscough (10th edn, Baillière, 1982). An American publication is *Douglas and Stromme's Operative Obstetrics* by E. J. Quilligan and F. Zuspan (4th edn, Appleton-Century-Crofts, 1982).

THERAPY

Two of the earliest texts published specifically on this topic during the past decade are P. J. Lewis' *Therapeutic Problems in Pregnancy* (MTP, 1977) and *Obstetric Therapeutics* edited by D. F. Hawkins (Baillière, 1974) The latter author has also edited a companion volume, *Gynaecological Therapeutics* (Baillière, 1981). There is also *Clinical Pharmacology in Obstetrics* by P. J. Lewis (Wright, 1983). A useful small work is *Handbook for Prescribing Medications During Pregnancy* edited by R. L. Berkowitz, D. R. Coustan and T. K. Mochizuki (Little, Brown, 1981)

Female reproductive organs: normal and abnormal

UTERUS, ENDOMETRIUM AND CERVIX

The most recent general text available is R. M. Wynn's *Biology of the Uterus* (2nd edn, Plenum, 1977). Two other volumes largely dealing with the normal uterus are H. J. Norris, A. T. Hertig and M. R. Abell's *The Uterus by 23 Authors* (Williams and Wilkins, 1973), a comprehensive work containing numerous references and a historical section, and C. A. Finn and D. G. Porter's *The Uterus* (Elek Science, 1975) which covers both comparative and human reproductive biology and contains extensive bibliographies. The endometrium is dealt with more specifically in H. Schmidt-Matthieson's *The Normal Human Endometrium* (McGraw-Hill, 1968), translated from the original German version of 1963, and F. A. Kimball's *The Endometrium* (MTP, 1980) the proceedings of the 8th Brook Lodge workshop on problems in reproductive physiology, which includes material on comparative studies. Information on the normal cervix can be found in J. A. Jordan and A. Singer's *The Cervix* (Saunders, 1976) and in *The Biology of the Cervix* edited by R. J. Blandau and K. Moghissi (Chicago University Press, 1973), which also contains a historical introduction. Two recent, more specialized books are *The Cervix in Pregnancy and Labour* edited by D. A. Ellwood and A. B. M. Anderson (Churchill Livingstone, 1981) and *Dilatation of the Uterine Cervix: Connective Tissue Biology and Clinical Management* edited by F. Naftolin and P. G. Stubblefield (Raven Press, 1980).

Books on uterine disorders and their management include: S. G. Silverberg's *Surgical Pathology of the Uterus* (Wiley, 1977); J. L. Bennington's *Surgical Pathology of the Uterine Corpus* (Saunders, 1980); P. Malpas' *Genital Prolapse and Allied Conditions* (Harvey and Blythe, 1955); S. Joel-Cohen's *Abdominal and Vaginal Hysterectomy* (2nd edn, Heinemann, 1972) and C. F. Krige's *Vaginal Hysterectomy and Genital Prolapse Repair* (Witwaterstrand University Press, 1965). Radiotherapy is dealt with in *High Dose-Rate Afterloading in the Treatment of Cancer of the Uterus* edited by T. D. Bates and R. J. Berry (*British Journal of Radiology Special Report No 17,* 1980), the report of a workshop held in April, 1978. The diagnosis and treatment of endometrial disorders is dealt with in A. Blaustein's *Interpretation of Biopsy of Endometrium* (Raven Press, 1980); G. Dallenbach-Hellweg's *Histopathology of the Endometrium* (3rd edn, Springer, 1981), translated by F. D. Dallenbach; J. A. Chalmers' *Endometriosis* (Butterworths, 1975); *Endometrial Cancer* edited by M. G. Brush, R. J. B. King and R. W. Taylor (Baillière, 1978); and *Endometrial Carcinoma and its Treatment* edited by L. A. Gray Sr. (Thieme, 1977). Aspects of benign and malignant conditions of the cervix are covered in S. F. Patten's *Diagnostic Cytopathology of the Uterine Cervix* (2nd edn, Karger, 1978); E. Burghardt's *Early Histolo-*

gical Diagnosis of Cervical Cancer (Saunders, 1973); and vol 6 in the series *Major Problems in Obstetrics and Gynecology; Cervical Pathology and Colposcopy*, comprising selected papers from the Second World Congress of Cervical Pathology and Colposcopy edited by E. Burghardt, E. Holzer and J. A. Jordan (Thieme, 1978); F. A. Langley and A. C. Crompton's *Epithelial Abnormalities of the Cervix Uteri* (Heinemann, 1973); *Cancer of the Uterine Cervix* edited by E. C. Easson (Saunders, 1973); *Cervical Cancer* edited by G. Dallenbach-Hellweg (Springer, 1981); M. Coppleson and B. Reid's *Preclinical Carcinoma of the Cervix Uteri: its Nature, Origin and Management* (Pergamon, 1967); and *Pre-Clinical Neoplasia of the Cervix*, the proceedings of the 9th College Study Group, October, 1981 (RCOG, 1982).

OVARY

A full study is contained in the three-volume work by Professor Lord Zuckerman and B. J. Weir (2nd edn, Academic Press, 1977). Other recent books of interest are *Biology of the Ovary* edited by P. M. Motta and E. S. E. Hafez (Nijhoff, 1980) and vol 2 in the series *Developments in Obstetrics and Gynaecology; Endocrine Function of the Human Ovary* (Academic Press, 1976), which is vol 7 in the Serono Symposia series; *Dynamics of Ovarian Function* edited by N. B. Schwartz and M. Hunzicker-Dunn (Raven Press, 1981); *Functional Morphology of the Human Ovary* edited by J. R. T. Coutts (MTP, 1981) and *Comparative Morphology of the Mammalian Ovary* by H. Mossman and K. L. Duke (University of Wisconsin Press, 1973), which gives synoptic data on the ovaries of more than 65 families of mammals and contains over 30 pages of references. The following texts, among others, deal with various disorders of the ovary: D. Tacchi's *Ovarian Gynaecology* (Saunders, 1976) and J. Horsky and J. Presl's *Ovarian Function and its Disorders* (Nijhoff, 1981), the third volume in the series *Developments in Obstetrics and Gynaecology*. Material on the many and varied ovarian tumours can be found in H. Fox and F. A. Langley's *Tumours of the Ovary* (Heinemann, 1976); N. A. Janovski and T. L. Paramanandhan's *Ovarian Tumors* (Thieme, 1973); G. Teilum's *Special Tumors of Ovary and Testis* (2nd edn, Munksgaard; Lippincott; 1976); and S. F. Serov and R. E. Scully's *Histological Typing of Ovarian Tumours* (WHO, 1973), which is part of the *International Histological Classification of Tumours Series* produced by the World Health Organization. Cancerous tumours are the subject of H. R. K. Barber's *Ovarian Carcinoma: Etiology, Diagnosis and Treatment* (Masson, 1978); *Ovarian Cancer* edited by C. E. Newman, C. H. J. Ford and J. A. Jordan (Pergamon, 1980), comprising the Proceedings of an International Symposium held in 1979; and *Biology of Ovarian Neoplasia* (UICC, 1980), Report No 11 in a series of workshops.

FALLOPIAN TUBES

Available texts include C. J. Pauerstein's *The Fallopian Tube: a Reappraisal* (Lea and Febiger, 1974); J. D. Woodruff and C. J. Pauerstein's *The Fallopian Tube: Structure, Function, Pathology and Management* (Williams and Wilkins, 1969); and *The Oviduct and its Functions* edited by A. D. Johnson and C. W. Foley (Academic Press, 1974), which is primarily a comparative study of mammals. Material on fallopian tube surgery is largely devoted to techniques of sterilization and reversal and is detailed on page 419.

VULVA AND VAGINA

C. M. Ridley's *The Vulva* (Saunders, 1975) forms vol 5 in the series *Major Problems in Dermatology* and contains sections on history as well as on anatomy and dermatology. Benign diseases are the subject of E. G. Friedrich's *Vulva Disease* (Saunders, 1976) which is vol 9 in the series *Major Problems in Obstetrics and Gynecology;* H. L. Gardner and R. H. Kaufman's *Benign Diseases of the Vulva and Vagina* (2nd edn, Hall, 1981); and *Diseases of the Vulva* by N. A. Janovski and C. P. Douglas (Harper and Row, 1972). The following deal largely with malignant tumours: M. Stening's *Cancer and Related Lesions of the Vulva* (ADIS Press, 1980) and S. Way's *Malignant Disease of the Vulva* (Churchill Livingstone, 1982), while surgical aspects are covered in E. H. Copenhaver's *Surgery of the Vulva and Vagina: a Practical Guide* (Saunders, 1981); *Atlas of Vaginal Surgery* by G. Reiffenstuhl and W. Platzer (2 vols, Saunders, 1975), translated by E. J. Friedman and E. A. Friedman and edited by the latter; and *Vaginal Surgery* by D. H. Nichols and C. L. Randall (Williams and Wilkins, 1976). The normal vagina is the subject of *The Human Vagina* by E. S. E. Hafez and T. N. Evans (North Holland, 1978) and specific conditions are treated in two monographs, namely, J. C. Moir's *Vesico-Vaginal Fistula* (2nd edn, Baillière, 1967) and *New Advances in the Treatment of Candidial Vaginitis, No 7* in the *International Congress and Symposium Series* of the Royal Society of Medicine (Chairman Professor Rosalinde Hurley, RSM, 1979).

The reproductive process

REPRODUCTIVE PHYSIOLOGY

Reproductive physiology, both human and comparative, is well documented and the following are a representative selection. Two of the more substantial works are *Principles and Management of Human Reproduction* edited by D. E. Reid, K. J. Ryan and K. Benirschke (Saunders, 1972) and *Reproductive Biology* by H. Balin and S. Glasser (Excerpta Medica, 1972), which comprises a series of critical essays by specialists. General textbooks are well represented by two titles: R. P. Shearman's *Human Reproductive Physiology* (2nd edn, Blackwell, 1979) and E. W. Page, C. A. Villee and D. B. Villee's *Human Reproduction: Essentials of Reproductive and Perinatal Medicine* (3rd edn, Saunders, 1981). Shorter texts at an introductory level are *Human Reproduction: An Integrated View* by J. I. D. Sadow *et al.* (Croom Helm, 1980); *Human Reproduction and Developmental Biology* by D. J. Begley, J. A. Firth and J. R. S. Hoult (Macmillan, 1980); and, from America, *Human Reproduction: Physiology and Pathophysiology* edited by R. W. Huff and C. J. Pauerstein (Wiley, 1979). Papers in *Recent Advances in Human Reproduction* comprise the proceedings of the First International Congress on the subject and are edited by A. Campos da Paz *et al.* (Excerpta Medica; American Elsevier; 1976), while the proceedings of the Third World Congress, 1981, have since appeared as *Human Reproduction* edited by K. Semm and L. Mettler (Excerpta Medica, 1981).

The immunological aspects of reproduction are covered in a number of texts ranging from *Immunology of Reproduction* edited by J. S. Scott and W. R. Jones (Academic Press, 1976) to the more recent *Immunological Factors in Human Reproduction* edited by S. Schulman, F. Dondero and M. Nicotra (Academic Press, 1982). Neuro- and psychoneuroendocrinological aspects of this subject are of interest and *Neuroendocrinology of Reproduction: Physiology and Behavior* edited by N. T. Adler (Plenum, 1981) is probably the most recent text of note.

OVULATION, MENSTRUATION AND ASSOCIATED DISORDERS

Of the recent books available on ovulation, probably the most comprehensive is that edited by E. S. E. Hafez entitled *Human Ovulation: Mechanisms, Prediction, Detection and Induction* (North Holland, 1979); also important is *Follicular Maturation and Ovulation* edited by R. Rolland *et al.* (Excerpta Medica, 1982). More specific aspects are covered in *Control of Ovulation* by D. B.

Crichton *et al.* (Butterworths, 1978), which contains the proceedings of a conference; and *Induction of Ovulation* by R. B. Greenblatt (Lea and Febiger, 1979).

R. F. Vollman's *The Menstrual Cycle* (Saunders, 1977) is a useful general text and other relevant publications include S. L. Israel's *Diagnosis and Treatment of Menstrual Disorders and Sterility* (5th edn, Harper and Row, 1967); *Endocrine Causes of Menstrual Disorders* edited by J. R. Givens (Year Book Medical Publishers, 1978), the proceedings of a symposium; *Dysmenorrhea* edited by M. Y. Dawood (Williams and Wilkins, 1981); *The Premenstrual Syndrome* edited by P. A. Van Keep (MTP, 1981), the proceedings of a workshop; and, for the laywoman, K. Dalton's *Once a Month* (Fontana, 1978; Harvester Press, 1979).

The menopause has been the subject of a number of studies in recent years. The proceedings of a Serono Symposium were published as No 39 in the series in a volume entitled *The Menopause: Clinical, Endocrinological and Pathophysiological Aspects* edited by P. Fioretti *et al.* (Academic Press, 1982) and the proceedings of an international symposium held in Rome in 1979 were published as *The Menopause and Postmenopause* edited by N. Pasetto, R. Paoletti and J. L. Ambrus (MTP, 1980). The proceedings of the first three International Congresses on the Menopause have been published under various titles, all edited by P. A. Van Keep and various co-authors. These were published in 1976, 1979 and 1982 respectively. Other relevant titles include *The Menopause: a Guide to Current Research and Practice* edited by R. J. Beard (MTP, 1976); *The Management of the Menopause and Post-Menopausal Years* edited by S. Campbell (MTP, 1976) and *The Role of Estrogen in the Management of the Menopause* edited by I. D. Cooke (MTP, 1978). For the laywoman there is W. H. Utian's *The Menopause Manual: A Woman's Guide to the Menopause* (MTP, 1978).

FERTILIZATION

A good basic text is *Fertilization: Comparative Morphology, Biochemistry and Immunology* edited by C. B. Metz and A. Monroy (2 vols, Academic Press, 1967–1969), as is C. R. Austin's *Ultrastructure of Fertilization* (Holt, Rinehart and Winston, 1968), which is a volume in the *Biology Studies Series.* K. Yoshinaga, R. K. Meyer and R. O. Greep have edited *Implantation of the Ovum* (Harvard University Press, 1976) and the proceedings of an international workshop held in 1976 have appeared in a volume entitled *Human Fertilization* edited by H. Ludwig and P. F. Tauber (Thieme, 1978).

EMBRYOLOGY

The literature of this subject is extensive and only a small selection can be cited here. Standard texts of interest are J. Langman's *Medical Embryology* (4th edn, Williams and Wilkins, 1981); *Human Embryology: Prenatal Development of Form and Function* by W. J. Hamilton and H. W. Mossman (4th edn, Macmillan, 1972) and K. Moore's *The Developing Human: Clinically Orientated Embryology* (3rd edn, Saunders, 1982), which is intended for the use of undergraduates. M. J. T. Fitzgerald's *Human Embryology: a Regional Approach* (Harper and Row, 1978) contains a useful six-page glossary of embryologic terms. Finally, there is a monograph available on the blastocyst which is edited by R. J. Blandau and entitled *Biology of the Blastocyst* (Chicago University Press, 1971).

PREGNANCY

The most comprehensive text available is R. G. Edwards' *Conception in the Human Female* (Academic Press, 1980). Over a thousand pages long, it covers such topics as sexual differentiation, regulation of reproduction, human sexuality, fertilization and implantation, to name a random selection, and it also contains a section on legal and ethical aspects. A Ciba Foundation Symposium on *Maternal Recognition of Pregnancy* was published under that title as No 64 in their new series of Symposia (Excerpta Medica, 1979).

Among the fascinating illustrated texts available are D. Harvey's *A New Life: Pregnancy, Birth and Your Child's First Year* (Marshall Cavendish, 1979), with chapters by experienced obstetricians and paediatricians, and *The Book of the Child: Pregnancy to 4 Years Old* edited by S. C. Docherty (2nd edn, Scottish Health Education Unit, 1980), which is a booklet intended to provide an attractive source of instruction for parents, actual and prospective. A popular volume by the Swedish photographer Lennart Nilsson entitled *The Everyday Miracle: a Child is Born* (Faber, 1977) was produced in a revised edition in that year with the assistance of three co-authors. As well as illustrations produced by electron microscopy the volume contains a number of photographs of the fetus-in-utero, obtained by judicious use of optical lenses attached to a camera. Two titles on multiple pregnancy are *Human Multiple Reproduction* by I. MacGillivray, P. P. S. Nylander and G. Corney (Saunders, 1975) and *Twin Biology and Multiple Pregnancy*, which is Part A of *Twin Research 3* (3 vols, Liss, 1981), being the Proceedings of the Third International Congress of Twin Studies,

1980, edited by L. Gedda, P. Parisi and W. E. Nance. For pregnancy in the older woman and in the adolescent the reader is referred to page 403. The subject of antenatal care is covered in *Browne's Antenatal Care* by J. C. McClure Browne and G. Dixon (11th edn, Churchill, 1978).

It may be useful to note that books are available on the following subjects as they relate specifically to, or complicate, pregnancy: nutrition, neurology, psychology, endocrinology, urology, immunology and, more specifically, carbohydrate metabolism, proteins, steroids and prostaglandins. Also available are books dealing with pregnancy complications in relation to certain regions of the body such as the kidney, liver, thyroid and heart, and with certain conditions such as diabetes, septic shock, hypertension, trauma, epilepsy, drug dependence, genetic disease and coagulation disorders. A selection of the more useful monographs is:

The Pregnant Diabetic and Her Newborn: Problems and Management by J. Pedersen (2nd edn, Munksgaard, 1977)

The Diabetic Pregnancy: a Perinatal Perspective by I. R. Merkatz and P. A. J. Adams (Grune and Stratton, 1979)

Drug Abuse in Pregnancy and Neonatal Effects edited by J. L. Rementeria (Mosby, 1977)

Birth Defects and Drugs in Pregnancy by O. P. Heinonen, D. Slone and S. Shapiro (PSG, 1977), which contains numerous statistical tables

Maternal Nutrition in Pregnancy: Eating for Two edited by J. Dobbing (Academic Press, 1981), the proceedings of a workshop on the subject held the previous year

Trauma in Pregnancy by H. J. Bucksbaum (Saunders, 1979)

The Thyroid Gland in Pregnancy by G. N. Burrow (Saunders, 1972)

Liver and Pregnancy by N. A. M. Bergstein (Excerpta Medica, 1973)

Heart Disease and Pregnancy by P. Szekely and L. M. Snaith (Churchill Livingstone, 1974)

Tumor und Gravidität by A. Verhagen (Springer, 1974), which contains numerous references

Genetic Disease in Pregnancy: Maternal Effects and Fetal Outcome by J. D. Schulman and J. L. Simpson (Academic Press, 1981)

Endocrinology of Pregnancy edited by F. Fuchs and A. I. I. Klopper (Harper and Row, 1977)

Mental Illness in Pregnancy and the Puerperium by M. Sandler (Oxford University Press, 1978)

Septic Shock in Obstetrics and Gynecology by D. Cavanagh, P. S. Rao and M. R. Comas (Saunders, 1977)

Pregnancy Hypertension edited by J. Bonnar, I. MacGillivray and E. M. Symonds (MTP, 1980), which is one of the more recent of a number of books on the subject and comprises the proceedings of the First Congress of the International Society for the Study of Hypertension in Pregnancy

Neurology of Pregnancy by J. O. Donaldson (Saunders, 1978)

Kidney Function and Disease in Pregnancy by M. D. Lindheimer and A. I. Katz (Lea and Febiger, 1977)

Pathology of Toxaemia of Pregnancy by H. L. Sheehan and J. B. Lynch's (Churchill Livingstone, 1973), which contains an extensive bibliography

Epilepsy, Pregnancy and the Child by D. Janz *et al.* (Raven Press, 1982).

There are also more general works which review the various complications of pregnancy, and the oldest of these, yet one which is still useful, is *Medical, Surgical and Gynecologic Complications of Pregnancy* written by the staff of the Mount Sinai Hospital, New York City, and edited by J. J. Rovinsky and A. F. Guttmacher (2nd edn, Livingstone, 1965). Three later publications are *Medical Complications During Pregnancy* by D. M. Haynes (McGraw-Hill, 1969); *Medical Disorders in Obstetric Practice* by C. G. Barnes (4th edn, Blackwell, 1974); and *Medical Complications During Pregnancy* by G. N. Burrow and T. F. Ferris (2nd edn, Saunders, 1982). There is only one publication reviewing surgical cases in this context, *Surgical Disease in Pregnancy* by H. P. K. Barber and E. A. Graber (Saunders, 1971). Among several books covering infections in pregnancy is *Infections and Pregnancy* edited by C. R. Coid (Academic Press, 1977) and a certain amount of information can be gleaned from books on infections in gynaecological and obstetric practice cited earlier. Also cited in an earlier section are books on therapeutics in obstetrics and gynaecology.

FOETUS

In recent years there has been a tremendous increase in the output of literature dealing with the foetus, since the unborn child has, as a result of technological advances, become an object of investigation and treatment in its own right. Many texts on perinatal medicine as a general subject have appeared but they are largely of American origin. Examples are *Perinatal Medicine: Management of the High Risk Fetus and Neonate* edited by R. J. Bolognese and R. H. Schwarz (Williams and Wilkins, 1977) and *Current Developments in Perinatology: the Fetus, Placenta and Newborn* edited by F. P. Zuspan (Mosby, 1977).

Other useful books are:

Fetal Physiology and Medicine: the Basis of Perinatology edited by R. W. Beard and P. W. Nathanielsz (Saunders, 1976)
Fetal Endocrinology edited by M. J. Novy and J. A. Resko (Academic Press, 1981)
Fetal and Neonatal Pathology: Perspectives for the General Pathologist edited by A. J. Barson (Praeger, 1982)
Biological and Clinical Aspects of the Fetus edited by Y. Notake and S. Suzuki (Thieme; Igaku Shoin; 1977)
Foetus and Placenta by A. H. Klopper and E. Diczfalusy (Blackwell, 1969)
A Handbook of Pre-Natal Paediatrics for Obstetricians and Paediatricians by G. F. Batstone, A. W. Blair and J. M. Slater (MTP, 1971), which contains useful appendices including fetal growth charts
Laboratory Investigation of Fetal Diseases edited by A. J. Barson (Wright, 1981)
The Fetus and Newly Born Infant: Influences of the Prenatal Environment by R. E. Stevenson (2nd edn, Mosby, 1977)
Modern Management of the Rh Problem edited by J. T. Queenan (2nd edn, Harper and Row, 1977)

Human Embryonic and Fetal Death edited by I. H. Porter and E. B. Hook (Academic Press, 1980)
Human Fetal Endocrines by J. E. Jirasek (Nijhoff, 1980)
Perinatal Pathology edited by E. Grundmann (Springer, 1979)
Viral Diseases of the Fetus and Newborn by J. B. Hanshaw and J. A. Dudgeon (Saunders, 1978)

A large and fairly comprehensive monograph is *Neonatal-Perinatal Medicine: Diseases of the Fetus and Infant* by R. E. Behrman *et al.* (2nd edn, Mosby, 1977). Recent texts on foetal monitoring include L. A. Cibils' *Electronic Fetal-Maternal Monitoring: Antepartum, Intrapartum* (Nijhoff, 1981), while the Royal College of Obstetricians and Gynaecologists have published *The Current Status of Fetal Heart Rate Monitoring and Ultrasound in Obstetrics*, the proceedings of a scientific meeting held in December, 1977, edited by R. W. Beard and S. Campbell (RCOG, 1978). Finally, two useful standard textbooks dealing with fetal pathology are E. L. Potter and J. M. Craig's *Pathology of the Fetus and the Infant* (3rd edn, Year Book Medical Publishers, 1976), which is extensively illustrated, and J. E. Morison's *Foetal and Neonatal Pathology* (3rd edn, Butterworths, 1970).

PLACENTA, AMNION AND CHORION

The beautifully produced large-quarto volume entitled *The Human Placenta* by J. D. Boyd and W. J. Hamilton (Macmillan, 1970) is an authoritative work which also contains some historical information and an extensive bibliography. Also useful for reference is *The Pathology of the Human Placenta* by K. Benirschke and S. G. Driscoll (Springer, 1967), which is a translated reprint from *Handbuch der Speziellen Pathologischen Anatomie und Histologie* VIII/6. The normal placenta is the subject of E. M. Ramsey and M. W. Donner's *Placental Vasculature and Circulation: Anatomy, Physiology, Radiology, Clinical Aspects. Atlas and Textbook* (Saunders; Thieme; 1980); of *Placental Proteins* by A. I. I. Klopper and T. Chard (Springer, 1979); and of *The Human Placenta: Proteins and Hormones* edited by A. I. I. Klopper, A. Genazzani and P. G. Crosignani, the proceedings of the Serono Symposium No 35 (Academic Press, 1980). More specific texts are *Placental Transfer* edited by G. V. P. Chamberlain and A. W. Wilkinson (Pitman, 1979) and *Placental Function Tests* by T. Chard and A. Klopper (Springer, 1982). Apart from the volume by Benirschke and Driscoll already mentioned, H. Fox's *Pathology of the Placenta* (Saunders, 1978) is a useful study of that particular aspect, while the potential of the placenta for experimental work is discussed in P. Beaconsfield and C. Villee's *Placenta: a Neglected*

Experimental Animal (Pergamon, 1979). Texts on fetal membranes other than the placenta are few, but G. L. Bourne's *The Human Amnion and Chorion* (Lloyd-Luke, 1962) is worth noting, along with *Amniotic Fluid: Research and Clinical Application* edited by D. V. I. Fairweather and T. K. A. B. Eskes (2nd edn, Excerpta Medica, 1978). The section devoted to the prenatal diagnosis of genetic defects contains titles which cover material on amniocentesis.

TROPHOBLASTIC TUMOURS

A somewhat dated but still popular publication is K. D. Bagshawe's *Choriocarcinoma: the Clinical Biology of the Trophoblast and its Tumours* (Arnold, 1969). W. W. Park's *Choriocarcinoma: a Study of its Pathology* (Heinemann, 1977) also contains a brief historical introduction and R. Hertz's *Choriocarcinoma and Related Trophoblastic Tumors in Women* (Raven Press, 1977) contains material on hydatidiform mole as well as choriocarcinoma. A useful new work is *Trophoblastic Neoplasms: Clinical Principles of Diagnosis and Management* by D. P. Goldstein and R. S. Berkowitz (Saunders, 1982), vol 14 in the series *Major Problems in Obstetrics and Gynecology*.

LABOUR AND DELIVERY

Two textbooks relating to this subject are E. A. Friedman's *Labor: Clinical Evaluation and Management* (2nd edn, Appleton-Century-Crofts, 1978) and H. Oxorn's *Human Labor and Birth* (4th edn, Appleton-Century-Crofts, 1980). Related titles of interest are K. O'Driscoll and D. Meagher's *Active Management of Labour* (Saunders, 1980); *Endocrine Factors in Labour*, the proceedings of a symposium edited, on behalf of the Society for Endocrinology, by A. I. I. Klopper and J. Gardner (Cambridge University Press, 1973); and H. Weidinger's *Labour Inhibition: Betamimetic Drugs in Obstetrics* (Fischer, 1977). *Pre-term Labour*, the proceedings of the 5th Study Group of the Royal College of Obstetricians and Gynaecologists, October, 1977, is out of print but is useful for information. A sociological study based on the findings of a questionnaire circulated to representative samples of women and professionals throughout the country has been published under the title *The Dignity of Labour? A Study of Childbearing and Induction* by A. Cartwright (Tavistock Publications, 1979).

Apart from the information available in books on operative obstetrics cited earlier in the chapter, those dealing with more precise aspects are J. A. Chalmers' *The Ventouse: the Obstetric Vacuum Extractor* (Lloyd-Luke, 1971); E. Parry-Jones' *Kielland's Forceps* (Butterworths, 1952) and *Barton's Forceps* (Sector Publishing, 1972), by the same author. The proceedings of a scientific meeting held at the Royal College of Obstetricians and Gynaecologists in May, 1980, have been published as *Outcomes of Obstetric Intervention in Britain* edited by R. W. Beard and D. B. Paintin (RCOG, 1980).

The subject of pain relief in labour is well represented in the literature. One of the most comprehensive texts, although now a little out of date, is J. J. Bonica's *Principles and Practice of Obstetric Analgesia and Anaesthesia* (2 vols, Davis, 1967–1969). Two useful British textbooks are J. S. Crawford's *Principles and Practice of Obstetric Anaesthesia* (4th edn, Blackwell, 1978) and D. D. Moir's *Obstetric Anaesthesia and Analgesia* (2nd edn, Baillière, 1980), which contains a historical introduction. The latter author has also produced a handbook for midwives entitled *Pain Relief in Labour* (4th edn, Churchill Livingstone, 1982). *Epidural Analgesia in Obstetrics: a Second Symposium* (Lloyd-Luke, 1980) edited by A. Doughty contains some useful papers on that particular technique. Several American publications have recently appeared, of which E. V. Cosmi's *Obstetric Anesthesia and Perinatology* (Appleton-Century-Crofts, 1981) is notable for the comprehensive bibliographies contained in most of the chapters.

PUERPERIUM

Few publications are available on this subject. Apart from A. Sharman's *Reproductive Physiology of the Post-partum Period* (Livingstone, 1966), most works emphasize psychological aspects. Two recent titles are M. Sandler's *Mental Illness in Pregnancy and the Puerperium* (Oxford University Press, 1978) and W. A. Brown's *Psychological Care During Pregnancy and the Postpartum Period* (Raven Press, 1979). K. D. Dalton's *Depression after Childbirth* (Oxford University Press, 1980) is intended for the laywoman.

Fertility, infertility, sterilization, family planning and abortion

Material on fertility may, perhaps, be largely ignored in this chapter as it is of less interest to practising clinicians than, for example, to those engaged in population studies. However, it may be of interest to note two supplements to the *Journal of Biosocial Science*. Supplement 5 is entitled *Fertility in Adolescence* (Galton

Foundation, 1978) and comprises the proceedings of the Seventh Biomedical Workshop of the International Planned Parenthood Federation (IPPF) held in 1977. The proceedings of the Eighth IPPF Workshop, 1978, were published under the title *Fertility in Middle Age* (Galton Foundation, 1979).

Recent advances in techniques such as microsurgery and *in-vitro* fertilization are reflected in recent literature on infertility. Because of the significant contribution and changes these developments have made, earlier literature is not included here. Among general texts are *The Infertile Couple* edited by R. J. Pepperell, B. Hudson and F. C. Wood (Churchill Livingstone, 1980) and *Infertility: a Textbook Based on the Work of the Northern Hospital Philip Hill Parenthood Clinic* edited by E. E. Philipp and G. B. Carruthers (Heinemann, 1981), while recent topics of current interest are dealt with in *Modern Trends in Infertility and Conception Control* edited by E. E. Wallach and R. D. Kempers (Williams and Wilkins, vol 2, 1982); *Advances in Diagnosis and Treatment of Infertility* edited by V. Insler and G. Bettendorf (Elsevier; North Holland; 1981), contains symposium proceedings; and *Research on Fertility and Sterility: Proceedings of the Xth World Congress on Fertility and Sterility, 1980* edited by J. Cortes-Prieto, A. Campos da Paz and M. Neves-E-Castro (MTP, 1981). Other new publications worth noting include *Tubal Infertility: Diagnosis and Treatment* edited by G. Chamberlain and R. Winston (Blackwell, 1982) and Nos 1 and 2 of the proceedings of the Serono Clinical Colloquia on Reproduction, both edited by P. Crosignani and B. L. Rubin and entitled, respectively, *Microsurgery in Female Infertility* (Academic Press, 1980) and *Endocrinology of Human Infertility* (Academic Press, 1981). In-vitro fertilization is now an established technique and two of the first publications to be completely devoted to the subject are *In Vitro Fertilization and Embryo Transfer* edited by E. S. E. Hafez and K. Semm (MTP, 1982) and *Human Conception in Vitro: Proceedings of the First Bourn Hall Meeting* edited by R. G. Edwards and J. M. Purdy (Academic Press, 1982). The story of events which led to the birth of the first 'test-tube baby' is told in R. G. Edwards and P. C. Steptoe's book *A Matter of Life: the Story of a Medical Breakthrough* (Hutchinson, 1980) written to appeal to the general public. Sterility of the male partner is a subject treated in such texts as *Male Infertility* by R. D. Amelar, L. Dubin and P. C. Walsh (Saunders, 1977) and in J. Cohen and W. F. Hendry's *Spermatozoa, Antibodies and Infertility* (Blackwell, 1978).

Where the subject of female sterilization and its reversal is concerned, recent titles are A. J. Penfield's *Female Sterilization by*

Minilaparotomy or Open Laparoscopy (Urban and Schwarzenberg, 1980); H. P. Brown and S. N. Schanzer's *Female Sterilization. An Overview with Emphasis on the Vaginal Route and the Organization of a Sterilization Program* (Wright; PSG; 1982); and a volume of workshop proceedings entitled *Advances in Female Sterilization Techniques* edited by J. J. Sciarra, W. Droegmueller and J. J. Spiedel (Harper and Row, 1976). The reversal of both male and female sterilization is a topic which has recently captured a great deal of attention and both aspects are covered in the published proceedings of a workshop entitled *Reversal of Sterilization* edited by J. J. Sciarra, G. I. Zatuchni and J. J. Spiedel (Harper and Row, 1978), while *Reversibility of Female Sterilization* edited by I. A. Brosens and R. M. L. Winston (Academic Press; Grune and Stratton, 1978) confines itself to the female.

A basic knowledge of the theory and practice of contraception is essential to the practising clinician in obstetrics and gynaecology and also to general practitioners. *Human Fertility Control: Theory and Practice* by D. F. Hawkins and M. G. Elder (Butterworths, 1979) provides useful background reading and can be supplemented with any of a selection of available handbooks, such as S. Ramaswamy and A. J. Smith's *Practical Contraception* (Pitman, 1976); *Essentials of Family Planning* by Dame Josephine Barnes (Blackwell, 1976); *Family Planning Handbook for Doctors* edited by R. L. Kleinman (5th edn, IPPF, 1980) and a small booklet entitled *Handbook of Contraceptive Practice* by S. Carne, G. Chamberlain and J. McEwan (DHSS, 1979), prepared for the Standing Medical Advisory Committee of the Central Health Services Council. Two recent publications cover immunological aspects: G. P. Talwar's *Immunology of Contraception* (Arnold, 1980) and *Immunological Aspects of Reproduction and Fertility Control* (MTP, 1980). A study carried out for the DHSS within two Area Health Authorities, by I. Allen, is entitled *Family Planning, Sterilization and Abortion Services* (Policy Studies Institute, 1981) and new developments in the field of fertility control are the subject of *Recent Advances in Reproduction and Regulation of Fertility* (Elsevier; North Holland; 1979), the proceedings of a symposium edited by G. P. Talwar. Finally, there are numerous publications on individual methods of contraception, such as *Intrauterine Contraception* (4th edn, IPPF, 1977), a small booklet edited by R. L. Kleinman; J. Marshall's *Planning for a Family: an Atlas of Mucothermic Charts* (2nd edn, Faber, 1979), a paperback intended for the laywoman, as is J. Guillebaud's *The Pill* (Oxford University Press, 1980); and rather more substantial volumes are also available, such as D. A. Edelman, G. S. Berger and L. Keith's

Intrauterine Devices and Their Complications (Hall, 1979). As there is such a wealth of literature available on all aspects of family planning anyone desiring detailed information is best directed to such organizations as the International Planned Parenthood Federation, the Family Planning Association or the Margaret Pyke Centre.

Many of the available texts on abortion, especially those published in the years immediately following the passing of the 1967 Abortion Act, tend to concentrate on legal and sociological aspects rather than techniques and complications. *Abortion* by D. M. Potts, P. L. Diggory and J. Peel (Cambridge University Press, 1977) presents a fairly useful all-round view of the subject and other useful titles are *Abortion and Sterilization: Medical and Social Aspects*, edited by J. E. Hodgson *et al.* (Academic Press; Grune and Statton; 1981); S. Neubardt and H. Schulman's *Techniques of Abortion* (2nd edn, Little, Brown, 1977); *Pregnancy Termination: Procedures, Safety and New Developments* edited by G. I. Zatuchni, J. J. Sciarra and J. J. Speidel (Harper and Row, 1979); and a simple booklet entitled *Menstrual Regulation* edited by R. L. Kleinman (IPPF, 1976). Ethical problems are dealt with in texts such as D. Callahan's *Abortion: Law Choice and Morality* (MacMillan, 1970) and *Abortion: the Personal Dilemma* by R. F. R. Gardner (Paternoster Press, 1972), in which a Christian gynaecologist examines the medical, social and spiritual issues. One other title covers a very specific topic, namely *Septic Abortion* by R. H. Schwarz (Lippincott, 1968).

Human genetics, congenital abnormalities and prenatal diagnosis

A standard work on human genetics is J. L. Hamerton's *Human Cytogenetics. Vol 1: General Cytogenetics; Vol 2: Clinical Cytogenetics* (2 vols, Academic Press, 1971). Other titles of interest are A. I. Taylor's *Practical Human Cytogenetics* (Baillière, 1974); A. E. H. Emery's *Elements of Medical Genetics* (5th edn, Churchill Livingstone, 1979); E. H. R. Ford's *Human Chromosomes* (Academic Press, 1973); and *A Handbook of Medical Genetics* by J. S. and E. M. Fitzsimmons (Heinemann, 1980). A Ciba Foundation Symposium (No 66 in their new series) has been published as *Human Genetics: Possibilities and Realities* (Excerpta Medica, 1979). The subject of counselling is covered by A. C. Stevenson and Brigid C. C. Davison's *Genetic Counselling* (2nd edn, Heinemann, 1976) and S. Reed's *Counseling in Medical Genetics* (3rd edn, Liss, 1980). Other titles dealing with genetics in a special context are *Genetics and the Law* by A. Milunsky and G. J. Annas

(Plenum, 1976); *Genetic Disease in Pregnancy: Maternal Effects and Fetal Outcome* edited by J. D. Schulman and J. L. Simpson (Academic Press, 1981); and T. F. Thurmon's *Rare Genetic Diseases: a Guidebook* (CRC Press, 1974), which lists rare diseases with a frequency in the general population of less than 1 in 1000.

The subject of congenital malformations is covered in Chapter 20. From the standpoint of obstetricians and gynaecologists, apart from standard textbooks, there is one very comprehensive monograph of importance, J. Warkany's *Congenital Malformations: Notes and Comments* (Year Book Medical Publishers 1971), which contains over 1200 pages. Two books on genital abnormalities are *Selected Topics on Genital Anomalies and Related Subjects* compiled and edited by N. B. Rashad and W. R. M. Morton (C. C. Thomas, 1969) and C. M. Dougherty and R. Spencer's *Female Sex Anomalies* (Harper and Row, 1972). Also useful are H. W. Jones and W. W. Scott's *Hermaphroditism, Genital Anomalies and Related Endocrine Disorders* (2nd edn, Williams and Wilkins, 1971) and C. J. Dewhurst and R. R. Gordon's *The Intersexual Disorders* (Baillière Tindall, 1969). Anencephaly is covered in J. M. and J. H. Elwood's *Epidemiology of Anencephalus and Spina Bifida* (Oxford University Press, 1980) and R. J. Lemire, J. B. Beckwith and J. Warkany's *Anencephaly* (Raven Press, 1978).

The prenatal diagnosis of genetic disorders and the prevention of fetal abnormalities are topics which have recently engendered a great deal of interest. Books in this connection are:

Towards the Prevention of Fetal Malformation edited by J. B. Scrimgeour (Edinburgh University Press, 1978)

Prevention of Neural Tube Defects: the Role of Alpha Fetoprotein edited by B. F. Crandall and M. A. B. Brazier (Academic Press, 1978)

Antenatal Diagnosis of Genetic Disease by A. E. H. Emery (Churchill Livingstone, 1973)

Genetic Disorders of the Fetus: Diagnosis, Prevention and Treatment edited by A. Milunsky (Plenum, 1979)

Recent Advances in Prenatal Diagnosis edited by C. Orlandi, P. E. Polani and L. Bovicelli (Wiley, 1981)

Fetoscopy edited by I. Rocker and K. M. Laurence (Elsevier, 1981)

Plasma Hormone Assays in Evaluation of Fetal Wellbeing edited by A. Klopper (Churchill Livingstone, 1976)

Prenatal Diagnosis and Selective Abortion by H. Harris (Nuffield Provincial Hospitals Trust, 1974)

Prenatal Diagnosis of Genetic Disease by D. C. Siggers (Blackwell, 1978), a concise introduction to the subject.

Female endocrinology

Although a great deal of literature is available on the general topic of endocrinology, only material pertaining to the female is relevant here. Comprehensive general texts are *Textbook of Endocrinology* edited by R. Williams (6th edn, Saunders, 1981) and *Fundamentals of Clinical Endocrinology* by R. Hall *et al.* (3rd edn, Pitman, 1980). Two very large tomes which deal specifically with the female are *Gynecologic Endocrinology* edited by J. J. Gold and J. B. Josimovich with 59 contributors (3rd edn, Harper and Row, 1980) and J. Botella-Llusia's *Endocrinology of Woman* translated by E. A. Moscovic (Saunders, 1973). Titles worth noting on special aspects of the subject are:

Endocrinology of Pregnancy edited by F. Fuchs and A. Klopper (2nd edn, Harper and Row, 1977)

Fetal Endocrinology: an Experimental Approach by P. W. Nathanielsz (North Holland, 1976), which is vol 1 in the series *Monographs of Fetal Physiology*

Hormonal Disorders in Gynecology by P. J. Keller (translated by T. C. Telger, Springer, 1981)

Maternal-Fetal Endocrinology by D. Tulchinsky and K. J. Ryan (Saunders, 1980)

Reproductive Endocrinology: Physiology, Pathophysiology and Clinical Management by S. S. C. Yen and R. B. Jaffe (Saunders, 1978)

Hirsutism by P. Mauvais-Jarvis, F. Kuttenn and I. Mowszowicz (Springer, 1981)

Venereal diseases

One or two representative texts are required for the non-specialist in this field who, nonetheless, requires a fairly substantial knowledge of the subject for examination purposes or because the problem is encountered to some extent in clinical practice. The following are useful for general reference: A. King, C. S. Nicol and P. Rodin's *Venereal Diseases* (4th edn, Baillière Tindall, 1980) and *Recent Advances in Sexually Transmitted Diseases – 2* edited by J. R. W. Harris (2nd edn, Churchill Livingstone, 1981).

Female urology

Female urology is becoming more of an entity within the general context of obstetrics and gynaecology, a fact reflected in the increasing numbers of publications devoted to it. Two recent texts that give general coverage are *Gynecologic Urology and Urodynamics: Theory and Practice* edited by D. R. Ostergard (Williams and Wilkins, 1980) and H. J. Buchsbaum and J. D. Schmidt's *Gynecologic and Obstetric Urology* (Saunders, 1978). A recent scientific meeting at the Royal College of Obstetricians and Gynaecologists has been published as *The Incontinent Woman* edited by J. A. Jordan and S. L. Stanton (RCOG, 1981) and other titles on the subject of female incontinence and its management include S. L. Stanton's *Female Urinary Incontinence* (Lloyd-Luke,

1977); *Surgery of Female Incontinence* edited by S. L. Stanton and E. A. Tanagho (Springer, 1980); and *Incontinence and its Management* edited by D. Mandelstam (Croom Helm, 1980). R. F. Zacharin's *Stress Incontinence of Urine* (Harper and Row, 1972) is an older publication, but its opening chapter contains a good historical review. Finally, A. Kilmartin's little 'self-help' paperback *Understanding Cystitis* (Pan, 1975) is quite informative on a subject that is often overlooked in the literature.

Sexual medicine

Recent publications on the subject of human sexual behaviour include *Human Sexual Behaviour* by M. P. Feldman and M. J. MacCulloch (Wiley, 1980); *Sex, Hormones and Behaviour* (Excerpta Medica, 1979) and no 62 in the new Series of Ciba Foundation Symposia; *Human Sexuality* edited by C. P. Austin and R. V. Short (Cambridge University Press, 1980; Book 8 in the *Reproduction in Mammals* series intended for undergraduates); and *Progress in Sexology: Selected Papers from the Proceedings of the 1976 International Congress of Sexology,* edited by R. Gemme and C. C. Wheeler (Plenum, 1977). Two frequently quoted studies, both by W. H. Masters and V. E. Johnson, are entitled *Human Sexual Response* (Little, Brown, 1966) and *Human Sexual Inadequacy* (Little, Brown, 1970).

General coverage of the subject is given in E. J. Trimmer's *Basic Sexual Medicine: a Textbook of Sexual Medicine and an Introduction to Sex Counselling Techniques* (Heinemann, 1978) whilst a series of articles that appeared in the *British Medical Journal* have been published as *Aspects of Sexual Medicine* (British Medical Association, 1976). Other sources of information on sexual dysfunction and its therapy include D. Jehu's *Sexual Dysfunction: a Behavioural Approach to Causation, Assessment and Treatment* (Wiley, 1979); J. and L. LoPiccolo's *Handbook of Sex Therapy* (Plenum, 1978); H. S. Kaplan's *Disorders of Sexual Desire* (Baillière, 1979); and *The New Sex Therapy* (Penguin, 1978), by the same author.

Statistics

Statistical information is frequently required on various aspects of obstetrics and gynaecology, and to those unacquainted with relevant sources this can prove a formidable task. Reliable statistics on given topics are often unobtainable on a national basis and, indeed, may not even exist at all. On such occasions, individual hospital reports, or published studies of a series of cases in journal literature, may be the only sources of representative figures available. However, the researcher in this subject field should be made aware of the major sources of statistical information and a number are described here, based on experience of answering typical enquiries in a specialist library.

The publications of the Office of Population Censuses and Surveys are an obvious primary source of national statistics and are described elsewhere (Chapter 4, page 86). The sections of importance within the confines of this chapter are Series FMI (Births); DH1, DH2, DH3 (Mortality Statistics); MB1 (Cancer Statistics); MB3 (Congenital Malformations); and AB (Abortion Statistics). Series AB was previously published as *Supplement on Abortion to The Registrar General's Statistical Review of England and Wales,* and is a source of detailed figures back to April 1968, when the 1967 Abortion Act came into effect. *Population Trends,* which has been published quarterly by HMSO since 1975, contains a regular series of tables on subjects such as abortion and birth statistics, together with articles on various aspects of population studies some of which are of particular interest to obstetricians and gynaecologists, such as those dealing with perinatal mortality. Another official publication, and one of great importance, is a triennial report from the Department of Health and Social Security devoted to the detailed analysis of maternal mortality statistics. The latest to appear is entitled *Report on Confidential Enquiries into Maternal Deaths in England and Wales, 1976–1978* (HMSO, 1982) and is No 26 in the series *Reports on Health and Social Subjects.*

A survey of births in the UK took place for one week in April, 1970, and many of the results are analyzed in the two published volumes of *British Births 1970. A Survey Under the Joint Auspices of the National Birthday Trust Fund and the Royal College of Obstetricians and Gynaecologists.* Volume 1, entitled *The First Week of Life,* was published under the direction of R. Chamberlain *et al.* (Heinemann, 1975) and contains chapters, with detailed tables, on such topics as birthweight and length of gestation, illness of the baby, and stillbirths and first-week deaths. Volume 2, *Obstetric Care* by G. Chamberlain *et al.* (Heinemann, 1978), covers aspects indicated by the title such as antenatal care, labour and labour induction.

Finally, *Maternity Care in the World: International Survey of Midwifery Practice and Training. Report of a Joint Study Group of the International Federation of Gynaecology and Obstetrics and the*

International Confederation of Midwives (2nd edn, International Federation of Gynaecology and Obstetrics; International Confederation of Midwives, 1976) is a comprehensive source of international statistics, particularly on birth and infant mortality rates, although maternal and perinatal mortality figures are not given. Wherever possible figures for 1973 are quoted, but less recent or estimated statistics are substituted where 1973 figures have not been made available.

History and biography

Gynaecology and obstetrics, particularly the latter, are subject fields which readily lend themselves to historical documentation. Numerous histories now exist, although few are readily available except for reference in a limited number of libraries. In view of the level of interest in the subject it is helpful to be aware of the most useful sources of information which can quickly be traced at need in specialist or long-established large medical collections.

Ancient history is covered by W. J. S. McKay's *The History of Ancient Gynaecology* (Baillière, 1901) which deals with the Egyptian, Hindu, Greek and Roman periods; it contains a list of works consulted but lacks an index. Several anthropological studies are available of which the most comprehensive is easily H. H. Ploss, M. Bartels and P. Bartels' *Woman: An Historical, Gynaecological and Anthropological Compendium* translated and edited by E. J. Dingwall (3 vols, Heinemann, 1935), which covers all aspects of womanhood in all races and cultures. It contains over 1000 illustrations and an extensive bibliography, but unfortunately no index, although material is arranged in a logical sequence. A more recent text, also more readily available, is D. A. M. Gebbie's *Reproductive Anthropology – Descent Through Woman* (Wiley, 1981).

As far as British obstetrical and gynaecological practice is concerned the two basic information sources are H. R. Spencer's *The History of British Midwifery from 1650 to 1800* (Bale, 1927) which is continued by J. M. Munro Kerr, R. W. Johnstone and M. H. Phillips' *Historical Review of British Obstetrics and Gynaecology, 1800–1950* (Livingstone, 1954), a well-documented volume with indexes of personal names and subjects. A translation from Middle English of a medieval manuscript (Sloane 2463), so far the earliest known reference source in obstetrics in the vernacular to be made freely available in printed form, has recently been published. Translated by B. Rowland it is entitled *Medieval Woman's Guide to Health* (Croom Helm, 1981), although the original manuscript is often referred to as the *English Trotula*. For information on the development of midwifery as a profession, as distinct from obstetrics, a useful source is J. Donnison's *Midwives and Medical Men: A History of Inter-Professional Rivalries and Women's Rights* (Heinemann, 1977). J. Dewhurst's *Royal Confinements* (Weidenfeld and Nicolson, 1980) spans two centuries from the Restoration Stuarts to Queen Victoria and is a publication which has appealed greatly to the taste of both medical men and the lay public. The history of the specialty in America is the subject of H. Speert's *Obstetrics and Gynecology in America: a History* (American College of Obstetricians and Gynecologists, 1980).

As far as general histories of the subject are concerned H. Speert has produced *Iconographia Gyniatrica: a Pictorial History of Gynecology and Obstetrics* (Davis, 1973) in which there is rather more emphasis on illustrative material than text, and the same author has also produced an earlier volume entitled *Essays in Eponymy: Obstetric and Gynecologic Milestones* (Macmillan, 1958). J. V. Ricci's books are comprehensive studies with extensive lists of references, and quotations from original sources: *One Hundred Years of Gynaecology, 1800–1900* (Blakiston, 1945); *The Genealogy of Gynaecology. History of the Development of Gynaecology throughout the Ages. 2000 B.C. to 1800 A.D.* (2nd edn, Blakiston, 1950); and *The Development of Gynaecological Surgery and Instruments: A Comprehensive Review of the Evolution of Surgery and Surgical Instruments for the Treatment of Female Diseases from the Hippocratic Age to the Antiseptic Period* (Blakiston, 1949) while T. Cianfrani's *A Short History of Obstetrics and Gynecology* (C. C. Thomas, 1960) sets the subject in a background of social, economic and general medical history. A popular, readable narrative without documentation but with a selective bibliography was provided by I. H. Flack under the pseudonym H. Graham in *Eternal Eve* (Heinemann, 1950), of which a revised, abridged edition was published in 1960; a short but authoritative little book by W. Radcliffe called *Milestones in Midwifery* (Wright, 1967) has general appeal. On more specialized topics are the invaluable *Obstetric Forceps: its History and Evolution* (Art Press, 1929) by Sir Kedarnath Das and J. H. Young's *Caesarean Section: the History and Development of the Operation from Earliest Times* (Lewis, 1944), while the Chamberlen family and their famous forceps are the subject of W. Radcliffe's *The Secret Instrument (The Birth of the Midwifery Forceps)* (Heinemann, 1947) and J. H. Aveling's *The Chamberlens and the Midwifery Forceps. Memorials of the Family and an Essay on the Invention of the Instrument* (Churchill, 1882).

Various efforts have been made to document the life and work of some of the more notable obstetricians and gynaecologists, although few of these biographies are outstanding. Most worthy of mention are:

Memoir of Sir James Y. Simpson by J. Duns (Edmonstone and Douglas, 1873)
Simpson and Syme of Edinburgh by J. A. Shepherd (Livingstone, 1969)
Dr. William Smellie and his Contemporaries by J. Glaister (Maclehose, 1894)
William Smellie, the Master of British Midwifery by R. W. Johnstone (Livingstone, 1952), which is shorter but nonetheless authoritative
Spencer Wells. The Life and Work of a Victorian Surgeon by J. A. Shepherd (Livingstone, 1965);
Semmelweis: his Life and Doctrine by Sir W. J. Sinclair (Manchester University Press, 1909)
Mea Culpa and the Life and Work of Semmelweis by L. P. Celione (Little, Brown, 1937), translated from the French by R. A. Parker
Woman's Surgeon: the Life Story of J. Marion Sims by S. Harris (Macmillan, 1950)
The Story of my Life by J. M. Sims (Appleton, 1884 and 1888)

There is, as yet, no definitive biography of William Hunter (1718–1783), but the following studies may be useful:

William Hunter: Anatomist, Physician, Obstetrician . . . with Notices of his Friends Cullen, Smellie, Fothergill and Baillie by R. H. Fox (Lewis, 1901)
Two Great Scotsmen; the Brothers William and John Hunter by G. R. Mather (Maclehose, 1893)
Memoir of William and John Hunter by G. C. Peachey (privately printed, 1924)
James Douglas of the Pouch and his Pupil William Hunter by K. B. Thomas (Pitman, 1964)

In this connection a new biography by J. L. Thornton entitled *Jan van Rymsdyk: Medical Artist of the Eighteenth Century* (Oleander, 1982) documents what is so far known of the life and work of this great illustrator who was largely responsible for illustrating Hunter's *Gravid Uterus* (1774) and other eighteenth-century texts and papers. Finally, there is available a collection of short biographies of eminent figures of this century in the form of Sir John Peel's *The Lives of the Fellows of the Royal College of Obstetricians and Gynaecologists, 1929–1969* (Heinemann, 1976).

Other texts which should perhaps be mentioned are *Records and Curiosities in Obstetrics and Gynaecology* compiled by I. L. C. Fergusson, R. W. Taylor and J. M. Watson (Baillière Tindall, 1982); a history of the Royal College of Midwives, 1881–1981 entitled *Behind the Blue Door* (Baillière Tindall, 1981) by B. Cowell and D. Wainwright, and Sir William Fletcher Shaw's *Twenty-five Years: The Story of the Royal College of Obstetricians and Gynaecologists, 1929–1954* (Churchill, 1954), which has been updated by Sir John Peel in an article entitled *The Royal College of Obstetricians and Gynaecologists, 1929 to 1979* published in *the British Journal of Obstetrics and Gynaecology*, **86,** 673–692, 1979.

Conclusions

The above selection from the literature on each of the major topics associated with obstetrics and gynaecology emphasizes the fact that even the more specialized branches of medicine are now covered by extensive lists of publications, which are daily augmented. General medical libraries cannot hope to cover every field in depth, and this chapter is intended to reveal the extent of the literature and to aid in the selection of items on specific subjects.

20

Paediatrics

E. S. Brooke

Paediatrics is concerned with the diseases and disorders of infants and children and with the development, health and welfare of the normal child. Children are no longer treated as 'little adults', so paediatrics is now a branch of medicine in its own right. In recent years the development of a number of specialties within the field has produced a significant increase in the literature.

Indexes, abstracts and bibliographies

Paediatric literature is included in the *Index Medicus* and the *NLM Current Catalog* (*see* Chapter 3). For current awareness three of the sections of *Current Contents* may be useful, depending on the bias of the research; these are *Current Contents, Clinical Practice, Current Contents, Life Sciences,* and *Current Contents, Social and Behavioral Sciences.*

Excerpta Medica Section 7 covers *Pediatrics and Pediatric Surgery* from 1947. The International Children's Centre issues *Courrier* (Paris, 1950–) six times per year, which includes abstracts in French and English, and has annotated lists of recently published books and occasional articles. *International Abstracts of Pediatric Surgery* are published in the *Journal of Pediatric Surgery* (Grune and Stratton, 1966–). The development of the child is covered by *Child Development Abstracts and Bibliography* (Society for Research in Child Development, 1930–). Each year the

Bibliography of Developmental Medicine and Child Neurology appears as a supplement to *Developmental Medicine and Child Neurology* (Heinemann, 1962–).

Reference books

Most reference books, such as dictionaries, directories and pharmacopoeias, used by paediatricians are those that are used by all medical men, but S. I. Magalini and E. Scrascia's *Dictionary of Medical Syndromes* (2nd edn, Lippincott, 1981) is particularly useful. The British Paediatric Association has produced the *BPA Clasification of Diseases* (2 vols, BPA, 1979) which aids the standardization of diagnostic data. The *Catalog of Teratogenic Agents* by T. H. Shepherd (3rd edn, Johns Hopkins University Press, 1980) should be consulted when birth defects are being considered.

Reviews

With subject fields expanding so rapidly, review volumes are most helpful. Paediatric subjects appear in many such volumes, but the following should particularly be mentioned: *Advances in Pediatrics* (Year Book Medical Publishers, 1942–), *Progress in Pediatric Surgery* (Urban and Schwarzenberg, 1970–) and *Year Book of Pediatrics* (Year Book Medical Publishers, 1933–).

Periodicals

Articles on child health and disease appear in many general medical journals and also in journals for specific subjects, e.g. endocrinology or pathology. There are so many journals devoted specifically to children that only a select list can be included here.

Select list of periodicals

Acta Paediatrica Scandinavica (Almqvist and Wiksell, 1921–)
American Journal of Diseases of Children (American Medical Association, 1911–)
Archives of Disease in Childhood (British Medical Association, 1926–)
Child; Care, Health and Development (Blackwell, 1975–)
Child Development (Society for Research in Child Development, 1930–)
Clinical Pediatrics (Lippincott, 1962–)
Developmental Medicine and Child Neurology (Heinemann, 1962–)
Early Human Development (Elsevier–North Holland, 1977–)

European Journal of Pediatrics (Springer, 1976–; formerly *Zeitschrift für Kinderheilkunde*, 1911–1975)
Journal of Child Psychology and Psychiatry (Pergamon, 1960–)
Journal of Pediatric Surgery (Grune and Stratton, 1966–)
Journal of Pediatrics (Mosby, 1932–)
Journal of Tropical Pediatrics (Oxford University Press, 1955–)
Pediatric Clinics of North America (Saunders, 1954–)
Pediatric Research (Williams and Wilkins, 1967–)
Pediatrics (American Academy of Pediatrics, 1948–)

Series

There are several monographic series which are important to the paediatrician:

Birth Defects, Original Article Series (A. R. Liss, 1964–)
Clinics in Developmental Medicine (Heinemann, 1964–)
Major Problems in Clinical Pediatrics (Saunders, 1964–)
Modern Problems in Pediatrics (Karger, 1954–)
Monographs in Pediatrics (Karger, 1971–)
Topics in Paediatrics (Pitman, 1979–)
Topics in Perinatal Medicine (Pitman, 1980–)

Monographs

Paediatrics

There are many textbooks of paediatrics, some having gone through several editions. Particularly to be mentioned are *Pediatrics* edited by A. M. Rudolph, which is the 17th edition of *Holt's Diseases of Infancy and Childhood* (Appleton-Century-Crofts, 1982) and *Nelson's Textbook of Pediatrics* edited by V. C. Vaughan *et al.* (11th edn, Saunders, 1979). Probably the most important British title is *Textbook of Paediatrics* edited by J. O. Forfar and G. C. Arneil (2nd edn, Churchill Livingstone, 1978). Three volumes which appeal to undergraduate students are *Diseases of Children* by H. Jolly (4th edn, Blackwell, 1981), *Essential Paediatrics* by D. Hull and D. I. Johnston (Churchill Livingstone, 1981), and *A Colour Atlas of Paediatrics* by M. Dynski-Klein (Wolfe, 1975).

Postgraduate students find J. H. Hutchinson's *Practical Paediatric Problems* (5th edn, Lloyd-Luke, 1980) useful. In *Recent Advances in Paediatrics* edited by D. Hull (6th edn, Churchill Livingstone, 1981) each chapter is a good review of a subject. *Practice of Pediatrics* (4 vols and index, Harper and Row), now edited by

V. C. Kelley, is looseleaf in form, and is regularly revised with new chapters sent to subscribers to replace old ones. A textbook written for general practitioners by general practitioners is *Child Care in General Practice* edited by C. Hart (2nd edn, Churchill Livingstone, 1982). Other helpful texts are:

Scientific Foundations of Paediatrics edited by J. A. Davis and J. Dobbing (2nd edn, Heinemann, 1981)

Clinical Paediatric Physiology edited by S. Godfrey and J. D. Baum (Blackwell, 1979)

Water and Electrolytes in Pediatrics by L. Finberg *et al.* (Saunders, 1982)

Prevention in Childhood of Health Problems in Adult Life edited by F. Falkner (WHO, 1980)

Child Health in the Community edited by R. G. Mitchell (2nd edn, Churchill Livingstone, 1980)

Growth and development

The normal growth of the child has to be studied before the abnormal, and the three-volume work *Human Growth* edited by F. Falkner and J. M. Tanner (Baillière Tindall, 1978–1979) covers the subject in depth. G. H. Lowrey's *Growth and Development of Children* (7th edn, Year Book Medical Publishers, 1978) is for more general use, and J. M. Tanner's *Foetus into Man* (Open Books, 1978) is a basic and easily understood book. J. M. Tanner and R. H. Whitehouse's *Atlas of Children's Growth* (Academic Press, 1982) illustrates normal variation in growth, and also growth disorders. Normal data is presented for quick use by J. M. H. Buckler in *A Reference Manual of Growth and Development* (Blackwell, 1979). A child's height, whether too short or too tall, can be a problem, and in this context *Assessment of Skeletal Maturity and Prediction of Adult Height (TW2 Method)* by J. M. Tanner *et al.* (Academic Press, 1975) is useful. Two volumes on growth disorders are W. A. Marshall's *Human Growth and its Disorders* (Academic Press, 1977) and D. W. Smith's *Growth and its Disorders* (Saunders, 1977).

The Normal Child by R. S. Illingworth (7th edn, Churchill Livingstone, 1979) is a standard text. The development of the child is well illustrated by M. Sheridan in *Children's Developmental Progress from Birth to Five Years* (3rd edn, NFER Publishing Co., 1975) and supplemented by her *Spontaneous Play in Early Childhood, from Birth to Six Years* (NFER Publishing Co., 1977). *Developmental Paediatrics*, by K. S. Holt (Butterworths, 1977) and *Development of the Infant and Young Child* by R. S. Illingworth (7th edn, Churchill Livingstone, 1980) are basic texts. A brief and simple handbook for use in assessing the child in clinic or surgery is *Basic Developmental Screening: 0–4 years* by R. S. Illingworth (3rd edn, Blackwell, 1982).

Diagnosis and therapy

The screening of children for illness is becoming more important, and a relevant book edited by W. K. Frankenberg and B. W. Camp is entitled *Pediatric Screening Tests* (C. C. Thomas, 1975). Two other books to aid diagnosis are Caffey's *Pediatric X-ray Diagnosis* (7th edn, 2 vols, Year Book Medical Publishers, 1978) and *Pediatric Ultrasound* by J. O. Haller and M. Schneider (Year Book Medical Publishers, 1980).

Regularly revised editions are necessary in therapeutics, and there are two such that apply to children: *Current Pediatric Therapy* edited by S. S. Gellis and B. M. Kagan (10th edn, Saunders, 1982) and *Pediatric Therapy* edited by H. C. Shirkey (6th edn, Mosby, 1980). A pocket-sized book by P. Catzel and R. Olver is entitled *The Paediatric Prescriber* (5th edn, Blackwell, 1981). The third volume of the *Topics in Paediatrics* series is *Recent Advances in Paediatric Therapeutics* edited by H. B. Valman (Pitman, 1982), and each chapter covers a different subject.

Nutrition

Nutrition affects the welfare of the infant and the future of the child and A. W. Wilkinson has edited a book entitled *Early Nutrition and Later Development* (Pitman, 1976). *MacKeith's Infant Feeding and Feeding Difficulties* edited by C. B. S. Wood and J. A. Walker-Smith (6th edn, Churchill Livingstone, 1981) and *Textbook of Paediatric Nutrition* edited by D. S. McLaren and D. Burman (2nd edn, Churchill Livingstone, 1982) are valuable texts. A. Ashworth *et al.* have compiled the annotated bibliography *Infant and Young Child Feeding,* published as a supplement to the journal *Early Human Development* (vol 6, April 1982).

Breast feeding is being actively encouraged and an international symposium on the subject was published under the title *Human Milk; its Biological and Social Value* edited by S. Freier and A. I. Eidelman (Excerpta Medica, 1980). S. L. Bahna and D. C. Heiner have drawn together useful information in *Allergies to Milk* (Grune and Stratton, 1980).

The sick child needs special attention and D. Francis' book *Diets for Sick Children* (4th edn, Blackwell, in preparation) gives great help to doctors, especially where specialized dietetic advice is not available. *A Colour Atlas of Nutritional Disorders* compiled by D.

S. McLaren (Wolfe, 1981) gives a vivid picture of disorders caused by faulty feeding. Other books in this field are R. E. Olsen's *Protein–Calorie Malnutrition* (Academic Press, 1975), M. Winick's *Childhood Obesity* (Wiley, 1975) and H. Bruch's *Eating Disorders; Obesity, Anorexia Nervosa and the Person Within* (Routledge and Kegan Paul, 1974).

Pathology

Textbooks on pathology include C. L. Berry's *Paediatric Pathology* (Springer, 1981), J. M. Kissane's *Pathology of Infancy and Childhood* (2nd edn, Mosby, 1975), Potter and Craig's *Pathology of the Fetus and the Infant* (3rd edn, Lloyd-Luke, 1976) and L. P. Dehner's *Pediatric Surgical Pathology* (Mosby, 1975). A handbook of clinical tests and reference ranges has been compiled by B. E. Clayton *et al.*, *Paediatric Chemical Pathology* (Blackwell, 1980).

Hematology of Infancy and Childhood edited by D. G. Nathan and F. A. Oski (2nd edn, Saunders, 1981) is in two volumes, whilst *Smith's Blood Diseases of Infancy and Childhood* edited by D. R. Miller *et al.* (4th edn, Mosby, 1978) is a comprehensive text in one volume. The first volume in the *Topics in Paediatrics* series is by P. H. M. Jones and entitled *Haematology and Oncology* (Pitman, 1979). Cancer in childhood is covered by W. W. Sutow *et al.* in *Clinical Pediatric Oncology* (2nd edn, Mosby, 1977) and by P. G. Jones and P. E. Campbell in *Tumours of Infancy and Childhood* (Blackwell, 1976).

Immunology is a growing subject, and E. R. Stiehm and V. A. Fulginiti's *Immunologic Disorders in Infants and Children* (2nd edn, Saunders, 1980) is a standard text. C. W. Bierman and D. S. Pearlman have edited a book on *Allergic Diseases of Infancy, Childhood and Adolescence* (Saunders, 1980), and a guide to practical management is J. A. Kuzemko's *Allergy in Childhood* (Pitman, 1978).

Ciba Foundations Symposium No 10, *Intrauterine Infections* (Elsevier, 1973), is an important source of information about the effect of infections on the future infant. R. D. Feigin and J. D. Cherry's *Textbook of Pediatric Infections* (2 vols, Saunders, 1981) and S. Krugman and S. L. Katz's *Infectious Diseases of Children* (7th edn, Mosby, 1981) should also be mentioned.

Gastroenterology

Abdominal pain can be elusive to diagnosis and J. Apley's small book *The Child with Abdominal Pains* (2nd edn, Blackwell, 1975) is rather special in this context. Large books on gastroenterology are *Paediatric Gastroenterology* by C. M. Anderson and V. Burke (Blackwell, 1975) and *Pediatric Clinical Gastroenterology* by A. Silverman and C. C. Roy (3rd edn, Mosby, 1983). A concise volume is edited by J. T. Harries and entitled *Essentials of Paediatric Gastroenterology* (Churchill Livingstone, 1977). J. Walker-Smith's book *Diseases of the Small Intestine in Childhood* (2nd edn, Pitman, 1979) and A. P. Mowat's book *Liver Disorders in Childhood* (Butterworths, 1979) are written with a specific area in mind. Also useful is Ciba Foundation Symposium No 42, *Acute Diarrhoea in Childhood* (Elsevier–North Holland, 1976).

Nephrology and urology

Pediatric Kidney Disease edited by C. M. Edelman *et al.* (Little, Brown, 1978) is in two volumes: *Pediatric Nephrology* by M. I. Rubin and T. M. Barratt (Williams and Wilkins, 1975), a comprehensive one-volume work; and *Renal Disease in Childhood* by J. A. James (3rd edn, Mosby, 1976), a useful shorter text.

D. Innes Williams and J. H. Johnston edited *Paediatric Urology* (2nd edn, Butterworths, 1982) and H. B. Eckstein *et al.* edited *Surgical Pediatric Urology* (Thieme, 1977). *Bladder Control and Enuresis* is edited by I. Kolvin *et al.* (Heinemann, 1973).

Cardiology

A short textbook is *Heart Disease in Paediatrics* by S. C. Jordan and O. Scott (2nd edn, Butterworths, 1981). Two of the longer textbooks are *Heart Disease in Infants and Children* edited by G. Graham and E. Rossi (Arnold, 1980) and *Heart Disease in Infancy and Childhood* by J. D. Keith *et al.* (3rd edn, Macmillan, 1978).

Churchill Livingstone publish a series of volumes entitled *Paediatric Cardiology* (vols 1–5, 1978–1983). R. H. Anderson and A. E. Becker have written *Cardiac Anatomy* (Churchill Livingstone, 1980) and also *Pathology of Congenital Heart Disease* (Butterworths, 1981). J. R. Zuberbuhler stresses non-invasive diagnosis in his book *Clinical Diagnosis in Paediatric Cardiology* (Churchill Livingstone, 1981).

Other diseases

Books on diseases of the various systems of the body include:

Gynecology of Childhood and Adolescence by J. W. Huffman *et al.* (2nd edn, Saunders, 1981)

Clinical Paediatric Endocrinology by C. G. D. Brook (Blackwell, 1981)
Childhood Diabetes and its Management by J. O. Craig (2nd edn, Butterworths, 1981)
Clinical Pediatric Dermatology by S. Hurwitz (Saunders, 1981)
Paediatric Otolaryngology by J. F. Birrell (Wright, 1978)
Asthma in Children by J. A. Kuzemko (2nd edn, Pitman, 1980)
Respiratory Illness in Children by P. D. Phelan *et al.* (2nd edn, Blackwell, 1983)
Disorders of the Respiratory Tract in Children by E. L. Kendig and V. Chernick (4th edn, Saunders, 1983)
Pediatric Ophthalmology edited by R. D. Harley (2nd edn, 2 vols, Saunders, 1983)
Visual Handicap in Children edited by V. Smith and J. Keen (Heinemann, 1979)
Rheumatic Disorders in Childhood by B. M. Ansell (Butterworths, 1980)
Muscle Disorders in Childhood by V. Dubowitz (Saunders, 1978)

Tropical medicine

Diseases of Children in the Subtropics and Tropics edited by D. B. Jelliffe and J. P. Stanfield (3rd edn, Arnold, 1978) is the standard work in this field. R. G. Hendrickse has edited *Paediatrics in the Tropics* (Oxford University Press, 1981) which gives a current review of the subject.

The health of the child in the developing countries is particularly important. D. Morley's book *Paediatric Priorities in the Developing World* (Butterworths, 1973) outlines the problems that have to be faced and G. J. Ebrahim's *Paediatric Practice in Developing Countries* (Macmillan, 1981) discusses main issues in child health in developing countries. Basic books used by health workers include *Primary Child Care* by M. King *et al.* (Oxford University Press, 1978), *See How They Grow* by D. Morley and M. Woodland (Macmillan, 1979) and *Textbook of Paediatric Surgery in the Tropics* by F. A. Nwako (Macmillan, 1980).

Maternal and child health is an area of preventive medicine among a large proportion of the population of any country. Basic information is given by C. D. Williams and D. B. Jelliffe in *Mother and Child Health; Delivering the Services* (Oxford University Press, 1972). Experts share their experience in *Maternal and Child Health Around the World* edited by H. M. Wallace and G. J. Ebrahim (Macmillan, 1981), and *Advances in International Maternal and Child Health* edited by D. B. and E. F. P. Jelliffe gives up-to-date information with good reference lists (Oxford University Press, vol 1, 1981; vol 2, 1982).

Genetics and inherited disease

A short introduction to genetics is A. Emery's *Elements of Medical Genetics* (5th edn, Churchill Livingstone, 1979). Other books on genetics include F. Vogel and A. G. Motulsky's *Human Genetics: Problems and Approaches* (Springer, 1979) and H. Harris' *Principles of Human Biochemical Genetics* (3rd edn, Elsevier, 1980). An essential reference book is V. A. McKusick's *Mendelian Inheritance in Man; Catalogs of Autosomal Dominant, Autosomal Recessive, and X-linked Phenotypes* (5th edn, Johns Hopkins University Press, 1978).

Prenatal diagnosis of inherited disorders is covered by H. Galjaard in *Genetic Metabolic Diseases* (Elsevier–North Holland, 1980). Clinicians with little knowledge of genetics will find P. S. Harper's book *Practical Genetic Counselling* (Wright, 1981) helpful.

The standard work on inherited metabolic disease is edited by J. B. Stanbury *et al.* and is entitled *Metabolic Basis of Inherited Disease* (5th edn, McGraw Hill, 1982). A small introductory text, *Inborn Errors of Metabolism,* is edited by R. Ellis (Croom Helm, 1980) and a larger textbook is M. G. Ampola's *Metabolic Diseases in Pediatric Practice* (Little, Brown, 1982).

Malformations

Congential Malformations by J. Warkany (Year Book Medical Publishers, 1971) is a standard work and W. L. Nyhan and N. O. Sakati's *Genetic and Malformation Syndromes in Clinical Medicine* (Year Book Medical Publishers, 1976) and D. Bergsma's *Birth Defects Compendium* (2nd edn, Macmillan, 1979) are also important. D. W. Smith's *Recognizable Patterns of Human Malformation* (3rd edn, Saunders, 1982) and *Recognizable Patterns of Human Deformation* (Saunders, 1981) are both profusely illustrated.

The surgeon correcting malformations will find *Embryology for Surgeons; the Embryological Basis for the Treatment of Congenital Defects* by S. W. Gray and J. E. Skandalakis (Saunders, 1972) helpful. *Handbook of Teratology* edited by J. G. Wilson (4 vols, Plenum, 1977–1978) is an exhaustive work.

Surgery

A good introduction to paediatric surgery is *Essentials of Paediatric Surgery* by H. H. Nixon and B. O'Donnell (3rd edn, Heinemann, 1976), but the standard work is *Pediatric Surgery* edited by M. M. Ravitch *et al.* (3rd edn, 2 vols, Year Book Medical Publishers, 1979). Two atlases are H. H. Nixon's *Paediatric Surgery,* which is a volume in the third edition of *Rob and Smith's Operative*

Surgery (Butterworths, 1978), and *A Colour Atlas of Paediatric Surgical Diagnosis* edited by L. Spitz *et al.* (Wolfe, 1981). *Surgical Conditions in Paediatrics* by H. H. Nixon (Butterworths, 1978) is written by a surgeon for his medical colleagues and gives total management of the patient rather than operative technique; S. L. Gans' *Surgical Pediatrics; Non-operative Care* (2nd edn, Grune and Stratton, 1980) gives an overall picture. J. C. Mustarde edited a book entitled *Plastic Surgery in Infancy and Childhood* (2nd edn, Churchill Livingstone, 1979).

Orthopaedics is a branch of surgery which W. J. W. Sharrard covers in his book *Paediatric Orthopaedics and Fractures* (2nd edn, 2 vols, Blackwell, 1979). An introductory text has been written by G. C. Lloyd-Roberts, *Orthopaedics in Infancy and Childhood* (Butterworths, 1971). Two specific problems are covered by C. C. M. James and L. P. Lassman in *Spina Bifida Occulta* (Grune and Stratton, 1981) and by G. C. Lloyd-Roberts and A. H. C. Ratcliff in *Hip Disorders in Children* (Butterworths, 1978). *Physiotherapy in Paediatrics* by R. Shepherd (2nd edn, Heinemann, 1980) outlines the work of the physiotherapist.

Paediatric Emergencies edited by J. A. Black (Butterworths, 1979) aims to help in the treatment of a child injured or taken suddenly ill; it is a large book but has short concise entries. A practical manual for the general practitioner or casualty officer is by C. M. Illingworth, *The Diagnosis and Primary Care of Accidents and Emergencies in Children* (2nd edn, Blackwell, 1982). J. G. Randolph *et al.* edit *The Injured Child: Surgical Management* (Year Book Medical Publishers, 1979).

Naturally anaesthesia for children is different from that for adults and two books on the subject are *Anaesthesia for Children, Including Aspects of Intensive Care* by T. C. K. Brown and G. C. Fisk (Blackwell, 1979) and *Paediatric Anaesthesia, Trends in Current Practice* by G. J. Rees and T. C. Gray (Butterworths, 1981).

Psychology and psychiatry

Normal human development is contained in J. Kahn and S. E. Wright's *Human Growth and the Development of Personality* (3rd edn, Pergamon, 1980). An introduction to normal child behaviour is by T. J. Kenny and R. L. Clemmens, *Behavioral Pediatrics and Child Development* (2nd edn, Williams and Wilkins, 1980). Abnormal behaviour is the subject of R. and P. McAuley's *Child Behaviour Problems* (Macmillan, 1977).

Books on specific problems are numerous and a selection is given here:

Pica; a Childhood Symptom by D. J. Bicknell (Butterworths, 1975)
The Hyperactive Child edited by D. P. Cantwell (Spectrum Publications, 1975)
Lead Absorption in Children edited by J. J. Chisholm and D. M. O'Hara (Urban and Schwarzenberg, 1982)
Out of School; Modern Perspectives in Truancy and School Refusal edited by L. Hersov and I. Berg (Wiley, 1980)
Learning Disabilities and Related Disorders edited by J. G. Millichap (Year Book Medical Publishers, 1977)
The Development and Disorders of Speech in Childhood by M. E. Morley (3rd edn, Churchill Livingstone, 1972)
Dyslexia Research and its Applications to Education by G. T. Pavlides and T. R. Miles (Wiley, 1981)
The Child with Delayed Speech by M. Rutter and J. A. M. Martin (Heinemann, 1972)
Autism; a Reappraisal of Concepts and Treatment edited by M. Rutter and E. Schopler (Plenum, 1978)
Down's Anomaly by G. F. Smith and J. M. Berg (2nd edn, Churchill Livingstone, 1976).

An introduction to psychiatry is P. Barker's *Basic Child Psychiatry* (4th edn, Granada Publishing, 1983). From the large number of titles on child psychiatry, three have been selected: *Child Psychiatry* edited by M. L. Rutter and L. Hersov (Blackwell, 1976), *Psychopathological Disorders of Childhood* by H. C. Quay and J. S. Werry (2nd edn, Wiley, 1979) and *Scientific Foundations of Developmental Psychiatry* edited by M. Rutter (Heinemann, 1980). For non-psychiatrists, F. H. Stone's *Psychiatry and the Paediatrician* (Butterworths, 1976) aims to make psychiatric problems understandable. A. S. Gurman and D. P. Kniskern have edited *Handbook of Family Therapy* (Brunner–Mazel, 1981) and P. Barker has written an introduction to the subject in *Basic Family Therapy* (Granada Publishing, 1981).

Mental Handicap by B. Kirman and J. Bicknell (Churchill Livingstone, 1975) and *Pathology of Mental Retardation* by L. Crome and J. Stern (2nd edn, Churchill Livingstone, 1972) are useful in conjunction with each other. L. B. Holmes *et al.* have edited an excellently illustrated book, *Mental Retardation; an Atlas of Diseases with Associated Physical Abnormalities* (Macmillan, 1972).

Neurology and neurosurgery

The Practice of Pediatric Neurology by K. F. Swaiman and F. S. Wright (2nd edn, Mosby, 1982) is in two volumes that cover the subject extensively. A smaller book is J. H. Menkes' *Textbook of Child Neurology* (2nd edn, Lea and Febiger, 1980). H. F. R. Prechtl's *The Neurological Examination of the Full Term Newborn Infant* (2nd edn, Heinemann, 1977) is a practical guide. Books on specific conditions include:

Neurology of Hereditary Metabolic Diseases in Children by R. D. Adams and G. Lyon (McGraw Hill, 1982)
Neurologic Infections in Children by W. E. Bell and W. F. McCormick (2nd edn, Saunders, 1981)
Neurophysiological Basis for the Treatment of Cerebral Palsy by K. Bobath (2nd edn, Heinemann, 1980)
Neurodevelopmental Problems in Early Childhood edited by C. M. Drillen and M. B. Drummond (Blackwell, 1977)
Epilepsies of Childhood by N. V. O'Donohoe (Butterworths, 1979)
Epilepsy and Psychiatry by E. H. Reynolds and M. R. Trimble (Churchill Livingstone, 1981)

Atlas of Pediatric Neurosurgical Operations (Saunders, 1982) was conceived and begun by D. D. Matson, and completed by J. Shillito. *Neurosurgery of Infancy and Childhood* by D. D. Matson (2nd edn. Thomas, 1969) and K. Till's *Paediatric Neursurgery* (Blackwell, 1975) are recommended.

Newborn infant

Just as the child is not to be treated as a 'little adult', the newborn infant is not to be treated as a 'little child', and there is a literature especially for the neonate. G. B. Avery's *Neonatology* (2nd edn, Lippincott, 1981) and A. J. Schaffer and M. E. Avery's *Diseases of the Newborn* (4th edn, Saunders, 1977) cover the subject in depth. *Clinical Perinatology* edited by S. Aladjem *et al.* (2nd edn, Mosby, 1980) is useful to obstetricians as well as paediatricians. *Craig's Care of the Newly Born Infant* edited by A. J. Keay and D. M. Morgan (7th edn, Churchill Livingstone, 1982), *Medical Care of Newborn Babies* by P. A. Davies *et al.* (Heinemann, 1972) and *Neonatal Behavioral Assessment Scale* by T. B. Brazleton (Heinemann, 1973) are smaller and more practical in their approach.

A great deal of interest is now shown in the size of the infant and L. O. Lubchenco's book *The High Risk Infant* (Saunders, 1976) defines the risk in relation to low or high birth weight and gestational age. L. M. S. and V. Dubowitz have compiled a manual to aid the assessment of *Gestational Age of the Newborn* (Addison-Wesley, 1977). In *Born too Soon or Born too Small* (Heinemann, 1976) G. A. Neligan *et al.* have followed, for seven years, the development of a group of high-risk infants from Newcastle upon Tyne.

Improved care and technological advances have helped save many infants, but for the survivors there may be added problems. Other specialized books of the newborn include:

The Lung and its Disorders in the Newborn Infant by M. E. Avery and B. D. Fletcher (4th edn, Saunders, 1981)
Separation and Special-care Baby Units edited by F. S. W. Brimblecombe *et al.* (Heinemann, 1978)

Assisted Ventilation of the Neonate edited by J. P. Goldsmith and E. H. Karotkin (Saunders, 1981)

Neonatal Anaesthesia by D. J. Hatch and E. Sumner (Arnold, 1981)

Neonatal Orthopaedics by R. N. Hensinger and E. T. Jones (Grune and Stratton, 1981)

Hematologic Problems in the Newborn by F. A. Oski and J. L. Naiman (3rd edn, Saunders, 1982)

Neonatal Surgery by P. P. Rickham *et al.* (2nd edn, Butterworths, 1978)

The Neonate with Congenital Heart Disease edited by R. D. Rowe *et al.* (2nd edn, Saunders, 1981)

Physiology of the Newborn Infant by C. A. Smith and N. M. Nelson (4th edn, C. C. Thomas, 1976)

Neonatal Dermatology by L. M. Solomon (Saunders, 1973)

Neurology of the Newborn by J. J. Volpe (Saunders, 1981)

Social aspects

Much concern is now shown for the rights of the child and there is a wealth of legislation contained in Sir Clarke Hall and A. C. L. Morrison's *Law Relating to Children and Young Persons* (9th edn, Butterworths, 1977; 2nd cumulative supplement, 1981). A small book of interest is M. L. K. Pringle's *The Needs of Children* (2nd edn, Hutchinson, 1980), and an increasing problem is outlined in *Children of Immigrants to Britain* by E. de H. Lobo (Hodder and Stoughton, 1978). S. Wolkind edits a book entitled *Medical Aspects of Adoption and Foster Care* (Heinemann, 1979).

The relationship between child and parent is covered in *Parent–Infant Bonding* by M. H. Klaus and J. H. Kennell (2nd edn, Mosby, 1982). C. H. Kempe and R. E. Helfer edited the forerunner in child abuse, *The Battered Child* (3rd edn, University of Chicago Press, 1980). *Child Abuse and Neglect* edited by N. S. Ellerstein (Wiley, 1981) looks at the subject from a medical point of view, and *Sexually Abused Children and their Families* edited by P. B. Mrazek and C. H. Kempe (Pergamon, 1981) covers a newly recognized problem within this area.

The care of the handicapped and chronically-ill child involves much understanding of the child and the family. L. Burton has produced two books in this field, *Care of the Child Facing Death* (Routledge and Kegan Paul, 1974) and *The Family Life of Sick Children* (Routledge and Kegan Paul, 1975). Two small books about the everyday needs and care of sick children are *More than Sympathy* by R. G. Lansdown (Tavistock, 1980) and *The Other Side of Paediatrics* by J. Jolly (Macmillan, 1981). *The Child with Disabling Illness – Principles of Rehabilitation* edited by J. A. Downey and N. L. Low (2nd edn, Saunders, 1981), *Handicapped Children* by J. D. Kershaw (3rd edn, Heinemann, 1973) and *Handicaps in Childhood* edited by M. Manciaux (Karger, 1982) are all useful texts. Going into hospital can have dramatic effects on children and two books on this subject are *Emotional Care of Hospitalized Children* by M. Petrillo and S. Sanger (2nd edn, Lippincott, 1980) and *Beyond Separation* edited by D. Hall and M. Stacey (Routledge and Kegan Paul, 1979).

Surveys of groups of children, at birth and as they grow up, give much valuable information. In 1958 there was a British Perinatal Mortality Survey and from this came two reports, *Perinatal Mortality* by N. R. Butler and D. G. Bonham (Livingstone, 1963) and *Perinatal Problems* by N. R. Butler and E. D. Alberman (Livingstone, 1969). The National Child Development Study (1958 Cohort) has produced three reports, *From Birth to Seven* by R. Davie *et al.* (Longman, 1972), *11,000 Seven Year Olds* by M. L. K. Pringle *et al.* (Longman, 1966) and *Britain's Sixteen Year Olds* edited by K. Fogelman (National Children's Bureau, 1976). Under the auspices of the National Birthday Trust Fund and the Royal College of Obstetricians and Gynaecologists, the British Births Survey 1970 has been commenced on children born between 5th and 11th April 1970, called *British Births, 1970, Vol 1: The First Week of Life* (Heinemann, 1975), *Vol 2: Obstetric Care* (Heinemann, 1978). A report of the British Births Child Study (1970) is *The Prevalence of Illness in Childhood* by R. N. Chamberlain and R. N. Simpson (Pitman, 1979), which surveys approximately 10 per cent of the children in the original survey.

A study of health and illness in children in Newcastle has been the subject of three volumes, *A Thousand Families in Newcastle upon Tyne* by J. Spence *et al.* (Oxford University Press, 1954), and *Growing Up in Newcastle upon Tyne* (Oxford University Press, 1960) and *The School Years in Newcastle upon Tyne* (Oxford University Press, 1974) both by F. D. W. Miller *et al.* A study by a general practitioner in Brixton is recorded in M. Pollak's *Today's Three Year Olds in London* (Heinemann, 1972) and *Nine Years Old* (MTP Press, 1979), and gives an insight into the experiences of children, living side by side, but being reared in different cultural life styles.

History and biography

Specialized books on paediatrics did not appear until the sixteenth century, but earlier writers had made observations on children's diseases. J. Ruhräh's anthology *Pediatrics of the Past* (Hoeber, 1925) gives a fascinating glimpse into writings from Hippocrates (460–370 BC) to Friedrich Ludwig Meissner (1796–1860). J.

Ruhräh followed this with his *Pediatric Biographies,* reprinted from the *American Journal of Diseases of Children,* where they were originally printed between January 1928 and December 1931. The biographies continued to be published monthly in the *Journal* until the end of 1935.

G. F. Still wrote *The History of Paediatrics* (Oxford University Press, 1931) and this covers the subject from earliest times up to the end of the eighteenth century. Abt–Garrison's *History of Pediatrics* (Saunders, 1965) includes F. H. Garrison's *History of Pediatrics,* reprinted from *Pediatrics,* edited by I. A. Abt (vol 1, Saunders, 1923), with chapters on more recent times by A. F. Abt. T. E. Cone has written *History of American Pediatrics* (Little, Brown, 1979) and J. M. Tanner has written *History of the Study of Human Growth* (Cambridge University Press, 1981)

Pioneers in Pediatrics by A. Levinson (2nd edn, Froben Press, 1943) and B. S. Veeder's *Pediatric Profiles* (Mosby, 1975; originally published in the *Journal of Pediatrics*) give biographical sketches of many famous paediatricians.

The American Pediatric Society published a *Semi-centennial Volume* in 1938. This contains biographical sketches of the founders and members, as well as an historical sketch of the Society. The history of the British Paediatric Association is held in two volumes, H. C. Cameron's *The British Paediatric Association 1928–1952* (British Paediatric Association, 1955) and V. Neale's *The British Paediatric Association 1952–1968* (Pitman, 1970). G. Fanconi wrote on the international scene in *The History of the International Paediatric Association* (Schwabe, 1968).

The biographies of Abraham Jacobi (1830–1919) and Mary Jacobi (1842–1906), who were both professors of children's diseases, are told in R. Tonax's book *The Doctors Jacobi* (Little, Brown, 1952). W. Craig records the story of *John Thompson: Pioneer and Father of Scottish Paediatrics, 1856–1926* (Livingstone, 1968), and A. Dally writes about Cicely Williams (born 1893), famous for her work in tropical child health, in *Cicely: The Story of a Doctor* (Gollancz, 1968).

21

Dentistry

E. M. Spencer*; revised by M. A. Clennett

The modern literature of dentistry has developed since the mid-nineteenth century, when the dentist began to achieve professional status and to strive towards systematic instruction and qualification. Dental books had been published in increasing numbers since the sixteenth century, but such historical works are not mentioned in this chapter, which must be limited to books of current interest. Similarly, the periodical literature must be confined to those journals currently providing a means of communication between dentists and their co-workers.

Journals

General dental journals

All the developed countries have official bodies representing the national dental profession, and most issue a journal publishing scientific articles of importance on all aspects of dentistry.

The leading British dental periodical is the *British Dental Journal (BDJ)*, which is, since 1880, the official organ of the British Dental Association, a body that furthers the interests of all branches of the profession. The *BDJ* is published twice a month, and has papers describing research work, clinical cases and epidemiological surveys. Series of articles are regularly commissioned from leading authorities, on such subjects as orthodontics and occlusion.

* Formerly Librarian, British Dental Association

Foremost among foreign associations' periodicals is the *Journal of the American Dental Association* (US, monthly), other important titles being the *Australian Dental Journal* (bi-monthly), *New Zealand Dental Journal* (quarterly), *Journal of the Canadian Dental Association* (monthly) and *Swedish Dental Journal* (bi-monthly). Leading journals from Europe, publishing in their own language, are:

Österreichische Zeitschrift für Stomatologie (Austria)
Chirurgien-Dentiste de France
Tandlaegebladet (Denmark)
Deutsche Zahnärztliche Zeitschrift (West Germany)
Stomatologie der DDR (East Germany)
Nederlands Tijschrift voor Tandheelkunde
Norske Tannlaegeforenings Tidende (Norway)
Schweizerische Monatsschrift für Zahnheilkunde (Switzerland)
Stomatologija (USSR)

Although most other titles are in specialist fields, there is still a need and use for others general in scope. The *International Dental Journal* (quarterly) is the organ of the International Dental Federation (FDI), an organization whose annual congress produces a number of important papers, many of which are published in the *Journal*. An important contribution is made by the *Journal of Dental Research* (US, monthly), published under the auspices of the International Association for Dental Research (IADR). Special supplements are issued which contain abstracts of the IADR Annual Congress and other significant meetings.

The *Scandinavian Journal of Dental Research* (bi-monthly, Denmark) is published by Munksgaard, a firm renowned for the quality of its dental productions. Until 1970 known as *Odontologisk Tidskrift,* this journal chiefly comprises papers from Scandinavian authors, but has international interest, and is the official publication of the Scandinavian Division of the IADR.

Acta Odontologica Scandinavica (bi-monthly, Norway) publishes scientific and clinical papers in English and has issued over 70 supplements on specific topics, many of which have become classics.

In Britain, the *Journal of Dentistry* (bi-monthly) has successfully upheld the reputation of its predecessor, *Dental Practitioner*, which it replaced in 1973. *Dental Update* (bi-monthly) is of particular interest to the British clinician, excluding research material from its remit.

Specialist journals

Most titles appear under the auspices of specialist societies, being published either by a society itself or by a commercial publisher on the society's behalf.

CHILDREN'S DENTISTRY

The oldest established title is the *Journal of Dentistry for Children* (US, bi-monthly), but newer arrivals are other American titles such as *Journal of Pedodontics* (quarterly) and *Pediatric Dentistry* (bi-monthly). The *Proceedings of the British Paedodontic Society* (annual) is the only British publication.

ORTHODONTICS

The *American Journal of Orthodontics* (US, monthly) is the most longstanding title, while the *Angle Orthodontist* (US, quarterly) expounds a particular school of thought. The *British Journal of Orthodontics* (quarterly) is an excellent successor to the annual *Proceedings of the British Society for the Study of Orthodontics;* the *Transactions of the European Orthodontic Society*, formerly annual, is similarly replaced by the *European Journal of Orthodontics* (UK, quarterly).

ORAL SURGERY

The key periodicals in this field are *Oral Surgery, Oral Medicine, Oral Pathology* (US, monthly) and *Journal of Oral and Maxillofacial Surgery* (US, monthly), the latter adding its second adjective in 1982. The increased scope of this field is reflected by the addition of three new publications since 1972: *Head and Neck Surgery* (US, bi-monthly), *Journal of Maxillofacial Surgery* (Germany, quarterly) and *International Journal of Oral Surgery* (Denmark, bi-monthly). The *British Journal of Oral Surgery* (quarterly) is an important title reflecting practice in this country.

PERIODONTOLOGY

There is no British journal in this field. *Journal of Periodontology* (US, monthly) publishes case reports and scientific papers. The Scandinavian titles *Journal of Periodontal Research* and *Journal of Clinical Periodontology* (both from Denmark, bi-monthly) are complementary, and both regularly include important review articles.

RESTORATIVE DENTISTRY

Pre-eminent here is the *Journal of Prosthetic Dentistry* (US, monthly) with clinical and research papers. A research-orientated approach is found in *Journal of Oral Rehabilitation* (UK, bi-monthly).

OTHER SPECIALTIES

Important academic periodicals are *Journal of Oral Pathology* (Denmark, bi-monthly), *Archives of Oral Biology* (UK, monthly) and *Caries Research* (Switzerland, bi-monthly). *Journal of Endodontics* (US, monthly) and *International Endodontic Journal,* which was formerly the *Journal of the British Endodontic Society* (quarterly), both cater for the research worker and the clinician. *Community Dentistry and Oral Epidemiology* (Denmark, bi-monthly) gives international coverage in this field, while *Journal of Public Health Dentistry* (US, quarterly) has articles chiefly relating to America.

Non-dental journals

Some titles regularly include articles of dental interest. The *Annals of the Royal College of Surgeons of England* (bi-monthly) reflects the activities of the Faculty of Dental Surgery with scientific and historical papers, and the *Journal of the Royal Society of Medicine* (monthly) includes papers given before its Section of Odontology. *Calcified Tissue International,* formerly *Calcified Tissue Research* (German, bi-monthly) has included some important dental contributions.

Textbooks and monographs

Because of the rapid increase in specialization, general works on dentistry tend to be old or written for ancillary staff, such as dental surgery assistants. An example is H. Levison's *Textbook for Dental Nurses* (5th edn, Blackwell, 1978). A general book for students that provides introductory or revision material is *Essentials of Dental Surgery and Pathology* by R. A. Cawson (3rd edn, Churchill Livingstone, 1978), which stresses the clinical side of dentistry. *Scientific Foundations of Dentistry* edited by B. Cohen and I. R. H. Kramer (Heinemann, 1976), which is intended for those studying for higher dental qualifications, is a magnificent résumé of knowledge by nearly 70 authors. For the general dental practitioner J. Manning has edited *General Dental Practice* (Kluwer, 1978–1982), a two-volume, loose-leaf work. Volume A covers clinical aspects and Volume B practice management. An excellent introduction for the layman is J. Forrest's *The Good Teeth Guide* (Granada, 1981).

Anatomy, histology, physiology, microbiology

The most concise books on dental anatomy are J. H. Scott and N. B. B. Symons's *Introduction to Dental Anatomy* (9th edn, Churchill Livingstone, 1982) and J. H. Scott and A. D. Dixon's *Anatomy for Students of Dentistry* (4th edn, Churchill Livingstone, 1978). A larger, more detailed American work is *Oral Anatomy* by H. Sicher and E. L. Dubrul (7th edn, Mosby, 1980). For illustrations are recommended the pocket-sized *Dental Morphology: an Illustrated Guide* by G. C. Van Beek (2nd edn, Wright, 1983) and the comprehensive *Colour Atlas and Textbook of Oral Anatomy* by B. K. B. Berkovitz and B. J. Moxham (Wolfe, 1978). This book includes comparative anatomy within its scope, the only other current title on this topic being B. Peyer's *Comparative Odontology* (University of Chicago Press, 1968). Specialized aspects of morphology are dealt with in R. C. Wheeler's *Pulp Cavities of the Permanent Teeth* (Saunders, 1976) and D. R. Brothwell's *Dental Anthropology* (Pergamon, 1963), which has contributions on the oral structures and development of primates and primitive man.

A standard text on maxillofacial development is by D. H. Enlow, entitled *Handbook of Facial Growth* (2nd edn, Saunders, 1982). A smaller, British text is by D. H. Goose and J. Appleton, *Human Dentofacial Growth* (Pergamon, 1982), and a concise American text is D. M. Ranly's *Synopsis of Craniofacial Growth* (Appleton-Century-Crofts, 1980).

C. L. B. Lavelle's *Applied Physiology of the Mouth* (Wright, 1975) is an excellent book on this subject, as is *Physiology and Biochemistry of the Mouth* by G. N. Jenkins (4th edn, Blackwell, 1978). The encyclopaedic work edited by Professor A. E. W. Miles in two volumes, *Structural and Chemical Organisation of Teeth* (Academic Press, 1967) remains a standard work and emphasizes the histological aspects of anatomy and physiology.

The best known book on histology is *Orban's Oral Histology and Embryology* edited by S. N. Bhaskar (9th edn, Mosby, 1980). Briefer coverage is given by J. W. Osborn and A. R. Ten Cate in *Advanced Dental Histology* (4th edn, Wright, 1983), while the latter author has also written *Oral Histology: Development, Structure and Function* (Mosby, 1980). I. A. Mjor and J. J. Pindborg's *Histology of the Human Tooth* (Munksgaard, 1973) is a standard work.

Embryology is well described in *Development of the Human Dentition* by P. G. M. Van der Linden and H. S. Duterloo (Harper and Row, 1976). D. Permar's *Oral Embryology and Microscopic Anatomy* by R. C. Melfi (7th edn, Lea and Febiger, 1982) is an important text, while G. H. Sperber's *Craniofacial Embryology* (3rd edn, Wright, 1981) is a useful British book.

W. A. Nolte's *Oral Microbiology* (4th edn, Mosby, 1982) is a most detailed work on this subject, and a concise account is provided by T. H. Melville and C. Russell's *Microbiology for Dental Students* (3rd edn, Heinemann, 1981).

The growing significance of immunology is reflected by the publication of I. M. Roitt and T. Lehner's *Immunology of Oral Disease* (Blackwell, 1980) and of the briefer *Introduction to Oral Immunology* by A. E. Dolby, D. M. Walker and N. Matthews (Arnold, 1981).

Pathology and radiography

In pathology the most comprehensive work is *Thoma's Oral Pathology* edited by R. J. Gorlin and H. M. Goldman (6th edn, 2 vols, Mosby, 1970), while basic general texts are W. G. Shafer, M. K. Hine and B. M. Levy's *Textbook of Oral Pathology* (4th edn, Saunders, 1983) and J. B. Walter, M. C. Hamilton and M. S. Israel's *Principles of Pathology for Dental Students* (4th edn, Churchill Livingstone, 1981). J. J. Pindborg has written *Pathology of the Dental Hard Tissues* (Munksgaard, 1970), which deals with enamel lesions, and A. E. Dolby covers soft-tissue pathology in *Oral Mucosa in Health and Disease* (Blackwell, 1975). R. B. Lucas's *Pathology of Tumours of the Oral Tissues* (3rd edn, Churchill Livingstone, 1976) is a most authoritative work, giving accounts of neoplastic lesions with photographs and well chosen lists of references. The classification of tumours is expounded by texts in a series published by the World Health Organization: P. N. Wahi's *Histological Typing of Oral and Pharyngeal Tumours* (WHO, 1971) and *Histological Typing of Odontogenic Tumours, Jaw Cysts and Allied Lesions* by J. J. Pindborg and I. R. H. Kramer (WHO, 1971). There are good colour plates in *Colour Atlas of Oral Histopathology* by A. E. Marsland and R. M. Browne (HM&M, 1975). J. J. Pindborg discusses premalignant lesions in *Oral Cancer and Pre-cancer* (Wright, 1980).

There are a number of textbooks on dental radiography now available, a reputable work being A. H. Wuehrmann and C. R. Manson-Hing's *Dental Radiology* (5th edn, Mosby, 1981). For the student, *Dental Radiography* by N. J. D. Smith (Blackwell, 1980) is suitable, while practitioners will find R. Mason's *Guide to Dental Radiography* (2nd edn, Wright, 1982) a useful book. O. E. Langland, R. P. Langlais and C. R. Morris have produced an important work in a specialized field, *Principles and Practice of Panoramic Radiology* (Saunders, 1982).

Oral medicine, pharmacology

Authoritative works on oral medicine are J. J. Gayford and R. Haskell's *Clinical Oral Medicine* (2nd edn, Wright, 1979) and L. W. Burket's *Oral Medicine* edited by M. A. Lynch (7th edn, Lippincott, 1977). Clinical conditions are well illustrated in W. R. Tyldesley's *Colour Atlas of Oral Medicine* (Wolfe, 1978).

The dental implications of systemic disease are ably covered by C. Scully and R. A. Cawson in *Medical Problems in Dentistry* (Wright, 1982), while the wider significance of mouth lesions is discussed in *Oral Manifestations of Systemic Disease* by J. H. Jones and D. J. Mason (Saunders, 1980).

Drugs chargeable to the National Health Service which dentists may prescribe are listed in the *Dental Practitioners' Formulary 1982–84,* which is issued with the *British National Formulary No 4* (British Medical Association and Pharmaceutical Press, 1982). L. W. Kay gives an account of drugs in general in *Drugs in Dentistry* (2nd edn, Wright, 1972) and a full description is given by R. A. Cawson and R. G. Spector in *Clinical Pharmacology in Dentistry* (3rd edn, Churchill Livingstone, 1982).

Dental caries and preventive dentistry

L. M. Silverstone's *Dental Caries* (Macmillan, 1981) and E. Newbrun's *Cariology* (2nd edn, Williams and Wilkins, 1983) are general texts. The various means of using fluoride are described by J. J. Murray and A. J. Rugg-Gunn in *Fluorides in Dental Caries Prevention* (2nd edn, Wright, 1982) while the Royal College of Physicians' report *Fluoride, Teeth and Health* (Pitman Medical, 1976) endorses, after thorough investigation, the value of fluoride and its safety. E. Johansen, D. R. Taves and T. O. Olsen review the many studies published on fluorides in *Continuing Evaluation of the Use of Fluorides* (Westview Press, 1979).

J. O. Forrest's *Preventive Dentistry* (2nd edn, Wright, 1981) surveys the various methods available for the prevention of dental diseases, as also does R. E. Stallard in *A Textbook of Preventive Dentistry* (2nd edn, Saunders, 1982).

Restorative dentistry and endodontics

E. L. Hampson's *Textbook of Operative Dentistry* (4th edn, Heinemann, 1980) is a basic undergraduate book. F. J. Harty and D. H. Roberts have edited contributions from the staff of the Eastman Dental Hospital to produce *Restorative Procedures for the Practising Dentist* (Wright, 1974), an excellent text for the clinician. D. R. Kennedy's *Paediatric Operative Dentistry* (2nd edn, Wright, 1979) concentrates on the treatment of children. There are illustrations of operative procedures in J. R. Grundy's *Colour Atlas of Restorative Dentistry* (Wolfe, 1980).

In endodontics, L. I. Grossman's *Endodontic Practice* (10th edn, Lea and Febiger, 1981) is a standard work, but the most readable and practical book is F. J. Harty's *Endodontics in Clinical Practice* (2nd edn, Wright, 1982). For the reference library, there is the comprehensive *Endodontics* by J. I. Ingle and E. Beveridge (2nd edn, Lea and Febiger, 1976).

Occlusion and temporomandibular joint

The standard book on occlusion is P. E. Dawson's *Evaluation, Diagnosis and Treatment of Occlusal Problems* (Mosby, 1974). Other authoritative works are H. Thomson's *Occlusion in Clinical Practice* (Wright, 1981) and *Advances in Occlusion* by H. C. Lundeen and C. H. Gibbs (Wright, 1982).

An exhaustive text on the temporomandibular joint is *Temporomandibular Joint Function and Dysfunction* edited by G. A. Zarb and G. E. Carlsson (Munksgaard, 1979). A useful work is B. G. Sarnat and D. M. Laskin's *The Temporomandibular Joint* (3rd edn, C. C. Thomas, 1980), while H. D. Ogus and P. A. Toller's *Common Disorders of the Temporomandibular Joint* has the general practitioner's information needs in mind.

Oral surgery

An elementary text is J. R. Moore's *Principles of Oral Surgery* (3rd edn, Manchester University Press, 1982). The two-volume *Outline of Oral Surgery* by H. C. Killey and L. W. Kay is justly popular among clinicians (revised reprint, Wright, 1975) and N. L. Rowe and H. C. Killey's *Fractures of the Facial Skeleton* (2nd edn, Livingstone, 1968) is a classic work. For the reference collection or specialist surgeon, a comprehensive text is W. H. Bell, W. R. Proffit and R. P. White's *Surgical Correction of Jaw Deformities* (2 vols, Saunders, 1980).

Special aspects are discussed in T. J. Starshak and B. Saunders' *Preprosthetic Oral and Maxillofacial Surgery* (Mosby, 1980) and H. C. Killey and L. W. Kay's *Prevention of Complications in Dental Surgery* (2nd edn, Churchill Livingstone, 1977).

Anaesthesia

All methods used in dental practice are discussed in *Anaesthesia and Analgesia in Dentistry* by R. A. Green and M. P. Coplans (Lewis, 1973). P. Sykes has edited *Drummond-Jackson's Dental Anaesthesia and Sedation,* the standard work on intravenous anaesthesia. Good guides in local anaesthesia are *Local Analgesia in Dentistry* by G. L. Howe and F. I. H. Whitehead (2nd edn, Wright, 1981) and *Local Analgesia in Dentistry* by D. H. Roberts and J. H. Sowray (2nd edn, Wright, 1979). W. B. Jorgensen and J. Hayden's *Sedation, Local and General Anaesthesia* (3rd edn, Lea and Febiger, 1980) is useful for its presentation of the Jorgensen technique. The accepted work on conscious sedation is H. Langa's *Relative Analgesia in Dental Practice* (2nd edn, Saunders, 1976).

Periodontology

Essentials of Periodontology and Periodontics by T. MacPhee and G. Cowley (3rd edn, Blackwell, 1981) covers the topic for students and practitioners, as does J. D. Manson's *Periodontics* (3rd edn, Kimpton, 1980). There is more detail of techniques in H. M. Goldman and D. W. Cohen's *Periodontal Therapy* (6th edn, Mosby, 1980). Clinical conditions and therapy are illustrated in J. D. Strahan and I. M. Waite's *Colour Atlas of Periodontology* (Wolfe, 1978). M. J. Oringer's *Electrosurgery in Dentistry* (2nd edn, Saunders, 1975) remains the most useful book on this specialized technique.

Children's dentistry

There has recently been a spate of new, large books on this subject. Among the best are *Atlas of Pedodontics* by J. M. Davis, D. B. Law and T. M. Lewis (2nd edn, Saunders, 1981) and *Pedodontics: a Systematic Approach* by B. O. Magnussen (Munksgaard 1981). Standard, but more concise works, are P. J. Holloway and J. N. Swallow's *Child Dental Health* (3rd edn, Wright, 1982) and R. J. Andlaw and W. P. Rock's *Manual of Paedodontics* (Churchill Livingstone, 1982). R. Rapp and G. B. Winter have produced the excellent *Colour Atlas of Clinical Conditions in*

Paedodontics. The condition of children's teeth is surveyed in J. E. Todd's *Children's Dental Health in England and Wales, 1973* (HMSO, 1975). An important aspect of paedodontics is discussed in detail in J. O. Andreasen's *Traumatic Injuries of the Teeth* (2nd edn, Munksgaard, 1981) and more briefly in J. A. Hargreaves, J. W. Craig and H. L. Needleman's *Management of Traumatized Anterior Teeth of Children* (2nd edn, Churchill Livingstone, 1981).

Orthodontics

The most exhaustive work is that in two volumes by T. M. Graber and B. F. Swain, *Current Orthodontic Concepts and Techniques* (2nd edn, Saunders, 1975). Good British books are *A Textbook of Orthodontics* by T. D. Foster (2nd edn, Blackwell, 1982) and *Principles and Practice of Orthodontics* by J. R. E. Mills (Churchill Livingstone, 1982). The most detailed work on removable appliances is T. M. Graber and B. Neumann's *Removable Orthodontic Appliances* (Saunders, 1977), while a practical handbook is J. D. Muir and R. T. Reed's *Tooth Movement with Removable Appliances* (Pitman, 1979). A useful text for students and practitioners is *Introduction to Fixed Appliances* by K. G. Isaacson and J. K. Williams (2nd edn, Wright, 1978). Special techniques are discussed in R. C. Thurow's *Edgewise Orthodontics* (4th edn, Mosby, 1982), G. G. T. Fletcher's *The Begg Appliance and Technique* (Wright, 1981) and *Rapid Maxillary Expansion* by D. W. Timms (Quintessence, 1981).

Prosthetic dentistry, crown and bridgework

R. M. Basker, J. C. Davenport and H. R. Tomlin's *Prosthetic Treatment for the Edentulous Patient* (Macmillan, 1976) and *Partial Dentures* by J. Osborne and G. A. Lammie (4th edn, Blackwell, 1974) are standard British textbooks. The American viewpoint is given in C. O. Boucher's *Prosthetic Treatment for Edentulous Patients* (8th edn, Mosby, 1980) and W. L. McCracken's *Removable Partial Dentures* by D. Henderson and V. Steffel (6th edn, Mosby, 1981). Special types of prostheses are discussed in H. W. Preiskel's *Precision Attachments in Dentistry* (3rd edn, Kimpton, 1979), *Immediate and Replacement Dentures* by J. N. Anderson and R. Storer (3rd edn, Blackwell, 1981) and *Overdentures* by A. A. Brewer and R. M. Morrow (2nd edn, Mosby, 1980). Prostheses for cleft palate are discussed in *Maxillofacial Rehabilitation* by J. Beumer, T. A. Curtis and D. N. Firtell (Mosby, 1979).

A popular book on crown and bridgework is H. T. Shillingburg,

S. Hobo and D. Whitsett's *Fundamentals of Fixed Prosthodontics* (2nd edn, Quintessence, 1981), with D. H. Roberts' *Fixed Bridge Prostheses* (2nd edn, Wright, 1980) also being a standard work. Concise guidance is given in G. F. Kantorowicz's *Inlays, Crowns and Bridges* (3rd edn, Wright, 1979). A specialized book on porcelain and the associated techniques is J. W. McLean's *Science and Art of Dental Ceramics* (2 vols, Quintessence, 1979–1980).

Technical aspects are dealt with in two books by D. Stananought: *Laboratory Procedures for Inlays, Crowns and Bridges* (Blackwell, 1975) and *Laboratory Procedures for Full and Partial Dentures* (Blackwell, 1978).

Technology and materials

A standard British text is J. Osborne, H. J. Wilson and M. A. Mansfield's *Dental Technology and Materials for Students* (7th edn, Blackwell, 1979). N. Martinelli and S. C. Spinella's *Dental Laboratory Technology* (3rd edn, Mosby, 1981) is useful, despite its American bias.

Well-established textbooks dealing with both clinical and scientific aspects of materials are *Skinner's Science of Dental Materials* by R. W. Phillips (8th edn, Saunders, 1982) and *Restorative Dental Materials* edited by R. G. Craig (6th edn, Mosby, 1980). Briefer coverage is found in E. C. Combe's *Notes on Dental Materials* (3rd edn, Churchill Livingstone, 1977). The practical applications of specific materials are discussed in I. D. Gainsford's *Silver Amalgam in Clinical Practice* (3rd edn, Wright, 1976) and *Tooth Coloured Filling Materials in Clinical Practice* by L. W. Deubert and C. B. G. Jenkins (2nd edn, Wright, 1982). The American Dental Association's *Dentist's Desk Reference* (ADA, 1981) has much useful information.

Practice management, assistants

There has been a wealth of American books on this topic, but the most useful is H. C. Kilpatrick's *Work Simplification in Dental Practice* (3rd edn, Saunders, 1974). D. W. Crosthwaite has written the concise *Handbook of Dental Practice Management* (Churchill Livingstone, 1982), while J. E. Paul instructs on the best use of assistants in practice in his *Manual of Four Handed Dentistry* (Quintessence, 1980). There are several textbooks available for dental assistants, notably H. Levison's *Textbook for Dental Nurses* (5th edn, Blackwell, 1978) and S. Gelbier and M. A. H. Copley's *Handbook for Dental Surgery Assistants and Other Ancillary*

Workers (2nd edn, Wright, 1977).

J. E. Seear's *Law and Ethics in Dentistry* (2nd edn, Wright, 1981) is the standard book in its field. For foreign regulations and information about practice overseas the Fédération Dentaire Internationale (FDI) has published *Handbook of Regulations of Dental Practice* (2nd edn, FDI, 1976).

An excellent textbook on forensic dentistry is *Dental Identification and Forensic Odontology* by J. W. Harvey (Kimpton, 1976), while for an introductory text L. M. Cameron and B. G. Sim's *Forensic Dentistry* (Livingstone, 1974) is recommended.

For public health dentistry are recommended G. L. Slack's *Dental Public Health* (2nd edn, Wright, 1981) and J. M. Dunning's *Principles of Dental Public Health* (3rd edn, Harvard University Press, 1979). The findings of the national dental survey in England and Wales in 1978 appear in *Adult Dental Health* by J. E. Todd and A. M. Walker (HMSO, 2 vols, 1980, 1982), while the most recent for Scotland is *Adult Dental Health in Scotland 1972* by J. E. Todd and A. Whitworth (HMSO, 1974). The children's dental health survey has already been mentioned.

Indexes and abstracts

Index Medicus, although it includes the leading dental periodicals, is not the chief tool to be used in searching the literature for dental subjects. The *Index to Dental Literature* is similar in format, although it appears in quarterly instead of monthly parts, each cumulating with the previous issues for the year until the bound annual volume appears. The creation of the *Index* began in 1898 as the brain-child of Arthur Black, who worked retrospectively back to 1839, when the first regular dental journal made its debut. The *Index* covered five-year periods up to 1950, when the first annual volume was published; its subject arrangement was at first based on the Dewey Classification with an author index. An outline of and an index to the classification is printed on the centre pages. In 1939 the classified arrangement was abandoned in favour of author and subject entries published in one alphabetical sequence, but they separated once again in 1965 when the MEDLARS production methods of the National Library of Medicine were adopted. In addition to periodical publications, the *Index* now lists dental dissertations and theses, and also new dental books.

The principal abstracting journal in dentistry is *Dental Abstracts,* published monthly by the American Dental Association. Some 200 journals are covered, with dental titles from the US predominating, but with occasional excursions into medical and scientific periodicals and lay journalism. There are about 25 subject headings, each with four or five abstracts every month, and an annual index of authors and subjects. *Oral Research Abstracts,* which ceased publication in 1978, included about 7000 abstracts each year. It gave a more comprehensive coverage of research publications from a considerably wider range of sources, being particularly valuable for abstracts of foreign-language papers.

The *Year Book of Dentistry* (Year Book Medical Publishing) appears annually, giving a retrospective review of some 200 articles, one-third from non-American sources, under about 20 headings. The abstracts are signed and include brief comments by the abstractors, with illustrations, diagrams and tables reproduced from the original papers.

The *Journal of the Western Society of Periodontology Periodontal Abstracts* (US, quarterly) devotes about half the pages of each issue to a critical appraisal of the literature of one special subject, the rest comprising abstracts of articles in the specialty, grouped under various headings.

Until 1962, when foreign-language articles first began to be included, only articles in English were cited in the *Index to Dental Literature.* Articles published after 1934 in foreign journals may sometimes be traced in the bibliographical half of *Deutsche Zahn-, Mund- und Kieferheilkunde,* which still gives short abstracts of papers from the world's dental literature in subject groupings, with author and subject indexes. Foreign-language articles published between 1925 and 1933 may be traced in *Fortschritte der Zahnheilkunde,* which has a similar arrangement, and those published between 1902 and 1932 in *Index der Deutschen und Ausländischen Literatur,* which lists articles under authors in broad subject groups and has author and subject indexes but no abstracts. The 1902 volume notes articles published since 1847.

Reviews

Oral Sciences Reviews, published in Copenhagen by Munksgaard, is a series of 10 volumes published during the years 1972 to 1977. Each volume is devoted to a particular topic, and provides comprehensive analytical review articles, with extensive bibliographies, by leading authorities in each field. The *Dental Clinics of North America* (US, quarterly) may be regarded as a review journal, since it reports on current theories and practice, publishing 'state of the art' papers rather than original research. *Advances in*

Oral Surgery (Mosby) has appeared at three-year intervals, since 1974. The first two volumes are general in coverage, the third (1980) being devoted to problems of the temporomandibular joint.

Conferences

The International Dental Congresses, once separately published, have not appeared since 1936 in book form. The *International Dental Journal* now publishes selected proceedings of the Fédération Dentaire Internationale annual congress.

ORCA, the European Organisation for Research on Fluoride and Dental Caries Prevention published the proceedings of its 9th (1962) to 12th (1965) congresses as separate volumes, entitled *Advances in Fluoride Research and Dental Caries Prevention* (Pergamon). Latterly, the ORCA congresses have been reported as abstracts in the journal *Caries Research*.

The International Association of Dental Research annual meetings are abstracted in special issues of the *Journal of Dental Research*.

The 2nd (1965), 3rd (1968) and 4th (1971) congresses of the International Association of Oral Surgeons have been published as monographs (Munksgaard, 1967, Livingstone, 1970, Munksgaard, 1973), but the 5th (1974), 6th (1978) and 7th (1980) appeared as issues of the *International Journal of Oral Surgery*.

The 2nd to 5th International Conferences on Endodontics have been printed (University of Pennsylvania, 1958, 1963, 1968 and 1973), the 6th appearing as a monograph entitled *Mechanism and Control of Pain* edited by L. I. Grossman (Masson, 1979).

Bibliographies

Subject bibliographies

There has been a trend away from published bibliographies, but those compiled some while ago are, nevertheless, still valuable today. Two useful bibliographies on caries are by G. Toverud *et al. A Survey of the Literature of Dental Caries* (US National Research Council, 1952) and its update by J. F. Brislin and G. J. Cox, *Survey of the Literature of Dental Caries 1948–1960* University of Pittsburgh Press, 1964).

A. R. Catron and F. G. Evans have compiled a *Bibliography on the Mechanical and Physical Properties of the Teeth* (University of

Michigan, 1970). *Social Sciences and Dentistry, a Critical Bibliography* edited by N. D. Richards and L. K. Cohen (FDI, 1971) gives critical reviews of the international research literature for the years 1955 to 1970 in dentistry's social science aspects. Each chapter concludes with an impressive list of references. An author index would have enhanced the value of this work as a reference book.

Bibliographies: dental books

There are several useful works for identifying dental writings of historical interest. B. W. Weinberger compiled his *Dental Bibliography* (Part I, 1929; Part II, 1932) from his own library and that of the New York Academy of Medicine. Books, monographs, theses and reprints are in alphabetical order of authors and Part II has a subject index to both bibliographies. Part I lists dental periodicals by geographical subdivision as well as noting medical classics containing references to dentistry, while in Part II is found a list of dental books published between 1530 and 1810. Weinberger claimed to have included every important dental work to have been published and, although there are omissions, his work is highly regarded.

C. G. Crowley's *Dental Bibliography* (S. S. White Co, 1885) was a pioneer effort in comprehensiveness, listing dental books published from 1536 to 1885, chronologically arranged in five geographical groups.

A *Dental Bibliography* by J. Menzies Campbell (David Low, 1949), lists British and American dental books and pamphlets published between 1682 and 1880 in a chronological arrangement with an author index; it is widely used by collectors and historians. The *Catalogue of the J. Menzies Campbell Collection Presented to the Royal College of Surgeons of England* (RCS, 1970) lists pre-1860 books alphabetically by author.

H. L. Strömgren's *Index of Dental and Adjacent Topics in Medical and Surgical Works before 1800* (Munksgaard, 1955) is arranged in two sections, the first alphabetically by author, the second by subjects. In the author section annotations indicate the references of dental importance.

Current books are listed in a preliminary section of the *Index to Dental Literature*.

Dictionaries

There are three dictionaries of dental terminology available. The

Heinemann Modern Dictionary for Dental Students compiled by J. E. H. Fairpo and C. G. Fairpo (2nd edn, Heinemann, 1973) is an essential reference work for all British professionals, from surgery assistant to practising dentist. C. O. Boucher's *Clinical Dental Terminology* edited by T. J. Zwemer (3rd edn, Mosby, 1982) has longer explanations, but lists many words not of clinical relevance. S. Jablonski's *Illustrated Dictionary of Dentistry* (Saunders, 1982) includes many medical terms, also trade names and biographical entries, and gives more detail for dental entries than Boucher.

The British Standards Institution has issued a *Glossary of Terms Related to Dentistry* (BS 4492: 1983) listing terms and definitions for nine subdivisions of dentistry. Some terms are described as 'deprecated' where their use is considered undesirable.

English–foreign-language dictionaries are almost non-existent, but the FDI's *Lexicon of Dental Terms with their Equivalents in Español, Deutsch, Français, Italiano* (Sijthoff, 1966) is invaluable to the translator. A good English–German dictionary, *Dental Wörterbuch* compiled by H. Bucksch (Verlag Neuer Merkur, 1970), has filled one of the gaps in this field.

Miscellaneous reference works

The *Dentists Register* (General Dental Council, annual) lists all registered dental practitioners' and gives names, addresses, date of registration and qualifications. Similar lists exist for most developed countries; some, such as the American, provide considerable information. There is no dental equivalent to the *Medical Directory*.

The *Dental Laboratory Yearbook and Directory* (Morgan) gives much technical information. Particularly useful are the sections listing trade names, equipment or materials, manufacturers and suppliers. The *FDI Basic Fact Sheets* (FDI, 1981) give information about dentistry in 79 countries, with particular reference to manpower, education and licensure, surveys of oral and dental conditions, practice and fluoridation. WHO published a *World Directory of Dental Schools, 1963* (WHO, 1967) which gives particulars of dental education, curricula, examinations and qualifications. A complementary title is their *World Directory of Schools for Dental Auxiliaries, 1973,* (WHO, 1977).

History and biography

The classic text on history, although it stops at the end of the eighteenth century, is *A History of Dentistry* by V. Guerini (Lea and Febiger, 1909), a work of great accuracy and careful scholarship. The briefest accurate book on this subject is L. Lindsay's *Short History of Dentistry* (Bale, 1933). *A History of Dentistry* by A. W. Lufkin (2nd edn, Kimpton, 1948) gives a more detailed account which includes the history of dental anaesthesia. It tends to stress the contributions of America, as does B. W. Weinberger's two-volume work, *An Introduction to the History of Dentistry in America* (Mosby, 1948). An excellent text, with more emphasis on European developments and many illustrations, is W. Hoffman-Axthelm's *History of Dentistry* (Quintessence, 1981). H. Prinz's *Dental Chronology* (Kimpton, 1945) gives notes on persons and developments from ancient times to the mid-twentieth century. An important book for the study of British dental history is A. Hill's *The History of the Reform Movement in the Dental Profession in Great Britain during the last Twenty Years* (Trübner, 1877). The *Jubilee Book of the British Dental Association* (Bale, 1930) presents a chronological description of the BDA's achievements between 1880 and 1930, a period of immense importance in the profession's development, while its 100th anniversary saw the publication of *The Advance of the Dental Profession: A Centenary History, 1880–1980* (BDA, 1979). International aspects of the growth of dentistry are traced in *The Story of the Fédération Dentaire Internationale, 1900–1962* by J. Ennis (FDI, 1967) and, more briefly, by G. H. Leatherman in *The FDI – 1900–1980 (Quintessence, 1981). The History of the Royal Army Dental Corps* has been edited by L. J. Godden (RADC, 1971).

Two pictorial books of great interest are *The Dentist in Art* by J. J. Pindborg and L. Marvitz (Munksgaard, 1960), which depicts works of art with dental features, and *A Pictorial History of Dentistry* by C. Proskauer and F. H. Witt (Dumont Schauberg, 1962), which uses contemporary art to illustrate dental developments.

Sir Frank Colyer's *Old Instruments Used for Extracting Teeth* (Staples, 1952) is a well-illustrated and accurate work of great value to students of historical instruments. B. W. Weinberger's two-volume *Orthodontics: An Historical Review of its Origin and Evolution* (Mosby, 1926) covers this specialized subject up to 1870, but with some errors. *The Strange Story of False Teeth* by J. Woodforde (Routledge and Kegan Paul, 1968) gives an exact and entertaining history of prosthetic dentistry.

Biographical works of a dental nature are scarce. The supreme example is Sir Zachary Cope's *Sir John Tomes: A Pioneer of British Dentistry* (Dawson, 1961). J. Menzies Campbell's *Dentistry Then and Now* (3rd edn, privately printed, 1981), a revision of his

From a Trade to a Profession (privately printed, 1958), opens with
a description of the author's experience of 50 years of dental practice and continues with a fascinating miscellany of historical topics.

Conclusion

Despite the growth of specialization in the different fields of dentistry, its interactions with other medical and scientific disciplines
are many. Although not discussed here, these links must be
remembered and sources in other relevant areas should be used
when appropriate.

22

Historical, biographical and bibliographical sources

E. Gaskell*; revised by E. J. Freeman

History

There is obviously little hope of compressing a complete or even reasonably comprehensive survey of writing on the history of medicine into the space of a single chapter. All that is attempted here is to provide the neophyte, and particularly the amateur historian, with a bibliographical *entrée* to a fast-growing subject.

The major historiographical development in the subject since the last edition of this guide has been the increasing strength of the social history approach to medicine's past. This now dominant trend has largely resulted from the entry of academic historians and social scientists into the field. The work of these new professionals is, to a large extent, displacing the traditional monopoly of amateur historians usually trained in medicine and science.

No-one has yet produced a generally acceptable definition of what is, precisely, the social history of medicine. The product is easier to recognize than to describe. Its chief marks are the assumption that medicine is always relative to the society or culture that produces it. Further, that both medicine and society are best described in terms of patterns and structures which can be related to each other. Above all, the medicine of the past must not be described in categories derived exclusively from the science of the present day. 'History in context' is the basic slogan of the social historian of medicine. At its worst a verbal fashion (the 'constipation

* Formerly Librarian, Wellcome Institute for the History of Medicine

463

and society' mode, as one recent writer put it), the social history of medicine more usually sins by promising more than it can deliver. In the hands of its finest practitioners, however, the social approach to medical history can be an illuminating and exciting entry to the medicine of the past.

It has to be said that the standard source books for the history of medicine, such as Garrison and Morton's *Medical Bibliography* (4th edn, Gower Pub. Co., 1983) and Blake and Roos' *Medical Reference Works, 1679–1966* (MLA, 1967), *Supplement 1, 1967–68* compiled by M. V. Clarke (1970); *Supplement 2, 1969–72* and *Supplement 3,* 1973–74 both compiled by J. S. Richmond, do not as yet reflect the emphases of the social history of medicine in their selection of either primary or secondary sources. The student must take into account the bibliographies of general history and the social sciences in order to ensure contact with the latest and best work. (*See also* sections on Bibliography and Indexes below.)

General

Single-author general histories of medicine are now rare, the exceptions occasionally coming from continental Europe and, perhaps, reflecting the existence of large captive audiences of medical students. Professionalization has inevitably produced specialization and modern medical historians do not care to attempt single-handed the grand general syntheses of their forebears. The older English-language one-volume histories are now best avoided. The student needing a general introduction is better served by histories of science, such as S. F. Mason's *A History of the Sciences* (revised edn, Abelard-Schuman, 1962) or A. C. Crombie's *Augustine to Galileo,* last printed in a one-volume edition (Heinemann, 1979). Not a comprehensive history, W. P. D. Wightman's *The Emergence of Scientific Medicine* (Oliver and Boyd, 1971) is a trim, paperback masterpiece which traces the evolution of medical concepts from classical times to the seventeenth century. Written without a trace of condescension towards outmoded ideas, this book desperately needs reprinting. P. T. Durbin has edited *A Guide to the Culture of Science, Technology and Medicine* (Free Press, 1980), an invaluable introduction to current historical ideas supported by good bibliographies. Chapter 3 is on the history of medicine. An unusual approach is reflected in H. L. Coulter's *Divided Legacy: a History of the Schism in Medical Thought,* (3 vols, Wehawken Book Co., 1973–1977). The author maintains that 'medical thinkers in western culture may be divided into two traditions – those who attribute primary importance to the sensory data of experience being opposed to those who seek the reality assumed to lie behind the sensory data'. Readers of European languages should consider (in German) C. Lichtenthaeler's *Geschichte der Medizin* (2 vols, Deutscher Ärzte-Verlag, 1977), available also in French (A. Fayard, 1978); E. Fischer-Homberger's *Geschichte der Medizin,* (2nd edn, Springer, 1977); E. H. Ackerknecht's *Geschichte der Medizin* (4th edn, Enke, 1979); (in Italian) V. Busacchi's *Storia della Medicina* (2nd edn, Patron, 1978); A. Pazzini's *Storia dell' Arte Sanitaria dalle Origini a Oggi* (2 vols, Ed. Minerva Medica, 1973).

New varieties of history proliferate. J. Barzun's *Clio and the Doctors: Psycho-history, Quanto-history and History* (Chicago University Press, 1974) is an interesting survey. L. Demause has edited a collection of essays on a particularly controversial type of historical investigation, *The New Psychohistory* (Psycho-history Press, 1975).

Collections of essays can be suggestive alternatives to chronological surveys. An example is *The Double Face of Janus and Other Essays in the History of Medicine* (Johns Hopkins, 1977) by the doyen of medical historians, Owsei Temkin.

The gap left by the demise of one-volume histories has been filled, paradoxically, by multi-volumed, many-authored histories, affordable only by libraries and of value chiefly for their often magnificent illustrations. Recent examples are *Historia Universal de la Medicina* edited by P. Lain Entralgo (7 vols, Salvat, 1972–1975) and *Histoire de la Médecine, de la Pharmacie, de l'Art Dentaire, et de l'Art Vétérinaire* by J. C. Sournia *et al.* (A. Michel, etc., 1978), available also in German (8 vols, plus index vol, Andreas, 1980); and A. S. Lyons and R. J. Petrucelli's *Medicine: an Illustrated History* (Abrams, 1980).

Period histories

PREHISTORY

Diseases in Antiquity by D. Brothwell and A. T. Sandison (C. C. Thomas, 1967) may now be supplemented by D. Brothwell's *Digging up Bones. The Excavation, Treatment and Study of Human Skeletal Remains* (2nd edn, B. M. Nat. Hist., 1972). *Human Palaeopathology* by S. Jarcho (Yale University Press 1966) is the proceedings of a symposium and the findings described are mostly from digs in the US. *Bones, Bodies and Disease* by C. Wells (Thames and Hudson, 1964) comprises essays on different types of abnormalities, cannibalism, vital statistics, etc. *History of Medicine vol 1, Primitive and Archaic Medicine* by H. E. Sigerist (Oxford University Press, 1951) is still useful but needs supplementing by later work, such as *Mummies, Disease and Ancient Cultures* by A. and E. Cockburn (Cambridge University Press, 1980) and L. R. Binford's *Bones: Ancient Men and Modern Myths* (Academic Press, 1981).

ANCIENT

F. Köcher's *Die babylonisch–assyrische Medizin in Texten und Untersuchungen* (W. de Gruyter, 1963–) is a continuing series (6 vols to date, 1980), with reproductions of texts and commentary. A. P. Leca's *La Médecine Egyptienne au Temps des Pharaons* (R. Dacosta, 1971) is an attractively produced book as, on similar topics, is P. Ghaliounghi's *The House of Life. Magic and Medical Science in Ancient Egypt* (2nd edn, B. M. Israël, 1973). H. E. Sigerist's *History of Medicine, vol 2, Early Greek, Hindu and Persian Medicine* (Oxford University Press, 1961) encroaches on the classical period as do H. Peters' *Die Arzt und die Heilkunst in alten Zeiten* (4th edn, E. Diederichs, 1973) and G. Majno's *The Healing Hand: Man and Wound in the Ancient World* (Harvard University Press, 1975), an extraordinary *tour de force* by an eminent American surgeon.

CLASSICAL

Fine general introductions to Greek science and medicine are G. R. Lloyd's two volumes, *Early Greek Science: Thales to Hippocrates* (Chatto and Windus, 1970) and *Greek Science after Aristotle* (Chatto and Windus, 1972) which are supplemented by his later volume *Magic, Reason and Experience: Studies in the Origin and Development of Greek Science* (Cambridge University Press, 1979). Older but still indispensable is L. Edelstein's *Ancient Medicine* (Johns Hopkins, 1967), comprising collected essays by a profoundly learned man, now dead. Also useful is F. Kudlien's *Der Beginn des medizinischen Denkens bei den Griechen von Homer bis Hippokrates* (Artemis, 1967), which has a short appendix of texts. H. Flashar's *Antike Medizin* (Wissenschaftliche Buchgesellschaft, 1971) is a useful collection of reprinted papers by O. Temkin *et al.* J. Scarborough's *Roman Medicine* (Thames and Hudson, 1969) is the only general book on its subject in English, but should be used with caution. E. D. Phillips' *Greek Medicine* (Thames and Hudson, 1973) concentrates on the Hippocratic corpus to the neglect of Galen, but M. Tallmadge May's translation of Galen's *De usu Partum* (2 vols, Cornell University Press, 1968) has an excellent introduction on Greco-Roman anatomy and physiology. Recent scholarly work on Galen may be sampled in *Galen: Problems and Prospects* edited by V. Nutton (W.I.H.M, 1981), which comprises conference proceedings. The pervasive influence of classical medicine in later times can be studied in O. Temkin's *Galenism: Rise and Decline of a Medical Philosophy* (Cornell University Press, 1973) and W. D. Smith's *The Hippocratic Tradition* (Cornell University Press, 1979).

MEDIEVAL

In spite of the fact that George Sarton loathed everything characteristically medieval his *Introduction to the History of Science* (3 vols in 5, Williams and Wilkins, 1927–1948) is now, and is likely to remain, the basic, indispensable bibliographic guide to the period. The general histories in English all have their failings, the most general of which is an understandable reliance on British materials. The best are still C. H. Talbot's *Medicine in Medieval England* (Oldbourne, 1967) and S. Rubin's *Medieval English Medicine* (David and Charles, 1974). E. J. Keeley's *Medieval Medicus. A Social History of Anglo-Norman Medicine* (Johns Hopkins, 1981) is an attractively written book, marred by the author's use of anachronistic expressions. Two profoundly learned works are by B. Lawn, *Salernitan Questions* (Clarendon Press, 1963) and *The Prose Salernitan Questions* (Oxford University Press, 1979), which are brilliant analyses of medical disputations. Special topics are handled by S. N. Brody's *The Disease of the Soul: Leprosy in Medieval Literature* (Cornell University Press 1974) and P. Richards' *The Medieval Leper and his Northern Heirs* (D. S. Brewer, 1977). The standard work on plague, medieval and later, is J. N. Biraben's *Les Hommes et la Peste en France et dans les Pays Européens et Méditerranéans,* (2 vols, Mouton, 1975). The effect of the plague on British history may be studied with the help of J. Hatcher's *Plague, Population and the English Economy, 1348–1530* (Macmillan, 1977) and R. S. Gottfried's *Epidemic Disease in 15th Century England* (Leicester University Press, 1978). A fine study of a late medieval medical teacher is N. G. Siraisi's *Taddeo Alderotti and his Pupils* (Princeton University Press, 1981). Finally, the important topic of Arabic medicine is best studied in E. G. Browne's *Arabian Medicine* (Cambridge University Press, 1921, reprinted 1962), which is now rather old-fashioned, and M. Ullmann's *Islamic Medicine* (Edinburgh University Press, 1978).

RENAISSANCE TO THE EIGHTEENTH CENTURY

A useful taste of current scholarly research is offered by *Health,*

Medicine and Mortality in the 16th century edited by C. Webster (Cambridge University Press, 1979). J. O'Hara May's *Elizabethan Dyetary of Health* (Coronado Press, 1977) is a survey of ideas on regimen in health and sickness. A. G. Debus' *The Chemical Philosophy. Paracelsian Science and Medicine in the 16th and 17th Centuries* (2 vols, Neale Watson, 1977) offers a view of an important anti-Galenic movement. Anything by Walter Pagel is worth reading, although rarely easy going, e.g. his *Paracelsus: an Introduction to Philosophical Medicine in the Era of the Renaissance* (Karger, 1958) or his *William Harvey's Biological Ideas: Selected Aspects and Historical Background* (Karger, 1967). The latter study may be supplemented by a collection of essays edited by J. J. Bylebyl in *William Harvey and his Age* (Johns Hopkins, 1979). C. Webster's *The Great Instauration: Science, Medicine and Reform, 1626–1660* (Duckworth, 1975) is a good, though densely written, example of 'history in context' by the Reader in the History of Medicine of the University of Oxford. L. S. King's books are essential reading for students of eighteenth-century medicine, although there are clear signs of a swing away from his ideas and emphases. His *The Road to Medical Enlightenment, 1650–1695* (Macdonald, 1970) examines the transition from Galenism to iatrochemistry and iatrophysics, whereas *The Medical World of the 18th Century* (Chicago University Press, 1958, reprinted by Krieger, 1971) and *The Philosophy of Medicine: the Early 18th Century* (Harvard University Press, 1978) both develop King's ideas on the eighteenth century.

Foreign influences may be studied in E. A. Underwood's *Boerhaave's Men at Leyden and After* (Edinburgh University Press, 1977). L. Clarkson's *Death, Disease and Famine in Pre-industrial England* (Gill and Macmillan, 1975) attempts to place medicine in a wider social and economic context.

NINETEENTH AND TWENTIETH CENTURIES

Many general studies of the last two centuries draw their evidence from the histories of particular countries, so this section should be read in conjunction with those immediately following. Begin with the essays edited by C. Webster in *Biology, Medicine and Society, 1840–1940* (Cambridge University Press 1981). F. N. L. Poynter's *Medicine and Man* (C A. Watts, 1971) is 'a discussion of contemporary problems illuminated by references to some of their historical origins' and *Der Arzt und der Kranke in der Gesellschaft des 19. Jahrhunderts* edited by W. Artelt and W. Rüegg (F. Enke, 1967) records symposium proceedings, including articles documented from English, German and Russian novels.

Most of the following references draw their evidence from British or American sources:

Doctors and the State: the British Medical Profession and Government Action in Public Health, 1870–1912 by J. L. Brand (Johns Hopkins, 1965)

Health Care and Popular Medicine in 19th Century England edited by J. Woodward and D. Richards (Croom Helm, 1977) is a not entirely successful attempt to exemplify the social history approach

Half a Century of Medical Research by Sir A. L. Thomson (2 vols, HMSO, 1973, 1975) deals with the role of government funded research in terms of the history of the Medical Research Council

Antivivisection and Medical Science in Victorian Society by R. D. French (Princeton University Press, 1975)

The Division in British Medicine. A History of the Separation of General Practice from Hospital Care, 1911–68 by F. Honigsbaum (Kogan Page, 1979)

Profession and Monopoly: a Study of Medicine in the United States and Great Britain by J. L. Berlant (University of California Press, 1975)

The Return of the Plague: British Society and Cholera 1831–32 by M. Durey (Gill and Macmillan, 1979)

The Scientific Revolution in Victorian Medicine by A. J. Youngson (Croom Helm, 1979)

The People's Health 1830–1910 by F. B. Smith (Croom Helm, 1979) is a controversial but stimulating study notable for its 'anti-doctor' emphasis

By country and region

GREAT BRITAIN

The proceedings of symposia held by the British Society for the History of Medicine (Pitman, 1962–1971) include volumes on Cambridge, the Commonwealth, pharmacy, hospitals, and education. They are all now a little dated and should be used with caution. Sir George Clark's *History of the Royal College of Physicians* (3 vols, Clarendon Press, 1964–1972) is a gracefully written study of an influential British institution by a professional historian, and covers the period 1518 to 1948 (vol 3 is by A. M. Cooke). F. F. Cartwright's *A Social History of Medicine* (Longmans, 1977) is especially useful for students if its publishers will keep it in print. J. Cule's *A Doctor for the People. 2000 Years of General Practice in Britain* (Update Books, 1980) is an attractively written and illustrated account for the general reader. Two books chosen to demonstrate the importance of regional studies are D. Hamilton's *The Healers: a History of Medicine in Scotland* (Canongate, 1981) and *Wales and Medicine. An Historical Survey* edited by J. Cule (J. D. Lewis, 1975) contains papers given at the 9th British Congress on the History of Medicine held at Swansea and Cardiff in 1973.

US

Public Health in the Town of Boston, 1630–1822 by J. B. Blake (Harvard University Press, 1959)

Medicine and Society in America, 1660–1860 by R. H. Shryock (New York University Press, 1960)

American Medicine and the Public Interest by R. Stevens (Yale University Press, 1971), studies the effects of specialization and government medical care in the twentieth century

Medicine in New England 1790–1840 by B. Riznik (Old Sturbridge Inc, 1969)

Medical Men at the Siege of Boston, April 1775–April 1776: Problems of the Massachusetts and Continental Armies by P. Cash (American Philosophical Society, 1973)

Theory and Practice in American Medicine edited by G. H. Brieger (Science History Publications, 1976)

Two Centuries of American Medicine (1776–1976) by J. Bordley and A. M. Harvey (W. B. Saunders, 1976)

Advances in American Medicine: Essays at the Bicentennial edited by J. Z. Bowers and E. F. Purcell (2 vols, J. Macy, 1976)

Adventures in Medical Research: a Century of Discovery at Johns Hopkins by A. M. Harvey (Johns Hopkins, 1976)

The Healers: the Rise of American Medicine by J. Duffy (McGraw Hill, 1976)

The Therapeutic Revolution. Essays in the Social History of American Medicine edited by M. J. Vogel and Charles E. Rosenberg (University of Pennsylvania Press, 1979)

EUROPE

E. H. Ackerknecht's *Medicine at the Paris Hospital, 1794–1848* (Johns Hopkins, 1967) is on the rise of clinical medicine in Europe. *Medicine and Society in France* edited by R. Forster and O. Ranum (Johns Hopkins, 1980) contains translated essays from the famous French history journal *'Annales'*. Other titles are:

Histoire de la Médecine Belge by F. A. Sondervorst (Elsevier Librico, 1981)

Medical Revolution in France 1789–1796 by D. M. Vess (University Press of Florida, 1975)

Geschichte der medizinischen Wissenschaften in Deutschland by A. Hirsch was published as long ago as 1893, but reprinted by Johnson Reprint Corp., New York, 1966, and is a still useful and detailed history of the eighteenth and nineteenth centuries, with a brief review of earlier periods

The Vienna Medical School of the 19th Century by E. Lesky (translated by L. Williams and I. S. Levij, Johns Hopkins, 1976)

Historia Social de la Medicina en la España de los Siglos XIII el XVI, vol 1, La Minoría Musulmana y Morisca by L. Garcia Ballester (Akal, 1976)

Storia della Medicina Italiana by S. de Renzi (5 vols, Forni, 1966, reprinted from the original 1845–1848 edn)

AFRICA

Work on the pre-colonial, as well as the European-influenced, medical history of Africa is a growth industry:

Religion and Healing in Mandari by J. Buxton (Clarendon Press, 1973)

A Service to the Sick. A History of the Health Services for Africans in Southern Rhodesia, 1890–1953 by M. Gelfand (Mambo Press, 1976)

Body and Soul in Zulu medicine by H. Ngubane (Academic Press, 1977)

African Folk Medicine. Practices and Beliefs of the Bambara and Other Peoples by
P. J. Imperato (York Press, 1977)
Disease in African History. An Introductory Survey and Case Studies edited by G.
W. Martwig and K. D. Patterson (Duke University Press, 1978)
Pestilence and Disease in the History of Africa by J. N. P. Davies (Witwatersrand
University Press, 1979)

ORIENT

For Arabic medicine reference should be made to the titles listed
under the Medieval period above, supplemented by S. H. Nasr's
Islamic Science – an Illustrated Study (World of Islam, 1976),
which, along with other studies by the same author, presents an
interesting though controversial view of traditional Arabic medicine through the eyes of a prominent modern Islamic thinker.
Cyril Elgood's *Safavid Medical Practice* (Luzac, 1970) covers
medicine, surgery and gynaecology in Persia from 1500 AD to
1750 AD. D. Brandenburg's *Priesterärzte und Heilkunst im alten
Persien* (J. Fink, 1969) discusses medicine in the writings of Zara-
thustra and Firdausi, while vol 2, Part 2 of C. A. Storey's *Persian
Literature: a Bibliographical Survey* (Royal Asiatic Soc.,
1958–1971) is basic for the serious student.

For China P. Huard and Ming Wong's *Chinese Medicine* (World
University Library, 1968), translated from the French, emphasizes
the continuity of Chinese medicine down to modern times. R. C.
Crozier's *Traditional Medicine in Modern China* (Harvard University Press, 1968) looks at the relationship of medicine to cultural
and intellectual developments in China since 1800. Joseph
Needham's *Clerks and Craftsmen in China and the West* (Cambridge University Press, 1970) includes essays on protoendocrino-
logy in medieval China, elixir poisoning, hygiene and examinations. Needham's *Science and Civilization in China* (5 vols, Cambridge University Press, 1954–) is a definitive account by a brilliant
scientist and scholar leading a team of Chinese experts. *Modern
China and Traditional Chinese Medicine* edited by G. B. Risse (C.
C. Thomas, 1973) and *Medicine and Society in China* edited by J.
Z. Bowers and E. F. Purcell (J. Macy jnr. Fnd., 1974) are collections of essays with complementary emphases.

Japanese medicine is described in M. Wong, P. Huard and Z.
Ohya's *La Médecine Japonais des Origines à nos Jours* (R.
Dacosta, 1974).

Much writing on traditional Indian medicine is of disappoint-
ingly poor quality. J. Jolly's *Indian Medicine*, translated from the
original German and supplemented by C. G. Kashikar (2nd
revised edn, Munshiram Marshareal, 1977), although an old

book, is still one of the best accounts. O. P. Jaggi's *History of Science and Technology in India* (13 vols to date, Atma Ram, 1973–) will be the most extensive modern account, when complete.

Tibetan medicine is best studied in E. Finckh's *Foundations of Tibetan Medicine* (vol 1, Watkins, 1978) – second volume is at press.

Doubtfully part of the Orient, but indubitably there and important, is Australia. E. Fordis' *Bibliography of Australian Medicine, 1790–1900* (Sydney University Press, 1976) is the starting point for study.

Nursing

The history of nursing, as that of hospitals (*see* below), is cursed with dull narrative and anecdotal accounts. Two older works are worth consulting: M. A. Nutting and L. Dock's *A History of Nursing* (4 vols, (G. P. Putnam's Sons, 1907–1912) and I. M. Stewart and A. L. Austin's *History of Nursing* (5th edn, G. P. Putnam, 1962). Also useful is V. and B. Bullough's *The Care of the Sick: the Emergence of Modern Nursing* (Croom Helm, 1979). A. M. C. Thompson's *Bibliography of Nursing Literature, 1859–1960* (L. A., 1968; Supplement 1961–70, 1974) has sections on history and biography, and is supplemented by the quarterly bibliographies on nursing in general issued by the Royal College of Nursing. B. Ehrenreich and D. English's *Witches, Midwives and Nurses: a History of Women Healers* (Feminist Press, 1973) presents another side of nursing history. G. L. Deloughery's *History and Trends of Professional Nursing* has now achieved its 8th edn, (C. V. Mosby, 1977). R. White's *Social Change and the Development of the Nursing Profession. A Study of the Poor Law Nursing Service, 1848–1948* (H. Kimpton, 1978) and the volume of essays edited by C. Davies, *Rewriting Nursing History* (Croom Helm, 1980), in their different ways blow a fresh breeze into a musty corner of medical history.

Hospitals

The Evolution of Hospitals in Britain edited by F. N. L. Poynter (Pitman, 1964) includes a comprehensive bibliography of secondary works by E. Gaskell. B. Abel-Smith's *The Hospitals, 1880–1948* (Heinemann, 1964) has, as a companion volume, R. Pinker's *English Hospital Statistics* (Heinemann, 1966). G. M. Ayers' *England's First State Hospitals . . . 1867–1930* (WIHM,

1971) is massively documented. J. D. Thompson and G. Goldin's *The Hospital: a Social and Architectural History* (Yale University Press, 1975) is perhaps the best and most certainly the most beautifully illustrated general account, although D. Jetter's *Geschichte des Hospitals* (4 vols to date, F. Steiner, 1966–1980) is becoming the standard European history. J. Woodward's *To do the Sick no Harm. A Study of the British Voluntary Hospital System to 1875:* (Routledge, 1974) is a far better book than its silly, publisher-imposed, title would suggest.

Histories of individual hospitals are legion and almost always excruciatingly dull, except to ex-staff members. The following are noteworthy examples from a large field:

The General Infirmary at Leeds by S. T. Anning (2 vols, Livingstone, 1963–1966)

A Short History of the Radcliffe Infirmary by A. H. T. Robb-Smith (Church Army Press, 1970)

The Life and Times of a Voluntary Hospital. The History of the Royal Belfast Hospital for Sick Children by H. G. Calwell (The Hospital, 1973)

The Royal Hospital of Saint Bartholomew, 1123–1973 by V. C. Medvei and J. L. Thornton (St. Bart's, 1974)

The History and Traditions of the Moorfields Eye Hospital by F. W. Law (2 vols, H. K. Lewis, 1975)

University College Hospital and its Medical School: a History by W. R. Merrington (Heinemann, 1976)

London Pride. The Story of a Voluntary Hospital by A. E. Clark-Kennedy (Hutchinson Benham, 1979).

Medical education

T. Puschmann's *A History of Medical Education* was translated from the German edition of 1889 (H. K. Lewis, 1891) and is useful, as is C. Newman's *The Evolution of Medical Education in the 19th Century* (Oxford University Press, 1957). *The History of Medical Education* edited by C. D. O'Malley (University of California Press, 1970) contains papers (some now a little outdated) on each of the main countries. T. N. Bonner's *American Doctors and German Universities: a Chapter in Intellectual Relations 1870–1914* (University of Nebraska Press, 1963) examines a period when 'a high proportion of the most talented and ambitious of American medical men studied . . . in German universities'. *Oxford Medicine* edited by K. Dewhurst (Sanford, 1970) has papers on the rise of the Oxford clinical school. Also useful are M. Kaufman's *American Medical Education: the Formative Years, 1765–1910* (Greenwood Press, 1976) and W. S. Craig's *History of the Royal College of Physicians of Edinburgh* (Blackwell, 1976). M. J. Peterson's *The Medical Profession in mid-Victorian London* (University of California Press, 1978) is a sociological study of an important, formative period.

Biography

The shelves of historical medical libraries groan under an accumulated load of biographies built up by the strong hagiographical tradition which has afflicted medicine since the nineteenth century. At the present time the flow has shrunk to a merciful trickle, as the great man approach to medical history weakens.

The most useful general dictionary of medical biography is A. Hirsch's *Biographisches Lexikon der hervorragenden Ärzte aller Zeiten und Völker* (5 vols, with a supplement, Urban and Schwarzenberg, 1929–1935) which was continued in 2 vols covering fifty years more (1932–1933). Four of its predecessors which have not been entirely superseded are N. F. J. Eloy's *Dictionnaire Historique de la Médecine Ancienne et Moderne* (4 vols, H. Hoyois, 1778; reprinted Brussels, 1973), with good bibliographies and biased towards France, Belgium and Italy; J. E. Dezeimeris *et al. Dictionnaire Historique de la Médecine Ancienne et Modern* (4 vols, Béchet, 1828–1839); A. J. L. Jourdan's *Dictionnaire des Sciences Médicales: Biographie Médicale* (7 vols, Panckoucke, 1820–1825; reprinted Amsterdam, 1967), which supplements the two preceding titles; and A. L. J. Bayle and A. J. Thillaye's *Biographie Médicale* (2 vols, Delahaye, 1855; reprinted Amsterdam, 1967, the contents of which were gathered eclectically (from Eloy *inter alios*), then revised and rearranged in chronological order.

Within the last fifteen years three excellent works have appeared, each fulfilling a different role. A. G. Debus' *World Who's Who in Science* (A. N. Marquis, 1968) covers the full sweep of recorded history with brief entries. More selective is T. I. Williams' *Biographical Dictionary of Scientists* (3rd edn, A. and C. Black, 1982), but it contains longer entries. Authoritative, almost definitive, are the entries in *Dictionary of Scientific Biography* edited by C. C. Gillispie (16 vols, Scribner, 1970–80), written by professional historians of science and medicine.

Two books deal exclusively with the lives of medieval practitioners, namely C. E. A. Wickersheimer's *Dictionnaire Biographique des Médecins en France au Moyen-Age* (2 vols, Droz, 1936), of which a new edition (actually a reprint of the two basic volumes) has recently appeared under the general editorship of G. Beaujouan, with a supplementary volume by D. Jacquart (Droz, 1979) and C. H. Talbot and E. A. Hammond's *The Medical Practitioners in Medieval England: a Biographical Register* (WIHM, 1965).

For the period since 1518 there is W. Munk's *Roll of the Royal College of Physicians of London* (2nd edn, 3 vols plus 3 supplements, RCP, 1878–1982), a work which contains hundreds of short biographies of the British medical élite, a short history of the College and lists of office-holders, lecturers and prize-winners.

In the difficult period before the regular run of *Medical Directories* began in 1845, one has to rely on the irregularly produced volumes of the same general title published in 1779, 1780 and 1783. There are useful lists of apothecaries in C. Wall, H. C. Cameron and E. Underwood's *History of the Worshipful Society of Apothecaries of London, vol 1 1617–1815* (only one volume, Oxford University Press, 1963). Interested students may consult the unpublished typescripts of vol 2 in the Wellcome Institute for the History of Medicine, London.

Useful sources for the middle and lower social reaches of the healing professions are J. H. Bloom and R. R. James' *Medical Practitioners in the Diocese of London, Licensed . . . 1529–1752* (Cambridge University Press, 1935), J. H. Raach's *Directory of English Country Physicians, 1603–1643* (Dawson, 1962) and R. W. Innes Smith's *English-Speaking Students of Medicine at the University of Leyden* (Oliver and Boyd, 1932).

The nineteenth century is better served by biographical sources. Key events were the creation in 1800 of the College of Surgeons, leading to its first printed list of members in 1805 and the passing in 1815 of the Apothecaries' Act. The year 1840 saw the publication of a cumulated list of apothecaries who had passed the Society's new examinations. For the higher ranks of the surgical profession one should consult V. G. Plarr's *Lives of the Fellows of the Royal College of Surgeons of England* (2 vols, Wright, 1930), continued in three volumes compiled by Sir D'Arcy Power for the years 1930–1951 (RCS, 1953), by W. R. LeFanu and R. H. O. B. Robinson for 1952–1964 (Livingstone, 1970), and by Sir J. P. Ross and W. R. LeFanu for the years 1965–1973 (Pitman Medical, 1981). The Royal College of Obstetricians and Gynaecologists has a biographical record in Sir John Peel's *The Lives of the Fellows . . . 1929–1969* (Heinemann Medical, 1976).

For military medicine the basic works are D. G. Crawford's *Roll of the Indian Medical Service, 1615–1930* (Thacker, 1930) – an appendix and errata were issued in 1933; and W. Johnston, A. Peterkin and R. Drew's *Commissioned Officers in the Medical Services of the British Army, 1660–1960* (2 vols, WIHM, 1968).

For countries other than Great Britain, a good selection of references would be:

FRANCE

Les Biographies Médicales by P. Busquet and A. Gilbert (5 vols, Baillière, 1927–1936)

Biographies Médicales et Scientifiques edited by P. Huard, a promised series which has not, thus far, gone beyond *vol 1: 18th Century* (R. Dacosta, 1972).

ITALY

Profili Bio-bibliografici di Medici e Naturalisti Celebri Italiani del Sec. XV al Sec. XVIII (2 vols, Serono, 1925–1928); vol 1 only was reissued in 1932

GERMANY

Biographisches Lexikon by A. Hirsch (*see* page 474)

US

Dictionary of American Medical Biography by H. A. Kelly and W. L. Burrage (Appleton, 1928) which includes Canadians
Biography of Eminent American Physicians and Surgeons by R. F. Stone (2 edn, Carlon and Hollenbeck, 1898)
American Medical Biography by J. Thacher (2 vols, with a new introduction and a bibliography by W. J. Bell, Jr., Da Capo, 1967); this is a reprint of the first edition which appeared in 1828

In the sphere of collective biography H. E. Sigerist's *The Great Doctors* (Allen and Unwin, 1933, reprinted 1972) retains its status as a classic account of 'doctors' from Imhotep to Osler. Three older, British-centred works combine elegance and period charm: B. W. Richardson's *Disciples of Aesculapius* (2 vols, Hutchinson, 1900), T. J. Pettigrew's *Medical Portrait Gallery* (4 vols, Fisher, Whittaker, 1838–1840) and G. T. Bettany's *Eminent Doctors* (2 vols, (Hogg, 1885). A bibliography of the literature on diseases of famous persons and of descriptions of disease by eminent writers is provided by J. B. Gilbert's *Disease and Destiny* (Dawsons, 1962).

Students in search of biographies should consult J. L. Thornton's *A Select Bibliography of Medical Biography* (2nd edn, LA, 1970) and the New York Academy of Medicine's *Catalog of Biographies* (G. K. Hall, 1960).

Single-subject biographies which have achieved some lasting value are:

Ugo Benzi D. P. Lockwood (Chicago University Press, 1951)
The Life and Times of Gaspare Tagliacozzi, Surgeon of Bologna 1545–1599 by M. T. Gnudi and J. P. Webster (H. Reichner, 1950)
Andreas Vesalius of Brussels by C. D. O'Malley (University of California Press, 1964)
Paracelsus and *Harvey* both by W. Pagel (*see* page 468)
Beloved Son Felix by E. and T. Plater (translated by S. Kennett, F. Muller, 1963)
The Life of William Harvey by Sir Geoffrey Keynes (Clarendon Press, 1966)
Marcello Malpighi and the Evolution of Embryology by H. R. Adelmann (5 vols, Cornell University Press, 1966)
The Correspondence of Henry Oldenburg, 1641– edited by A. R. Hall and M. Boas Hall (10 vols to date, University of Wisconsin Press, 1965–)
Herman Boerhaave by G. A. Lindeboom (Methuen, 1968)
Lettsom by J. Johnston Abraham (Heinemann, 1933)
Sir Charles Bell by Sir G. Gordon-Taylor and E. W. Walls (Livingstone, 1958)

The Life and Times of Sir Charles Hastings by W. H. McMenemy (Livingstone, 1959)
Life and Times of Thomas Wakley by Sir S. Squire Sprigge (Longmans, 1897)
Sir John Simon by R. Lambert (MacGibbon and Kee, 1963)
Life of Louis Pasteur by R. Vallery-Radot (Constable, 1923)
Florence Nightingale by C. Woodham-Smith (Constable, 1950)
Elizabeth Garrett Anderson by J. Manton (Methuen, 1965)
Life of Sir William Osler by H. Cushing (2 vols, Clarendon Press, 1925, reprinted Oxford University Press, 1940)
Harvey Cushing by J. F. Fulton (C. C. Thomas, 1946)
Florence Nightingale. Reputation and Power by F. B. Smith (Croom Helm, 1982), a much needed, astringent treatment of the 'Nightingale myth' which will annoy the pious

Finally, not to be ignored are catalogues of portraits, often containing not only pictures but small masterpieces of biography based on meticulous research. The best known examples are:

Photographs of Eminent Men of all Countries by T. H. Barker (2 vols, Churchill, 1867–1868)
Royal College of Physicians of London: Portraits by G. E. W. Wolstenholme (2 vols, Churchill–Elsevier, 1964, 1977)
College Portraits . . . Royal College of Physicians of Edinburgh by R. Thin (Oliver and Boyd, 1927)
A Catalogue of the Portraits and Other Paintings, Drawings and Sculpture in the Royal College of Surgeons of England by W. R. LeFanu (Livingstone, 1960)
Catalogue of Engraved Portraits in the Royal College of Physicians of London by A. H. Driver (RCP, 1952)
Catalogue of Portraits in the Wellcome Institute by R. Burgess, (WIHM, 1973)
Portrait Catalog. New York Academy of Medicine (5 vols, plus supplements, G. K. Hall, 1959–1970)

Bibliography

If medicine cannot quite claim to be the oldest profession, it can certainly look back further than most to an exceptionally well recorded past, thanks to a long line of dedicated historians, bibliographers and librarians.

The first printed history-cum-bibliography of medicine was written by Symphorien Champier (1472–1539), a physician and polymath who devoted a large part of his energies to the rescue and transmission of classical scientific learning. His fifty-seven-leaf tract *De Medicinae Claris Scriptoribus* (Lyons, *ca.* 1506) is divided into five sections each of which has a chronological sequence of bibliographies. The story of Champier's pioneering efforts and accounts of those later bibliographers whose work is still of importance to the medical historian may be read in J. F. Fulton's *The Great Medical Bibliographers: a Study in Humanism* (University of Pennsylvania Press, 1951) and E. Brodman's *The Development of Medical Bibliography* (MLA, 1954; reprinted 1981).

The principal older bibliographies still useful to the historian include Conrad Gesner's *Bibliotheca Universalis* (3 vols, and an appendix, Zurich, 1545–1555). The section on medicine was planned but never appeared, but the other *libri* contain much of relevance to medicine. J. A. Van Der Linden's *De Scriptis Medicis* (Amsterdam, 1637; 2nd edn, 1651; 3rd edn, 1662) set a new style in medical bibliographies by combining a main alphabetical sequence of entries with subject indexes. The revision of this work by Mercklin, *Lindenius Renovatus* (Nuremberg, 1686) includes entries for articles in periodicals and produces a useful list of the individual treatises of Galen and Hippocrates. Martin Lipenius' *Bibliotheca Realis* (Frankfurt, 1679–1685) was printed in admirably clear double columns. This subject bibliography covers the writings of *ca.* 20 000 authors and has an effective system of indexes and cross-references. Cornelius à Beughem compiled two bibliographies in the late seventeenth century, both of which cover literature produced in the decades prior to publication: *Bibliographia Medica et Physica Novissima* (Amsterdam, 1681) lists books published between 1651 and 1681 while *Syllabus Recens Exploratorum in Re Medica* (Amsterdam, 1696) indexes articles in the early volumes of such periodicals as then existed (e.g. *Journal des Sçavans*).

Albrecht von Haller (1708–1777) produced an extraordinarily rich collection of bibliographies in a noble series of folio volumes. All his great *Bibliothecae* (on botany, 2 vols, London 1771–1772; on surgery, 2 vols, Basle, 1774–1775; on anatomy, 2 vols, Zürich, 1774–1777; and on medicine, 4 vols, Berne, 1776–1788) are remarkable for their thoroughness and accuracy.

Towards the end of the eighteenth century the flow of medical literature quickened. More monographs appeared and the periodical began to make its now characteristic contribution to scientific and medical publishing. Quite clearly, if scientists or doctors wished to keep abreast of the latest information in their field, they would be more likely to find it quickly and easily in a bibliography arranged by subject, rather than in the traditional author form. Two early works that fall into this category are C. W. Kestner's *Bibliotheca Medica* (Jena, 1746), which has sections on pathology, therapeutics, materia medica, dietetics, etc., supplemented by an author index; and Stephanus H. de Vigilliis von Creutzenfeld's *Bibliotheca Chirurgica* (2 vols, Vienna, 1781), in which annotated entries are grouped under an alphabetical sequence of heads representing the different branches of surgery.

For the same period, the best example of a subject bibliography is Wilhelm G. Ploucquet's *Literatura Medica Digesta, sive Repertorium Medicinae Practicae, Chirurgiae atque Rei Obstetricae*, (4 vols, Tübingen, 1808–1809).

A work that complements Ploucquet's is J. D. Reuss' *Repertorium Commentationum a Societatibus Litterariis Editarum* (16 vols, Göttingen, 1801–1821; reprinted Burt Franklin, 1961). This splendid guide to the contents of learned society journals is clearly printed and well designed. Volumes 10 and 16 deal with science and medicine.

One of the finest achievements in the history of medical bibliography is Adolph C. Callisen's *Medicinisches Schriftsteller-Lexicon*. Published in thirty-three indifferently printed volumes (Copenhagen, 1830–1845; reprinted B. de Graaf, 1962–1964), this marvellously compendious and accurate guide names and identifies (by their places of residence) hundreds of authors active in the period from about 1750 to 1830. Under each name are given particulars of that person's literary output – journal articles included – even down to the different editions and translations. For good measure, Callisen gives references to book reviews and lists the contents of contemporary periodicals, volume by volume, from their beginnings. The reprinting of this indispensable tool of research was one of the more intelligent actions of a section of the modern publishing industry not noted for its rational choices.

Some of the new journals produced cumulative indexes and these can be useful to the historian. Four especially good examples are *London Medical and Physical Journal*, 1799–1818; *Edinburgh Medical and Surgical Journal* (and its predecessors), 1731–1823, annexed to which is a list of Edinburgh theses from 1726 to 1823; *Medico-chirurgical Review*, 1820–1834; and *Journal de Médecine, Chirurgie et Pharmacie*, 1754–1826. All four are indexed by subject and author.

A. Hiersemann, an enterprising German publishing house, has embarked on a series of volumes ambitiously aimed at indexing German natural history and medical periodicals for the years before 1850. Entitled *Indices naturwissenschaftlich–medizinischer Periodica bis 1850*, the first volume, edited by A. Geus, covers the journal *Der Naturforscher*, 1774–1804, and has indexes for authors, subjects and illustrations. Volume 2 of this excellent series, edited by D. von Engelhardt, appeared in 1974, on the chemical journals of Lorenz von Crell.

When one considers the mountain of medical literature created during the nineteenth century, it becomes obvious why no single bibliography – not even that remarkable creation the *Index-Catalogue of the Library of the Surgeon General's Office, United*

States Army: Authors and Subjects. (1st–5th series in 61 vols, Government Printing Office, 1880–1961) – has succeeded in mapping out the terrain completely. Current medical bibliography owes almost everything to the *Index-Catalogue* and its National Library of Medicine successors. We must also give credit to the Royal Society of London's *Catalogue of Scientific Papers, 1800–1900* which, in 19 volumes (various publishers, 1867–1925; Johnson Reprint Corporation and Kraus Reprint Corporation, 1965) lists alphabetically by author thousands of periodical articles on most branches of science, including the pre-clinical, but excluding clinical medicine. It has been continued for material published after 1900 as the *International Catalogue of Scientific Literature.*

The Royal Society's deficiencies in the listing of medicine are only partly made good by R. Neale's very selective *Medical Digest,* a bizarrely classified index to the contents of fewer than twenty journals for the period 1850 to 1877 and beyond that (in two subsequent editions) up to 1899. In E. J. Waring's *Bibliotheca Therapeutica* (2 vols, New Sydenham Soc., 1878–1879) there are references to over 10 000 books 'arranged under 600 separate headings or articles'.

A natural response to the growth in periodical literature was the attempt to monitor it by means of abstracts. This new trend gathered force from the middle of the nineteenth century. The most important abstracting journals were Schmidt's *Jahrbücher der in- und ausländischer gesammten Medicin* (1834–1922), proof-sheets of which were furnished to the New Sydenham Society to act as a basis for its own annual survey of the literature, *Year Book* (London, 1860–1879); W. Braithwaite's *Retrospective of Practical Medicine and Surgery* (Simpkin and Marshall, 1846–1901); and Ranking's *Half-yearly Abstract of the Medical Sciences* (London, 1845–1873). There are many other similar publications.

Students interested in the history of the scientific and medical periodicals should consult B. Houghton's *Scientific Periodicals: their Historical Development, Characteristics and Control* (C. Bingley, 1975) and D. A. Kronick's *A History of Scientific and Technical Periodicals, 1665–1790* (2nd edn, Scarecrow Press, 1976).

Library catalogues

It would be wrong to consider printed catalogues as mere book-finding instruments when, at their best, they can be singularly agreeable to read and browse among.

The *Bibliotheca Osleriana* (Clarendon Press, 1929; reprinted McGill University Press, 1969) is the key to the older part of the historical collections of the Osler Library at McGill University, Montreal. In spite of the current reaction against the 'Oslerian view' of medical history, this catalogue retains much interest for biblio-philes and book-dealers.

The *Bibliotheca Walleriana* (2 vols, Almqvist and Wiksell, 1955) is, likewise, a monument to a private collection, now housed in the Royal University, Uppsala. It records over 20 000 items, including many rare classic texts on medicine and related subjects. Volume 2 has useful sections on secondary works of medical history, bio-graphy, and bibliography.

The Wellcome Institute for the History of Medicine's library is one of the richest collections in the world and its catalogues are much used by librarians, researchers and the trade. Still incom-plete, its *Catalogue of Printed Books . . . (until) 1850* consists, so far, of one volume on *Incunabula* (1954), one volume on books (including incunabula) printed before 1641 (1962), and two volumes for the period 1641 to 1850 as far as the letter L (by authors' names) published in 1966 and 1976 respectively. In addition, the Institute has published catalogues of Western and Arabic manu-scripts, the former in two volumes (1962, 1973) and the latter in one (1967). The Institute's *Subject Catalogue* of (largely) secondary literature has been published in 18 vols (comprising three series – subject, topographical and biographical) by Kraus International Publishers (1980).

The older portions of the National Library of Medicine's collec-tions are dealt with in R. J. Durling's *A Catalogue of Sixteenth Cen-tury Printed Books*, (NLM, 1967) with a supplementary volume issued in 1971, edited by P. Krivatsy. D. M. Schullian's *A Catalogue of Incunabula and Manuscripts* (H. Schuman, 1948) is from the same institution, and has an appendix on oriental manuscripts by F. E. Sommer. More recently the NLM has produced *A Short-title Catalogue of Eighteenth Century Printed Books* (NLM, 1979).

Other related guides are:

Incunabula Scientifica et Medica by A. C. Klebs (St. Catherine Press, 1938)
Incunabula Medica, 1467–1480 by W. Osler (Bibliographical Society, 1923)
Deutsche Medizinische Inkunabeln by Karl Sudhoff (Barth, 1908)
The Awakening Interest in Science during the First Century of Printing, 1450–1550 by M. B. Stillwell (Bibliographical Society of America, 1970), about half of which covers medicine and natural science
A Catalogue of the Medieval and Renaissance Manuscripts and Incunabula in the Boston Medical Library by J. F. Ballard (privately printed, 1944)
The Morris H. Saffron Collection of Books on Historical Medicine: a Short-title Catalogue (New Jersey College of Medicine and Dentistry, 1981)
Author–Title Catalog of the Francis A. Countway Library of Medicine for Imprints through 1959 by Harvard Medical Library (10 vols, G. K. Hall, 1973)

Verzeichnis medizinischer und naturwissenschaftlicher Drucke 1472–1830 Wolfen-büttel, Herzog August Bibliothek, (14 vols, Kraus-Thomson, 1976–1978)

Other medical library catalogues and some of their characteristics are, in summary form.

LONDON

Royal College of Physicians (1912): author entries (occasionally annotated), lists of Harveian Orations and Lumleian Lectures, no serial publications

Royal Medical and Chirurgical Society (now *Royal Society of Medicine*) (3 vols, 1879): author entries in vols 1 and 2, including serial titles by country, subject index in vol 3, list of Jacksonian Prize Essays

Royal College of Surgeons (1831): author entries with additional headings for 'Journal', 'Midwifery', 'Hospital', 'Academy', etc.

English Books Printed before 1701 (Royal College of Surgeons, 1963): author entries with coverage of English-language books by British authors published abroad

Medical Society of London (1829): drastically short author entries

Manuscripta Medica: W. Dawson (Medical Society of London 1932)

Society of Apothecaries (1913): author entries for 1700 items

University College, London (1887): author entries, including sections for Reports, Academies and Periodicals

EDINBURGH

Royal College of Physicians (2 vols, 1898): author entries (many of them analytical), with headings for reports and journals, includes a chronological list of librarians and a catalogue of medical portraits, engravings, etchings and busts

A Catalogue of the 16th Century Medical Books in Edinburgh Libraries by D. T. Bird (1982)

GLASGOW

Faculty of Physicians and Surgeons (2 vols, 1885–1901): author entries preceded by an index of subjects, includes periodicals and reports (by subject) and a two-page list of MSS

Hunterian Museum in the University of Glasgow (1930); author entries with a topographical index of books printed before 1600 and a one-page list of items in Chinese

ENGLISH PROVINCES

Manchester Medical Library (1890): author entries, with reports arranged by subjects

Manchester Medical Library (1972): extremely detailed author entries for the period 1480 to 1700, with indexes to match

Liverpool Medical Institution (1968): author entries up to the end of the nineteenth century, excludes serials

York Medical Society (1961): author entries

Cole Library, Reading University (1969): Part 2 plus supplement (1975), author entries, in a rough chronological order, with a good subject index and a generous amount of reference material

Pybus Collection, University of Newcastle Library (1981): includes letters and engravings, 15th-20th centuries, as well as medical books.

US

Harvey Cushing Collection, Yale University (1943): author entries, including separate sections for MSS, incunabula and orientalia

H. Winnett Orr Collection, American College of Surgeons (1960): in four parts, including one for rare books and classics and one for life and literature

Reynolds Library, University of Alabama (1968): author entries, with sections on incunabula and MSS.; well illustrated

University of Oklahoma Libraries: sciences collections (1976)

FRANCE

Bibliothèque Nationale (3 vols, 1859–1889): classified, no index but good table of contents

HOLLAND

Nederlandsche Maatschappij tot Bevordering der Geneeskunst (2 vols, 1930–1959): a remarkably good collection, classified with sections for manuscripts and autograph letters

AUSTRIA

Josephinisches Bibliothek: history of medicine (1974)

Encyclopaedias and dictionaries

It was only in the eighteenth century that dictionaries of medicine came permanently upon the scene as the most potent means yet discovered for diffusing the elements of medical knowledge among the profession and the educated public. The three best examples are S. Blankaart's *Lexicon Medicum Graecolatinum* (Amsterdam, 1679), of which seven editions appeared between 1684 and 1726 under the title *A Physical Dictionary: in which all the Terms relating either to Anatomy, Chirurgery, Pharmacy, or Chemistry, are . . . explain'd;* J. Quincy's *Lexicon Physico-medicum* (London, 1719), which began its long career in the heyday of iatrophysics and ended it at the time of Lavoisier (11th edn, 1794); and R. James's *Medicinal Dictionary* (3 vols, 1743–1745), an exhaustive work to which Dr Johnson contributed a preface. As for encyclopaedias, one thinks immediately of Diderot and D'Alembert's *Encyclopédie* (published variously in the 1770s) by reason of its magnificent illustrations and substantial sections on surgery and medicine.

For the nineteenth century a good choice of dictionaries would be R. Hooper's *Lexicon Medicum* (London, 1802), which continues on from where Quincy left off, reaching an 8th edn in 1848; J. Copland's *Dictionary of Practical Medicine* (3 vols, London, 1832–1858), which contains 'prescriptions, bibliography and formulae'; New Sydenham Society's *Lexicon of Terms used in Medicine and the Allied Sciences* edited by Power and Sedgwick (5 vols, London, 1881–1899), which includes long accounts of medicine, surgery, midwifery, and pathology, and 'accurate information [on] the drugs and preparations of the Indian and of the several European pharmacopoeias, with the doses, etc.'.

The following encyclopaedias are of the first importance. *Dictionaire* [sic] *des Sciences Médicales* (60 vols, Paris 1812–1922) has a two-volume subject index and *Encyclopädisches Wörterbuch der medicinischen Wissenschaft* (37 vols, Berlin, 1828–1849) has a subject index. *Cyclopaedia of Practical Medicine* edited by Forbes, Tweedie and Conolly (4 vols, London, 1833–1835) claims to 'rescue ancient literature from oblivion and to present the latest knowledge acquired by the French, German and Italian pathologists'. *Nouveau Dictionnaire de Médecine et de Chirurgie* (40 vols, Paris, 1864–1886) presents 'articles d'ensemble' under general headings in an alphabetico-classed order and has a complete index of subjects in the final volume where there is also a long addendum on microbes. *Dictionnaire Encyclopédique des Sciences Médicales* edited by Dechambre (100 vols, Paris, 1864–1889) has extraordinarily good bibliographies and numerous biographical articles, and in vol 1 an overall survey of dictionaries.; *British Encyclopaedia of Medical Practice* edited by Sir H. Rolleston (12 vols, London, 1936–1944); 2nd edn, by Lord Horder (12 vols, plus index, London, 1950–1952) has historical notes scattered throughout; *see* especially Rolleston's introduction.

Dictionaries of eponyms, syndromes and quotations should be taken into account. The leading ones are:

Die Eigennamen in der Krankheitsterminologie by I. Fischer (M. Perles, 1931)
Die klinische Eponyme by B. Leiber and T. Olbert (Urban and Schwarzenberg, 1968)
Die klinische Syndrome by B. Leiber and G. Olbrich (5th edn., Urban and Schwarzenberg, 1972)
Illustrated Dictionary of Eponymic Syndromes and Diseases and their Synonyms by S. Jablonski (W. B. Saunders, 1969)
Dictionary of Medical Syndromes by S. I. Magalini (2nd edn, Lippincott, 1981)
Anatomical Eponyms by J. Dobson (2nd edn, Livingstone, 1962)
Familiar Medical Quotations by M. B. Strauss (Little, Brown, 1968)

A growing trend in modern publishing is the production of dictionaries of concepts. For the history of medicine two of the most useful are *Dictionary of the History of Ideas: Studies of Selected Pivotal Ideas* edited by P. P. Wiener (4 vols, Scribner, 1973) and *Dictionary of the History of Science* edited by W. F. Bynum, E. J. Browne and R. Porter (Macmillan, 1981), a desk-top volume, even more accessible since it is now (1983) available in paperback.

Indexes to the historical literature

As medical history, as a subject, has grown and expanded so, paradoxically, has it become more and more necessary for the student to look beyond those sources concerned specifically and narrowly with the subject itself. Recourse must be had to the indexes and serial bibliographies produced for general history, the social sciences, classics, linguistics, and so on, if the careful researcher is not to miss significant work. To list even a selection these would, however, be beyond the scope of the present book.

Current Work in the History of Medicine is issued quarterly by the Wellcome Institute for the History of Medicine, London. Its editorial core is a MEDLINE printout to which are added entries derived from non-medical sources. New and forthcoming books are also listed. No cumulation has been published but all the entries in the series (117 parts to date) are included in the Wellcome Institute Library *Subject Catalogue* described above (page 481).

Complementary to *Current Work* is the National Library of Medicine's annual *Bibliography of the History of Medicine*. Published since 1965, it has an alphabetical arrangement of topics under general headings such as 'Statistics and Demography' and 'Tropical Medicine', preceded by a substantial section devoted to biographies. Cumulations appear at five-yearly intervals, the latest of them being in 1979.

From the very start of its long life *Isis*, founded by George Sarton in 1913, and now the leading international journal in the history of science, has regularly given over one part of each annual volume to a 'critical' (i.e. annotated) bibliography of newly published work in its field. Cumulations of these have been published as follows: *Isis Cumulative Bibliography. A Bibliography of the History of Science formed from ISIS Critical Bibliographies 1–90, 1913–65* edited by M. Whitrow: *Vol 1 (Part 1): Personalities A–J; Vol 2 (Part 1): Personalities K–Z; Part 2: Institutions; Vol 3: Subjects; Vol 4: Civilizations and Periods – Prehistory to Middle Ages; Vol 5: Civilizations and Periods – 15th to 19th Centuries* (Mansell, 1971–1982). The same cumulation occurs for *ISIS Critical Bibliographies 91–100, 1966–1975* edited by J. Neu: *Vol 1: Personalities and Institutions* (Mansell, 1981). Further volumes are to come.

The European counterpart to the *Isis* bibliographies is the French *Bulletin Signalétique: Histoire des Sciences et des Techniques* produced by the Centre de Documentation: Sciences Humaines, Paris.

For work in particular countries, one may have recourse to (for

Spain) *Indice Historico Médico Español,* an author list, published since 1962 as an off-shoot of the periodical *Cuadernos de Historia de la Medicina Española* and (for North America) to G. Miller's *Bibliography of the History of Medicine of the United States and Canada, 1939–1960* (2nd edn, Johns Hopkins, 1964).

Of the bibliographies that are defunct or that lie fallow we need mention *Index zur Geschichte der Medizin und Biologie, etc.,* for the years 1945 to 1952 edited by W. Artelt (vol 1, 1953) and J. Steudel (vol 2, 1966), these two volumes are crammed with nearly 20 000 entries and arranged in a way that tends to impede quick reference. J. Pagel's *Historisch-medicinische Bibliographie für die Jahre 1875–1896* (Berlin, 1898) is classified but without the indexes that this arrangement demands; it is good, however, for biographies and local histories. F. A. Pauly's *Bibliographie des Sciences Médicales* (Tross, 1874, reprinted D. Verschoyle, 1954) has excellent detailed sections on hospitals, epidemics, institutions, etc. *Mitteilungen zur Geschichte der Medizin und der Naturwissenschaften* (Leipzig, 1902–1942, 1961–64) is an abstracting journal rather than a true bibliography; and all the more valuable for that reason.

Finally, the age of electronics and the ubiquitous 'chip' is upon us. Films and tapes, etc., are listed in B. Eastwood's *Directory of Audio-visual Sources: History of Science, Medicine and Technology* (Science History Publications, 1979).

Automated data bases have yet to make their real contribution to historical studies. Enormously successful in the sciences and technology, these new sources of information suffer at the present time from the shortness of their memories and the relative expense of using them. The most useful ones for the historian of medicine with access to a terminal or subscription agency may be selected from the many services listed in J. L. Hall's *On-line Retrieval Handbook* (ASLIB, 1977, revised frequently).

Readings

Books of readings containing reprints of, or substantial extracts from medical classics appear to fulfil two main consumer needs. First, they help to feed the collective nostalgia of the health professions by providing a sort of *cordon bleu* cook-book of all the 'recipes' which, from the modern point of view, appear to have stood the test of time. As such, they undoubtedly nourish the progressionist, upwards-and-onwards view of medicine's past which professional historians spend much time combatting. Secondly, teachers of medical history seek to provide their pupils with easily assimilative gobbets of text in an accessible language, usually English, for the purposes of course work.

Whatever we may think of these motives, anthologies of medical classics exist and may be consulted with considerable profit as introductions to further study.

A selection of the many available titles is:

Classic Descriptions of Disease by R. H. Major (3rd edn, C. C. Thomas, 1945)
Selected Readings in Pathology by E. R. Long (2nd edn, C. C. Thomas, 1961)
A History of Medicine: Selected Readings by I. S. King (Penguin Books, 1971)
Hippocratic Writings by G. R. Lloyd (Penguin Books, 1978)
Medical America in the 19th Century: Readings from the Literature by G. H. Brieger (Johns Hopkins, 1972)
Greek Medicine: being Extracts Illustrative of Medical Writing from Hippocrates to Galen by A. J. Brock (E. P. Dutton, 1929)
Selected Readings in the History of Physiology by J. F. Fulton and L. G. Wilson (2nd edn, C. C. Thomas, 1966)
Source Book of Medical History by L. Clendening (Dover, 1960), a convenient paperbacked collection
Three Hundred Years of Psychiatry, 1535–1860 by R. Hunter and I. Macalpine (Oxford University Press, 1963) English scene from Bartholomaeus Anglicus to 1860, with lucid and often witty editorial comments on texts which range widely beyond any narrow definition of 'psychiatry'
Readings in Pharmacy by P. A. Doyle (J. Wiley, 1962)
Readings in Pharmacology by B. Holmstedt and G. Liljestrand (Macmillan, 1963), from the Ebers Papyrus and by way of the 'School of Salerno' into sections headed e.g. 'experimental pharmacology', 'local anaesthesia', etc
Milestones in Modern Surgery by A. Hurwitz and G. Degenshein (Hoeber-Harper, 1958)
Classics of Cardiology by F. A. Willius and T. A. Keys (2 vols, revised edn, Dover, 1961)
Sickness and Health in America: Readings in the History of Medicine and Public Health by J. W. Leavitt and R. L. Numbers (University of Wisconsin Press, 1978)

Reprints

The buyer of reprints and facsimiles needs a deep purse and endless patience, since this part of the publishing field has grown into an undisciplined jungle. Although publishers continue to deny it, it is clear that the retail price of reprints is geared to a strict consideration of what the potential market will bear, with perhaps an eye on the secondhand value of the original, rather than on the cost of manufacture plus a reasonable profit-margin. This, perhaps, accounts for the irritating frequency of titles announced but never finally published.

The essential guide to current reprints is *Guide to Reprints* published annually by Guide to Reprints Inc., in both author and subject listings.

University Microfilms International also publish annually an *Author/Title/Subject Guide to Books on Demand*. The guide itself is now (1982) available on microfiche, and the books listed may be purchased either in book (bound xerox) or film/fiche form.

The older reprints (up to 1967) are listed in Renate Ostwald's *Nachdruck-Verzeichnis* (2 vols, G. Nobis, 1965, 1969).

The librarian or collector needs to watch the often bulky, seasonal catalogues of the main reprint publishers; for Britain, Mansell, Gregg International and, until recently, Dawson; for the USA, Johnson Reprint Corp. and Kraus-Thomson; for Germany and Austria, Müller, G. Olms of Hildesheim, and the Akademische Druck of Graz; for Italy, Olschki. Points to be noted are:

(1) Is the reprint merely a tarted-up and hence overly-expensive product aimed specifically at the rich doctor market?
(2) Does it have any kind of critical introduction? This point is particularly important when buying reprints for student use.
(3) For early books particularly, is there a note in the reprint denoting the copy actually used?
(4) Is the reproduction clear and free from smudging and printed on good quality paper?

The wonderful techniques of modern colour-printing have made possible many beautiful but expensive facsimiles of manuscripts. These are really collectors' pieces and it is difficult to see much use for them in working libraries. They are as inaccessible as the originals to the untrained and scholars will generally need to see the originals in any case.

Finally, we need to look forward to a not too distant future when virtually instantaneous facsimile transmission and other electronic marvels will, at least in theory, and of course at a price, make the contents of great libraries available almost anywhere.

Periodicals

A generous selection of the current periodicals in the history of medicine and related fields is arranged in alphabetical order in the list below.

The student of medical history cannot afford to neglect the major periodicals in general history and the social sciences. A growth area in recent years has been the number of new titles devoted to non-western or 'alternative' medical systems. Also to be sought out are the numerous *Newsletters*, often distributed free or at very low cost, by institutions, societies and research groups, particularly in the US but also in the UK and continental Europe.

Ambix. The journal of the Society for the Study of Alchemy and Early Chemistry (London, 1937, vol 1–)

Annals of Science. A quarterly review of the history of science since the Renaissance (London, 1936, vol 1–)

Archives Internationales d'Histoire des Sciences (Paris, 1947, vol 1–)

Boletín de la Sociedad Española de Historia de la Medicina (Madrid, 1961, vol 1–)

British Journal for the History of Science (London, 1962, vol 1–)

Bulletin of the History of Medicine. Organ of the American Society for the History of Medicine (Baltimore, John Hopkins, 1933, vol 1–)

Bulletin et Mémoires de la Société Internationale d'Histoire de la Médecine. (Brussels, 1954–1961, vols 1–8)

Bulletin de la Société Française d'Histoire des Hôpitaux (Paris, 1959, vol 1–)

Clio Medica (Oxford, now Amsterdam, 1965, vol 1–)

Comparative Medicine – East and West. Formerly *American Journal of Chinese Medicine.* This original title resumed in 1979 (New York, 1973, vol 1–)

Cuadernos de Historia de la Medicina Española (Salamanca, 1962, vol 1–)

Culture, Medicine and Psychiatry Dordrecht and Boston, 1977, vol 1–)

Dynamis. Acta Hispanica ad Medicinae Scientiarumque Historiam Illustrandam (Granada, 1981, vol 1–)

Gesnerus. Organ of the Swiss Society for the History of Medicine and Science (Aarau, 1943, vol 1–)

Histoire des Sciences Médicales, Organ of the French Society. Before 1967 the Society's official organ was called *Histoire de la Médecine* (Paris, 1967, vol 1–)

Historia Hospitalium. Mitteilungen der Deutschen Gesellschaft für Krankenhausgeschichte (Düsseldorf, 1966, vol 1–)

History of Science. An annual review of literature, research and teaching(Cambridge, 1962, vol 1–)

Indian Journal of the History of Science (Madras, 1956, vol 1–)

Isis. An international review devoted to the history of science and its cultural influences (Philadelphia, 1913, vol 1–)

Janus. Archives Internationales pour l'Histoire de la Médecine, etc (Amsterdam, 1896, vol 1–)

Journal of Ethnopharmacology. An interdisciplinary journal devoted to bioscientific research on indigenous drugs (Lausanne, 1979, vol 1–)

Journal of the History of Arabic Science (Aleppo, 1977, vol 1–)

Journal of the History of the Behavioral Sciences (Brandon, 1965, vol 1–)

Journal of the History of Biology (Cambridge 1968, vol 1–)

Journal of the History of Medicine and Allied Sciences (New York, 1946, vol 1–)

Journal of Medicine and Philosophy (Chicago, 1976, vol 1–)

Journal of Psychohistory. Until 1976 known as *History of Childhood Quarterly (New York, 1973, vol. 1–)*

Koroth. A quarterly journal devoted to the history of medicine and science, Organ of the Israel Society (Jerusalem and Tel Aviv, 1952, vol 1–)

Medical History. Published by the Wellcome Institute, London (London, 1957, vol 1–)

Medicina Tradicional. Instituto Mexicana para el Estudio de las Plantas Medicinales (Mexico, 1977, vol 1–)

Medizin Historisches Journal (Hildesheim, 1966, vol 1–)

NTM Scriftenreihe für Geschichte der Naturwissenschaft, Technik und Medizin (Berlin, 1960, vol 1–)

Pagine di Storia della Medicina (Rome, 1957, vol 1–)

Pharmaceutical Historian. Newsletter of the British Society for the History of Pharmacy (London, 1967, vol 1–).

Pharmacy in History. American Institute for the History of Pharmacy. Before 1965 called *A.I.H.P. Notes.* (Madison, 1955, vol 1–)

Psychohistory Review. Before 1976 called *Group for the Use of Psychology in History, Newsletter* (Springfield, 1972, vol 1–.

Rivista di Storia della Medicina. Organ of the Italian Society. Before 1958 under a slightly different title (Rome, 1910, vol 1–)

Sudhoffs Archiv. Began life as *Archiv für Geschichte der Medizin* (Leipzig 1908, vol 1–

Tibetan Medicine (Dharamsala, 1980, vol 1–)

Traditional Medical Systems (Calcutta, [1980?], vol 1–).

Veterinary History. Organ of the Veterinary History Society (London, 1973, vol 1–).

23

Audio-visual materials

M. C. Jones

The importance of audio-visual aids in medicine has long been recognized – as Sir John McMichael, then Chairman of the Postgraduate Medical Federation, said in 1970 'We have always been the first to demand any new advances which come along in illustrative techniques, to use them in medical education. Other sciences, even the physical sciences, lag well behind, and in fact the initiatives in developing audio-visual aids are stemming out from medicine. . .' (McMichael, 1970). Although the absence of copyright libraries or legal deposit regulations for non-book materials has led to some difficulty in tracing and selecting suitable audio-visual aids, increasing numbers of useful selection guides are becoming available. This chapter concentrates on the situation in the UK, mentioning foreign materials only where they are of significant help to the British user.

History

Most historical information about the development and early use of audio-visual materials comes in the form of journal articles describing the development of particular audio-visual collections – e.g. Engel (1970a), Graves and Graves (1979) – and in the descriptive leaflets distributed by such collections.

However, general surveys of how departments of medical illustration developed into audio-visual resource centres are given by

Engel (1969, 1974) and Beard (1982). Townsend and Heath (1977) looked at the history of educational technology as applied to nursing. The report (Jones 1965) of the working party chaired by Sir Brynmor Jones in 1963 not only described the history of audio-visual aids in scientific education, but also played a significant role in making it!

One of the first specialist film libraries was that established by the British Medical Association in 1946 (Engel, 1970a; 1970b) which took over 16 mm films formerly held by Kodak. This library is now administered by the British Life Assurance Trust for Health Education in collaboration with the British Medical Association. The Royal College of General Practitioners was the first in the medical field to set up, in 1957, a library of audiotapes and slides (Graves and Graves, 1970). It was not until 1970 that another of the Royal Colleges – the Royal College of Obstetricians and Gynaecologists – established an audiotape/slide library (Roberts, 1970). The growing use of videotape in medicine is well documented by Paegle *et al.* (1980), Dranov *et al.* (1980) and Van Son (1982).

From the earliest days of audio-visuals in medicine, users have formed themselves into societies and organizations to facilitate discussion of common problems. The Institute of Medical and Biological Illustration was founded in 1968 to bring together all those professionally engaged in audio-visual communication in the life sciences to stimulate the study and application of all aids to communication in medicine and biology.

The Association of Programmed Learning and Educational Technology was developed in 1969 from the Association for Programmed Learning to reflect changing interests, and then in 1979 it became the Association for Educational and Training Technology. The Association's main aim is to promote communication amongst educational technologists and those of various disciplines who are interested in the subject.

The Scientific Film Association (*The Lancet,* 1982) established a Medical Committee in 1944 to encourage the use of film for education, information and research, the publication of catalogues and of reviews of medical films, and the provision of advice to film-makers. The Committee is now planning to disband, as its work is being done by other more appropriate bodies. The Scientific Film Association amalgamated with the British Industrial Film Association in 1967 to become the British Industrial and Scientific Film Association (BISFA), and its interests are now directed more towards industry than science.

A fuller list of such organizations and their addresses (including organizations outside the UK) is given in each edition of the *International Yearbook of Educational and Instructional Technology*, published for the Association for Educational and Training Technology by Kogan Page Ltd (Osborne, 1982) and in its American counterpart, the *Educational Media Yearbook* (Brown and Brown, 1982).

But why use audio-visuals at all? One of the shortest and clearest arguments is an article written by McArthur (1982) for health professionals in developing countries. For lengthier explanations *see* Romiszowski (1974), Jones (1965), or almost any book on educational technology. It has been suggested that audio-visual media are becoming more familiar than books – e.g. A. H. Thompson (1981) quotes a survey showing 'that 77% of the Swedish population watch television, 30% listen to audiocassettes and 29% read books'.

Audio-visual formats

Very often the terms 'audio-visual' and 'non-book' are used synonymously. They are not synonyms. An item in *Educational Technology* (1982) says 'In a day of computers and videodiscs, 'AV' smacks of filmstrip projectors and slide shows.' This is not necessarily a disadvantage if 'audio-visual' is to be seen as 'a sub-group within the area of non-books' (Liebenow, 1981). Liebenow, writing on behalf of the section on statistics for the special audio-visual materials issue of the *IFLA Journal*,* continues

> It is assumed that criteria for audiovisual materials are that they need some sort of equipment for them to be made perceptible for the human being. For this reason, pictures, for example, regardless of whether they are paintings, graphics or photographs, should not necessarily be counted as being AV material, since they are directly perceivable to the naked human eye and are also present as pictures in books. Nevertheless, the opinions on this are divided.
>
> A very broad classification for AV materials is proposed, which nevertheless partially separates things which are closely related. This broad classification is based upon the human organ which perceives this material. Thus: auditory material, which reproduces only those things which are heard, visual material which is seen, and then the truly audiovisual material which is perceived by both the eye and the ear.

The first category covers records, tapes and cassettes; the second slides, transparencies and silent films; the third sound films, sound slide series, videocassettes, magnetic tapes with picture-tone records and picture records. Microforms however

* International Federation of Library Associations

'are not audiovisual material. They are nothing more than a reduced form of the printed book and are merely found in another form than is usual'. The same reasoning may be applied to exclude computer software from this account of audio-visual materials.

The above paragraph lists all the most common formats. Useful definitions of each and its respective advantages or disadvantages are given by Boucher *et al.* (1973), Barker (1981), McArthur (1982) and Pinion (1982). Forget (1978) also provides brief definitions, as used to describe the different formats for library catalogue cards.

The use of videocassette as one of the newer media is particularly well documented, e.g. Dranov *et al.* (1980) and Van Son (1982). The drawback at present is the mutual incompatibility of the four formats most widely available. Some teachers/lecturers make use of different audio-visual media in one presentation, utilizing qualities special to each. Proponents of the latest audio-visual type to enter the market, the videodisc, claim that it has all the advantages of a multi-media presentation in one easy-to-use disc. The first videodiscs and their players went on sale in the UK during 1982, in direct competition with the pre-recorded videocassettes for home use. But it is the videodisc's capacity for information storage that has attracted most attention (Grills, 1981; McArthur, 1982). Grills also provides what is perhaps the best definition to date 'an iridescent 12-inch disc containing microscopic images imbedded in the disc for video and audio information'.

Storage

Advice on storage varies between the user-orientated, with emphasis on ease of access to materials – Rydesky (1980), Barker (1981), Pinion (1982) – and the highly technical, requiring careful control of temperature and humidity levels. Cockburn (1982) has found, in a review of the literature, only seven accounts of medical slide storage and retrieval systems, and he goes on to describe a method he has used successfully. Barker and Harden (1980) also write at length on the subject.

Drawing on her experience as Media Librarian at the Open University, Harrison (1980) explains methods of storage, cleaning, use, and long term preservation of film, video, and sound recordings.

Verny and Heider (1982) present a few tips on handling and storing videotape. Forget (1978) looks at different types of storage equipment.

Selection

Producers and distributors

A substantial proportion of audio-visual materials for medicine have traditionally been produced in the audio-visual departments of large hospitals and medical schools, and kept for internal use. Gradually, as these departments have grown in size and importance, so the reputation of their products has spread, and other organizations have wanted to acquire them. In some cases, problems of copyright and the ethics of patient privacy have meant that the programmes have had to remain available to a restricted audience only. But some centres, like the University of Newcastle Regional Postgraduate Institute for Medicine and Dentistry and the University of Southampton Department of Teaching Media are able to sell or hire programmes they have produced. Others, like the University of Aberdeen and the University of Glasgow, distribute materials through a commercial company.

As well as producing their own materials, large hospitals and medical schools hold collections of audio-visual aids produced elsewhere, e.g. Charing Cross Hospital Medical School Library and St. Bartholomew's Hospital Audio-Visual Teaching Department. Normally these are available only to their own staff and students, but a certain amount of interlending with other institutions takes place.

The full extent of audio-visual interlending was explored in British Library Research and Development Report 5526 (Pinion, 1980a) and a short account of its findings was published in *Interlending Review* (Pinion, 1980b).

Mention has already been made of the founding of the British Medical Association Film Library in 1946 (Engel, 1970a; 1970b) and the Graves Medical Audiovisual Library in 1957 (Graves and Graves, 1979). Both act as distributors of audio-visual materials produced elsewhere, but whereas the BMA (now BMA/BLAT) Film Library has encouraged film development by stringent testing of all titles submitted and by internationally recognized competitions, GMAL has grown by commissioning and co-producing programmes to fill perceived needs. Other non-profit making audio-visual distributors include the MSD Foundation, which is sponsored by the pharmaceutical company Merck, Sharp and Dohme, and specializes in tape-slide and videocassettes for general practitioners (Sabbagh, 1979); the Higher Education Film Library; the Scottish Central Film Library; and the Foundation for Teaching Aids at Low Cost – TALC (Lunnon 1979).

Foremost among the commercial distributors of medical audio-visuals must be Oxford Educational Resources Ltd, which holds over 2000 titles in health and medicine, many originating from medical schools in the UK and overseas. Concord Films Council, Guild Sound and Vision, the BBC, and Camera Talks also number important medical titles amongst their stock.

Of the many significant audio-visual collections outside the UK, the largest must be the National Library of Medicine Audiovisual Center, described in a new history of the National Library of Medicine (Miles, 1982). The US Academy of Health Sciences holds over 800 videotapes which are made available to recognized organizations submitting a blank tape for each programme required.

Some overseas collections have UK agents, e.g. the Sandoz Pharmaceutical Company (Switzerland) and the World Health Organization distribute their films through the BMA/BLAT Film Library, and prints of films from the French Scientific Film Library are available through the Scottish Central Film Library.

There are far too many audio-visual libraries and distributors to list in this short chapter. Appendix 2 lists the major directories of audio-visual suppliers in the UK and overseas.

Catalogues and directories: UK

The process of finding suitable audio-visual materials does not end with the identification of the major distributors and there are a number of guides to help the newcomer to the field to find his or her next step: Barker (1981), Pinion (1982), Rydesky (1980) and Van Son (1982) have already been cited. The *International Yearbook of Educational and Instructional Technology* (Osborne, 1982) is invaluable, as is the *Educational Media Yearbook* (Brown and Brown, 1982). A shorter guide which assumes no previous knowledge of any aspect of audio-visual materials is *Module 9* of the *Practical Documentation* series produced by the International Planned Parenthood Federation (Forget, 1978).

Like book publishers, producers and distributors of audio-visual materials print catalogues of items available. The best of these are updated regularly and provide very full details of each programme – author, running time, number of slides or frames where appropriate, date, intended audience and a brief synopsis of contents. The catalogue of the Graves Medical Audio-visual Library, produced both in paper and microfiche, is an outstanding example. GMAL makes available, in addition, shorter catalogues listing tape-slide programmes relevant to specific audiences, e.g. remedial therapists, nurses, etc. Titles are arranged by *MeSH* headings. BBC Enterprises, the MSD Foundation, Oxford Educational Resources and the University of Newcastle Regional Postgraduate Institute for Medicine and Dentistry also produce extremely helpful catalogues. Regrettably, some audio-visual distributors still supply nothing better than title lists and in some cases even the format is not given.

It is not surprising that the need has been felt for a *Medical Books in Print* of the audio-visual world. Perhaps the first British attempt was the catalogue published in 1948 by the Medical Committee of the Scientific Film Association and the Royal Society of Medicine, which gave details of some 200 films. The 1970 edition of this catalogue, *Medical Films Available in Great Britain,* produced with the assistance of the British Life Assurance Trust (Engel, 1970a) listed over 2100 titles. Since 1973 the BMA/BLAT Film Library has published, at regular intervals, an extensive catalogue, *Medical Films* (BMA/BLAT Film Library, 1980) to describe its own holdings – now approximately 800 films – and all winners of the BLAT Certificate of Educational Commendation (*see* below). Contents are arranged under broad subject headings, supplemented by a title index. A more detailed subject index would make the catalogue an even more useful tool.

In 1974 the Council for Educational Technology, assisted by the Department of Audio Visual Communication of the British Medical Association and the British Life Assurance Trust for Health Education (which were soon to become one body – the British Life Assurance Trust Centre for Health and Medical Education), produced *HELPIS – Medical,* * a directory of over 960 medical audio-visual materials (Council for Educational Technology, 1974) produced in institutions of higher education. Mostly films and videocassettes, the contents were arranged by Universal Decimal Classification (UDC) divisions with comprehensive subject and title indexes. This was an invaluable aid, but is now sadly out of date. There are no plans for a new edition because medical programmes are now incorporated in the general *HELPIS* catalogue.

For health education materials, the *Health Education Index* (Edsall, 1980) is unequalled. Aimed at schoolteachers, it describes books and audio-visuals listed by health topic, and the directory of suppliers at the beginning is a useful guide to organizations working in the health education field. The Index is fully revised every two to three years.

The Medical Information Service of the British Council was,

* Higher Education Learning Programmes Information Service

until spending cuts forced it to merge into the British Council's Central Information Service, a very useful source of information about new audio-visual materials in medicine, publishing details in its journal *British Medicine* (taken over in May 1980 by Pergamon Press, who prepare it with assistance from the Royal Society of Medicine) and in occasional resource lists on special subjects. Two *British Medicine* supplements *Non-book Materials in Medicine* (British Medicine, 1978a) and *Non-book Materials in Nursing and Medical Ancillary Subjects* (British Medicine, 1978b) were very helpful for locating materials and it would be extremely useful if the new publisher were to produce updated editions.

There are several major multidisciplinary sources of information about audio-visuals. *HELPIS,* already mentioned, has been published since 1971, firstly by the Council for Educational Technology and since 1976 by the British Universities Film Council (BUFC). The 7th edn appeared in print and microfiche in November 1982 (BUFC, 1982). Its medical content is much expanded – medicine was excluded from the early editions, when it was still unclear how much duplication there would be with the BMA/BLAT film catalogue. Like *HELPIS – Medical,* it is arranged by UDC with impressive subject and title indexing. For economic reasons, future editions will probably be published on microfiche only. Another important directory published by the British Universities Film Council is *Audiovisual Materials for Higher Education* – the 1979–1980 edition (Ballantyne, 1979) is in four parts: *History and the Arts; Social Sciences; Biology, Medicine and Life Sciences;* and *Physical Sciences and Technology;* with a fifth volume, the *Update Edition 1981–82* published in 1981. Again, this edition is available in print or microfiche, but the next edition, probably 1983–1984, may appear on microfiche only. The British Universities Film Council is considering offering subscribers a complete database (i.e. *Audiovisual Materials for Higher Education* and *HELPIS* plus regular updates) on microfiche. Entries in the two directories are already in uniform style, classified by UDC, and the distinction between audio-visual programmes produced *for* or *by* higher education no longer seems as important as the need for easy retrieval of useful items.

As the British Universities Film Council has so much experience in the provision of useful and up-to-date catalogues it is hardly surprising that they were among the bodies approached for help when the British Library decided to launch its own audio-visual directory, the *British Catalogue of Audiovisual Materials* (British Library, 1979). Inspired by the British Library/ILEA* Learning

* Inner London Education Authority

Materials Recording Study (Ferris, 1981) the experimental edition, in 1979, was compiled from the collections held by the Reference Library of the ILEA's Central Library Resources Service, and the Higher Education Film Library and from selected publishers' catalogues. The catalogue used Dewey classification and provided title and subject indexes similar to those used by the British Universities Film Council. Entries were rather brief and the catalogue was of greatest importance in that it signalled the British Library's willingness to cater for the needs of users of audio-visual materials. There was very little coverage of medical topics. The supplement, published in 1980, drew additionally on information supplied by commercial and other distributors, and item entries were noticeably more detailed. This seemed to herald a significant advance in the bibliography of audio-visuals. Unfortunately, it now seems that spending cuts within the British Library may prevent further editions.

The British Film Institute (BFI), which maintains an archive collection of 16 mm films and television programmes, published in 1980 a catalogue of its non-fiction holdings (BFI, 1980). This is disappointing as a record of medical titles.

The *Video Source Book – U.K.* (2nd edn, Professional Volume, 1982), which lists over 5000 programmes, is also rather low in medical titles. It is probably safe to say that it would be rare to find in either of these directories a medical film or video not mentioned in any of the locations already cited.

Catalogues and directories: overseas

American directories of medical audio-visuals are dominated by the *National Library of Medicine Audiovisuals Catalog,* published quarterly since 1978, with an annual cumulation, to list and describe items held in the National Library of Medicine Audiovisual Center as well as relevant new materials. Prior to 1975 some audio-visuals had been included in the *National Library of Medicine Current Catalog.* In 1977 the Library published a separate volume, the *AVLINE Catalog* covering items catalogued in 1975 and 1976. The first *NLM Audiovisuals Catalog Annual Cumulation* was published for items new in 1977. Since 1978 the NLM no longer includes any audio-visual materials except serial titles in the *NLM Current Catalog.* The *Audiovisuals Catalog* is arranged so that films, videocassettes and tape-slide programmes are easy to find under title or *MeSH* subject heading.

Apart from this there are numerous directories covering medicine as one of many educational topics. For example, Drolet (1981) suggests fifty reference sources for answering enquiries on audio-visuals in any subject.

The *Educational Film Locator* (1980) lists university rental sources for more than 40 000 films. Films are arranged by title, with additional indexes by subject and audience level.

The three *Videologs* (Business and technology; General interest and education; Health sciences) provide extensive coverage of US videotape production. The *Health Sciences Videolog* (Videolog, 1981) lists over 7000 specialist videotapes and cassettes by title, cross-referenced in a *MeSH* index.

Audiocassettes may be located through a much more modest publication, the *Audiocassette Directory* (McKee, 1979), published by Cassette Information Services. It is not, however, the easiest of publications to use: cassettes are arranged by name of the producer/distributor, and subject access is achieved through a 10-page index. The updating service is excellent: subscribers are sent the *Audio-Cassette Newsletter,* describing any titles newly available.

A few years ago Bowker planned to make available on microfiche a compilation of audio-visual catalogues from English-language producers. The first instalment of the resulting *World AV Programme Directory* was published in 1979 (Videofilm Centre, 1979). For an annual fee of £170 subscribers were entitled to receive twenty-three producers' catalogues on forty-one microfiches in a binder, and three further mailings of microfiches to cover a total of 30 000 indexed entries, plus facilities for ordering items from the London office of the compilers, a preview plan and custom searching. Some early subscribers were disappointed with both the currency of the contents and the quality of reproduction, e.g. Macartney and Jordan (1980) recommended that would-be purchasers with satisfactory catalogue collections should wait to see how further instalments developed.

Online services

The major online service for locating medical audio-visual materials is AVLINE, developed in 1973 as a component of MEDLARS and becoming operational in 1975. A full account of its background and development is given by Suter and Waddell (1982). The user's point of view is presented by Bridgman and Suter (1979). Access is through the MEDLARS online system or in printed catalogue form (i.e. the *National Library of Medicine Audiovisuals Catalog*). UK users have access to AVLINE and other MEDLARS services through the British Library BLAISE- LINK service (British Library, 1982).

To complement its experimental printed edition, the *British*

Catalogue of Audiovisual Materials, the British Library introduced AVMARC, which contains over 5000 audio-visuals available in the UK. Entries follow the standard MARC format with additional information for physical description. This is accessible to users of BLAISE-LINE (British Library, 1982). Unlike AVLINE, AVMARC is not restricted to medical topics. The British Universities Film Council is hoping to be able to put its complete database on BLAISE in the near future.

For a description of the other online services listing audio-visuals on various aspects of health and medicine, *see* the excellent review by A. Van Camp (1980).

Information services

Just as there are libraries prepared to compile bibliographies on specialist topics so there are information centres which will provide resource lists (sometimes, lamentably, called mediagraphies) of audio-visual materials. These centres co-exist with audio-visual libraries in institutions and societies which are able to provide services only to their own members.

The Centre for Medical Education at the University of Dundee provides two information services for the location of audio-visual aids. The Medical Audio-Visual Aids Information Service (MAVIS), established in 1976 (Barker and Harden, 1979), is an information retrieval service on medical and dental audio-visual material available in the UK. Initially funded by the Wellcome Foundation Ltd and Update Publications Ltd, MAVIS was at one time able to carry out searches free of charge, but users are now charged a fee. Demand on MAVIS led to the establishment of a parallel Health Education Materials Information Service (HEMIS) sponsored by the Scottish Health Education Unit to perform searches on health education topics. The future of HEMIS is now in some doubt as the Scottish Health Education Group (formerly Unit) announced in 1982 its intention of withdrawing the funding. The information banks for both services consist of details of individual programmes, taken from publishers' catalogues, stored on 8×5 inch cards. The cards are filed in classified order using the National Library of Medicine classification system. For each request a photocopy of all relevant cards is made and sent to the enquirer.

The Library of the British Life Assurance Trust Centre for Health and Medical Education also compiles resource lists on request, usually at no charge. The service is based on a collection of catalogues supplied by producers of English-language audio-visual materials (mostly from the UK and US), subject-indexed on 5×3 inch catalogue cards. With the assistance of the staff of the BMA/BLAT Film Library, lists can be compiled of slides, sound recordings, films, videocassettes, etc, on almost any medical topic. Searches for details of particular programme titles are also attempted. Visitors to the BLAT Library are welcome to browse through the catalogues or the subject index.

The audio-visual needs of nurses are met by AV-MINE at the National Health Service Learning Resources Unit, Sheffield Polytechnic (Heath, 1982). Details of relevant items are stored on 8×5 inch cards in a carousel unit. Since the first list was prepared in 1976, eleven resource booklets on wide subject areas, e.g. community nursing, have been produced. Telephone and postal enquiries are also handled. At present, AV-MINE relies on grants from outside, e.g. the King's Fund Centre, London, but it hopes to be incorporated on a permanent basis into the work of the Learning Resources Unit.

The British Universities Film Council (BUFC) information service is prepared to answer postal or telephone queries about the availability, production and use of audio-visual materials in higher education. For an annual subscription, users are entitled to various BUFC publications, information during the year on new materials in up to four subject areas, reduced prices at certain BUFC events and use of the information service.

The Health Education Council resources centre publishes, from time to time, lists of materials on different health topics, e.g. smoking, personal relationships, and will answer individual queries.

Reference centres

Some organizations maintain reference centres where would-be purchasers can preview materials they may wish to use. The Audio-Visual Reference Centre at the British Universities Film Council was established with financial assistance from the Nuffield Foundation as a preview and research facility for audio-visual materials produced in universities, polytechnics and other institutions of higher education. It now holds approximately 650 items.

Health education audio-visuals may be consulted in the resources centre of the Health Education Council.

Evaluation

Although reference centres such as those mentioned above exist and some distributors of materials offer preview facilities, it is of more help to the would-be purchaser/user to see a published review of the item, considering it in relation to its intended audience.

Journals

An increasing number of journals are devoting space to listing and reviewing new materials, e.g. *British Medicine, British Universities Film Council Newsletter, Information* (from the BLAT Centre), *Journal of Audiovisual Media in Medicine* and *Journal of Family Practice* (Geyman, 1979). For comprehensive lists see the *International Yearbook of Educational and Instructional Technology* Osborne, 1982); the *Audiovisual and Microcomputer Handbook* (Henderson and Humphreys, 1982); or the *Educational Media Yearbook* (Brown and Brown, 1982). A few major journals are listed in Appendix 3. The *Media Review Digest* publishes compilations of reviews of any audio-visual media. It has recently extended its coverage to take in review publications from outside the US: the only drawbacks are its price (120 dollars in 1980) and the fact that medical topics are greatly outnumbered by fiction and other non-fiction titles.

Assessment schemes

In 1970 the British Medical Association Film Library undertook the critical assessment of all its holdings so that a new catalogue could be issued with sufficient information to help potential users in their selection (Engel, 1970a). At the same time the British Life Assurance Trust Certificate of Educational Commendation was instigated so that all films could be assessed by a special review panel made up of appropriate specialists according to the stated audience and purpose of the film. During the first twelve months over seventy films were assessed, but fewer than forty certificates could be awarded. This certification scheme is still in operation and BLAT Certificates are highly valued by medical film producers. The BMA/BLAT Film Library also administers film competitions leading to various prizes for outstanding merit. Reviews of all award-winning films are published in the BMA/BLAT catalogue *Medical Films* (BMA/BLAT Film Library, 1980). For the first time in 1980 this appeared in two volumes – one for films held in the Library and another listing films held elsewhere. As new editions of *Medical Films* appear only every two to three years, reviews are also printed as available in *Information* from the BLAT Centre. The evaluation process was explained in a publication

Film in Medical Education (1973), produced by a special working party.

Films held in the French Scientific Film Library are reviewed by the British Universities Film Council before being made available for hire: reviews are printed in the *BUFC Newsletter*.

Suter and Waddell (1982) explain how and why materials are reviewed before incorporation into AVLINE – the reviews may be seen both in the computer print-outs and the *National Library of Medicine Audiovisuals Catalog*.

Finally, Van Son (1982) includes a very helpful chapter on user-evaluation of videocassettes that could well be applied to other formats.

Equipment

Audio-visual equipment becomes out of date even more rapidly than the contents of films. Each user develops a fondness for particular makes or models, learns its 'foibles' and becomes an expert on its use and maintenance.

Newcomers to the field need unbiased advice on what to buy and how to look after it. Certain published guides have already established themselves as indispensable, for example the USPECs produced by the Council for Educational Technology. USPECs (or User Specifications) are a series of regularly updated pamphlets intended as a means of providing information to educational users on the selection and operation of equipment for teaching and learning. Technical Assessment Reports are also published for equipment covered by those USPECs containing technical specifications' (Council for Educational Technology, 1982). USPECs published so far, free of charge (in quantities up to 100) and of copyright, include *No 3 Overhead Projectors* (2nd edn, 1976); *No 4 Cassette Audio Tape Recorders and Playback Units (monophonic)* (2nd edn, 1978); *No 7 Projection Screens* (1980); and *No 23 Magazine Slide Projectors for 50×50 mm slides* (1979). An *Index of Audio Visual and Associated Equipment and Systems* is currently in preparation, and USPEC No 15 on *Videocassette/Cartridge Recorders and Playback Units* is to be revised to cover video systems generally, for publication in 1983/1984.

Other serial publications that assist with equipment selection include: *AV Equipment Directory* (National Audio Visual Association (1980) which contains photographs, specifications and prices for every type and model of equipment offered by members of NAVA; *Audiovisual Market Place* (1982) which lists 600 equipment dealers with products for rental or purchase; *Audio-visual and Microcomputer Handbook* (Henderson and Humphreys, 1982) which advises on choosing and hiring equipment; *International Yearbook of Educational and Instructional Technology* (Osborne, 1982) which carries a list of manufacturers of particular categories of hardware; *Media Equipment: A Guide and Dictionary* (Rosenberg and Doskeg, 1976) which provides checklists for evaluating equipment and a glossary of audio-visual hardware terms; *Video Register* (Gardiner, 1981) which lists manufacturers, consultants and dealers; and the *Video Yearbook* (Robertson, 1981) which describes equipment and services. Of the many relevant journals, *Audiovisual* deserves special mention for its annual directory of equipment suppliers.

Two useful non-serial publications describing equipment and how to use it are *Non-book Materials in Libraries: A Practical Guide* by Fothergill and Butchart (1978) and K. Bale's contribution to the International Planned Parenthood's Module on audiovisual materials (Forget, 1978).

Until recently the National Audio-Visual Aids Centre ran a Technical Information Service to test and evaluate equipment and maintain a permanent exhibition for visitors to examine. Evaluation results were published in *Technical Reports* and the Educational Foundation for Visual Aids acted as a supplier of the approved equipment. In 1981, Government cuts in educational spending led to the closure of the Technical Information Service, and the Educational Foundation for Visual Aids became more commercial in outlook. A new organization arose to replace the Technical Information Service – the Training and Educational Systems Testing Bureau (TEST) (Crocker, 1982). This TEST Bureau, staffed by the team from the National Audio-Visual Aids Centre, assesses equipment in its own laboratory and publishes bimonthly *Technical Reports on AV equipment*, plus a newsletter, *Technical News*, both available on subscription. The Bureau also provides services to the Council for Educational Technology by offering technical facilities and consultancy to the Council's Support Group on Equipment Standards, Specification and Operation.

Conclusion

Finally, what happens next for audio-visual aids in medicine? An editorial in *Video* (1982) claimed that the videodisc is already obsolete because of plans to produce a new standard 8 mm videocassette by 1984.

The Department of Medical Illustration at the John Radcliffe Hospital in Oxford is working on a new project to 'set video alongside photography as an established and respected medium for the presentation of physical signs and symptoms' – tentatively called the Oxford Video Dictionary of Medical Syndromes (Metcalfe, 1982). In other words the role of audio-visuals in medicine is continuing to grow in importance, and would-be users will have to learn to locate them even in the absence of a British National Mediagraphy or Audio-Visuals in Print. It is to be hoped, however, that the British Library's initiative in preparing the *British Catalogue of Audiovisual Materials* and AVMARC will lead to a national system for recording new materials. And it is not beyond possibility that the BMA/BLAT scheme for systematic evaluation of new films could be emulated by some other organization with regard to different audio-visual formats.

Acknowledgements

I should like to thank Mr J. Ballantyne of the British Universities Film Council and Mr P. Bell of the BMA/BLAT Film Library for their help in supplying information.

References

Audiovisual Market Place (1982), Ann Arbor, MI, Bowker

Ballantyne, J. (1979), *Audio Visual Materials for Higher Education 1979–80,* 4 vols, 4th edn British Universities Film Council: Also, *Update Edition 1981–82,* London, BUFC, 1981

Barker, V. F. (1981), Audiovisual stock and services. In: *Medical Librarianship,* p. 122, ed. M. Carmel, London, Library Association

Barker, V. F. and Harden, R.McG. (1979), *J. Audiov. Media Med.,* **2,** 60

Barker, V. F. and Harden, R. McG. (1980), *The Storage and Retrieval of 35 mm Slides,* Dundee, Association for the Study of Medical Education (ASME Medical Education Booklet No. 11); also published in *Med. Educ.,* **14** (1), January 1980

Beard, L. F. H. (1982), *Media in Education and Development,* **15,** 28

Boucher, B. G. *et al.* (1973), *Handbook and Catalog for Instructional Media Selection,* Englewood Cliffs, New Jersey, Educational Technology Publications

Bridgman, C. F. and Suter, E. (1979), *J. Med. Educ.,* **54,** 236

BFI (1980), *National Film Archive Catalogue. vol 1. Non-fiction films,* London, BFI

British Library (1979), *British Catalogue of Audiovisual Materials,* London, British Library Bibliographic Services Division (1st experimental edition): Also, *Supplement,* London, B.L. Bibliographic Services Division, 1980

British Library (1982), *British Library Bibliographic Services Division Newsletter* No **25,** 1

BMA/BLAT Film Library (1980), *Medical Films Selected for their Educational Value,* 2 vols, London, BLAT

British Medicine (1978a), Non-book materials in medicine, *British Medicine,* **7,** Supplement I

British Medicine (1978b), Non-book materials in nursing and medical ancillary subjects, *British Medicine,* **7,** Supplement II

British Universities Film Council (1982), *HELPIS 1982–83.* Audio-Visual Materials from British Institutions of Higher Education, 7th edn, London, BUFC

Brown, J. W. and Brown, S. N. (1982), *Educational Media Yearbook,* Littleton, Libraries Unlimited Inc

Cockburn, N. (1982), *J. Audiov. Media Med.* **5,** 27

Council for Educational Technology (1974), *HELPIS – medical,* 1st edn, A catalogue of audiovisual and other educational materials in medicine and allied fields produced by institutions of higher education in the UK, London, Councils and Education Press Ltd

Council for Educational Technology (1982), *User Specifications,* News Sheet, August 1982, 1

Crocker, T. (1982), *C.E.T. News,* No **15,** 12

Dranov, P. *et al.* (1980), *Video in the 80's: Emerging Uses for Television in Business, Education, Medicine and Government,* White Plains, New York, Knowlege Industry Publications Inc

Drolet, L. L., Jr. (1981), *American Libraries,* **12,** 154

Edsall, B. (ed.) 1980), *Health Education Index and Guide to Voluntary Social Welfare Organisations,* London, B. Edsall

Educational Film Locator, 2nd edn (1980), . . . of the Consortium of University Film Centers and R. R. Bowker, Ann Arbor, MI, Bowker

Educational Technology (1982), **22,** (7) 7

Engel, C. E. (1969), *Br. J. Hosp. Med.,* **17,** Equipment supplement November

Engel, C. E. (1970a), *Update,* May, 647

Engel, C. E. (1970b), Some innovations and investigations in medical education. In: *Aspects of Educational Technology, vol IV* p. 26, edited by A. C. Bajpai and J. F. Leedham, London, Pitman

Engel, C. E. (1974), *Med. Biol. Illus.,* **24,** 174

Ferris, D. J. (1981), *Learning Materials Recording Study: Report of a Study Funded by the British Library,* London, Council for Educational Technology

Film in Medical Education – Production and Use (1973). A document for discussion by an International Working Party established by the Audio Visual Communication Panel, Board of Science and Education, British Medical Association with the Medical Committee, British Industrial and Scientific Film Association, London, Council for Educational Technology/British Life Assurance Trust

Forget, J. P. (1978), *Audio Visual Materials Storage and Information Processing,* London, International Planned Parenthood Federation (Practical documentation. A training package for librarians. Module 9)

Fothergill, R. and Butchart, I. (1978), *Non-book Materials in Libraries: a practical guide,* London, Bingley

Gardiner, E. (ed.) (1981), *Video Register 1981–82,* White Plains, New York, Knowledge Industry Publications

Geyman, J. P. (1979), *J. Fam. Pract.,* **8,** 985

Graves, J. and Graves, V. (eds) (1970), *3rd Conference on the Use of Audiotape in Medical Teaching, 14th October 1970,* p. 2, Chelmsford, Medical Recording Service Foundation

Graves, J. and Graves, V. (1979), *J. Audiov. Media Med.,* **2,** 95

Grills, C. M. (1981), *Videodisc/Teletext,* **1,** 14

Harrison, H. P. (1980), *Art Libraries Journal,* **5,** 13

Heath, J. (1982), *Audiovisual Librarian,* **8,** 129

Henderson, J. and Humphreys, F. (eds) (1982), *Audiovisual and Microcomputer Handbook*, 3rd edn, London, Kogan Page

Jones, B. (Chairman) (1965), *Audio-visual Aids in Higher Scientific Education*, Report of the Committee appointed by the University Grants Committee, the Department of Education and Science and the Scottish Education Department in February 1963, London, HMSO

The Lancet (1982), **1,** 919

Liebenow, P. K. (1981), *IFLA Journal*, **7,** 335

Lunnon, R. J. (1979), *J. Audiov. Media Med.*, **2,** 112

McArthur, J. R. (1982), *J. Audiov. Media Med.*, **5,** 21

Macartney, N. and Jordan, D. A. (1980), *Audiovisual Librarian*, **6,** 27

McKee, G. (1979), *Audiocassette Directory*, Glendale, California, Cassette Information Services

McMichael, J. (1970), Have we proved the effectiveness of tape? In: *3rd Conference on the use of audiotape in medical teaching, 14th October 1970*, p.54, edited by J. Graves and V. Graves (*op. cit.*)

Metcalfe, J. (1982), *IMBI News*, No **72,** 8

Miles, W. D. (1982), *A History of the National Library of Medicine*, Ch. XXIV, Washington DC, US Government Printing Office

National Audio Visual Association (1980), *AV Equipment Directory 1980–81, 26th edn*, Fairfax, Virginia, NAVA

National Library of Medicine Audiovisuals Catalog, Published quarterly, with the 4th issue being the annual cumulation, Bethesda, National Library of Medicine.

Osborne, C. W. (1982), *International Yearbook of Educational and Instructional Technology 1982/83*, London, Kogan Page

Paegle, R. D. *et al.* (1980), *Med. Educ.*, **14,** 387

Pinion, C. F. (1980a), *The Interlending and Availability of Audiovisual Materials in the U.K.: Report of a Survey Conducted in 1979*, Boston Spa, British Library (B.L R & D Report 5526)

Pinion, C. F. (1980b), *Interlending Review*, **8,** 55

Pinion, C. F. (1982), Audiovisual materials. In: *Handbook of Special Librarianship and Information work* p.128, 5th edn, edited by L. J. Anthony, London, ASLIB

Roberts, D. W. (1970), The Royal College of Obstetricians – audiovisual aids – present position and plans for the future. In: *3rd Conference on the use of audiotape in medical teaching, 14th October 1970*, p.18, edited by J. Graves and V. Graves (*op. cit.*)

Robertson, A. (ed.) (1981), *Video Yearbook 1981*, 6th edn, Poole, Blandford Press

Romiszowski, A. J. (1974), *The Selection and Use of Instructional Media*, London, Kogan Page

Rosenberg, K. and Doskeg, J. S. (1976), *Media Equipment: a Guide and Dictionary*, Littleton, Libraries Unlimited Inc

Rydesky, M. M. (1980), Audiovisual media: special library asset or bane? In: *Special librarianship: a new reader*, p. 521, edited by Eugene B. Jackson, London, Scarecrow

Sabbagh, K. (1979), *J. Audiov. Media Med.*, **2,** 114

Suter, E and Waddell, W. H. (1982), *J. Med. Educ.*, **57,** 139

Thompson, A. H. (1981), *IFLA Journal*, **7,** 325

Townsend, I. and Heath, J. (1977), Is educational technology infectious? In: *Aspects of Educational Technology, vol XI. The Spread of Educational Technology*, p. 189, edited by P. Hills and J. Gilbert, London, Kogan Page

Van Camp, A. (1980), *Database*, **3** (3), 17

Van Son, L. G. (ed.) (1982), *Video in Health*, White Plains, New York, Knowledge Industry Publications Inc

Verny, R. G. and Heider, M. (1982), Selecting and using video programs In: *Video in Health*, p. 97, edited by L. G. Van Son (*op. cit.*)

Video (1982) **8** (5), 3

Video Source Book U.K., 2nd edn (1982), Professional volume, Godalming, Bookwise Video

Videofilm Centre (1979), *World AV Programme Directory*, London, Videofilm Centre (microfiche only)

Videolog (1981), *The Health Sciences Videolog*, 2nd edn, New York, Video-Forum

Appendix 1

Addresses of organizations mentioned in the text

University of Aberdeen Television Service, King's College, Aberdeen AB9 2UB

Association for Educational and Training Technology, c/o BLAT Centre, BMA House, Tavistock Square, London WC1H 9JP

BBC Enterprises Film and Video Sales, Room 503, Villiers House, The Broadway, London W5 2PA

British Film Institute, 81 Dean Street, London W1V 6AA

British Industrial and Scientific Film Association, 26 D'Arblay Street, London W1V 3FD

BLAISE Marketing, British Library Bibliographic Services Division, 2 Sheraton Street, London W1V 4BH

British Life Assurance Trust Centre for Health and Medical Education, BMA House, Tavistock Square, London WC1H 9JP

BMA/BLAT Film Library, BMA House, Tavistock Square, London WC1H 9JP

British Universities Film Council, 81 Dean Street, London W1V 6AA

Camera Talks Ltd, 31 North Row, London W1R 2EN

Charing Cross Hospital Medical School Library, The Reynolds Building, St. Dunstan's Road, London W6 8RB

Concord Films Council Ltd, 201 Felixstowe Road, Ipswich, Suffolk IP3 9BJ

Council for Educational Technology, 3 Devonshire Street, London W1

Educational Foundation for Visual Aids, Paxton Place, Gipsy Road, London SE27 9SR

Foundation for Teaching Aids at Low Cost, Institute of Child Health, 30 Guilford Street, London WC1N 1EH

University of Glasgow, Audio-Visual Service, 64 Southpark Avenue, The University, Glasgow G12 8LB

Graves Medical Audiovisual Library, Holly House, 220 New London Road, Chelmsford, Essex CM2 9BJ

Guild Sound and Vision Ltd, Guild House, Oundle Road, Peterborough PE2 9PZ

Health Education Council Resources Centre, 78 New Oxford Street, London WC1A 1AH

Higher Education Film Library, c/o Scottish Central Film Library, Dowanhill, 74 Victoria Crescent Road, Glasgow G12 9JN

Institute of Medical and Biological Illustration, 27 Craven Street, London WC2N 5NX

John Radcliffe Hospital, Department of Medical Illustration, Headington, Oxford OX3 9DU

MSD Foundation, Tavistock House, Tavistock Square, London WC1H 9JZ

MAVIS, Centre for Medical Education, University of Dundee, Ninewells Hospital and Medical School, Dundee DD1 9SY

National Audio-Visual Aids Centre, Paxton Place, Gipsy Road, London SE 27 9SR

N.H.S. Learning Resources Unit, Sheffield City Polytechnic, 55 Broomgrove Road, Sheffield S10 2NA

National Library of Medicine Audiovisual Center, 8600 Rockville Pike, Bethesda, Maryland 20209, US

University of Newcastle Regional Postgraduate Institute for Medicine and Dentistry, The Medical School, The University, Newcastle upon Tyne NE1 7RU

Oxford Educational Resources Ltd, 197 Botley Road, Oxford OX2 0HE

St. Bartholomew's Hospital Audio Visual Teaching Department, The Robin Brook Centre for Medical Education, West Smithfield, London EC1A 7BE

Scottish Central Film Library, Dowanhill, 74 Victoria Crescent Road, Glasgow G12 9JN

University of Southampton Department of Teaching Media, Highfield, Southampton SO9 5NH

Training and Educational Systems Testing Bureau, Vauxhall School, Vauxhall Street, London SE11 5LG

US Army Academy of Health Sciences, Attn: HSA-SMD, Fort Sam Houston, Texas 78234, US

Appendix 2

Directories listing producers/distributors of audio-visual aids

Ballantyne, J. (1981), *Audio Visual Materials for Higher Education. Update Edition 1981–82*, London, British Universities Film Council

BMA/BLAT Film Library (1980), *Medical Films Selected for their Educational Value*, vol 2, London, BLAT

British Universities Film Council (1982), *HELPIS 1982–83*, 7th edn, London, BUFC

Brown, J. W. and Brown, S. N. (1982), *Educational Media Yearbook*, Littleton, Libraries Unlimited Inc

Dyke, R. (ed.) (1979), *Audio-visual Centres in Institutions of Higher Education in Europe*, Warwick, University of Warwick/UNESCO

Dyke, R. (ed.) *Audio-visual Centres in Institutions of Higher Education in Asia and Australasia* (in press)

Gardiner, E. (ed.) (1981), *Video Register 1981–82*, White Plains, New York, Knowledge Industry Publications

Geddes, G. and MacKechnie, J. (1981), *AVSCOT Checklist of U.K. Audio Visual Software Producers*, Glasgow, AVSCOT

Kodak (1981), *Directory of Audiovisual and Film Producers 1982/83*, Hemel Hempstead, Kodak

Oliver, E. (ed.) (1981), *Researcher's Guide to British Film and Television Collections*, London, British Universities Film Council

Osborne, C. W. (1982), *International Yearbook of Educational and Instructional Technology 1982/83*, London, Kogan Page

Appendix 3

A select list of journals concerned with audio-visual aids in medicine

Those marked * carry reviews of new materials

Biomedical Communications
British Medicine
Feedback (Sheffield, NHS Learning Resources Unit)
Graves Medical Audiovisual Library Newsletter
* *Information* (London, BLAT Centre)
Institute of Health Education Newsletter
IMBI News (London, Institute of Medical and Biological Illustration)
* *Journal of Audiovisual Media in Medicine*
* *Journal of Family Practice*
Medical Teacher
The Health Services (Oxford, Pergamon)

The following, although not specifically concerned with medicine, frequently carry items of interest to medical readers. For lists of other journals on the use of audio-visual aids generally and on audio-visual aids generally and on audio-visual equipment, *see* sources cited in the text.

Audiovisual Librarian
British Journal of Educational Technology
* *British Universities Film Council Newsletter*
Screen Digest

24

The organization of personal index files

D. C. Roberts

The young doctor, no matter what branch of medicine he will pursue during his career, will be a perpetual student, trying, as best he can, to increase the sum of his understanding of established fact, and to become aware of new developments as they are reported.

As an undergraduate, the bulk of his knowledge came either by word of mouth from his teachers, or from textbooks which dealt with a whole subject (or a defined part of a subject) in what appeared to be a comprehensive manner. To retrieve any of this information required but little organization: his lecture notes were in exercise books or loose-leaf folders, one to each subject; his textbooks were clearly titled and contained indexes, while his teachers were at all times available with answers to those questions he could not resolve for himself. As a graduate his pattern of instruction tends to change. Much more of his effort to be informed is now expended on reports of original research, on review articles and on reports of proceedings of conferences. The sources of his knowledge are becoming both diverse and scattered, and he will be well advised to consider the organization of a personal index file before memory proves to be not enough to recall the sources of his knowledge. Setting up such a file is not difficult and need not be particularly time-consuming. This chapter is intended to be an elementary guide for the young reader of the medical literature to ways in which he may, by the use of personal index files, store and retrieve the information he gains by his reading. Some of the simpler methods of indexing are briefly described and discussed in relation to the specific needs of the medical scientist.

An introduction to the mechanics of indexing

The main sources of written information are books, periodicals, reports and letters. The discrete unit of information, in the case of the book, is the *chapter* or, sometimes, the book itself. In a periodical, it is the *article* (whether a signed research report, a review article, or a leading or other unsigned article). These units of information are, for the purposes of indexing, known as *documents*.

When every document (either in the original or as a facsimile copy) belongs to the reader, it is possible to use these documents as the actual objects to be stored and searched. This is the *document index file*. Thus, all papers on epilepsy are stored in a file labelled EPILEPSY. Most documents, however, contain more than one concept of interest. A paper on epilepsy may detail the clinical findings, deal with methods of treatment and compare the toxicity of therapeutic agents. Deeper indexing is required if all these concepts are to be recalled. This is usually achieved by using not the document itself as the object of search, but some representation of the document in its place. Files constructed on this basis are known as *surrogate files*. Each document is identified by a unique descriptor, which may be the bibliographic citation (which will usually, in addition, give information about the contents of the document as well as identifying it) or an uninformative descriptor, such as a number, which will lead, by reference to another file, to the bibliographic citation itself.

Index terms

Each concept of interest within a document is described by a single word or phrase (the *index term*) and these are grouped in an author index or a subject index, depending on whether they are concerned with the authorship or the text of the document. There is no choice of index terms in an author index, except that forenames may be represented by their initial letter. Thus, Jones, Sidney Charles may become Jones, S. C.; Jones, S., Jones, S. C. and Jones, S. C. A. must, however, be treated as three different people.

A subject index term may consist of a single concept (a *primary term*) or may have added to it a simple or a complex qualifying phrase (e.g. *Steroid. Steroid: in asthma. Steroid: change by of properties of acid ribonuclease*). The selection of appropriate primary index terms is essential for the production of a useful index file.

Selection of primary index terms

The professional indexer, working as one of a team, will use a predetermined list of acceptable index terms (a thesaurus). Anything he indexes must be under one or more of these terms: no other indexing terms may be used. This ensures identity of indexing between the members of the indexing team, but at the cost of the preparation of the thesaurus, its periodical revision, and continuing consultation to ensure that the term he wishes to use is, in fact, in the list. Fortunately, the individual, constructing an index for his own use is not so constrained. In any but the most widely based personal indexes, and in some of those where the total number of index terms permitted is rigidly restricted, he will be able to dispense with a formal, preconstructed thesaurus and choose his primary index terms as he goes along. The problem of the synonym and, to a lesser extent, of the homograph, must, however, be considered by him at all times.

Homographs are words with identical spelling but with different meanings. Thus, *induction* may mean different things to an obstetrician and to an embryologist. In personal indexes, however, these are not much of a problem and, provided their existence is borne in mind, rarely cause difficulty.

Synonyms are alternative ways of naming something, and are common in medical nomenclature. The professional indexer, as we have seen, decides between synonyms by reference to a thesaurus, and the individual wishing to set up a widely based index file or one in which the total number of index terms is restricted may wish to do the same. Probably the most useful, widely available thesaurus is *Medical Subject Headings* compiled by the National Library of Medicine of America. It is the thesaurus used for *Index Medicus* and appears with the January issue each year as well as in the *Cumulated Index Medicus*. Separate copies may be obtained from the US Government Printing Office, Washington, DC 20402, USA. There are, however, ways to deal with synonyms less formally. In many cases the reader will have become used to thinking of one particular synonym as the correct name for something, although aware that others call it by other names. Thus, he may invariably think of an *argentaffin cell,* while knowing that others may call it a *Kultschitsky cell,* a *basiogranular cell* or an *enterochromaffin cell.* When considering the tumour derived from this cell, he may reject the obvious name of *argentaffinoma,* having already been imprinted with one of the other names, *carcinoid* or *enterochromaffinoma*. The apparent inconsistency of his choice does not matter in a personal index file provided that his imprinting is sufficiently strong to ensure consistency in his indexing. He will, however, have to deal with a number of synonyms which evoke in him no automatic choice. *Chromosomes, Karyotype* and *Cytogenetics* may be an example. There are several ways to deal with this. He may make a firm choice, determining to index under this term only; he may decide to make no choice; or he may leave his final choice until later. In the first case let us assume that he chooses *Karyotype*. To ensure that he does not next time choose *Chromosomes* he will make two extra entries in his index: *Chromosomes* SEE *Karyotype* and *Cytogenetics* SEE *Karyotype*. If he decides to make no choice he will either enter the item under each of the three index headings or will enter under one only, but will search under all synonyms at the time of retrieval. If he decides to delay his choice, he will enter under one heading only, but will, from time to time, search his index for synonymous entries and eliminate them.

Conventional and co-ordinate indexes

The conventional index used in personal index files usually consists of a file of index terms each consisting of a primary term and, where desirable, a secondary term, which may achieve considerable subtlety of expression as:

> Antigenicity
> tumour, and ploidy, lack of correlation
> Radioactivity
> selective localization in tumour

The object is to make each term self sufficient, and the whole concept to be found in one place in the index.

In the co-ordinate index, the index terms are usually simple, but the file is designed to permit searching for complex concepts by combining a number of terms at the time of search. In general, conventional indexes are more bulky than co-ordinate indexes and, if manually produced, require more physical effort in their generation. It has been argued that the conventional index requires also more intellectual effort in its use, because of the relative complexity of its indexing terms. In some cases, at least, however, the relative ease of producing a co-ordinate index is outweighed by the intellectual effort required to retrieve complex concepts.

Types of personal file

As we have already seen, there are two types of index file: the document file and the surrogate file. The document file has only very limited application for the reader of the medical literature, so we will discuss here a number of types of surrogate files only.

The document to be represented is usually a paper in a periodical, a chapter in a book (or the book itself) or a letter containing a personal communication. All these are usually represented by a bibliographic citation thus:

> Millis, R. R. Correlation of hormone receptors with pathological features in breast cancer. *Cancer,* 1980, **46,** 2869–2871

> Peto, J., The incidence of pleural mesothelioma in chrysotile asbestos textile workers, In: *Biological Effects of Mineral Fibres,* vol 2, ed Wagner, J. C., pp 703–711, Lyon, IARC, 1980

> Cheng, T. C. (ed), *Current Topics in Comparative Pathobiology,* vol 1, *Academic Press,* New York and London, 1971

> Smith, J., Personal communication (Fluorescence microscopy: choice of filters), 1982

The title of any published communication is sacrosanct and may not be altered. In the case of personal communications, it is best to make up a descriptive title, since the original communication will be untitled. The names of journals are best written in full, since some editors require them in this form, some in one of several of the official systems of abbreviation, and others in esoteric variants of their own. It is easier to abbreviate from the complete, original name, particularly when dealing with unfamiliar journal titles.

Bibliographic citations may be used (as in the document index file) as the actual physical objects stored and searched, or may be used as a reference file to which other files (author and subject) refer. Let us now examine a number of systems of surrogate file, and consider their usefulness to the reader of the medical literature. In describing these systems we shall speak of the bibliographical file and the index file. When we speak of an index file we refer primarily to a subject index file, but a separate author index file may, of course, be added to any of the systems.

The loose-leaf file

This is a flexible and useful system, and one in which considerable depth of indexing can be achieved. The units of the index are entered on loose-leaf pages and kept in binders. The author uses those manufactured by Moore's Modern Methods Ltd, 37, Fleet Lane, London, EC4; the most useful page sizes being 3×6.25 inches and 5×8 inches. The binders are by no means cheap, but are extremely well made, and should last a lifetime. Two systems of indexing may be used.

The one-book system

Here the primary index terms are entered on separate sheets on index tabs attached to the right-hand margin or to the top of the sheet. These tabbed sheets are used as separators between which all bibliographic citations, entered one to a sheet, are placed. The sheets holding the citations are titled at the head or, if preferred, across the right-hand margin with both the primary and the qualifying index terms, and are then filed under the appropriate primary term in alphabetical order according to the qualifying term. A summary, or other notes, or a list of indexing terms used for that document may be added, if desired. The main disadvantage of the one-book loose-leaf system is that a separate sheet containing heading, citation, summary and indexing terms has to be made out for each index entry. If the reader has access to an appropriate form of duplication, this is only a small problem: the index headings are entered individually, and then the information on the body of the sheet is added by duplication. If no suitable method of duplication is available, and the effort of manual duplication is too great, the two-book system may be used.

The two-book system

The two-book system consists of a bibliographic file and an index file. The bibliographic citations are entered, one to a sheet (together with any additional information such as a summary or a list of indexing terms to be used) in the order they are received, and numbered consecutively. The index file has its index terms added as in the one-book system, but the individual sheets, instead of showing the full bibliographical citation, contain only the number assigned to the document in the bibliographical file. Because the citations in the index file are represented by numbers only, all entries under one indexing term may be entered on a single sheet (with continuation sheets, if necessary). The numbers may either be entered in sequence or in the arrangement used in Uniterm files (we shall be discussing Uniterm files later). The two-book system is, however, not very convenient when used as a Uniterm index and it is usually better to look upon it as a means to reduce the clerical effort required to produce a loose-leaf index rather than a means to obtain a more sophisticated index file.

The outstanding advantage of the loose-leaf file is its portability. It is particularly suited to those who do their work in a variety of places or, even, when travelling. For those who have a permanent base in which to work, the related card index file has positive advantages.

The card index file

The card index file is similar in conception to the loose-leaf file, but the units are entered on plain cards which are stored in filing drawers or cabinets. The most useful sizes of card are 125×75 mm (5 × 3 in) (the international library card) and 150×100 mm (6 × 4 in).

A convenient way to proceed is to use the larger card to record the bibliographical citation, a summary and a list of indexing terms to be used. The index terms can then be transferred at leisure to international library cards and the bibliographical citations added by duplication. The larger cards are then stored separately in alphabetical order by senior author and the smaller cards by index terms (as in the loose-leaf file) using tabbed index cards to indicate the position of the various subjects. An even more convenient way (provided local copyright laws permit and the facilities are available) is to place the full text of the paper on microfiche, and to use these in place of the larger card.

A duplicating machine designed specifically for international library cards may already be available in the library of institutions or may be considered for departmental use. An excellent machine of this type is the Minigraph, manufactured by Weber Marking Systems Ltd, Macmerry Industrial Estate, East Lothian, Scotland and 711 Algonquin Road West, Arlington Heights, Illinois 60005, USA. In the absence of duplicating facilities, the suggestions already made in the section on loose-leaf files are applicable.

The card index file has many advantages. Index cards are easier to file and to retrieve than sheets in loose-leaf binders and the whole index file is in a single place. When portability as a whole is not required, it is a simple way to index an unlimited number of documents to any required depth.

The Uniterm file

The Uniterm file is, essentially, a variant on the two-book loose-leaf filing system. A normal filing card is made out for each document with bibliographical citation and other details, given an accession number, and stored by number in a bibliographical file. These citations are retrieved by the use of Uniterm cards. The

Uniterm card is a special card with a space at the top for an index term and ten vertical columns filling the rest of the card numbered 0 to 9 from left to right. To post a document using Uniterm cards, the card with the appropriate index term is withdrawn from the file (or a new card titled) and the accession number of the document entered according to its terminal digit, in ascending order: thus the numbers 34, 74 and 184 will all be entered in the column 4. The Uniterm cards are filed alphabetically according to their index terms. Uniterm indexes are usually used as co-ordinate indexes: they carry, normally, simple index terms only, and searches for complex concepts are made by withdrawing cards for the constituent parts of the concept and searching them for identical numbers. The posting of accession numbers in vertical columns assists this searching, as it is easier to match numbers in one column on one card against numbers in the corresponding column on another card than it is to match any number on one card against any number on another.

Advantages of a Uniterm index are that it is more compact than the corresponding card index file and requires much less writing when duplication facilities are not available. Disadvantages are that the bibliographical citation is only arrived at by reference to a second file and that reducing a complex concept to its constituent parts for indexing may be difficult: co-ordinate indexes tend to lose delicate shades of meaning. The use of numbers instead of words may be an advantage or a disadvantage according to the constitution of the individual: some have difficulty in matching numbers, others in recognizing, at a glance, the meaning of a complex index term.

The optical coincidence card

We have seen, in the Uniterm index, that it is possible to refer to citations in a bibliographical file by means of numbers on a card. If these numbers, instead of being posted one by one in columns are preprinted on the card, each number has a unique position on a single card, and an identical position on each card. This is the optical coincidence card (also known as the peek-a-boo card).

The optical coincidence index is also a co-ordinate index, and the information recorded on the card is the same as in the Uniterm index (index term and document number only). It is the method of use that is different: the document number to be entered is punched out of the card, so that the preprinted number is now represented by a hole in the card. To retrieve the citations for a simple single-term concept, the card bearing the appropriate index term is drawn from the index and held up to the light. The numbers which have been punched refer to the document numbers in the bibliographical file. Similarly, complex concepts are retrieved by withdrawing the cards bearing the constituent parts of the concept, superimposing them, and again holding them to the light. The positions where the light shines through all the cards represents the numbers of the documents containing the complex concept.

The optical coincidence card provides a very compact index. It has the built-in disadvantage of all co-ordinate indexes of the difficulty of expressing subtle differences of meaning in simple index terms and, since the numbers are preprinted on the card, only that number of references to bibliographical citations can be entered: if more are required, a complete new stack of cards must be started, and searched separately. Optical coincidence cards are available in a variety of sizes bearing from about 400 to 20 000 numbers per card. The larger sizes, however, are not usually used in personal files owing to the size of the card and the sophisticated (and expensive) punches required for accurate posting. With fewer numbers the card is smaller and (usually) the numbers are more widely spaced, making possible the use of a simple hand punch. Probably the best way for readers of the medical literature to utilize optical coincidence cards is to use a card with about 500 numbers and to subdivide their index into main areas of interest, maintaining a separate section of their subject index and of their bibliographical index for each.

Thus far we have been considering systems of indexing in which the number of index terms which may be used is unlimited and in which the index terms may usually be selected as the file is built up. We shall now consider a system of indexing where the number of documents is unlimited, but the number of index terms is limited, and have to be decided upon before the file is built up. This is indexing with edge-notched cards.

The edge-notched card

Edge-notched cards consist of thin cards with one or more rows of numbered holes round the edges. They are available in a variety of sizes, the larger cards having, of course, more holes. The centre of the card is clear, and may be used for the bibliographical citation, notes and/or a list of indexing terms to be used for that document. The indexing terms are predetermined, each being represented by one or more of the holes at the edge of the card. To enter an index term, in the case of cards with a single row of holes, the cardboard between the hole and the edge of the card is removed with a special punch and, in cards with more than one row of holes, the cardboard between the required hole and the one directly above it is removed. If a needle is passed through a particular hole in a pack of cards, and these are fanned out and gently shaken, all the cards which have been notched at that hole will fall. If the needle is passed through an inner hole, all the cards will remain on the needle, but those punched at that hole will be lowered by the height of the notch. These lower cards may be collected by passing a second needle through a hole in the corner of the lower cards only. The first needle is then withdrawn, leaving the wanted cards on the second needle. To translate index terms into notches on the card, each index term must be allotted a number. If each numbered hole is allotted a single index term, search for that term is achieved by needling at that one hole, while co-ordinate searches may be made by needling at the holes representing the component parts of the complex concept. This system is known as direct coding and ensures that only the cards wanted are retrieved. This is achieved, however, by limiting the number of index terms which may be used to the number of holes on the card. The number of index terms which may be used can be increased beyond the number of holes in the card only by a system of indirect coding. Indirect coding is probably not for the beginner and both normal indirect coding and superimposed random coding can result in a number of unwanted cards being withdrawn (false drops) since codes may not be unique. If the reader requires further information on these sophisticated methods for the use of edge-notched cards, he is referred to Foskett (1967).

The main advantages of an indexing system using edge-notched cards are that there is no limit to the number of documents that may be accommodated, that the system is very compact and that each card carries a full bibliographical citation. The main disadvantages are that the number of index terms is limited and must be defined before the system is set up, that (in the more complicated systems) a separate file of codes must be maintained and that, since only about 250 to 300 cards can conveniently be sorted at one time, searching a large file can be very time consuming. The present author believes (though not everyone would agree) that edge-notched cards can most usefully be employed for small, discrete files on limited subjects, using a direct coding system.

Computerized index files

It is impossible, within a short chapter, to consider computerized personal index files in detail, and only a few general observations will be presented here. The hardware for such a system will be a micro-, mini- or mainframe computer, with appropriate storage facilities, which may be tape, or floppy or hard discs. In all cases it is essential that appropriate software (programmes) are available. Such programmes should permit the entry of bibliographical references, without restriction to their format or length, into files devoted to particular subjects and their retrieval as discrete, complete records either by record number or by the use of character strings. The terminal used is best with a screen (a visual display unit, VDU) and, if any of the contents of a file are to be used away from the terminals, a printer must be provided.

If suitable apparatus is available, computerized personal index files can be worthwhile and sometimes be very useful, but the reader is urged to consider carefully the pros and cons for his own circumstances before embarking on this type of file. He will often find that, in terms of accessibility, portability or effort expended, the manual file is more efficient in preparation or in use, and he should only adopt computerization if he can demonstrate superior efficiency for his particular purposes.

Conclusion

We have now considered a number of ways in which the reader of the medical literature may maintain a personal index file. It may not be out of place to offer a few general suggestions to the beginner:

(1) Choose the most simple system which you believe will suit your needs.
(2) Do not be afraid to experiment or to use a variety of systems for a variety of purposes.
(3) Never index a term if you do not know what it means.
(4) Restrict access to your personal file to people you really can trust.
(5) It is better to spend time looking things up for others than to lose part of your records.

Finally, this chapter is intended only as an elementary guide for the young reader. Two books recommended for further reading are:

Jahoda, A. *Information Storage and Retrieval Systems for Individual Researchers* (Wiley-Interscience, New York and London, 1970)
Foskett, A. C. *A Guide to Personal Indexes Using Edge-notched and Peek-a-boo Cards* (Bingley, London; Linnet Books, Hamden, Connecticut, 1967)

Index